vivian m. culver, r. n., b.ed., m.ed.

Formerly Consultant, Practical Nursing Education, State Department
of Education, Florida; Education Director, Florida State Board
of Nursing; Executive Secretary and Educational Consultant, North
Carolina Board of Nurse Registration and Nursing Education;
Director of Nursing Education, Broadlawns Hospital School of Nursing,
Des Moines, Iowa; Educational Director and Instructor, Christ Hospital
School of Nursing, Topeka, Kansas

modern bedside nursing

eighth edition

w. b. saunders company

philadelphia   *london*   *toronto*

W. B. Saunders Company: West Washington Square
Philadelphia, Pa. 19105

12 Dyott Street
London, WCIA 1DB

833 Oxford Street
Toronto, Ontario M8Z 5T9 Canada

Modern Bedside Nursing   ISBN   0-7216-2782-4

Last digit is the print number: 9   8   7   6   5   4   3   2

PREFACE

The response to the previous edition of MODERN BEDSIDE NURSING has helped to shape this, the eighth edition. The preface to the seventh edition stated that the book "...is designed to be as helpful as possible to both the student and the teacher of practical nursing...to make learning easier...to help the student be as self-directing as possible...and furnish [the teacher] some choices in curriculum planning." These purposes continue to be the basic intent of this edition. Therefore, not all is new.

The *six self-directing study features* of each chapter are retained: (1) *Objectives for the Student;* (2) *Suggested Study Vocabulary;* (3) *Chapter Introduction;* (4) *Chapter Summary;* (5) *Guides for Study and Discussion;* (6) *Suggested Situations and Activities.*

The basic belief that the patient and not the procedure should be at the heart of all nursing action prevails in this edition through the continued use of the "ten basic needs" approach involving all age groups in varying states of dependency and in a variety of illness conditions.

All content in this edition has been reviewed; much has been revised. New and up-dated content has been added. Most chapter objectives have been rewritten. The intention is that the student strive harder to use chapter content beyond the level of memorization to improve understanding. To support the learner in this effort, most end-of-the-chapter study guides and many of the suggested activities have been revised to relate more closely to chapter objectives. Charts are provided to help the student organize content to see its relationship to appropriate nursing action.

New information has been added relative to The Body as a Unified Whole, The Nervous System, Drug Abuse, Growth and Development Factors Related to Nutrition, and Illness Detection.

Coverage of medical-surgical nursing has been revised in three general ways: (1) Some content has been condensed. (2) Some content has been expanded to be more inclusive. (3) New content has been added; most noticeable are the additions related to the musculoskeletal disorders, digestive and endocrine disorders, stroke, heart and circulatory disorders, cancer treatment, and genitourinary disorders.

Greater attention has been given to the use of diagnostic tests, therapeutic measures and surgical treatment, with emphasis on the role and the responsibilities of the licensed practical/vocational nurse.

Several new tables introduce content in a compact form. Examples include: *Eight Wonders of the Human Body* (mechanisms of adaptation and control), *Pituitary Gland Hormones, Some Drugs for Specific Conditions,* and *Types of Surgical Treatment* with respect to the genitourinary systems.

The chapter, The Elderly Patient, has become a part of Unit IX, Nursing Care in General.

Nursing fundamentals are threaded throughout nursing content, and Appendix III, with its own table of contents, is again included for reference to some specific nursing measures with suggestions for modifications when age of the patient and individual circumstances make a difference.

Emphasis continues to be placed on the signs and symptoms of illness, and it

v

is pointed out how much is common in nursing of patients even when they have differing disease conditions. Age, state of dependency, and the disease condition of the patient are used to show how and why changes and adjustments are essential in medical management and nursing care.

A teacher's manual is available from the publisher; its purpose is to help the teacher use the text in a variety of curriculum patterns, offering ideas for teaching and for more effective learning.

I wish to express my gratitude to the many teachers who have used the previous edition with satisfaction and who have continued to encourage me in the preparation of this one. In particular, I am grateful to Louise C. Egan for the many hours she has given to assist me in the preparation of the manuscript.

My family and friends need mention for their understanding and encouragement during the many months of writing.

A special word of thanks to the staff of the W. B. Saunders Company for their help and suggestions, and to Robert E. Wright, Nursing Editor, my sincere appreciation for his assistance.

I accept responsibility for any errors or inaccuracies in this edition and will appreciate having them called to my attention.

Winter Haven, Florida   VIVIAN M. CULVER

CONTENTS

Unit IV
HUMAN DEVELOPMENT: THE LIFE SPAN

Unit V

HEALTH: INDIVIDUAL, FAMILY, AND COMMUNITY

Unit VI

NUTRITION: ITS RELATION TO HEALTH AND ILLNESS

Unit VII

INTRODUCTION TO ILLNESS

Unit VIII

DRUGS: THEIR ADMINISTRATION AND ACTION

Unit XI
NURSING THE MOTHER, NEWBORN, CHILD, AND ADOLESCENT

Unit XII
MENTAL DISORDERS AND TREATMENT

APPENDICES

TABLES

PRACTICAL NURSING –
THE LEARNER, THE WORK
AND THE ABILITIES

Being a student can be a rewarding and exciting experience. To learn is to add new dimensions to living. Our changing times call upon people to learn more and to continue to learn longer. It must become a lifetime habit for the person who wants to keep up with things happening around him, especially as these things relate to his work.

The student and practitioner of practical nursing are no different in this respect from anyone else. Learning must continue for a working lifetime.

The licensed graduate practical nurse is a well-recognized member of the nursing team. Her importance increases as the demands for more and improved nursing care multiply with increased numbers of people living longer and more healthful lives.

Unit I focuses on three main things:
1. How to become a better learner, a lasting learner.
2. A look at who the practical nurse is and the development of practical nursing education.
3. A consideration of some personal qualities which influence one's working and living with himself and with others.

Content in Unit I can be called foundation *information;* it will become foundation *knowledge* as you reuse it. In time, with use and reuse, this knowledge will help shape values and attitudes as well as understandings.

CHAPTER 1

LEARNING HOW TO LEARN

OBJECTIVES FOR THE STUDENT: Be able to:

1. Compare the activities of the learner with the activities of the teacher by giving three examples.
2. Explain this statement: "Learning is a personal, private matter."
3. Give two examples of how a student can assume responsibility in the learning process.
4. List four ways to improve study-learning habits.

SUGGESTED STUDY VOCABULARY*

learning	capacity	teacher role
involvement	attitude	student role
pursuit	image	vocabulary
accumulate	teaching-learning process	self-discipline

*Look for any terms you already know.

INTRODUCTION

You are here seeking *learning*—not education. Education is *the process by which you learn.* This educational program is made up of a series of planned learning experiences; it is an educational process that goes on for as many months as the program is long, and you live this process with your classmates and your teachers. The process will help you discipline your mind to permit learning to take place more rapidly. It guides you toward a prescribed goal; the goal is to become a licensed practical nurse.

To become a licensed practical nurse, the process will require much from you. You will be involved with *people* (teachers, classmates, hospital personnel, the patient, the public, etc.), *things* (books, course outlines, objectives, films, models, charts, notebooks, class schedules, clinical assignment schedules, etc.), and *activities* (conferences, class sessions, study, writing, talking, thinking, etc.).

Learning is the "product" you will come to own as you live the process.

Chapter I is designed to help you understand how to become involved in the process so that you will possess as many "learning products" as possible by the end of the program.

WHAT IS LEARNING?

Learning is a lifelong pursuit; it goes hand in hand with living whether in school or out. Everyone continues to accumulate facts, information, understanding, feelings, and opinions about things, people, and happenings about him as he goes along. Some people are more curious than others and pursue their learning by reading more, questioning more, seeing more, listening more, and thinking more deeply.

Learning is a personal matter; it happens inside, so to speak. The mind is often called the "seat of learning" and the brain houses it. The mind is actually power: power to memorize, to remember, to call back something past, to wish with; power to build feelings and attitudes and power to think.

The brain has an almost limitless capacity to "take in messages." What it does with all these messages is not clear to scientists at this time. The point here is that *you have a mind* and it has tremendous capacity to work for you.

Many factors influence the power of the mind. The owner can push that power or obstruct it; this is one reason why learning can be called a personal matter. You have a lot to "say" about your mind-power; it can flourish or it can linger along at a snail's pace.

Learning is an accumulative process that takes time. To accumulate means to bring together. Bringing together related facts and information takes time. Some people can accumulate and use more rapidly than others; some take longer to accumulate and use, but retain their accumulations longer than others. Some people do a rapid action accumulation (cramming for a test) for a specific purpose and have no intention of using it after the purpose is served.

A student realizes more fully the true meaning of "accumulation" as he nears the end of a well-organized program of studies. Students well along in a program have said "I can still remember the first time I had to.... Now I wonder why I thought it was such a big task." "As for ... it seemed to mean so much to everyone but me. I felt like saying,

"It's Greek to me" but after these months of using it, it is important because it now has meaning for me."

Keep in mind that learning is a slow accumulation of *fact* upon *fact*, which cluster together and become *knowledge*. Knowledge used and reused in one situation and then another produces *understanding* and shapes attitudes and values.

Learning does not occur in single-file order. The mind can take in facts, relate one fact to another, and reuse these combinations in endless ways. While this is happening the mind also has "feelings" about what is being learned — it can be called a "frame of mind." To say it another way: as thoughts trip across the mind, they do not travel in a single file; they are accompanied by feelings and attitudes. The learner's "frame of mind" has a lot to do with the learning he accumulates for himself.

To learn is to "discover" the meaning of things. The learner and the teacher discover together. This does *not* mean that the teacher has no store of knowledge or experiences or techniques to use during this discovery process. Quite the contrary, an apt teacher has all of these things in generous amounts in her "kit of tools." She uses them to guide you in the pursuit of knowledge so you can discover the meaning of things for yourself. She knows the direction she wants you to travel (she needs to be sure you know that direction too), but she does not put up a sign post at every turn telling you what to do. This would be far from "discovery." The teacher is the "thought provoker" and not the "answer provider" when learning is discovering. In this sense, learning becomes a motivating experience for the student; the teacher and the learner discover together.

Learning, then, is the product you gain from doing certain things and carrying out certain activities. As you proceed you gain mental products, which are yours because they are a part of you. Here are some examples of learning products:

1. A better understanding of something.
2. New facts never before known.
3. A new skill you can use.
4. An improvement of an old skill you have long had.
5. A new way to appreciate something or someone.

Learning changes you. As you start to own and use these new products you are not quite the same person you were before, because your interests change and so do your abilities and attitudes.

In the learning process new products replace old ones. For example, let us say that a particular student always has hurt feelings when he is criticized; he has difficulty accepting criticism of any kind. This "hurt" feeling gets in his way and prevents him from using the criticism to better himself. Finally someone (or he may do it for himself) helps him to use the criticism to examine what it is that he has done so that his work might improve. The student begins to understand that criticism can be useful to him and gradually the old product of "hurt" is replaced by a new product—"acceptance."

Another good example of replacing old products with new ones might be that as you study the pregnant woman, you learn that some old wives' tales you have heard about for years are not based upon facts; they are "hand-me-downs" which, when compared to actual facts, are not true. Hence you replace misinformation with correct information.

How does a learning product come about? Most often it is a combination of activities at work within the student. For example: Let us say that the learning product is *knowing how to take a temperature by mouth.* This product includes: knowing the equipment to use, proper handling of it, proper conditions for taking it, knowing how to read the thermometer, accurate recording of the temperature, and proper care of the equipment after use. But that is not all that happens in the mind of the nurse taking the temperature. Assume that the thermometer registered 103°F.: the nurse knows that the normal body temperature (taken by mouth) is about 98.6°F., so that as she compares that with the thermometer reading of 103°F. she realizes the patient has a higher than normal temperature. In her "thinking process," the nurse was *doing, comparing,* and *reasoning.*

In the learning process, one thing leads to another. For example, if the nurse above were you (a student) just beginning to understand fever, questions such as these might well be raised in your mind: What causes body temperatures to rise? How high can a temperature go and the patient survive? To get your answers you might search books, ask questions, or not be truly interested enough to do anything about getting answers.

Questions in your mind come from thinking. One bit of knowledge can serve as a mental springboard to seek more and new knowledge for the inquiring mind. In this way, moving from what you know to what you want to know helps you "learn how to learn." While the teacher is there to guide, assist, and direct you, you must realize that *you* have responsibility for being very active in doing certain things yourself if you are to learn.

WHAT DOES IT MEAN TO BE A LEARNER?

It takes involvement to be a learner. As stated earlier, you will be involved with people, things, and activities which will absorb your time, energies, and mind-power in a manner quite new for some. Willingness to become involved (and stay involved) and to surrender some things to make other things possible is a necessary quality for a learner. This is especially true when taking an intensive course such as practical nursing because knowledge accumulates at a fairly rapid rate. Your learning experiences are planned so that you can put new knowledge to work in short order, if you permit it.

It may further help you to understand what it means to be a learner, by saying "you and the teacher are involved in a transaction, a deal (of sorts) which leads to an accomplishment." The teacher is there to teach; you are there to learn. It is a process—a teaching-learning process. You are an important half of that process; the image you have of yourself and of the teacher can make quite a difference in the learning products you accumulate as time goes on.

First, a look at the teacher's role in the transaction: the teacher plans and directs your activities. The teacher has something that teaching machines, films, books, charts, or models can never have; that something is humanness. She brings feeling, tone, and expression to the process. If, in the past, you have thought that all you were supposed to do was to be present, listen, perhaps ask questions, take notes, read what you were told to read and expect the teacher to "tell you what you were supposed to know," you have missed a good share of the transaction. The teacher is there to create within you the purpose for getting information so you will want to learn; she is there to "lecture," yes; but more important her role is to provoke thought—your thought so that new mental substance has meaning for you.

Next, the student's role: as you become involved with people, things, and activities, you will do things with your body and your mind. Physically, you will get yourself where you need to be when you need to be there—classroom, clinical situation, library, study location at home, or a field trip. Mentally, you will be very active too. It will be necessary to cope with all manner of new words, ideas, and truly puzzling learning experiences.

The teacher will help you, but you are the personal owner of your thoughts and it is up to you to be sure you are "thinking straight." *This requires you to search for meaning.* Each person does this in his own way; the teacher watches for clues to see how you are getting along, but neither she nor anyone else can do it for you, because *learning is a personal matter.*

WHAT CAN A STUDENT DO TO MAKE LEARNING EASIER?

At best, learning is work. A student must decide for himself how much he will do to get it. Following are some suggestions which may prove useful to you.

1. *Attitude* affects your learning progress. Your outlook or attitude directly influences how you get along in the student role. A favorable mood is one of encouragement; success in some small or large activity makes one eager to proceed. While discouragement is apt to take over when success is slow in coming, patience and determination to stick with "the assignment" can push discouragement aside. You need to feel "good" about yourself and what you are pursuing. A feel of confidence will nurture a "feeling for learning."

2. *Build a new vocabulary.* Words—the substance books, questions, answers, tests, lectures, conversations and thoughts are made of—are vehicles for carrying messages. The more words you have at your command the more meaning you can "see" in your mind's eye. Words are the means for passing along information; they convey ideas and set up images in the mind. It has been said, "Man's greatest invention was language."

You will be exposed to many new words. Learning new words can be a difficult task, sheer drudgery for some. Medical terminology has been painstakingly built over the centuries. Many of the terms are made up of "combining forms." Appendix II in this text is a means to help you "unlock" medical terms to make learning them easier.

Your word-power is related to your reading, note taking, outlining, questioning, answering, oral and written reporting, test taking, listening, comparing, reasoning, and remembering. Devise your own personal means for building your vocabulary.

3. *Listening is an activity.* You need to know *how* to listen and how to *use* what you hear (see Fig. 1–1). To listen means to be alert

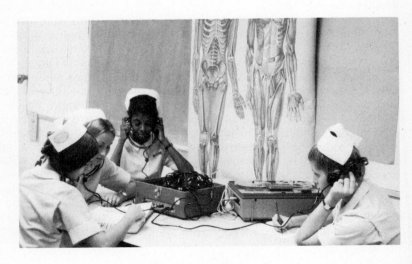

FIGURE 1–1 Listening is a learning activity. (Courtesy of Broward County School of Practical Nursing, Fort Lauderdale, Florida).

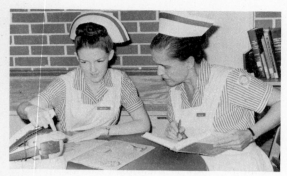

FIGURE 1–2 Students learn by asking each other questions. (Courtesy of Pensacola Junior College Practical Nursing Program, Pensacola, Florida.)

and give full attention to what is being said; until one trains himself to give full attention the mind wanders very easily to something else. As you listen, other things are going on. You think; you take some notes. And you try to see with your mind's eye what is meant. To help you understand something that is unclear, you raise questions mentally. You ask questions of yourself, the teacher, or a classmate (see Fig. 1–2). As things begin to fit together, facts and knowledge start to work for you, but *you* are the one who either makes them work or prevents them from working.

4. *Note-taking* is essential to remembering, some say. Taking notes serves several useful purposes: keeps you alert and listening; furnishes a ready review to refresh your memory; saves time when reviewing for a test. Keep in mind these things about note taking:

a. Be prepared. Study the assignment ahead of time. Then you will be familiar with what is being discussed.

b. Have material on hand. Each subject should have its special section in your notebook. This helps you to organize your notes and in the long run saves you time.

c. Be ready and have a plan. Start taking notes when the class begins. Some instructors are easier to follow than others. It will be up to you to notice how the instructor presents the material. During the following study period review and rearrange your notes if you need to while this material is fresh in your mind.

d. Keep notes brief, but include main points. Make headings of things to be remembered. Under such headings list the important facts. Do not try to copy every word spoken;

devise your own system of short cuts so you can capture the thought and not the whole sentence. Gaps can be filled in later. The ability to take useful notes improves as you work at it. Note-taking is a good habit if the notes are readable and in order. Notes have to make sense if they are to be helpful, so be sure your system of short cuts and abbreviations has meaning for you.

5. *Reading* is an essential learning activity. It helps produce learning but it does not guarantee learning. These guides should be helpful:

a. Read with a purpose. Select the chief facts to be learned and remembered.

b. Read and then try to recall what you have read. You may have to repeat this process several times before you learn the facts you have selected.

c. Practice to improve your skill. Reading is somewhat like "silent talking." To improve your speed avoid lip movements. Let your eyes do the muscular work.

d. If a reading laboratory is available and you need to improve your reading skills, make arrangements to use it.

e. Improve your thinking as you read. Sometimes it helps to pause and read a sentence more slowly. You will need to know the meaning of the words if you are to understand them, so use your dictionary as often as you need to. As you learn to concentrate better while you read, your thinking will improve. Study one idea at a time. Think about it. "See it" in your mind's eye.

6. *Outlining* helps you organize content *in your own words* under headings and subheadings. Use it to organize notes taken in class and during study. Putting information into your own words helps you to understand it better. Under each heading, try writing in your own words what it is about. This will force you to "think through" the topic. You may find that you know more than you thought you did, or you may have to re-read the text, check your notes, utilize the library, or discuss the work with the instructor.

7. *Underlining* serves to help you spot important ideas, whether single words, phrases, or whole sentences in your textbook. You can return and locate them easily during a review or a class. Remember, you want only to highlight the important ideas and facts.

8. *Using the library* is a "must." No instructor can or should try to provide all that

you need or want to know. A learner is a searcher. You will carry on your own search activities, for the most part. Today a library is often called an *instructional resource center* because it contains a great variety of materials and equipment besides books, pamphlets, and journals. These new materials include tape recordings, film strips, films, transparencies, and slides. Machines to use these materials are likewise there or close at hand. Make it your business early to get well acquainted with the library. The more you know about what it contains, the more time you will save using it, *and* you will use it more.

9. *Discuss what you have read with classmates.* Raise questions, try to explain your answers to them (or others) to see whether you have understood the work. (See Fig. 1–2).

10. *Preparing to take a test and earn a grade* disturbs some people, but not others, because some feel prepared while others do not. Preparation for a test takes effort. One of the easiest ways to put forth this effort is—do it daily. "Day to day" learning is better preparation by far for short quizzes, and for weekly, unit, or final tests than frantic cramming the night before. Since learning comes from your daily activity, you defeat your purpose by relying solely on last-minute cram-ming. It is known that it is easier to keep up than it is to catch up.

A word about tests: they are tools for learning that serve as a review and a means of organizing content. We tend to overlook this. When you have mastered the content, the pieces fit together and have meaning. Taking a sampling of that knowledge is not a painful task, but a challenge. Tests also serve as yard-sticks to measure learning. You will be graded, and your grade(s), along with other evidence, will be accumulated to assess your progress.

11. *Arrange materials, a time, and a place for study.* This saves time. Interruptions during study and the lack of a planned time for study are the two greatest "time thieves" known to students. The place should be quiet, materials should be at hand, and your study posture should be comfortable enough to avoid strain but not so comfortable as to invite sleep. Self-discipline is required: this means you must "get at it." Periods of about an hour (or even less) with a short break and a return to study are more beneficial than longer periods with no break. Learn what suits your study needs and arrange your time schedule accordingly. You are seeking learning. The products will be yours, so produce as much for yourself as you can.

SUMMARY

Learning goes hand and hand with living. We learn as we live. Education is a process by which one learns in a systematic or an organized way.

Learning is a personal matter; each individual carries on his activities (sometimes alone, sometimes with others) in a way that has meaning for him.

How a person feels about learning is as important as what he learns. Feeling can promote or impede the learning process.

There are ways to help make learning easier and each individual student must decide for himself what he must do to make his learning as easy as possible.

GUIDES FOR STUDY AND DISCUSSION

1. How do you know when you have learned something?
2. In your opinion, what do you think "feeling good about yourself" means?
3. A fact is a piece or bit of information. Understanding is something bigger. What is understanding?
4. What is meant by the term "frame of mind"?

5. It is said "learning changes one." Imagine it is 12 months from now. In what ways do you expect to be changed?

6. What is the role of the teacher in the teaching-learning process? What is the role of the learner?

7. How can you improve your study habits?

SUGGESTED SITUATIONS AND ACTIVITIES

1. Including any and all responsibilities you now have, draw up a reasonable weekly time plan for yourself. Try it out for a period of time. Review and modify it if necessary; make a plan that works for you.

2. Complete this chart. Check (✔) if it pertains to your study habits.

Factors which help learning   (✔)   If yes
1.
2.
3.
4.
5.

INTRODUCTION TO PRACTICAL/VOCATIONAL NURSING

TOPICAL HEADINGS

Introduction
The Licensed Practical
  Nurse
The Historical Basis of
  Practical Nursing

Practical Nursing
  Education
Summary

Guides for Study
  and Discussion
Suggested Situation
  and Activity

OBJECTIVES FOR THE STUDENT: Be able to:

1. Describe the two roles of the practical nurse.
2. Name three types of nursing personnel in today's hospital.
3. Trace the history of licensure laws for practical nursing in this country by starting with the first law.
4. State some reasons why practical nursing has made such rapid growth since World War II.
5. Name three present-day factors which influence the practice of the practical nurse.

SUGGESTED STUDY VOCABULARY*

waiver
optimum
observing

Role I
Role II
restoration
team effort

integral
sequence
stipend
articulation
self-directed learning

*Look for any terms you already know.

INTRODUCTION

To look ten, 12, or 15 months ahead and imagine yourself assisting in the care of the sick should be an exciting thought. You are enrolled in a program of studies which is designed to equip you with certain skills and understandings which, in turn, will produce some attitudes and values toward yourself and your work. You will develop feelings about what you are doing and about the group of workers you expect to join as a licensed or certified practitioner.

Perhaps, at this point, your innermost expectations are somewhat vague in terms of detail, but quite clear in the over-all direction you want to go. This is understandable because you have not yet "experienced" the preparation process.

Chapter 2 is designed to help you get acquainted with the work of the practical nurse, the development of the vocation as an identifiable part of nursing, and the educational programs preparing this member of the nursing team.

For the purpose of clarification, the title "practical nurse" is but one of several titles referring to the same worker-person. Titles such as "Nursing Assistant" commonly used in Canada and "Vocational Nurse" used in some states refer to the same type of prepared person as does the title "Practical Nurse" which is in wide use in the United States.

THE LICENSED PRACTICAL NURSE

The licensed practical nurse today is a person who holds a license (some type of registration or certification issued by the appropriate legal agency) gained by one of several means:

1. A license gained on the basis of experience, originally issued when a state passed a law to control the licensure of persons practicing as "practical nurses." This person is said to be licensed by *"waiver,"* meaning that educational requirements set forth in the new law have been "waived" or set aside for this person who had been practicing and who had furnished satisfactory proof of such practice.

2. A license gained on the basis of experience and passing an examination. In this instance, as above, experience was substituted for a program of study.

3. A license gained on the basis of having successfully completed a state approved practical nurse program and passing the state licensure examination. The common title for this practitioner is "licensed graduate practical nurse." The legal title *Licensed Practical Nurse* (LPN) is used by each of the three categories (provided, of course, that a license is current and the individual is in "good standing" with the licensing authority). If the state or jurisdiction uses the title vocational nurse, the legal title is *Licensed Vocational Nurse* (LVN). In the case of the title nursing assistant, the legal title is *Registered Nursing Assistant* (RNA) or *Certified Nursing Assistant* (CNA). The current law in the jurisdiction specifies the title to be used.

In terms of numbers, in the United States (1970) there were approximately 500,000 licenses issued to practical nurses; of this number, about 370,000 were employed. In Canada (1970) licenses were issued to 44, 924 (including 1,864 males) nursing assistants.

In terms of female versus male, it is predominantly a female vocation; however, there are tremendous numbers of employment possibilities for male practical nurses. As you will come to know, there is an ever-widening scope of employment possibilities for the licensed practical nurse. Men can fill many of these positions as well as or better than women.

Licensed practical nurses, as a working group, have good "staying" records; they tend to continue employment in a given location. Perhaps this is due, in part, to the fact that many students entering the program are somewhat older and have established homes. The factor of work stability is an important one to the employer. The community respects the person who makes a continued, worthwhile contribution (whatever the work may be) to the mainstream of community life. Community respect and job security play a real part in a person's satisfaction with his work and within himself. An effective licensed practical nurse is no exception; this work, well done, holds many satisfactions for the practitioner.

As you near the completion of your program, you will become more directly interested in employment possibilities and should have ample opportunity then to examine them in detail. At this point, it may be of interest to know that while many LPN's work in general hospitals, a growing number are found working in doctors' offices, public health agencies, nursing homes, intermediate care centers, and special care facilities for retarded individuals and the physically handicapped. In the field of mental illness, there is need for more LPN's.

For work safely and effectively done, the licensed practical nurse is an acknowledged and respected member of the nursing team.

The answer to the question "What does the licensed practical nurse do?" would depend upon who answered it. Some would say "she does everything the registered nurse does," "she does more than she is trained to do," "she wants to do more than she is prepared to do." Others would say, "she is an essential, well-trained person who assists in the care of patients," "she fills a much needed place in the health field," "she performs responsible tasks as a nursing staff member."

It is impossible to describe, task by task, exactly what the practical nurse does for the reason that conditions surrounding her employment fashion and shape her responsibilities. This may be cause for concern, for when taken to unrealistic extremes, such situations can be and often are much less than desirable. Carrying responsibilities beyond preparation for such practice is dangerous for the patient and leads to "over-stretching" the limits of the license to practice. (See *Malpractice* in Chapter 4.)

In 1940 the American Nurses Association issued a pamphlet called *Subsidiary Workers in the Care of the Sick*. Since that time the functions, qualifications and preparation of the practical nurse have been reviewed and revised periodically (1947, 1951, 1957, 1964, 1972).

The National Federation of Licensed Practical Nurses (NFLPN) and the American Nurses Association (ANA) worked together in 1957 and in 1964 to prepare a *Statement of Functions of the Licensed Practical Nurse*. It was published in the American Journal of Nursing, March, 1964.

One section of the statement, *Role Description,* describes the work of the LPN with respect to supervision and nursing situations as follows:

"The work of the LPN is an integral part of nursing. The licensed practical nurse gives nursing care under the supervision of the registered nurse or physician to patients in simple nursing situations. In more complex situations the licensed practical nurse functions as an assistant to the registered professional nurse." The statement goes on to define the "simple nursing situation" and the "more complex situation." These two types of situations have lent themselves to what is frequently called "roles," namely: Role I and Role II.

Role I: To function in this role requires limited "scientific" knowledge to meet the patient's needs. His condition is relatively stable, and not apt to fluctuate. The required nursing measures and the medical orders are based on a more limited or fixed set of scientific facts which follow a "1-2-3" (step-by-step) manner of proceeding. The focus in Role I is to help meet the daily living needs of the patient (all ages) taking into account his ability or inability to help himself (sometimes called "state of dependency"). His condition may be

stable, he may have no complicated equipment attached to him, he may be well on the way to recovery, he may be blind, or have both hands in casts. Or he may be a well and happy person two days old.

Role II: To function in this role requires the LPN to be of direct assistance to the registered professional nurse by carrying out selected tasks (even to completion in some instances) as well as directly assisting her with some nursing measures and doctor's orders.

The complexity of the patient situation can be influenced by many things: age and size of patient, nature of his disorder, severity of disorder, extent of disorder (how much of the body is involved and to what degree), the type and amount of equipment used to maintain and sustain the patient, the "power" of the drug therapy involved, etc. These factors increase the degree of scientific knowledge required to make patient-care judgments. The LPN is not prepared to make such judgments.

Role II includes gathering equipment, assisting in preparation for use, and involvement in the immediate environment while it is being used by the registered professional nurse or the doctor or both. This role calls for observing—"noticing with a purpose"—and reporting to the registered professional nurse the things which seem to indicate change, e.g., something different in the appearance of a patient, the amount and nature of body discharges, whether or not equipment is functioning properly.

Mention should be made that a "simple nursing situation" may abruptly become a "most complex nursing situation" and alter completely *who* should be doing *what* for the patient. Likewise, your role as "task performer" in a complicated nursing situation may gradually become a Role I situation (more stable and predictable) where you function more totally with the patient to help him meet his daily living needs.

Your success as a practitioner can be influenced by your clear understanding and acceptance of your functions as they fall within first one role and then the other.

NFLPN PUBLISHES STATEMENT

In June, 1970, the National Federation of Licensed Practical Nurses came out with its own *Statement of Functions and Qualifica-*

tions of the Licensed Practical Nurse. It was revised April, 1972, as follows:

PURPOSE

To identify the role of the Licensed Practical Nurse and serve as a guide to:

- The maximum utilization of the licensed practical nurse in nursing services.
- Self-evaluation of nursing practice by the licensed practical nurse.
- Development and evaluation of educational standard for the professional preparation of the licensed practical nurse, and
- The interpretation of licensing legislation.

ROLE AND RATIONALE

The work of the licensed practical nurse (LPN/LVN) is an integral part of nursing. Under the direction of a qualified health professional, the licensed practical nurse is a recognized member of the health-care team and performs nursing functions commensurate with his education and demonstrated competencies. On a selective basis, this will include the performance of a wide range of nursing activities. For purposes of this statement, nursing activities encompass situations ranging from:

- providing direct patient care at the bedside in relatively stable nursing situations such as hospitals, extended care units, nursing homes, private homes and other health care facilities and agencies;
- to performing nursing functions in semi-complex situations, such as hospital nursing service units, recovery rooms and labor rooms;
- to more complex situations, such as hospital nursing service units, intensive or coronary care units and emergency rooms;
- to the promotion of personal and community health—an important function of all well prepared members of the health-care team; to promoting and carrying out preventive measures in community health facilities such as well-baby clinics, out-patient clinics and services.

In semi-complex and complex nursing situations a greater depth of knowledge and a higher level of judgment are required of the LPN, and a closer working relationship with, and the greater the degree of direction by, the health professional.

The determination of the capabilities of the LPN in complex nursing situations should be arrived at through:

- An evaluation of the nursing needs of the patient;
- a realistic appraisal of the elements within the situation (e.g. the complexity of scientific principles underlying the functions and techniques to be carried out);
- the ability of the LPN to perform in the situation based on his knowledge, skills and previous nursing experience;
- the amount and character of the direction

needed by, and available to, the LPN in the performance of the functions and procedures.

EDUCATION

The LPN should be qualified for nursing practice through:

1. Preparation in a formal education program in practical nursing approved by the appropriate nursing authority in a state.
2. Initial orientation within the employing institution.
3. Inservice and continuing education for all nursing practitioners to maintain competencies, and for those who qualify, to gain additional competencies which will enable them to broaden their scope of nursing practice within the employing agency by the performance of specialized activities.

LEGAL STATUS

1. The LPN must be currently licensed to practice practical nursing according to state law, and
2. Must perform within the limits of preparation and experience.

PERSONAL QUALIFICATIONS

The LPN/LVN—

1. Recognizes and has a commitment to meet the ethical, moral and legal obligations of the practice of practical nursing.
2. Maintains and promotes good health practices.
3. Actively promotes and participates in nursing organizations, inservice education programs, workshops, institutes and other educational and community activities.

FUNCTIONS

The LPN is prepared to function as a member of the health-care team by exercising sound nursing judgment based on preparation, knowledge, skills, understanding and past experiences in nursing situations. The LPN participates in the planning, implementation and evaluation of nursing care in all settings where nursing takes place. The following illustrates the types of activities performed:

1. **Direct Patient Care**

    (In hospitals, extended care units, nursing homes, private homes and other related health facilities.)

    a. Provides for the emotional and physical comfort and safety of patients through:

    (1) The understanding of human relationships between and among patients, families and other health-care personnel.

    (2) Participation in the development, revision, and implementation of policies and procedures designed to insure comfort and safety of patients and other health-care personnel.

    (3) Assisting the patient with activities of daily living and encouraging appropriate self-care.

    (4) Recognizing and understanding the ef-

fects of social and economic problems upon patients.

(5) Protecting patients from behavior that would damage their self-esteem or relationship with families, other patients, or persons.

(6) Recognizing and understanding cultural backgrounds and spiritual needs, respecting the religious beliefs of individual patients.

(7) Considering needs of the patient for an attractive, comfortable and safe environment.

b. Observes, records and reports to the appropriate persons:

(1) General and specific physical and mental conditions of patients, and signs and symptoms which may be indicative of change.

(2) Stresses in human relationships between patients, patients' families, visitors and health-care personnel.

c. Performs more specialized nursing functions for which the LPN is prepared, such as:

(1) Administration of medications and therapeutic treatments prescribed for the patient.

(2) Preparation and care of patients receiving specialized treatments.

(3) Carrying out first aid, emergency and disaster measures.

d. Assists with rehabilitation of patients, according to the patient care plan, through:

(1) Knowledge and application of the principles of prevention of deformities (e.g., the normal range of motion exercises, body mechanics and body alignments).

(2) Encouragement of patients to help themselves within their own capabilities.

(3) Awareness of and encouraging the fulfillment of the special aptitudes and interests of patients.

(4) Utilizing community resources and facilities for continuing patient care.

2. **Community Health**

The licensed practical nurse contributes to community health through nursing activities usually performed outside patient-care institutions, e.g., visiting nurse associations, well-child and other public health clinics, and industrial nursing units.

3. **Individual Citizen of the Community**

The licensed nurse participates in activities which promote the community's attitudes and welfare in health care. As a private citizen, the LPN:

a. Utilizes community resources to promote a better understanding of the health services among the general public, and

b. Promotes and participates in community health projects and other health-oriented activities.

CONTINUING EDUCATION

Continuing Education is essential to prepare the LPN for her expanding role and to keep her informed of changes in nursing and medicine. It includes those organized educational experiences which are planned to help licensed practical nurses achieve more productive and satisfying fulfillment of their role as health workers. Improved patient care is the primary goal of all continuing education for the licensed practical nurse.

With additional preparation, the LPN is qualified to assume greater responsibility in:

a. Patient Care Management, such as:

(1) Serving as Team Leader, Charge Nurse or Unit Manager, and

(2) Supervising other nursing and health related personnel.

b. Specialized areas such as intensive care, coronary care, emergency, rehabilitation, operating room, obstetrics, pediatrics, health clinics and geriatrics.

UTILIZATION OF THE LPN

The Licensed Practical Nurse is prepared to administer patient care under the direction of health professionals. As a member of the nursing team, she participates in the development of the patient care plan. Administrative and supervisory personnel, responsible for total nursing service, assist each LPN to serve at her highest potential.

The *purpose* of nursing always remains the same: the sick need care and the helpless need protection. But *how* to meet the health needs of so many in a growing, changing world is posing challenging problems. The reasons are rather clear. Scientists release new knowledge, new equipment, and new techniques at a fast rate. Old questions are answered, new questions are raised, and the search for improved health care continues. All of this effort calls for people with specialized training to carry on some facet of work which in turn must be coordinated with the work of many other specially trained workers. This requires teamwork up and down the line in business and industry, including health care of people living in such a society. Today's hospital is as specialized as any other business or industry. Many different types of workers provide a vast number of services (some old and some new) which help detect the cause of illness, promote cure and restore people to optimum health. These workers provide food, maintain the equipment, "run" the laboratory tests, "do" treatments in special departments, keep the hospital clean, collect the money and pay the bills, fill prescriptions for medicines the doctor orders, maintain supplies of linen, etc.

The patient is under the medical management of the physician who must depend upon many such services to help him. One not mentioned above, but as important as any, is *nursing* service.

Nursing service today involves a group of people with various types of preparation (Fig. 2–1)—the registered professional nurse, the licensed practical nurse, the nurse aide and orderly (attendant). They use team effort. The patient, dependent upon so many to get what he needs while he is hospitalized, can feel like a "forgotten person" unless there is good planning among all concerned, and perhaps more importantly, unless *each* worker makes his attempt to help "humanize" the patient's hospital stay.

Division of activities among personnel is essential. A high order of professional leadership and decision-making is an absolute necessity in today's highly complex hospital situation. Less-trained personnel such as the licensed practical nurse require this type of working climate if they are to function within the limits of their preparation and do it effectively and safely.

THE HISTORICAL BASIS OF PRACTICAL NURSING

Nursing is as old as man. Through the centuries its progress has been slow and uneven, though recent years have brought rapid change and steady growth. Practical nursing has been a part of patient care through the years, but during the past 20 years or so the practical nurse has become a trained, licensed person prepared to give able assistance to the sick.

Nursing is defined in many terms, some much more complex than others. For less than the professional level practitioner, nursing may be defined as the process of assisting a person to do those things which he would ordinarily do for himself but is unable to because of some health disability. Primarily, this assistance is in relation to helping him meet his daily living needs. See Chapter 32 for essential needs of all patients.

The word *nursing* comes from a variety of

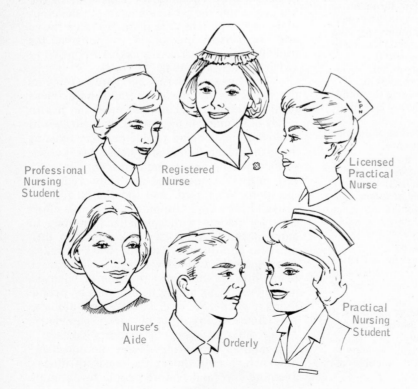

Professional Nursing Student

Registered Nurse

Licensed Practical Nurse

Nurse's Aide

Orderly

Practical Nursing Student

FIGURE 2–1   The nursing team.

meanings such as to nourish, to attend and take care of during helplessness, to comfort and protect. In the early family the mother was the nurse. Later, families joined together for help and protection and the one in the group who seemed to have the courage and supposed "luck" in helping the sick was given that responsibility, although others helped. This care continued for centuries. Some of the early knowledge was later lost, and new things were discovered.

There are many early stories about disease and suffering, and the Bible makes frequent reference to it. Nursing was very much a part of these past civilizations and it progressed as civilization progressed. People, time and events have always influenced nursing because nursing is an integral part of society (see Fig. 2–2).

Table 2–1 includes some of the factors which have shaped nursing since time began. The emergence of "practical nursing" is threaded throughout the table, with attention directed by the use of italics.

PRACTICAL NURSING EDUCATION

Growth in the numbers of recognized schools and of graduate practical nurses was very slow until World War II made demands for more nursing personnel. This need has continued, and from about 1950, there has been rapid growth in the number of practical nurses and the number of approved programs to prepare them.

As pointed out in Table 2–1, *early schools* offered short courses of a few weeks to train women to perform simple nursing tasks and assist their families during illness. These courses stressed the care of the invalid, the feeble elderly people, and sick children in the home, and included appropriate household assistance.

Today the practical nurse is prepared to function in quite a different way. Both "statements" (1964 and 1972) point up the wide range of functions of this nurse.

Practical nursing programs pose a real challenge to the learner and the teacher alike. There is no way to "teach all" or to "learn all," yet to function effectively the practical nurse needs certain fundamental (basic) skills, knowledges, and understandings. A challenge

exists in the selection of what is *basic*. What kinds of knowledges, skills, and understandings constitute a sound foundation for practice at a time when each day brings new knowledge and makes some knowledge out of date? Programs are more educationally sound than they have ever been. Perhaps the two most important "symptoms" of educational soundness are:

1. The learner is beginning to realize he is as much involved as the teacher.
2. The teacher is beginning to guide the learner in a cooperative sort of venture that leads to more self-direction for the learner. These two factors make many things possible in any program.

In respect to programs, as a whole, several important changes are gradually occurring:

1. Fewer students are paid stipends.
2. Better articulation exists between "theory and practice."
3. Students are doing things for and with patients sooner.
4. The "hard" line between "preclinical" and "clinical" learning is giving way to "continuousness"—a continuum of learning with a built-in relationship that is more meaningful to the learner.
5. Library resources are improving. Some include all manner of resource materials and are called "Instructional Resource Centers." Provisions are made for individual students to "go on their own" and review a technique that was taught with the help of a short film strip, a transparency, or a tape recording. This important change leads to self-directed learning.

Table 2–2 indicates current trends in the numbers of programs, admissions, and graduations in Canada and the United States.

Some *factors* which have promoted practical nurse education are: money; work of organized groups in nursing and outside; a growing population needing more health care; and expanding facilities for providing such care.

1. *Money* from public and private sources has been made available to promote practical nursing programs, and the federal government has given financial and other support for more than 20 years. Since 1956, the United States Office of Education has administered vocational education money to help states promote practical nurse education pro-

FROM TEMPLE TO MEDICAL CENTER

Highlights in the History of Hospitals

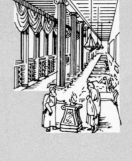

TEMPLES were used by the ancient Greeks to house their sick. Dedicated to Asclepius, the Greek god of medicine, these temples were often built near medicinal springs in which patients were ritually bathed and massaged. Treatment also included rest, special diets, and recreation.

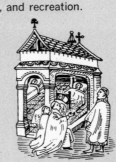

FIRST CHURCH HOSPITAL was built in A.D. 369 at Caesarea (now part of Turkey) by St. Basil, a father of the early Christian church. As Christianity spread, the sick became the concern of the church, and monasteries established hospitals for lepers, cripples, the blind, and the poor.

MEDIEVAL HOSPITALS were elaborate institutions that provided extensive care for the sick and the poor although little treatment for their diseases. In France, the Hôtel-Dieu de Beaune was typical. Architecturally beautiful, it offered privacy, cleanliness, and the opportunity for patients to attend Mass in bed.

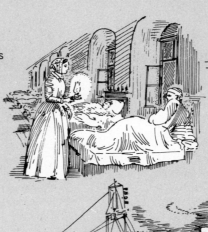

HOSPITAL REFORMS were started in 1853 by Florence Nightingale, who was appalled at the neglect into which hospitals had fallen. With 38 nurses, she scrubbed clean the British military hospitals in the Crimea and washed all the linen the patients wore. She was called The Lady with the Lamp because every evening she walked with a lantern among the hospital buildings, making her inspections.

MOBILE HOSPITALS were developed during both World Wars. Doctors, nurses, and supplies followed troop movements and set up field hospitals near the front lines. After emergency treatment, wounded soldiers were evacuated by airplane, ship, or train.

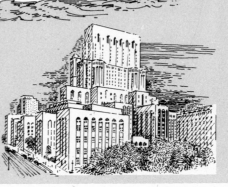

MEDICAL CENTERS that combine hospital, research, and teaching facilities are a modern development. These centers not only provide excellent medical care, but also train many doctors and do important research in the prevention and treatment of disease.

FIGURE 2–2 From temple to medical center. (Courtesy of Western Publishing Company.)

TABLE 2.1.   NURSING: FIVE PERIODS OF DEVELOPMENT

PERIOD	GENERAL INFORMATION
Period I: to 1860	*Period I*

(Pre-Nightingale Era) Sickness was a mystery as were birth, life, and death.

Period I

The care of the sick prior to the influence of Florence Nightingale (1820-1910). The "Pre-Nightingale Era" begins with the dawn of mankind and extends to about 1860. Early man's greatest mysteries were birth, life, disease, and death. Sickness was shrouded with superstitions (some persist to this day) and considered the work of some evil spirit. The medicine man pounded the patient's body, plunged him into hot and cold water baths, burned out the spirits with hot tools, and employed (trial and error) potions made from selected herbs, berries, and barks to purge the inside of the body. The local "medicine man" emerged as the person to "drive out the evil spirits."

Ancient man was kind and hospitable, despite the methods used during sickness. As people became more civilized, strangers were cared for in community inns.

Religious beliefs influenced the care of the sick among such people as the Egyptians, Assyrians, Indians, Chinese, Jews, Greeks, and Romans.

Christianity, the teachings of Christ, brought forth the "service to others" concept of helping the sick, the crippled, the destitute. This concept had great appeal for women; they began to take an active part in social service efforts. This effort continues to this day.

Inventions and discoveries marked the latter part of this period: the microscope and the thermometer (17th Century), discoveries in chemistry and physics and the inoculation for small pox (18th Century), the stethoscope (1818), and the discovery of anesthetics (1846).

By the time this period was drawing to a close, nursing was experiencing some "dark days"; the care of the sick in hospitals was wretched.

Period II: 1860-1900

Period II

(Nightingale Period) First Schools
England—Nightingale School of Nursing in London, 1860
United States—Bellevue Hospital in New York City, 1873
Canada—St. Catherine's General and Marine Hospital, 1873
First Practical Nursing School: Brooklyn YWCA, 1897

Period II

Nursing was recognized as work for women. Florence Nightingale opened a school of nursing in London (1860) and set forth ideas and "standards" which reached this country and influenced early efforts for "training nurses." Miss Nightingale is generally thought of as the originator of "modern nursing."

Schools of nursing opened rapidly at the end of this period. By 1900 more than 400 schools were established, while only ten years earlier there had been 35. This rapid expansion was due to the tremendous increase in hospitals where surgery was just beginning to take hold. Cheap labor was the reason for starting many schools. While some were superior, many schools were not. There were no state laws to regulate the practice of nursing or set educational standards for schools.

Despite the rapid increase in hospitals, the sick were generally cared for in their homes and babies were born there. Hospitals had questionable reputations and were thought of as "a place to go to die."

The *first practical nursing school* in the United States was organized by the YWCA, Brooklyn in 1897

(Table continued on following page)

TABLE 2.1. Continued.

Period III: 1900-1920
(Growth)

First law to register nurses—North Carolina, 1903
First law to license practical nurses—Florida, 1913
Earliest Practical Nursing Schools
Brattleboro, Vermont—the forerunner to *Thompson School for Practical Nursing* started in 1907 and renamed as such in 1917.
Detroit, Michigan—*The Bureau for Organizing Care of the Sick in the Home* program was started in 1913. Since 1937 it has been a part of the Detroit Public School System; today it is known as *Detroit Practical Nursing Center.*
Boston, Massachusetts—*Household Nursing Association School for Attendant Nursing* started in 1918. Today it is known as *Shepard-Gill School of Practical Nursing.*
Minneapolis, Minnesota—*Girls' Vocational High School* started the first practical nursing program financed by a public school system in 1919.

Period III

Professional nursing organizations started and became very active. Efforts to establish laws to regulate nursing got results. Forty-seven of the now 50 states and the District of Columbia enacted laws between 1903 and 1920. Regulations and standards for conducting schools to prepare "qualified" nurses were initiated. It was due to the lack of such standards that nurse leaders vigorously promoted efforts to get laws enacted.

One state, Florida, enacted in 1913 a law for practical nurse licensure. World War I made heavy demands on the supply of registered nurses and few trained practical nurses were available.

This period began to point up the need for someone to assist in the care of the sick in the home and help with housekeeping duties. In the handful of practical nursing schools, classes were small (by today's standards) and instruction was directed primarily toward the home care of chronic invalids, the feeble elderly) and little children; general housekeeping duties were also included.

Period IV: 1920-1940

(Between World War I and World War II)
All states (except Alaska, 1941) and the District of Columbia were using laws to control professional nursing practice by 1940.
Practical nurse licensure continued—four more states enacted laws to license practical nurses.

Period IV

Nursing was recognized around the world as being vital to defense at home and abroad. War (from ancient times on) always brings into focus the need for people to care for the injured and sick both on the battlefield and on the home front.

Schools of nursing (professional) and hospitals continued to increase until the Depression. Between 1930 and 1940 more than 400 hospitals closed and about 600 schools went out of existence.

During this period schools of practical nursing numbered less than 50.

Period V: 1940 to the present

Often called the "Scientific Age." A chief hallmark of this period is *change*—fast and constant.
Practical Nurse Licensure Moves Ahead
Practical nurse licensure laws enacted in every state and the District of Columbia by 1960. Most laws were passed from the mid forties to the mid fifties. Canada (Manitoba) enacted its first law in 1945. By 1971, 9 of 10 Canadian Provinces had licen-

Period V

From World War II on events in nursing have moved with the times. This period has several rather distinct yet overlapping eras: World War II, its demands and aftermath; acceleration of efforts to improve education; space exploration; the explosion of new knowledge and technologies due to scientific research.

Better communication media produced better informed citizenry. Demands for health care increased with a growing population and a "growing older" population. Prepaid hospital insurance plans made hospital care available to multitudes. Federal legislation provided for Medicare and Medicaid.

Efforts and emphasis included research related to

TABLE 2.1.   Continued.

sure laws for Nursing Assistants/ Practical Nurses.

Licensure laws were passed by Puerto Rico (1946), Guam (1952), Virgin Islands (1952).

Practical Nursing Programs Increase Rapidly
In the United States between the years 1961 and 1971 the number of programs increased from 739 to 1291: During this same period the number of graduates increased from over 18,000 to more than 38,500. By 1966 Canada's 101 schools graduated 3712 students, in 1970 111 schools graduated 4697.

mental retardation, mental illness, environmental pollution, and the use of atomic energy for detection and treatment of illness. Body organ transplants and organ substitutions along with equipment to sustain life when regular body parts fail are products of this era.

Period V, among many other things, can be called *a rapid growth period for practical nursing:* law enactment, large increase in number of schools and graduates, the beginning of organizations for the advancement of the group (and individual) and concerted efforts to improve practical nursing education.

Federal government assistance and private foundation support gave and continue to give momentum to practical nursing education. Federal monies are distributed through state departments of vocational education.

Since about 1964 there has been an increasing effort (federal and state) to promote additional health occupations programs to help meet the tremendous demand for health services. One program of first-hand importance to the practical nurse is the short, intensive course to train nurse aides and orderlies to do many of the tasks commonly included in the practical nurse curriculum.

Efforts are underway to make it possible for the graduate LPN to move up the nursing career ladder with some credit for previous study.

grams, while private organizations such as the W. K. Kellogg Foundation, the Kress Foundation, and the Avalon Foundation have provided money to assist states, nursing groups, and schools for specific purposes.

About three-fourths of the present programs are vocational programs (in vocational high schools, junior or community colleges, four-year colleges); others are administered by hospitals; and a few are sponsored by private agencies.

2. *Organized groups* within nursing and outside of nursing have worked separately and

together to guide and direct practical nursing education. Nursing groups include: the National League for Nursing (NLN), the American Nurses' Association (ANA), the National Federation of Licensed Practical Nurses (NFLPN), and the National Association for Practical Nurse Education and Service (NAPNES). See Chapter 5. Other agencies include the United States Office of Education, the United States Public Health Service, and private organizations such as those mentioned above.

3. *A rapidly-growing population,* aware

TABLE 2.2.   PROGRAMS, ADMISSIONS, GRADUATIONS

COUNTRY	YEAR	NUMBER PROGRAMS	NUMBER ADMISSIONS	NUMBER GRADUATIONS
Canada°	1966	101	4732	3712
	1970	111	5154	4697
United States‡	1966	1081	38,775	25,688
	1971	1291	60,057	38,556

°Statistical data secured from: Research Unit, Canadian Nurses' Association. Ottawa, Canada. June 1971.

‡Statistical data secured from: National League for Nursing. New York, N.Y. October 1971.

of health needs, will continue to protect itself with sickness insurance and will have the means to seek care (preventive and rehabilitative as well as remedial). Medicare and Medicaid make health care available to untold numbers. Those without protection will get help through public and private agencies.

More people needing care brings about the need for more health workers.

4. *More facilities* of all kinds are needed. Nursing homes, convalescent homes, intermediate care centers, clinics, and hospital beds have increased in number and will continue to expand as the population grows.

SUMMARY

More change has occurred in nursing since World War II than in all other periods combined. This period has been one of rapid growth for practical nursing education and the licensure of practical nurses.

The 1972 (revised) Statement of Functions and Qualifications of the LPN was prepared by NFLPN to describe the work of the LPN today.

The practical nurse has individual responsibilities for her part in the growth and acceptance of herself and her group. Being expert in the skills of patient care and knowing how to work with others in a cooperative, responsible way will go far to help this group to grow and progress.

GUIDES FOR STUDY AND DISCUSSION

1. Imagine yourself nursing during any one of the first four periods in nursing discussed in this chapter. What would it be like?

2. Who is involved in nursing the patient today?

3. What factors have made practical nursing grow so rapidly in the last 20 years?

4. The patient's needs determine the type of skilled nursing care he requires. What does this mean? Give examples.

5. Today we say the practical nurse is prepared for two main roles. What are they? Be ready to discuss the differences between them.

6. Table 2–1 includes the growth of practical nursing. Trace this growth starting with the first practical nursing school in this country.

SUGGESTED SITUATION AND ACTIVITY

1. Using the 1964 Statement (AJN March, 1964) and the 1972 Statement, compare them by locating things that are similar and things that are different. Be ready to discuss your findings.

2. See if you can complete this chart.

Nursing Organizations	Who May Become Members	Name of Official Journal	Functions
1. NFLPN			
2. NLN			
3. NAPNES			
4. ANA			

UNDERSTANDING THE NEEDS OF SELF AND OF OTHERS

TOPICAL HEADINGS

Introduction	Relationships	Guides for Study and
Self	Communications	Discussion
Self to Others	Summary	Suggested Situations
		and Activities

OBJECTIVES FOR THE STUDENT: Be able to:

1. Tell why self-direction is necessary in reaching individual goals.
2. Name and give examples of the two basic needs of man.
3. Explain the meaning of the term "behavior" as it pertains to self and to others.
4. Name eight factors which are essential to "good relationships."
5. Give two examples of how communications favorably influence relationships.

SUGGESTED STUDY VOCABULARY*

acceptance	ethics	physical need
relationships	ethical behavior	social need
communications	stimulus	self concept
"frame of mind"	belief	specialization
behavior	value	nursing team
	attitude	health team

---

*Look for any terms you already know.

INTRODUCTION

One meaning for the word "acceptance" is "well-received." Being *well-received* is a two-way road that leads from self to others and back to self. Nursing offers an unusual opportunity for practicing acceptance of others. Imagine for a moment how many different people you will be working with, caring for, and meeting in the years ahead. The number is limitless; but each such human experience will contain an "exchange" of feelings, reactions, moods, and the like. You present yourself to someone and this exchange takes place; likewise it happens when someone presents himself to you. There are ways to help make these exchanges be "well-received."

Chapter 3 is designed to help you consider how you present yourself to others so that you will be well-received, and in this "exchange," they will be, too. The chapter starts with "self" and the needs of "self" and continues on from self to others. Two main factors, relationships and communications, are included.

SELF

When you complete this program and have a license to practice, what will you take with you to your work? In almost all instances, you will not be required to take materials with you except for the traditional watch, pen and scissors because the employing agency will provide them. You will take YOU; your being holds the "human tools" you will use. It is this "inner kit of tools" the employer expects you to use, and he has agreed to pay you for using them effectively with the other humans involved.

A person's inner capabilities are made up of knowledge and understanding, skills and a "frame of mind." These inner dimensions are influenced by circumstances and produce all manner of behavior—action and interaction with others. You know (and have a right to expect) that your program will provide you opportunities to learn many new things: words, fingertip skills, ideas, and ways to do things, including the equipment needed to do them. Knowledge and understanding which you do not presently have will be yours. As you acquire these "learning products," you will experience feelings about what you are learning; you will place values on what you are doing and the people involved. Moods and feeling tones will be present; in fact, they are present as you read these words.

An effective worker, besides having "know how," is one who gets along with others and who feels "good" about himself. It has been said that more people lose their jobs because of the inability to get along with others than for any other single reason.

To nurse effectively is to be aware of the needs of other humans and respond (behave) accordingly; a nurse's behavior should show that she accepts people as they are, realizing that each human (self included) behaves as he "sees" fit to behave under the circumstances. A person acts according to the way he "sees" things or the way things seem to be to him.

Consider yourself in this example: you have been told that on Friday of next week you will be having a "big" unit test on Body Structure and Function. As you "see" it, you need to ready yourself as you go along. You study hard; you listen carefully. You ask questions of yourself and others; you answer them. You turn things over in your mind until they have meaning for you. In other words, you behave in ways to prepare yourself as well as you can for the test. When the appointed hour comes, you approach the task with assurance because you met your needs (behaved) as you saw fit under the circumstances. Standing to one side in this instance and looking at your own behavior during the time prior to the test and while taking the test itself, you observe a person carrying on activities in keeping with certain circumstances.

Patients are humans first and behave as they see fit under the circumstances, too.

The word *behavior* used here means the way a person responds to something that rouses the mind (stimulus). The human response may be "ordinary," "usual," "expected"; it may include shades or tints of the not-so-expected; it may be a response that the other person(s) finds quite jarring and upsetting.

To give you more insight into your own behavior (and hence others'), some basic terms are described. Keep in mind as you ponder them that they are not all as clear-cut as they appear in print. They somehow overlap in "real life situations."

It can be said that an individual has *beliefs, values, attitudes, needs,* and *a concept of himself,* all of which influence how he "sees something in his mind's eye" and behaves accordingly. Here they are briefly described:

1. *Belief*—a habit of the mind or a persuasion that something is "true." Where do beliefs come from? They come from faith, knowing something, assuming something, or from superstition.

2. *Value*—something one "sets store by" or rates highly; something treasured and prized. It is something important to an individual such as a particular friendship, material things, a particular experience.

3. *Attitude*—this part of one's inner self is closely related to belief; in a sense it is a belief acted out in the privacy of one's thoughts or displayed for others to see. Attitudes are related to one's values too. An attitude is the bent or turn of mind one has about something or somebody. Does that something or somebody have worth or lack worth? Like-

wise, an attitude might be thought of as a habit of the mind through which things are sorted out and judged.

4. *Basic needs** — these may be subdivided into two main groups:

   a. Physical (physiological)
     air
     food
     water
     shelter
     sleep
   b. Social (enhancement of self)
     approval
     acceptance
     status
     prestige
     power

5. *Concept or idea of self (self-concept)* — how a person sees himself and feels about himself. Does he like what he sees and feels? Does he want to be something other than he is? Does he feel content with the role(s) he plays? How does he "see" others? How does he think others "see" him?

While these questions may sound confusing, taken one at a time, a person can step aside and look at himself. Everyone has flashes of looking at himself. For example, something occurs and a person hastily utters a remark that he immediately realizes he should not have said. It was hurtful to someone and the owner of the remark is uncomfortable. He does not like what he feels and wishes he could withdraw the statement.

Be Well-received

Knowing that an individual has a social need for approval and acceptance, a nurse should be someone who accepts herself and who will be acceptable to others, who feels right about herself and will be well-received by others. To accomplish this requires *a basis for right action called ethics.*

Ethics is a standard or a rule of what is fitting or proper. An organized group very often has a written code of ethics or a set of moral standards to guide its members so that they will be well-received as people rendering their particular service to other people.

Following is the Code of Ethics for Li-

---

*Chapter 22, Health of the Individual, discusses nine specific daily living needs as they relate to you or any individual.

censed Practical Nurses developed by the National Federation of Licensed Practical Nurses, Inc.

1. The licensed practical nurse shall practice her profession with integrity.

2. The licensed practical nurse shall be loyal to the physician, to the patient, and to her employer.

3. The licensed practical nurse strives to know her limitations and to stay within the bounds of these limitations.

4. The licensed practical nurse is sincere in the performance of her duties and generous in rendering service.

5. The licensed practical nurse considers no duty too menial if it contributes to the welfare and comfort of her patient.

6. The licensed practical nurse accepts only that monetary compensation which is provided for in the contract under which she is employed, and she does not solicit gifts.

7. The licensed practical nurse holds in confidence all information entrusted to her.

8. The licensed practical nurse shall be a good citizen.

9. The licensed practical nurse participates in and shares responsibility of meeting health needs.

10. The licensed practical nurse faithfully carries out the orders of the physician or registered nurse under whom she serves.

11. The licensed practical nurse refrains from entering into conversation with the patient about personal experiences, personal problems, and personal ailments.

12. The licensed practical nurse abstains from administering self-medications, and in event of personal illness, takes only those medications prescribed by a licensed physician.

13. The licensed practical nurse respects the dignity of the uniform by never wearing it in a public place.

14. The licensed practical nurse respects the religious beliefs of all patients.

15. The licensed practical nurse abides by the Golden Rule in her daily relationships with people in all walks of life.

16. The licensed practical nurse is a member of the National Federation of Licensed Practical Nurses, Inc., and the state and local membership associations.

17. The licensed practical nurse may give credit to a commercial product or service, but does not identify herself with advertising, sales, or promotion.

The meaning of this code (each statement) can be something for you to search for as a student. Discover how it can operate for you. One could select terms from the code (with adaptation) and apply them to living in general. Terms such as integrity, loyalty, sincerity, trust, good citizenship, appropriateness of attire, respect, belief in the Golden Rule serve as guides for living as a person and likewise as a basis for ethical conduct for a nurse. You will note several items such as numbers 3, 5, 6 and 13 (among others) which are specifically for the practitioner.

Each nursing program points out what is expected of the student in relation to ethical behavior. The school handbook is generally a source of such information and can serve as a guide to help the student. But more important is the ability of the student to gradually become her own source of appropriate habit and social custom. With guidelines to follow and a willingness to discover the meaning of new aspects of behavior appropriate to a practical nurse, the student can become self-directing in this effort. This is a way ethical behavior becomes a way of living and experiencing things.

SELF TO OTHERS

Working in our culture calls for a high degree of cooperative effort. More and more people are trained to be specialists of one kind or another. A good example of this is found in the automobile repair industry. Almost any significant part of an automobile (radiator, wheels, brakes, motor, gears) has specialists who work on that particular part. The specialist becomes expert in his work and is constantly learning new things to help *keep* him expert.

The same circumstances exist in the health professions. Knowledge is increasing so rapidly that people must be trained in special aspects of health care so that the public can receive the best possible treatment and care.

Today, patient care involves many individuals who work together providing for patient comfort and well-being. More than anyone else, the patient is involved. When so many are doing things for and with him, it is necessary that each of these people gets along with the others, carry his responsibilities, and

be an acceptable person in the group—in other words, be well-received.

RELATIONSHIPS

What They Are

Good human relationships are good will applied with common sense. *Relationship means the various ways one person regards and responds to another person.* Often one is perplexed about why another person behaves the way he does; it is difficult to understand why he did what he did. At times you can shrug off this uncertainty without too much second thought, and go on; but sometimes a person's behavior really captures your attention and possibly your anger or sympathy or your assistance.

Good relationships are present, when the humans involved seem to regard one another favorably. They "get along together." Understanding, cooperation, and communications suffer when relationships are poor or undesirable. The "atmosphere" lacks such things as acceptance, warmth, and respect.

Importance

Nursing, a service that involves working *for* and *with* people, heartily needs a climate of good relationships. At best, it is difficult at times because immediate needs and pressure of time get in the way, but people working agreeably together can and do accomplish much despite the work load.

More often than not, when a former patient writes a note of appreciation to a hospital, he mentions human factors such as kindness and consideration for his individuality. This is an index to the worth of good feeling shared between patient and personnel.

Requirements

Good relationships are due to the people involved. Figure 3–1 shows some of the qualities they possess and the practices they follow. Nursing has no first claim to these qualities, but those who nurse need them and need to practice them.

As a person joining the nursing group, you have a responsibility to sharpen your rela-

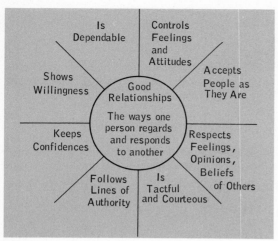

FIGURE 3–1   Some essentials in maintaining relationships.

tionship skills and develop new ones if necessary, because they are as important to your work as the nursing skills you learn.

Control of feelings and attitudes takes effort, more at some times than others, because under certain pressures one is inclined to press personal ideas or feelings on others, and they do not always take this too kindly. It helps to accept people as they are and to use good judgment in respecting their feelings, opinions, and beliefs, whether you agree with them or not.

Many times a relationship is not so dependent upon what is said as it is on such things as the tone of voice, a facial expression, or a body movement. Any of these can indicate understanding and acceptance or lack of it.

In nursing there are contacts with many different types of people. Good relationships are as much the responsibility of the practical nurse as of anyone else. This role calls for a warm, friendly, and willing individual who is sensitive to the needs of others and expresses these qualities through acceptable attitudes. The quality of care given will be measured not by fingertip skill alone, but also by the ability to accept and understand others, patients and family members as well as workers.

Barriers

The presence of certain factors may hinder good relationships and serve as an obstacle. Some stem from the nurse herself; some from the patient. They may include: erroneous ideas of patients about some illness and the feeling of the nurse that she must debate the issue with the patient; fixed ideas of a nurse about certain "types" of patients (i.e., the private room patient being more demanding, or the "uncooperative" label so quickly pinned to some); borrowed opinions with no factual bases; language and nationality differences; disapproval of act(s) leading to patient's condition (i.e., the unwed mother, the patient with syphilis); repulsive odors, unsightly wounds, unusual physical appearances, blindness, or deafness. Other factors which tend to cramp patient relationships include age, habit, vocabulary, education, and a person's general lack of well-being.

Regardless of circumstances surrounding the patient, the nurse has a responsibility to maintain the best possible relationships. When barriers arise, help is sometimes needed to cope with them. The help of the registered nurse or the physician should be sought because guidance often is needed to overcome some barriers. With continued experience, the practical nurse becomes more effective in caring for patients because she develops the ability to accept the patient as a person who needs assistance. She understands that she is there to aid him in a helpful, nonjudging way.

Barriers to good relationships arise between co-workers; some of the above examples apply. One all too frequent barrier is the lack of common courtesy and good manners—a matter of practice and habit. There is always time for courtesy.

THOSE INVOLVED IN RELATIONSHIPS

The Patient: As He Sees It

Sickness changes a person's outlook; his viewpoint is altered and he has time to think about his own circumstances. Many times he worries about things that never happen. A person who is sick is apt to be more aware of his own feelings then than when he is well and busy.

A person's usual ability to get along and cope with things is dulled when sick. Patience is in short supply. The patient can be worried, restless, anxious and even tearful. What he looks for is for someone to pay attention to his plight and be sympathetic to his needs.

If the patient is hospitalized he reacts to

the people and things around him. His outlook is distorted by physical discomfort, strange-looking equipment, regulations and the seemingly impersonal actions of the people coming and going in his surroundings.

Time permits thinking and watching for hopeful clues. The patient is on the alert for people friendly to human need and may make some unusual request in his search for people who care.

The idea of being captive (in the hospital) and not permitted freedom of heretofore ordinary choices can cause a patient to tailor-make his actions to suit his needs and protect his interests. This loss of independence leaves him with uncertainty as to what to do when he needs help.

The patient feels lost. The activity around him seems impersonal and he may wonder what is happening to him. He may even find it difficult to feel that someone knows about his plight because everything seems so geared to a system. The system may appear more important to the worker than the patient.

The patient senses his dependence upon others so he tries to get along. Perhaps for selfish reasons he wants to have a good image so that when he needs something personnel will respond. He wants to be sure that he receives those things the doctor has ordered, on time and without error.

What the patient wants is to feel secure about his needs and that they will be met safely and when required.

The patient observes personnel, watching for clues of carefulness and indications of interest in him and his well-being. Security improves when the patient believes that personnel are genuinely interested in him because they show by their actions (and work) that they like what they are doing and display some dedication to their work.

Favorable relationships between the patient and "his nurse" are helpful to his well-being because he feels more secure about what is happening to him.

What can the nurse do to strengthen relationships with the patient? Knowing what concerns the patient and what he seeks, the following practices will help.

1. Accept the patient as a person who has habits, likes and dislikes, fears, worries, and his own opinions, and who is part of a family. He is an individual who needs acceptance and respect for his individuality. This allows for flexibility in at least some aspects of his nurs-

ing care. Small adjustments that can be made in helping him meet his needs should be made to help him feel like a person first and a patient next.

2. Personal bias, prejudices, or problems of the nurse are kept to herself. The patient may have more than enough of his own to cope with.

3. Be a good listener.

4. Offer to help. Sometimes this means seeking the team leader or supervisor for specific directions, referring the problem to the appropriate person.

5. Be pleasant and show interest in the patient; these attitudes make him feel more secure.

6. Perform acts with care and thoughtfulness. Careless acts (and remarks) raise doubts in the patient's mind.

The Physician

In many situations, the practical nurse works under the direct supervision of a licensed physician and not under the supervision of a professional nurse. For example, in doing home nursing or office nursing, she will receive her directions from the physician; in turn, she is responsible to him for carrying out his orders and providing nursing care.

The physician, in directing the medical management of the patient, delegates some tasks to the nurse. At times these may include tasks the practical nurse is not prepared to carry out nor legally permitted to do, and she has a responsibility to remind him why she is unable to do so. The sincere manner in which this is done helps him to understand and accept her position in the matter and further to respect her as an honest person and as a dependable nurse—one who is primarily concerned with the safety of the patient.

The Professional Nurse

The practical nurse works more directly with the professional nurse than any other person. Each has responsibilities to the other in their respective but different roles. Chapter 2 points out the two chief roles of the practical nurse, and in each the professional nurse plays a part. Because of this, no two members of the health team need better understanding and acceptance of each other.

Good relationships exist when one nurse respects the other's ability and her contribution to patient care and is not threatened by them. In today's health care each nurse is needed, and the solutions to problems arising between the two should be sought and found by them, primarily. Employment opportunities are abundant; there is work for all qualified nursing personnel. The chief concern is one of using each nurse within her role and capacities. This calls for the best possible relationships between them.

Other Personnel

Nurse aides, orderlies, and ward secretaries (auxiliary personnel) perform tasks for patients. Some relate directly to their care and others do not. This large group of people represents an important helping hand to nursing. They need the climate of good relationships to make their best contribution. The practical nurse has a distinct responsibility to help them feel that they are important to a job well done.

Other professional workers in today's health care team include dietitian, pharmacist, cleric, social worker, physical therapist, occupational therapist, laboratory technician. With so many specialized workers, the matter of understanding and accepting the contributions of each is vital. Nothing breaks down relationships any faster than the attitude of a department that feels it is the most important and that everything must revolve around it. Hospital care today is the result of a high degree of cooperation among many people with many labels.

As an employee, you will find that while your contribution is needed, the same is true of all the others working in the same agency or institution, including the vast army of volunteer workers who render such a wide variety of services without pay.

The Nursing Team

The purpose of the "team" is to provide nursing care; it is a method or means of using nursing personnel to do things for and with patients. The several different workers (professional nurse, practical nurse, aide, and orderly) are grouped and their work is organized so that each team member performs the duties he or she is prepared to do. The team carries responsibility for the safe care of a group of patients. The needs of the patient determine who (on the team) assists him, and this requires planning and leadership which are the responsibility of the professional nurse.

Each team has a leader, and the members are responsible to her. She makes the assignments and performs nursing functions, yet serves as the coordinator of her group to see that patients' needs are met safely and by those capable of giving such care.

The size and membership of the team vary, not only from one place to another but within the same institution at different times of the day. Students (practical and professional) are members; on occasion a professional student may be the team leader. Assignments change with patients' needs and available personnel. The key to the success of the nursing team is cooperation, once the care plan is made. And cooperation depends upon giving and sharing, tolerance and understanding, and acceptance of each worker as an individual with a function to perform in the best interest of the patient.

COMMUNICATIONS: A PART OF RELATIONSHIPS

Communications may be described as any means used to convey or get across an idea, a feeling, or a thought. To communicate means to pass meanings or feelings from one person to another. This may involve listening, paying attention, tone of voice, writing, how a person looks (facial expression, grooming, posture), mood and touch.

Importance of Communications

Communication is a key to good relationships. People need to understand each other, their ideas, thinking, and feelings. This is extremely important between the nurse and the patient because each contact is a ready-made, self-starting situation for thoughts, impressions, observations, and feelings. Such a giving and receiving process may use the spoken or the written word, or it may take place without words at all.

Communication is stressed, but not because this is your first encounter with it. You have been communicating since birth and no doubt have developed considerable skill. The concern in your role as a practical nurse should be to realize how much depends upon your ability to communicate effectively with patients and others and to sharpen your skills and develop any needed new ones.

Skills in Communications

A patient may "get the message" just by looking at the nurse, or vice versa. While the spoken word is one of the most commonly used means for giving or receiving ideas, it is not the only one, nor the most important one at times. Consider how facial expressions show (or tell) a person's feelings, or how body posture, gestures, touch, and even mannerisms tell the story.

Skill in communications depends upon such things as ability to speak in understandable terms and to listen attentively in such manner that the speaker is aware you are listening. This means giving indication by facial expression, or by facing the speaker or giving verbal indication that you hear what is being said.

Sometimes words have different meanings for different people, and they fail to understand or respond. In nursing, nontechnical terms should be used in talking with most patients. These are the terms they are most apt to understand and, even then, an explanation may need to be restated. However, today the public is well informed through mass communication media (press, radio, television), and words previously uncommon to them are now in general use; judgment must be used in conversation with the patient to avoid "talking down" to him.

Opinions are formed as people communicate. The patient does this as he listens and watches; the nurse does this, also. One worker to another forms opinions too. Improvement in skill comes as one pays attention to the appropriateness of tone of voice, terms used, facial expressions, gestures, and body posture. Effective communications play a part in good relationships.

SUMMARY

People "behave"; that is, they respond to things that rouse the mind. A person responds according to the way things "seem" to be to him; therefore, he behaves as he "sees" fit under the circumstances. This basic fact should be remembered when dealing with self or with others, be they classmates, patients, teachers, or family.

Humans have basic physical and social needs; they have beliefs, values, and attitudes as well. These factors influence how a person "sees himself" (self-image) and how he feels about himself and his relationships with other people.

Ethics is a standard or a rule of proper behavior. It may be a written or an unwritten rule. Regardless of its being written or not, if it guides one's actions, it produces ethical behavior. The individual has the final say-so and the responsibility for conducting himself or for failing to conduct himself in an ethical manner. Ethical behavior is a matter of self-direction and is an essential part of nursing practice.

Specialization is common in our culture. Many types of skilled workers join efforts to provide services and produce goods. The same is true of patient care. Because it takes an increasing number of variously skilled people to handle health services, the concern for good human relationships becomes more pronounced than ever. The practical nurse needs to know and practice those types of behavior which promote sound, effective relationships with others. The value of using effective communication skills is as high for the practical nurse as it is for any other human. These skills can make the difference between effectiveness and ineffectiveness.

GUIDES FOR STUDY AND DISCUSSION

1. As you understand it, what does the word *behavior* mean?
2. See if you can describe (to your own satisfaction) the meaning of belief, value,

attitude, self-image. If you cannot, be ready to ask a question(s) which you feel may help clarify these meanings for you.

3. What are the two main groups of basic needs? Give examples of each.

4. People communicate. What means do they use?

5. Give examples (those existing in your classroom) of how people communicate without speaking (non-verbal).

6. Communications play a role in relationships. What other factors are involved? See Figure 3–1 and be ready to give an example of each factor.

7. Select at least five general terms of conduct (such as integrity) included in The Code of Ethics for The Licensed Practical Nurse and list an example of behavior you believe would fit each term.

SUGGESTED SITUATIONS AND ACTIVITIES

1. Devise a situation you (and classmates) can role play that will depict unethical conduct of a student in your program.

2. Imagine a nursing situation that would fit point number 7 in the code. Be ready to describe it to your classmates to see if they agree with you.

3. Select an item (statement, idea, etc.) in this chapter which was new to you when you studied it. Consider how you can use it for self-improvement.

4. If your program has a handbook of policies, review it and check (✔) those policies that pertain to ethical behavior.

THE LICENSED GRADUATE PRACTICAL NURSE

This two-chapter unit is concerned with two prominent aspects of nursing practice. *Chapter 4* is concerned with *legality or practice,* and what it means to the public and to the licensed practical nurse as far as her responsibilities and privileges are involved. *Chapter 5* discusses the *need for vocational growth* of the practitioner and her *responsibilities to self and her respective group*.

Together these chapters are designed to bring into focus some factors which will help provide the practitioner with a basis for sound judgments, prudent actions and a continued interest in self growth in a rapidly changing society.

CHAPTER 4

THE LEGAL ASPECTS OF NURSING PRACTICE

OBJECTIVES FOR THE STUDENT: Be able to:

1. Describe how a nurse practice act (law) protects the public; give two examples.
2. Describe how a nurse practice act helps the licensed practical nurse; give two examples.
3. Tell what it means to be held accountable for one's acts of negligence.
4. Explain the statement "a license to practice is a privilege which carries with it certain responsibilities."
5. Distinguish between the purpose of a mandatory law and a permissive law.

SUGGESTED STUDY VOCABULARY*

aspect
law
jurisdiction
libel
society

revoke or revocation
suspend or suspension
endorsement
negligence
malpractice

tort
crime
mandatory
permissive
waiver
prudent

*Look for any terms you already know.

INTRODUCTION

Laws are passed to safeguard the *public welfare*. Public welfare means that which is concerned with the social betterment of society or a group within that society such as *child welfare*.

Few aspects of our lives are left untouched by laws (directly or indirectly). Think for a moment of such things as health, travel, food, clothing, housing, schools, property, buying and selling, and consider how laws control or influence these necessities of life.

The practice of nursing is very much a

part of patient well-being. Patient welfare is the concern of the public at large; thus, the legal regulation of the practice of nursing is as necessary as the legal regulation of any other services rendered to society. It is essential that the sick receive care from persons capable of rendering *safe, effective* care.

Chapter 4 includes basic information which will become more meaningful as you begin to relate it to your actions and practices. Keep in mind that Chapter 3 relates to Chapter 4. One's values and attitudes influence behavior in uniform the same as in "street clothes." A conscience toward right conduct knows no particular attire. It is there or it is absent regardless of how one is garbed. Earning the right to use the initials LPN or LVN or CNA after one's name adds unique responsibilities as far as conscience, integrity, and the respect for the rights of others are concerned. This chapter points out what some of these additional responsibilities are and emphasizes the fact that the individual nurse is responsible for knowing the meaning of her license so as to conduct herself in such manner as to avoid misunderstandings, libel, and lawsuits.

THE LAW ITSELF

The letter "L" in LPN or LVN or "C" in CNA signifies to all that the person using these initials after her name has met and continues to meet some types of requirements. These requirements have their basis in a law controlling the practice of practical nursing in the jurisdiction (state, province) where the nurse is using them.

It will benefit you to *begin to know the purpose of "the law"* now, so that by the time you complete your program, you will have some meaningful guidelines to assist you in your future practice.

The word "law," as used here, refers to written rules of conduct enforced by a controlling authority; these rules come into being as a result of the lawmaking process within a jurisdiction.

Chapter 2 points out that by 1960 each state and the District of Columbia had a "law" to control the practice of practical nursing. Canada, by 1970, had such laws in nine of its ten provinces. A point to remember: *regulations to control practice have a legal founda-*

tion; much as a person may complain or fret about "what the law is," he must comply with (obey) it until it is changed (amended). As to those who plead ignorance of the law, defy or ignore it, or as is commonly said, "take the law into their own hands," society — through the court system — brings these persons to justice. This means that the courts hold persons accountable for their acts and determine whether they are innocent or guilty as charged.

It is within such governmental framework that a law to control the practice of nursing exists: namely, those who hold a license are required to live up to the terms of that license or be subject to "explaining" their actions to the courts.

A law undergoes change (is amended) as years go by because time and circumstances alter public welfare. This fact should be kept in mind during your working lifetime because you, as a citizen, and as one certified to practice, will be held accountable for "knowing the law" wherever you practice. This fact disquiets some; they say, "tell us *what* the law allows or disallows so we can learn it." "We want to know what it means so that when we practice we will be practicing legally."

At best, one can only use the jurisdiction's *present-day* regulations and interpret them. Even this can require legal explanation when the law is written in general terms, and there appear to be "gray areas" needing interpretation. Add to this the fact each jurisdiction writes its own law (there is no national law). It is entirely possible that the law in one jurisdiction may differ from the law in another. When you are told that it will be your responsibility to know what is allowable and what is not allowable under the terms of your license in a particular state or province, it means that *you must assume responsibility for informing yourself.* Be mindful, too, that laws change as time goes by; this places additional responsibility on you just as it does when driver's licensure laws change or tax laws change. You have an on-going responsibility for knowing what your license permits you to do.

To acquaint yourself with the law (commonly called Nurse Practice Act) in your jurisdiction, examine and discuss it and the regulations for carrying it out. Determine what is *specific* (spelled out) and what is *implied* (not spelled out but the intention is there). The current rules and regulations of the enforcement authority (commonly known as the State

Board of Nursing, or a similar title) are rules which must be followed because they are, in fact, based upon the current Nurse Practice Act.

WHAT DOES A NURSE PRACTICE ACT INCLUDE?

The law to control the practice of practical nursing is commonly called the "Nurse Practice Act." In some states it is a separate law and in others the provisions for practical nursing are a part of a general law which covers both professional and practical nursing practice. Twelve jurisdictions have separate laws while the others have combined laws. In Canada, five of the nine provinces (with laws) have separate laws. In some instances, having a separate law requires that there be a separate "board" to administer the law.

To control the practice of nursing, a nurse practice act usually provides for the following:

1. Use of the title licensed practical nurse (LPN), licensed vocational nurse (LVN), or certified nursing assistant (CNA used in some Canadian Provinces).

2. Licensure examination(s).

3. Issuing of licenses, their revocation and suspension.

4. Endorsement of candidates for out-of-state licensure.

5. Setting of standards for conducting pre-service programs to prepare practitioners.

6. Appointment of a board or a committee (commonly called State Board of Nursing in the U.S.; Canada uses various agencies: e.g., Department of Health, Province Nurses' Association, Boards) to see that the provisions of the law are carried out.

7. The definition of practical nursing may or may not be included (the limits of practice are interpreted by the Board).

The State Board of Nursing is a legally constituted body. Membership (who shall qualify to serve), tenure (how long they may serve), and general functions and duties of the Board are defined in the law. It is their responsibility to establish all specific rules and regulations as they relate to carrying out the stated provisions of the law. This legal body may not set rules and regulations that are in any way contrary to the intent of the law itself. The law is the basis for all action and control.

To fulfill responsibilities such as issuing licenses, the Board maintains vast systems of records to protect the public from someone getting an unwarranted license and to preserve the records of those who qualify for and receive licenses. They likewise maintain records of practical nursing schools in their jurisdiction.

The State Board of Nursing conducts hearings concerned with licensure to determine eligibility for licensure in some instances. They may revoke or suspend a license for just cause. Just cause includes those acts performed that were not in keeping with the law. Instances which may provoke the revocation or suspension of a license include gross incompetency, negligence while on duty, the commission of a serious crime (i.e., treason, murder, robbery, arson, etc.), habitual drunkenness, addiction to the use of drugs, or any other habit rendering a nurse unfit to care for patients.

Nurse practice acts vary from state to state in many ways; this fact may make interstate (from state to state) licensure difficult and time-consuming. Under our present system of states' rights, it cannot be expected that uniform nursing practice acts can be enacted, yet more uniform policies and procedures may be gained by voluntary cooperation between states.

Mandatory Versus Permissive Laws

In some states the law is *mandatory*. This means that all who nurse "for hire" must be licensed. However, in many states the law is *permissive*. This means that the law applies only to those persons who *represent* themselves as licensed nurses or who use the initials of RN (registered nurse) or LPN (licensed practical nurse) or LVN (licensed vocational nurse) or use some other signs or devices to indicate to the public that they are licensed. The trend is toward mandatory laws; such a move tends to provide more effective, safe care at the hands of those who do qualify for licensure.

The nurse needs to realize her license is a legal permit issued to her to allow her to practice nursing under the terms of that state's laws. A license is not considered a permanent or everlasting right to practice. It is usable only under the terms of the law and should be protected and respected; this requires the holder to respect the limits of the license and to be responsible for keeping it current as required by law.

A license issued in one state is not usable as such in another state. It is possible under certain conditions to procure a license in another state without taking this licensure examination in that state; this is called *endorsement*. For information about licensure in another state, write directly to the Board of Nursing of that state.

Licenses to practice nursing need to be renewed the same as other types of licenses. When a license is not renewed as required, it is considered lapsed (not active), and it becomes necessary to reinstate it or bring it up-to-date if the nurse wishes to continue to practice.

Once a license has been issued, the nurse needs to know how often and at what time the license needs to be renewed. Each state enacts its own regulations governing the renewal of a license and the fee to be charged for this. *The nurse is responsible for keeping her license active.* The Board of Nursing will always need to know when the address or the name of a licensee (the holder of the license) changes. Each licensed nurse is responsible for keeping them informed.

The State Board of Nursing provides consultative and supervisory services to schools of practical nursing in its jurisdiction to see that the rules and regulations for conducting these programs are met. It has the authority to approve or disapprove the opening of new schools and from time to time publishes lists of approved schools.

Another legal function of the Board is to provide for and conduct licensure examinations. It furnishes application forms and processes them to see that only qualified candidates are permitted to take the examinations. Successful candidates are issued certificates and licenses. All candidates are notified of their results.

One can readily see from the long list of responsibilities that the State Board of Nursing in each jurisdiction is not only an essential body, but one that is *important to the student and the LPN as well as to the public.* In brief, this is the agency which will conduct your licensure examination, issue the license, notify you of the need to renew your license (if they have your current address), and endorse you for licensure in another jurisdiction. *The current address of each State Board of Nursing is*

published in the January and July issues of the American Journal of Nursing. This is a fact worth remembering as you may need to use this information many times in the years ahead.

THE LEGAL STATUS OF THE PRACTICAL NURSE

As stated previously, holding a license to practice as a practical nurse carries rights and responsibilities. Every practical nurse needs to know what these rights and responsibilities are. Several such facts are briefly included.

Contract for Employment

This may be a written contract or a verbal (oral) one. In whatever form, a legal contract includes these three things: *an offer, an acceptance,* and *a consideration.* The breaking of a legal contract by either party establishes the basic right of the injured party to pursue the remedy available at law for the damages caused. This serves as a protection to the rights of the practical nurse and to her employer as well.

The *offer* or terms of work (hours, salary, days off, etc.) in an employment contract should be clearly stated and understood. The *acceptance* of such offer should likewise be understood and clearly stated. The *consideration* (in such an employment contract) is the doing of the work as agreed to under the offer and the *acceptance* of the contract in exchange for wages and other stipulated benefits (meals, laundering of uniforms, etc.).

In cases where the offer and the acceptance are not clearly stated and there is a breaking of the contract, the matter may be taken to court to determine the offending party.

Many factors enter into the making of a legal contract, and if there is any doubt in the mind of the nurse or the other party, legal counsel should be sought.

Status of the Practical Nurse in Performance of Her Services

The LPN may be employed by one of many different agencies (hospital, nursing home, physician's office, public health department, industrial plant, etc.) or do private duty caring for a patient in the home, hospital, nursing home, etc. In doing private duty she is employed by the patient or his family but works under the supervision of a physician or a registered professional nurse. The hospital is not her employer even though she may care for the patient there. Whether employed by a private patient, by a hospital, or by another agency, it is *essential* to remember that one is personally liable for his or her own negligent or wrongful acts. If employed in a hospital, for example, a nurse may involve her employer and make him liable in addition to herself, but *each person is responsible for his own negligence.*

Any individual acting as a nurse has certain duties to perform, and negligence may be involved if these duties are not carried out or if they are carried out without using a reasonable amount of cautious judgment or prudence. This includes any nurse, professional, practical, or student.

The individual who undertakes work requiring a degree of skill is considered by law to have promised that he *has* the degree of skill necessary to perform his work efficiently. This means that, with reference to the performance of some task involved in the care of a patient (or nonperformance of some task for à patient), the nurse should show better judgment in dealing with a nursing situation than would a schoolteacher or bricklayer. Knowing "right from wrong" takes on different shades of meaning under different circumstances.

The practical nurse is not excused from negligence or her own wrongful acts, any more than a student nurse or professional nurse. She is authorized by law to practice nursing under certain conditions, one being that she work only under direct orders of a licensed physician or under the supervision of a registered nurse. Another is that she can be held liable for unauthorized practice of medicine.

A legal yardstick that a nurse, professional, practical, or student, may use to measure the extent of her duties is simply this: *no one can give a nurse the right to assume greater responsibilities than the law authorizes her to assume.* As stated before, the practical nurse may involve her employer and make him liable in addition to herself in the course of her employment. To know the limits of one's license and to practice within these limits are a basic necessity and a personal responsibility of every nurse.

LEGAL FACTS RELATED TO PRACTICE

This is a day of lawsuits. It seems almost no one is immune from being sued by someone for something. Workers in the health field are particularly liable in this respect. Licensed practical nurses come within this group and have need to be familiar with some general facts which relate to legal and illegal practice. The following discussion includes *negligence, malpractice, tort, crime, witnessing.* Any one of these legal factors can serve as a basis for claims against a licensed practical nurse.

NEGLIGENCE

Everyone in society is subject to the basic rule of the law of negligence, which requires that we so handle our lives and our property as to avoid injury to any other person or his property.

Negligence is one of the most common causes for lawsuits involving nurses. Negligence may be defined as the failure to do something which a reasonable person would *do* under the same circumstances, or doing something which a reasonable person would *not do* under the same circumstances.

In rendering nursing care there are several examples of negligence which provoke lawsuits more frequently than others. One of the most common is burns. It does not take special training to know that an object that is too hot will cause a burn, and if a nurse applies such an overheated object to a patient, she can be held liable. Special care should be observed in using hot water bottles, heating pads, heat treatment equipment, solutions for treatment, and baths of all sorts.

The careless handling of sponges in the operating room is responsible for many suits against hospitals, physicians, and nurses. Here the nurse must be alert to her responsibilities as they relate to the handling and counting of sponges, lest one or more be left in the patient by error.

Common sense would seem to direct the nurse in preventing patients from falling out of bed. Some hospitals have routine orders concerning the use of side rails under certain conditions. A nurse should not only know what the hospital regulations require, but she should always use reasonable judgment to protect her patient from falling out of bed when his safety requires that type of protection. Suits for damages against nurses and hospitals all too frequently arise as a result of injuries caused when patients fall out of bed.

Negligence in identifying, preparing, and administering medications is still another common cause for lawsuits. A nurse cannot be too careful in preparing and giving medicines. Practical nurses may or may not be engaged in this, but if they are, they may be held liable for their own negligence or wrongful acts the same as professional nurses.

If equipment has been carelessly used or is defective, the patient may find cause for a suit for damages. Sometimes infections start from contaminated syringes and needles, or a patient is injured by faulty or defective equipment. The nurse may be held for negligence if it is proven to the satisfaction of the court that she did not perform her duties as a careful nurse would have performed them under the same circumstances.

The practical nurse needs to be aware of her responsibilities in caring for a patient's belongings, such as jewelry, money, dentures, clothing and the like. Hospitals have regulations for handling these possessions and they should be observed in every detail.

MALPRACTICE

Malpractice is described as conduct in a manner contrary to accepted rules, with injurious results to patients; this means misconduct or unreasonable lack of skill in performing professional and trustworthy duties.

When applied to physicians and nurses, the term malpractice includes such things as wrong or harmful treatment leading to injury of the patient, or some act of ignorance or carelessness that causes undue suffering or death. The term also includes lack of proper training or skills to do a task or carry out a function which results in harm to the patient. The act may proceed from reckless conduct and criminal intent (deliberate intention to commit an unlawful act).

Patients (or their family) who are dissatisfied with the results of their treatment and feel that they have been unduly harmed because of unskilled care are the most likely to sue. In some instances they sue the hospital (governmental or voluntary charitable hospitals in some states cannot be held liable) or the physician or the nurse. The patient seeks damages for such things as pain, suffering, loss of time, loss of ability, and personal inconvenience. The court must determine whether or not malpractice was involved. Increasing numbers of court cases involve nurses in malpractice lawsuits.

The patient's chart may be taken into the courtroom to furnish evidence of a patient's treatment and a record of his care. If for no other reason (and there are others) than this one important fact, accurate recording and reporting on the patient's chart make it an invaluable record.

The nurse's conduct should be without question in the keeping of confidences, practicing integrity in the pursuit of responsibilities, and her manner of relating to patients. Careless talk to a patient about what is being done for him or talking about one patient to another patient can be a breeding ground for patient discontent and dissatisfaction.

Information concerning malpractice insurance is something every practicing nurse should seek for her personal protection.

TORT

A *tort* is a wrongful act (does not include breaking a contract) against someone or something (property) which makes the person committing the act liable for damages (civil action). Some types of torts which nurses experience include *negligence, malpractice, holding a person against his will unjustifiably* (i.e., locking him in a room), *assault* (threatening to or touching another person unjustifiably), and *battery* (beating a person or causing him physical harm in an unlawful manner).

A person has a right to refuse some act of personal contact by another person if he chooses. A patient may refuse to have a bed bath or allow a nurse to cut his toe nails. He may refuse to have an arm soak ordered by the physician. These are examples of situations that can lead to a charge of battery against the nurse who proceeds to carry out the orders anyway.

Self-defense is the right of the nurse (or of anyone) in the event a patient strikes out and attacks her. Self-defense is a right, but it extends only to those measures that are necessary to protect oneself; such measures should be reasonable and appropriate to the situation.

Another wrongful act could be using *undue restraint to limit movement.* Hospitals have regulations concerning the use of side rails to protect patients from injury; likewise, there are regulations concerning the use of restraining equipment. The reasons for such regulations are two-fold: (1) to protect the patient's safety, and (2) to protect the hospital from employees who might not use proper judgment in applying them. The best advice concerning restraining any patient is to know the regulations established by the agency and follow them with care.

A person has the *right of privacy*. If this right is unlawfully invaded, it is grounds for a lawsuit to recover damages. Reasonable good judgment should guide one's actions in nursing patients. Permitting "outsiders" so to speak, to observe something happening to a patient may be cause for suit for damages.

CRIMES

A person may be prosecuted for crime through an act that the law calls a crime *or* by not doing something that is called for by law and declared to be a crime if it is not carried out. One common example is the law a state may have concerning a license to drive a car. If a license is required and a person drives without a license, he is criminally liable if the law states it is a crime to drive without it.

The same would apply to a nurse who practices nursing without a license in a jurisdiction with a mandatory law which states that those who nurse for hire must be currently licensed.

It is illegal to have narcotics in one's possession under certain circumstances. Illegal possession constitutes a crime because there are laws to control the handling and use of narcotics.

Crimes relate to public welfare. When some action is against the public welfare (state), it becomes a criminal action; these offenses range from small, petty acts (misdemeanors) to serious acts (felonies).

A *felony* is a grave crime, and serious in nature. A person convicted of a felony is subject to imprisonment in a state prison or in some cases, death.

BEING A WITNESS

At times, nurses are called upon to testify as to facts and circumstances in a court.

Under oath, they are expected to give true, factual information as it relates to the case at hand. Opinions and "hearsay" evidence are not wanted or permissible as far as evidence is concerned.

The knowledge that a patient's chart may be used in court makes accuracy in recording any chart entry of profound importance to the nurse. As a nurse, witnessing a will is an act to be avoided if at all possible. The patient should use an attorney to seek legal advice. Accurate charting of any such event is an ethical responsibility.

RESPONSIBILITIES IN EMERGENCY SITUATIONS

Some states have laws requiring a person involved in an automobile accident to give aid to any other person injured in the accident. If there is such a law, it must be obeyed. Beyond that there is no legal obligation for an individual to render care to a person in an emergency situation unless the individual chooses to do so. However, once this obligation is undertaken, it then becomes necessary to render help in keeping with the needs of the situation. One should know that under *emergency* circumstances a nurse, like any other person, may give care to save a life and, as such, this medical care would not be considered as coming under the practice of medicine. But in a case involving a so-called emergency situation, the person who claims she did not violate a medical practice act because she acted in an emergency situation must sustain the burden of proof that it was in fact an emergency situation.

"Good Samaritan Act"

People are sometimes reluctant to stop and give emergency aid to the injured for fear of being sued for services rendered. Some states have passed a law commonly known as the "Good Samaritan Act" which provides immunity from civil liability. Most generally under the terms of a "Good Samaritan Act" a person (any person, doctors included) may render emergency care, in good faith, at the scene of an accident (e.g., highway, street, etc., but not in a hospital or place where there is medical equipment) if the victim has no objection; the passer-by may render emergency care under these circumstances without the possibility of being held liable for any civil damages providing that the service given is reasonable and done with care under the circumstances.

SUMMARY

Laws are passed to safeguard the public welfare. In the case of nursing practice, practical or professional, the laws protect the public by setting standards for practical and professional nursing education and for licensure: they define who shall be licensed and under what terms.

Knowing about the license, what it means, how it is acquired, what it permits the nurse to do (or not do), and that it can be revoked or suspended under certain circumstances—all are the responsibility of the nurse.

A person is liable for his or her own acts of negligence. While others may be involved (administrator, supervisor, physician) the person who commits the act is held accountable for what was done. And no one can give a nurse the right to perform greater responsibilities than the law allows her to perform.

Under the law, the nurse has rights as well as liabilities and responsibilities. She is protected in the legal use of her license and against hazards in relation to her work in certain instances. Her rights of legal contract are protected. She may sue for payment of fees, for example, if a contract is broken by the other party.

The nurse does not need to fear the law, but rather she needs to understand and respect it in relation to her rights, privileges, and responsibilities.

The content in this chapter will be emphasized in many different clinical learning situations throughout the program. The intent and meaning will become more useful and clear as you apply it in your day-to-day practice and discussion.

GUIDES FOR STUDY AND DISCUSSION

1. Imagine that you held a license to practice nursing in this state and that you are moving to a neighboring state and plan to practice nursing there.
   a. How would you go about getting a license in that state?
   b. How will you become informed about the legal requirements and aspects in that state in order to take employment and to practice nursing legally?
2. Some state laws are mandatory and others are permissive. What is the difference between these two types of laws?
3. What is negligence? List some common causes of lawsuits that involve negligence in nursing practice.
4. The nurse practice act (law) protects the nurse as well as the public. How or in what way is this true?
5. Laws are amended by state law-making bodies. Knowing that ignorance of the law excuses no one, how can an individual keep abreast of the changes in the law regulating the practice of nursing? Think of ways this can be done.

6. *Legal Factors*	*Define it*	*Give an example*

Negligence
Malpractice
Tort
Crime
Felony

7. The Board of Nursing has many responsibilities. List as many as you can from your reading.

8. Some states have a law often called "Good Samaritan Act." What is the purpose of this law?

SUGGESTED SITUATIONS AND ACTIVITIES

1. Plan an employment situation (for role playing with classmates) in which you, an LPN, are expected to perform a service to a patient which appears to be "beyond the limits" of your license. Show how you ethically resolve this situation.

2. Examine the Nurse Practice Act in your jurisdiction.
   a. Is it a mandatory or permissive law?
   b. Does it specifically define the "acts" you may perform? If not, how do you know what you may or may not do? If uncertain, how would you proceed to find out?
   c. Does it define, in general terms, what is practical nursing?
   d. Search for other requirements such as renewal of license, fee for renewal, terms of revocation and suspension of license, etc.

CHAPTER 5

THE PRACTITIONER: OPPORTUNITIES AND RESPONSIBILITIES

TOPICAL HEADINGS

Introduction
Employment Opportunities
Seeking Employment
Continuing to Learn

A Citizen and Community Member
Nursing Organizations and Publications

Summary
Guides for Study and Discussion
Suggested Situations and Discussion

OBJECTIVES FOR THE STUDENT: Be able to:

1. Identify five different employment opportunities in the community for licensed practical nurses.
2. Describe three factors which have influenced practical nursing employment in recent years.
3. State two reasons why it is necessary to continue to learn.
4. List the main factors to consider when seeking employment and when leaving employment.
5. Name the nursing organizations open to LPN membership.
6. Explain two values of being a member of a national nursing organization(s).
7. Describe several ways an LPN can serve the community.

SUGGESTED STUDY VOCABULARY*

therapy
therapeutic
convalescing
mandatory

overextension
intensive care facility
intermediate care facility
extended care facility

personnel policies
self-improvement
constituent association

---

*Look for any terms you already know.

INTRODUCTION

Today there are some 375 different titled health workers involved in servicing the health needs of this country. Health workers represent one of the nation's fastest growing service groups. From 1969 to 1970 this group increased from 3.9 to 4.4 million persons.

Practical nursing emerged as a recognized member of the health team during the late 50's and the early 60's. It has rapidly continued its growth in numbers and in quality since then.

41

Chapter 2 pointed out some general over-all factors which have been influential. This chapter furnishes more specific information by pointing out practitioner responsibilities and employment opportunities.

EMPLOYMENT OPPORTUNITIES AND RESPONSIBILITIES

Today the licensed practical nurse works in all types of agencies involved in nursing. Chapter 2 pointed out (Table 2–1, Nursing: Five Periods of Development) how rapidly licensure laws were enacted following World War II and how schools or programs grew in numbers. If one is to appreciate present employment opportunities and responsibilities, it will help to examine two sets of factors: (Table 5–1)

1. The things (events and circumstances) which have promoted the use of the practical nurse.

2. The things (events and circumstances) which have raised questions concerning the use of the practical nurse.

Where Are Licensed Practical Nurses Working?

It might be simpler to list where they do not work because LPN's are employed in almost every conceivable situation involved with patient care. Employment opportunities are found in governmental and non-govern-

TABLE 5.1.   FACTORS WHICH INFLUENCED PRACTICAL NURSE EMPLOYMENT

PROMOTED	*RAISED QUESTIONS*
1. In early years, the need for someone to care for the sick in the home and carry out housekeeping activities.	1. Fear that a non-trained or less able person might take employment away from the "trained nurse."
2. World War I generated the need for auxiliary workers in military hospitals.	2. The Great Depression found many registered nurses without employment.
3. World War II generated the increased need for auxiliary nursing personnel in civilian hospitals— "the home front."	3. The fear that lesser trained personnel (less than the familiar three year "trained nurse") were not safe practitioners.
4. Federal money provided for practical nurse education: 1956—Temporary funds authorized. 1962—Manpower Development and Training Act. 1963—Vocational Education Act made funds permanently available according to appropriations by Congress.	4. The fear that lesser trained personnel might take employment opportunities away from the registered nurse.
5. Federal money for hospital expansion. Social legislation to provide hospital care, extended care, insurance to pay costs, etc.	5. The hit and miss approach to setting up practical nursing schools with few standards and great variations among them.
6. Population changes: increased numbers of people living longer.	6. Some practical nurses licensed by "waiver," while others by education and examination, created a supply of workers with different backgrounds.
7. Shortage of trained personnel propelled the LPN into all types of employment situations.	7. Concern that the practical nurse was doing more than basic prepration warranted.
8. More programs, better teaching, improved student selection.	8. Concern that practical nursing programs were trying to be "miniature" diploma programs and "be all things to all people."
9. LPN less mobile; stays in a locality.	9. Lack of understanding on the part of employing agency on how/where to use the graduate licensed practical nurse.
10. High percentage remain active or return to work.	10. Lack of direction on the part of registered nurses to delegate nursing tasks and functions to LPN according to the needs of patients.
11. Highly motivated as a group. Mature individual senses work satisfaction.	11. Overextension of responsibilities for the LPN; carrying on tasks and functions calling for a higher degree of judgment with limited registered nurse supervision.

mental situations including hospitals, nursing homes, public health nursing agencies, private duty, Armed Services, Veterans Administration, Peace Corps, industry and doctors' offices. LPN's work in agencies caring for the mentally ill and the retarded, with patients who have long term physical illnesses, and in rehabilitation centers.

Changing Patterns of Patient Care Influence Employment Opportunities

Increased demands for health care by all people are changing the facilities providing this care. *General hospitals* are filled with very sick patients who need the life-saving benefits of the latest equipment and therapy, elderly patients (eight out of ten have more than one disorder), and patients who need various laboratory tests and special treatments not available in the physician's office or outpatient clinics.

Special units and departments are equipped to care for the critically ill (for example, Intensive Care Unit). Teams of specially trained personnel work in these units and departments providing close observation and immediate therapy as needed.

Intermediate care facilities provide care for patients who are convalescing or who do not need the benefit of the highly technical equipment in the hospital.

Extended care facilities or *nursing homes* provide care for long-term patients (chiefly elderly persons) who require nursing care and attention. Some of these facilities are first-rate and meet a real need for society while others lack features (safety, sanitation, recreation, and diversional activities) which contribute to the patient's security, and physical and mental well-being.

Home health services have been available for many years to the sick who remain at home. Public health agencies (voluntary and official) have provided nursing services by having the nurse visit the home on a regular basis. Overcrowding of hospitals and other facilities, increased costs of away from home care, and the desire to be at home and enjoy familiar surroundings all play a part in determining the numbers of people who receive nursing services in their homes.

Neighborhood health clinics are appearing in large cities to bring health care closer to the people. The idea is that people will use the clinics if they are conveniently located.

All of these agencies provide employment opportunities for the licensed practical nurse. The years ahead may show further changes as population increases and people live longer. To meet the changing needs of society, one might foresee the time when the amount of home health services would be greatly increased and provide employment opportunities for the licensed practical nurse.

Special hospitals, special departments in general hospitals, day care centers, half-way houses, and out-patient clinics concerned with the emotionally disturbed patient need vast numbers of prepared workers. High on that list of workers are nursing personnel. This field of practice offers employment opportunities to the licensed practical nurse. Preparation for beginning employment starts in the basic program in some instances; there is need to include appropriate learning experiences in more schools so that the student comes to know this patient and his special needs.

SEEKING EMPLOYMENT

Obtaining employment is easy when the demand for workers is high. Such is the case in the health services today. For example, an effective LPN usually has no problem seeking and securing employment in centers of population.

The employer has every right to expect you to have basic skills and abilities appropriate for the license you possess. In addition, he is interested in your ability to get along well with other people and "be well-received."

Impressions start with first contacts, including your letter of application and your personal appearance and conduct during the interview.

A letter of application is a business letter; it should be typed or neatly written in ink on plain, business stationery and follow the form of a business letter with proper headings and appropriate opening and closing phrases. The contents of the letter should include a statement of inquiry about position openings or the reason for writing the letter, a statement(s) concerning your preparation and record of work experience, plus the names of persons who may be contacted for reference. Secure permission to use a person's name for reference beforehand.

Keep in mind that the letter of inquiry is the employer's first introduction to you, the sender. It creates an impression; it should be a good impression.

The interview, a meeting of two (or more) people by appointment, is often used by a person seeking work or a person seeking a worker. Interview time is face to face impression time. Important things to keep in mind are that you should make an appointment, keep it, and be on time. Employers often form poor impressions of people who walk in "off the street" seeking employment. Make preparations ahead of time by listing questions you would like to have answered. For instance, you will want to know the conditions of work as they relate to the *personnel policies* of the agency (hours of duty, sick leave, vacation, holidays, pension plans, group insurance, salary scale). Some agencies have personnel policy handbooks which serve as reference during and following the interview. In addition to personnel policies, you should determine what will be expected of you in the work situation. Prepare a list of your past employment (where and during what period of time) arranged in order as to dates. Likewise, list several persons the employer might contact to secure information about your work record; here again, get permission to use names ahead of time.

Personal appearance speaks for itself and plays a very real part in the employer's first impression. In one sentence—dress appropriately and have a well-groomed look about you. This takes into account good personal hygiene, and the sensible use of cosmetics and jewelry.

During the interview you will form impressions and so will the employer. As he asks and answers questions, he tries to judge your fitness (or lack of it) for employment, including your manner and attitude toward work. For instance, he is alert to the type of questions asked and what things seem most important. If salary and days off seem to be of first importance, the employer might have reason enough to wonder about the applicant's interest in the work itself. No one denies the importance of an adequate salary; it is a very real part of job satisfaction. But during the interview, why not wait with your questions about salary, days off, and other benefits until you have had (or made) opportunity to discuss the requirements of the work? It is another way to "put your best foot forward." Get answers to

questions about the work itself. Find out what is expected. The role of the licensed practical nurse varies from one place to another, and it will help to know ahead of time what the agency expects you to do. In relation to salary and other benefits, be sure to acquaint yourself with such things as salary range, social security and tax withholding plan, insurance provisions and retirement plans, if any.

As you ask and answer questions, you will be sizing up the person interviewing you and he will be sizing you up. The main thing to remember is that he will be getting acquainted with you, your abilities and interests, and you will be getting acquainted with the agency, the work expectations, and the policies regulating your employment. Do not hesitate to ask any questions you may have, but use good judgment in what you ask and when you ask it. This is why you should list your questions ahead of time.

A certain amount of time has been set aside for the interview and this calls for promptness at the beginning and in closing when matters of business are over.

Joining a professional registry has employment advantages when the nurse is on private duty. The registry is open 24 hours a day and is staffed by nurses who are available for conference when needed. Each applicant must meet certain requirements to have her name listed and to be called. Physicians, hospitals, nursing homes, and families call when they need a nurse, and the first one on call who is best suited for the case is sent. Special abilities of nurses are considered when such selections are made because it is better for both the patient and the nurse if the nurse is suited to the needs of the patient.

In communities without such a registry, the nursing office in the nearest hospital often serves as a center for private duty employment.

Resigning and Leaving

Circumstances cause people to change employment, but one should leave a position in such a way that he or she could return at some future time if conditions were favorable.

The private duty nurse discusses termination of employment with the patient (or family) and the physician, agreeably setting the last day of duty.

Leaving employment in a hospital (or other agency) is more complicated. Remembering that it is as important to resign and leave in the proper way as it is to seek employment, the nurse makes an appointment with the appropriate person and tells him or her of the decision. A reason or reasons for leaving should be honestly stated, and judgment and tact should be used if the work situation has been an unhappy one.

If it is known ahead of time that a letter of resignation is expected, it may be presented at the close of the appointment or may follow soon after. The policy of the hospital should be followed, but at least two weeks' notice should be given, if at all possible, to allow the employer time to make other arrangements. The difficulty of finding or training a replacement should be considered in setting the last day of employment.

The decision to leave a place of employment can be a difficult one. It is a mark of poor judgment to walk in, resign, and leave the same day; only under extreme conditions should this ever happen. A person's reputation, good or bad, follows him. Moving from place to place or staying only a short time in each frequently leads to employment difficulty. The prospective employer looks at such a record and wonders why this has happened.

CONTINUING TO LEARN

Earning a diploma and a license does not mean the end of learning. These two necessary items are your passports to practice as a licensed practical nurse. If things did not change, keeping up-to-date would be a rather simple matter. But this is not the case; things related to your practice not only change, they change rapidly. New knowledge, new equipment, and new therapies are constantly appearing, and these facts make it necessary for the LPN to continue to learn.

It has never been true that a person stops learning when he "graduates." We learn as long as we live. But today calls for something more with respect to continuing to learn. Today the individual must do something he has not done too well in the past—and that is plan for and carry out, on his own initiative, a continuing means for self-improvement. This takes effort and determination. For some people, this is a new responsibility because up to this point in life they have looked to others to

promote, encourage, and even pay them to attend classes. In addition, some have been unwilling to get involved in the learning situation once they have signed up for it. At this point in history, it is misleading to say it any other way: *individuals must assume more direct and continuous responsibility for their self-improvement in the world of work.* Opportunities for self-improvement are abundant. Whether one lives in a city or rural community, opportunities to learn are as close to an individual as his television set (in many instances), his mail box, or the local adult education course offered wherever there is an interest and need.

In-service education programs in institutions are found in increasing numbers because employers are becoming aware of the need to help keep employees up-to-date. One question you might ask during interview could be about provisions for in-service education. Institutions vary in this respect; some provide on-the-job time to participate and make attendance mandatory. Others provide the opportunity but leave it up to the individual whether or not she will attend on her own time. Other approaches are used, too.

The most important single factor in any type of self-improvement is the individual worker's attitude toward self-improvement. It pays (many times over) to be honest with yourself and cultivate the habit of being involved in activities which extend one's abilities, understandings, and interests. To do this includes more than simply taking a refresher course for LPN's now and then. For instance, just about anyone can profit from experiences which polish up his ability to get along with others so that he will "be well-received."

As stated in Chapter 3, more people lose their jobs due to inability to get along with others than for any other single reason. Many types of courses (e.g., communications, human relations) and group experiences help; they are not necessarily courses in nursing.

Educational television is available to thousands of people; as facilities improve and expand, it is all but impossible to imagine a person not being able to avail himself of some type of educational experience by this medium.

Another opportunity for learning, appearing in the home, will be an electronic unit or console which will permit the resident to "dial" or "switch" into instructional programs of his choice. Here again, the individual's attitude toward learning and his willingness to get and stay involved will be a key factor in his success with this opportunity.

The LPN, like anyone else, can expect change in work responsibilities and functions. As patterns for health care change and more people require more health services, the years ahead will call for people flexible in attitudes and abilities. Willingness to learn will be a necessity rather than a choice if one is to keep up-to-date, and perform effectively.

A CITIZEN AND COMMUNITY MEMBER

With the right attitude toward making an effective contribution while working, one is, in fact, performing as a responsible citizen. Ours is a culture where people are interdependent for food, clothing, shelter, health care, and services of all types. The work of one is important to the work of the other.

Communities are made up of people who are governed by laws, standards, and regulations. Communities are regulated and exist for the good of the whole. A good citizen takes seriously his responsibilities and privileges in such a society. He is involved in voting to help elect able public servants; he works to promote better schools and other needed commu-

nity services such as adequate provisions for health care, recreational facilities, libraries, and housing. Some of these community needs are met through taxes, others through voluntary efforts.

Opportunity for serving the community is everywhere. For instance, there is almost no limit to the variety of volunteer organizations which promote good things for people—rural and city dwellers alike. In our society, everyone can get involved in community betterment. As a licensed practical nurse, you will have unique opportunities to share in this challenge; as a citizen, it is your responsibility to do so.

NURSING ORGANIZATIONS AND PUBLICATIONS

While many groups and agencies have contributed to the growth and improvement of practical nursing, and some continue to do so, there are four nursing organizations which deserve special mention. These organizations are the National Federation of Licensed Practical Nurses, Inc. (NFLPN); National Association for Practical Nurse Education and Service (NAPNES); National League for Nursing (NLN); and the American Nurses' Association (ANA) (see Table 5–2).

TABLE 5.2. FOUR NURSING ORGANIZATIONS

NAME	MEMBERSHIP—JOURNAL
National Federation of Licensed Practical Nurses (NFLPN); 250 West 57th Street, New York, N.Y. 10019.	Open only to licensed practical nurses. The only one of the four organizations made up entirely of LPN's. Publishes *Bedside Nurse*
National Association of Practical Nurse Education and Services, Inc. (NAPNES); 535 Fifth Avenue, New York, N.Y. 10017.	Open to all interested citizens. Publishes *The Journal of Practical Nursing*
National League for Nursing (NLN); 10 Columbus Circle, New York, N.Y. 10019.	Open to all interested citizens. Publishes *Nursing Outlook*
American Nurses' Association (ANA); 2420 Pershing Road Kansas City, Missouri 64108.	Open only to registered nurses. The only one of the four organizations made up entirely of R.N.'s. Publishes *American Journal of Nursing*

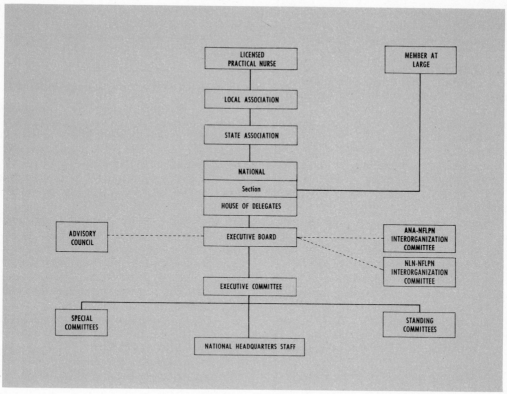

FIGURE 5–1   NFLPN membership organization chart. Reprinted with permission of the National Federation of Licensed Practical Nurses.

National Federation of Licensed Practical Nurses, Inc.

The National Federation of Licensed Practical Nurses (NFLPN), founded in 1949, is the organization whose membership is made up entirely of licensed practical/vocational nurses. Members join NFLPN in one of two ways: (1) through constituent state associations, or (2) directly as members-at-large if living in a state which has no constituent state association. (See Fig. 5–1.)

A constituent state association means a state organized (with by-laws, officers, committees, and divisional associations) and belonging to a federation or a group of such state organizations united for a common purpose. Members join the state association by paying annual dues, a small part of which are sent to the national office of NFLPN in New York City. Thus, a licensed practical nurse joins both the state and the national organizations.

The general *purpose* of NFLPN, as stated in its publication *NFLPN Philosophy*, is "to provide an opportunity for licensed practical nurses to meet and work together in the interest of their general welfare and for the improvement of patient care. All its activities are planned to carry out these objectives to the end that licensed practical nurses are prepared to give good nursing care."

NFLPN states its basic *function* is to serve its members in the following ways:

1. Promotes continuing education of licensed practical nurses.

2. Establishes principles of ethics for licensed practical nurses.

3. Offers every member an opportunity to participate in the activities of the organization.

4. Keeps its members informed on matters of interest through letters, bulletins, speakers and programs, and its official bimonthly publication, *Bedside Nurse*.

5. Makes available to its members the services of skilled specialists and consultants on organizational, legal, and nursing problems.

6. Enables its members to apply for the best type of low cost insurance.

7. Represents and speaks for LPN's in Congress when considering federal legislation affecting licensed practical nurses.

8. Encourages fellowship among licensed practical nurses.

9. Develops mutual understanding and goodwill between its members, other allied health groups, and the general public.

10. Trains its members to work effectively and cooperatively in organization.

11. Recruits men and women for the profession.

The NFLPN works cooperatively with other agencies. It is a member of an Advisory Council which includes representation from the National League for Nursing, American Nurses Association, American Hospital Association, American Medical Association, American Nursing Home Association, U. S. Office of Education and the National Health Council.

The state associations, working together with NFLPN, have accomplished a great deal toward bringing practical nursing to a place of recognition: members have benefited from improved licensure laws, enactment of laws in areas where none had existed, promoted workshops and continuing education efforts, improved working conditions, and better understanding of what is expected of the practical nurse. (See also Figure 5-1.)

The NFLPN realizes that the strength of the organization (as in any other group) lies in its members and their interest in working together toward the general welfare of the group. Improved welfare for the group and the individual makes membership important to every licensed practical nurse.

The National Association for Practical Nurse Education and Service, Inc.

The National Association for Practical Nurse Education and Service, Inc. (NAPNES), started in 1941, is an organization whose efforts are entirely devoted to practical nursing education and the practical nurse as practitioner. Membership is open to all interested citizens. This national organization has state and local constituent associa-tions and promotes a variety of efforts in practical nursing education.

Table 5-3 points out some of the events in the history of this organization.

National League for Nursing

The National League for Nursing (NLN) came into being in 1952 as a result of a merger of seven national committees and organizations. Membership in this organization is open to all interested citizens.

The object of the NLN is stated as follows in the NLN Bylaws (as amended May, 1971): "The *object* of this organization shall be to foster the development and improvement of hospital, industrial, public health, and other organized nursing service and of nursing education through the coordinated action of nurses, allied professional groups, citizens, agencies, and schools to the end that the nursing needs of people will be met."

The *functions* of the NLN according to Article I, Section 1, NLN Bylaws (as amended May, 1971) are:

1. To identify the nursing needs of society and to foster programs designed to meet these needs.

2. To develop and support services for the improvement of nursing care and nursing education through consultation, testing, accreditation,* evaulation, and other activities.

3. To work with the American Nurses' Association for the advancement of nursing.

4. To work with voluntary, governmental, and other agencies and groups toward the achievement of comprehensive health care.

5. To respond in appropriate ways to universal nursing needs.

In 1967, NLN reorganized its structure into two divisions: (1) *Division of Individual Members*, and (2) *Division of Agency Members*.

The Council of Practical Nursing Programs is the one (of six councils) in the *Division of Agency Members* which is concerned with school accreditation and program inprovement.

---

*NLN or NAPNES accreditation of practical nursing programs establishes institutional eligibility for participation in the National Vocational Student Loan Insurance Act.

TABLE 5.3. NAPNES: BEGINNING AND DEVELOPMENT

WHEN	WHAT
1941	*Association of Directors and Instructors in Schools of Practical Nursing.* Organized with some 20 schools as charter members.
1942	Name changed to *National Association for Practical Nurse Education, Inc. (NAPNE).*
1944	Approved a school accreditation service. States without laws to set standards for practical nurse education needed guidelines and standards for individual school development.
1947	Started to implement the school accreditation service which had been approved three years before.
1950	Extended its efforts to further promote practical nursing education and practical nursing.
1951	Published *Practical Nursing* magazine (bimonthly).
1955	*Practical Nursing* published monthly. Prepared and published course outlines for two extension courses for practical nurses who were not graduates from approved schools.
1959	S added to NAPNE changing the name to *National Association for Practical Nursing Education and Service, Inc.* This change was due to structure reorganization which created two departments—Department of Education and Department of Service to State Practical Nurse Associations.
1963	Changed the name of its magazine to *The Journal of Practical Nursing.*
1967	Approved by the U. S. Office of Education as one of two (NLN the other) nationally recognized accrediting agencies* for practical nursing programs for an initial two-year period. Following this initial period, progress made by NAPNES reviewed to determine its future role in practical nurse program accreditation.

*NAPNES or NLN accreditation of practical nursing programs establishes institutional eligibility for participation in the national Vocational Student Loan Insurance Act.

SUMMARY

In the past decade there has been vigorous growth in practical nursing in both the United States and Canada. Many things have promoted practical nursing education and the increased use of LPN's, LVN's, and RNA's in both countries. Likewise, many questions have been raised concerning the overextension of this nursing practitioner in meeting the health needs of citizens; they are employed in all types of agencies.

With the wide range of employment opportunities open to the LPN, it seems important to emphasize that a license to practice is limited, and one would be wise to determine the requirements of the work before accepting employment.

People learn as long as they live, but today calls for additional individual effort to keep abreast of rapid changes taking place in our society. This fact places important responsibilities on the shoulders of the LPN the same as anyone else.

Three national nursing organizations open to LPN/LVN membership are NFLPN, NAPNES, and NLN. Of these three, NFLPN is the only organization made up entirely of LPN's/LVN's.

GUIDES FOR STUDY AND DISCUSSION

1. Overextension of nursing care responsibilities for the LPN is a common happening. Why does this take place?
2. Why might an employer be doubtful about hiring a person who walks in "off the street" seeking employment?
3. What are the opportunities in your community for employment as an LPN? Select one and outline your plan to seek information about it.
4. Think of at least five ways you can continue to extend your education after you become a licensed practical nurse.
5. Be ready to agree or disagree with this statement: "Education today is a lifelong process."
6. Why should you become a member of one or more nursing organizations?
7. Study Table 5–2. Figure out which organizations an LPN could join and which official journals she could get.

SUGGESTED SITUATIONS AND ACTIVITIES

1. Role play an interview showing how best to represent one's self during an interview of employment.
2. Write a letter of application for your first job. Next, write a letter of resignation from that position after two years of employment.
3. Make an appointment for a conference with the person in charge of in-service education in an agency where you are having clinical learning experiences. Prepare a list of questions you will want to discuss concerning the in-service program so you will be well-informed about what it is and how it serves employees.
4. Prepare an exhibit of information about nursing organizations you can join and support as an LPN.

THE HUMAN BODY: NORMAL STRUCTURE AND FUNCTION

The main purpose of this unit is to provide general knowledge about the normal functions of the human body and the structures related to these functions.

The unit consists of 11 chapters; each chapter (except the first one) discusses some particular part of the body and its function. You will note that Chapter 12, *The Process of Metabolism*, is discussed "by itself" simply to assist you in seeing the relationship of this vital process to several systems. The process of metabolism cuts across the functions of a number of body systems and because of this it is sometimes difficult for the student to understand *what* it is and *why* it is. Metabolism is most directly related to the following systems: circulatory, respiratory, and digestive. Therefore, Chapter 12 immediately follows the discussion of these three systems.

Health depends upon cooperation between the body structure and its functions; it likewise depends upon cooperation among the systems working one with the other and a unified whole.

Unit III deals with normal body structure and function only. Abnormal conditions, disorders, and diseases affecting the various parts of the body are discussed, along with treatment and nursing care, in other parts of the book.

The knowledge you gain from this unit will be *your beginning understandings* about the body; you will use this foundation knowledge over and over. It will broaden and extend as you put it to work in one course after another, in one situation after another. Realizing this, you should not expect to know "everything" from the start. You will find yourself returning to this unit time after time to recall and to reestablish this basic information firmly in your mind.

Keep in mind that as scientists find new knowledge about the structure and function of the human body, what is truth today may not necessarily be truth tomorrow. The history of man is a story of constant change. New knowledge helps explain old facts and may even replace them.

CHAPTER 6

THE BODY AS A UNIFIED WHOLE, AND ITS PARTS

TOPICAL HEADINGS

Introduction
Some Wonders of
  the Human Machine
The General Plan of
  the Human Body
Structural Parts of
  the Human Body
    Protoplasm

Cells
Water and Body
  Fluids
Tissues
Membranes
Organs
Glands
Systems

Skin and Accessory
  Organs
Summary
Guides for Study and
  Discussion
Suggested Situations
  and Activities

OBJECTIVES FOR THE STUDENT: Be able to:

1. Given a list of eight wonders of the human body, describe one value of each.
2. Give an example of how the body performs as a unified whole.
3. State three functions of the cell.
4. List four factors which influence water balance in the body.
5. Distinguish between intracellular fluid and extracellular fluid.

SUGGESTED STUDY VOCABULARY*

anatomy	protoplasm	gland
physiology	tissue	system
ventral cavity	membrane	intracellular
dorsal cavity	organ	extracellular

---

*Look for any terms you already know.

INTRODUCTION

No machine compares with the wonders of the human body. While some comparisons can be made, there are many unique differences. Like other machines the body is made up of parts which work together. Like other machines the body needs something to furnish power and a means for waste removal.

Like other machines it requires reasonable care and proper maintenance to keep it in running order. There are spare parts for machines but only in recent years have there been spare parts (human and man-made) for some portions of the body.

There are matchless differences between the human body and the machine. For instance, man can continue himself through reproduction. The body has power to keep itself going, to restore itself and to make do under less than desirable conditions. It constantly carries on a repair service and with help it often overcomes serious disorders.

Man has a mind and is capable of action guided by inner forces. When hungry, food is sought. When tired, he sleeps. Man experiences joy, sorrow, disappointments and has the capacity to learn, create, imagine and feel, among other things.

The term "human anatomy" means the scientific study of body structures; what types of tissues the body is made of; how special cells make up bones, nerves, muscles, layers of the skin, membranes, hair, nails, etc. Anatomy also includes the study of body systems and the organization of the various organs and glands.

The term "human physiology" means the scientific study of the functions of the body; what functions are carried on and how they take place (if known); the work of special tissues (i.e., thyroid tissue) and their contributions are examined. Physiology delves into the secrets of the cell to try and find out why this very small piece of life seems to control so much and to influence so many things.

The purpose of this chapter is to introduce you to the body-machine, its wonders and its general plan. It provides a reference system of terms for acquaintance with locations, sides, positions, and cavities of the body. It deals with parts of the body, starting

---

TABLE 6.1. EIGHT WONDERS OF THE HUMAN BODY

1. *Adjustments to environmental changes—heat, cold, air pressure.* Body temperature—same (within a degree or so) for all people under normal conditions. Built-in means to promote heat loss and heat gain.	Brain area (hypothalamus brain stem) regulates heat reducing, heat promoting and shivering. Body temperature altered by: the time of day, physical activity, the body location of thermometer. Body heat reduced by more blood brought to dilated surface blood vessels to cool before returning to center of body. Sweating and decreased muscle activity also lower body heat. Body heat increased by surface blood vessel constriction allowing less blood to the surface, thus more blood remains within the center of the body. Body heat increased due to body chemistry. Upon signal certain hormonal substances released into tissue cells and carried by blood to other cells to increase their food-burning activity (increased metabolism) producing more heat.
Adjustments to air pressure—changes come more slowly than adjustments to heat and cold.	The more severe the air pressure change the more slowly the adjustments must be made, often requiring assistance. As air pressure lowers there is less oxygen and red blood cells pick up only a partial load of oxygen to take to the lungs and on to body tissues.
	Adjustment is made by increasing ventilation power of the lungs (sometimes four or five times the normal amount). Another adjustment takes several weeks. High altitude living causes body to gradually increase the number of red blood cells to help make up oxygen loss. Immediate assistance needed in high barometric situations (i.e., helmet diving).
2. *Built-in reserves.* **Liver:** Storehouse for ready to use fats, sugar, some proteins and some vitamins. A reservoir for holding back blood until needed. Cleans up the blood by removing wastes. If "blood pollution" is beyond removal ability of usual number of special liver cells, the liver has capacity to produce more special cells to take care of wastes. **Balanced Internal Environment.** A necessity for proper body functioning.	When special demands are made (more sugar, more blood, more oxygen, etc.). Body reserve capabilities go into action as mentioned in increased ventilation power.
	Body has ability to pull fluids or to push fluids to maintain a fluid balance, up to a point. If fluid loss is rapid or with prolonged vomiting or diarrhea the body draws fluid first from the spaces surrounding cells (interstitial spaces). If this fluid is not replaced, the body draws fluid from within the cells. This creates a serious fluid imbalance.

with living matter, called protoplasm, discusses the cell and briefly looks at main body structures.

SOME WONDERS OF THE HUMAN MACHINE

It is difficult to imagine how some one hundred trillion body cells (each with its own work to do) work together in harmony, but they do when a person is healthy. They work together in a highly organized fashion carrying out the many functions the body must perform from minute to minute, day in and day out. When some of these cells do not perform as they should a person begins to have complaints and to show signs of not feeling well. The purpose of health care is to prevent this from happening and to help restore cell harmony when illness occurs.

Checks and Balances

The body has a number of ways to keep it functioning within normal limits. They could be called *systems and mini-systems of checks and balances* which safely keep the body working properly. Healthful living habits help maintain this built-in system of checks and balances. Medical care during illness strives to return the imbalances back to normal or as near normal as possible. Table 6–1 describes eight capacities the body possesses to function within normal limits.

TABLE 6.1. EIGHT WONDERS OF THE HUMAN BODY (Continued)

3. *Sleep, rest, exercise.*
   A person must sleep regularly. Why there is a regular cycle of wakefulness and sleep is unknown. It may somehow be related to fatigue of nerves and muscles.

   Amount of sleep varies. Most require from six to eight hours a day. It is possible to go without sleep for two or three days. No one is known to have survived without sleep for much beyond nine days. Body needs to be restored—destroyed cells are replaced to keep the body in cell balance; heart and lungs work more slowly and other organs are less active, except perhaps some parts of the brain (dreaming, sleepwalking).

   Exercise
   In one form or another a person exercises from birth on. Play recreates the mind/body and is called recreation.

   Exercise is related to physical fitness because it improves blood circulation, breathing, body flexibility, and muscle firmness and strength.

4. *The body is a chemical laboratory.*
   Some few chemicals affect the body in general (i.e., growth). Many select to serve only certain tissues sometimes called "target tissues."

   Chemical action takes place in tissue cells and is responsible for producing heat and energy. It also influences growth and development and the rate at which these take place. Chemical action makes it possible for man to continue himself through reproduction; one remarkable chemical success is changing foodstuffs into body heat and energy. Chemicals influence the rate(s) the cells use food and absorb it through cell membranes.

5. *The body reproduces itself.*
   Cell reproduction up to a prescribed limit is a mystery but it is felt to be related to precoding within the genes.

   Within certain limits the body can replace some tissue and maintain about the same cell count at all times. Worn and dead cells are replaced by new cells. Certain tissues replace themselves rapidly (liver, bone marrow, glands); some not at all (nerve).

6. *The body heals, fights disease and calls attention to itself.*

   It has all manner of means to protect itself and keep it functioning: heals a wound and repairs the skin; clots the blood in a wound; destroys harmful organisms; has some powers of immunity and indicates distress (pain, fever, vomiting, etc.).

7. *Alert to surroundings and the need for safety.*

   The body has many ways to automatically trigger action to protect itself (i.e., blinking an eye, regarding balance when slipping). It has ability to sense the position of a body part, proper balance, etc.

8. *Man has powers all his own.*
   Certain wonders of the human body cannot be duplicated.

   Man has the ability to feel, experience, think, imagine and create. He makes decisions, renders judgments and learns from experience.

THE GENERAL PLAN OF THE HUMAN BODY

The body is designed according to the laws of living matter and for the work it performs. It is a delicate balance of many trillions of cells working in unison. Thus the body-plan must make it possible for these cells to live, function and divide.

Body structures are designed according to the work performed. For example — the human hand: What purposes does it serve? What is there about the structure of the hand that makes it so useful?

Even though a particular structure has its own identity and its own work to do, (i.e., nerves), it always carries on its work in relation to other body structures. One could call the healthy body an orchestration of all systems and parts.

To study the design of the human body it is necessary to use a reference system. The terms in this system are those uniformly used to describe the body. They serve as guide-posts to *position, planes* (imaginary lines passing through it) and *body cavities.*

To help you become acquainted with this general reference system use Table 6–2 along with Figure 6–1, checking one against the other.

STRUCTURAL PARTS OF THE HUMAN BODY

The body has many parts; each part is necessary and useful to the rest of the body. Separate a part from its place in this highly organized machine and it does not serve a purpose. The same is true of a wheel once it is removed from an automobile. But if one wants to know how a human body or an automobile is structured and functions, its parts need to be examined and studied.

To talk about the *structure* of the human body one needs a reference system too. This system includes:

protoplasm (living substance)
cells
water-body fluids
tissues
membranes
organs
glands
systems
skin and accessory organs

Protoplasm

A logical place to start examining body structure is with the building material found in every living cell; it is called *protoplasm.* Protoplasm is a living substance. The saying goes, "Where there is life, there is protoplasm." This is true for all plants and animals. This life-giving substance is a colorless, transparent, sticky material made up chiefly of water and food matter plus a small amount of dissolved salts.

Protoplasm fills a large portion of a body cell. The word itself is a general term including more precise terms. For example, examine Figure 6–2. Point to B (nucleoplasm) and F (cytoplasm) to locate protoplasm in two parts of a cell. Notices that most of the cell's protoplasm is called *cytoplasm;* this is a precise term for protoplasm when located in this particular part of a cell. A useful fact to remember about protoplasm is that it is a life-giving substance made up in great measure (60–90 per cent) of water.

Cells

The cell is the smallest "package" or unit of living matter in the body. Each cell has thickness, width, and length, but is too small to be seen without a microscope. It takes trillions of cells to make up the human body, and so it seems understandable that cells vary in form, size, and shape according to their location and work.

A cell is always at work; it is never idle. It *produces growth* by dividing and redividing according to the growth needs of the normal body. A cell is a *receiving, using,* and *storing unit;* it takes in, uses, and stores food substances. In a sense it might be called a "mini-factory" because a single cell produces energy from the food substances it receives and sends off the waste products.

No normal cell works in isolation and therefore cells must be in communication with one another to work together. This communication consists of sending substances (water, food, salts, oxygen, and wastes) back and forth. The process within a cell could be explained as follows. Look again at Figure 6–2. Note the membrane wall (G) around the cell. Anything entering (or leaving) the cell must pass through this membrane. In the instance of food substance, for example, a particle is too large to pass through the tiny pores

TABLE 6.2. BODY DIRECTIONS, PLANES, AND CAVITIES

TERM	*DESCRIPTION*
Direction	
Anatomic position	The standing body facing forward; arms at the sides and palms turned toward the front. Any reference to position (or direction) assumes that the body is in this (anatomic) position.
Anterior or Ventral	Toward the front, e.g., the lips are anterior to the mouth cavity.
Posterior or Dorsal	Toward the back, e.g., the spinal column is posterior to the lungs and the stomach.
Superior (Cranial)	Above, e.g., the crown of the head is superior to the ears.
Inferior (Caudal)	Below, e.g., the knee is inferior to the hip.
Medial	Midline of the body or nearest that midline, e.g., the breast is medial to the arm pit.
Lateral	Relates to a side or away from the midline, e.g., the arm pit is lateral to the breast.
Proximal	Closer to (nearer) point of attachment, e.g., the elbow is proximal to the wrist.
Distal	Farther from point of attachment, e.g., the wrist is distal to the elbow.
Planes*	
Sagittal (Vertical)	Dividing the body (up and down) into left and right sides. If exactly a midline division it is called *midsagittal*.
Transverse (Horizontal)	Dividing the body (across) into superior and inferior portions.
Coronal	Dividing the body into anterior and posterior portions.
Cavities	
Ventral (Anterior)	The space anterior to the spinal column. It is divided into superior and inferior parts by a muscular partition called the *diaphragm*. The superior space (above) is called the *thoracic* cavity. The inferior space (below) is called the *abdominal* cavity. Note that the lowest portion of the general abdominal cavity is known as the *pelvic* cavity.
	Most of the large body organs are located in these two cavities as follows:

	Thoracic Cavity *Abdominal Cavity*
	 lungs (2) stomach
	 heart and great vessels intestines
	 trachea and bronchi liver and gallbladder
	 esophagus pancreas
	      spleen
	      kidneys
	      urinary bladder
	      rectum
	      sex organs

Dorsal (Posterior)	This cavity consists of two main parts. The *cranial* part houses the brain and the *spinal* part houses the spinal cord.

*Note that in Figure 6-1 the imaginary lines are at right angles to each other.

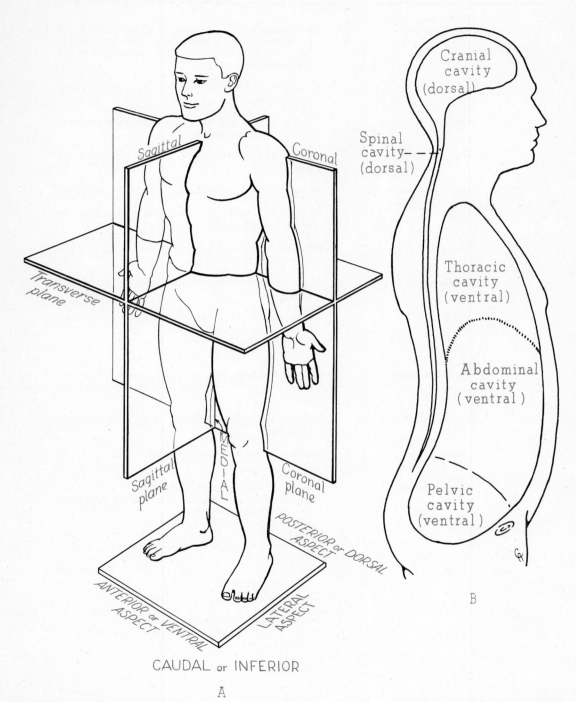

FIGURE 6–1 A, Anatomic position of body (anterior view, palms forward). B, Ventral and dorsal cavities. (Jacob and Francone: Structure and Function of Man).

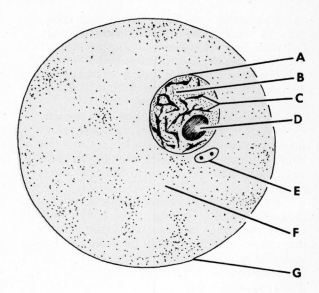

FIGURE 6–2 A body cell and its parts. A, nuclear membrane; B, nucleoplasm; C, chromatin; D, nucleolus; E, centrosome; F, cytoplasm; G, cell membrane. (Manner: Elements of Anatomy and Physiology.)

in the membrane, it is dissolved and then carried through. Once inside the cell, the food becomes part of the cytoplasm. To produce heat and energy, the cell needs oxygen; this too passes through the membrane and joins the food substance in the process. Food is the fuel and oxygen makes it burn. Burning produces wastes. One is carbon dioxide; it leaves through the membrane (diffusion) and is carried by the blood back to the lungs where it is expelled as we breathe out (exhale). Other wastes also exit through the membrane and find their way out of the body through the kidneys and the skin.

The actual passing of *water* substance through the cell wall is called *osmosis*. When a *gas* (oxygen, carbon dioxide) passes through, it is called *diffusion*. A cell can pick and choose the substance it will permit to enter (selective permeability); one cell may reject something that the next one accepts and uses. Scientists are trying to find out more about communications among cells. If and when they do, this knowledge may help to diagnose and possibly treat some disease conditions.

The main parts of a cell are (Fig. 6–2):

Membrane—a thin, flexible outer wall which permits molecules of substances to move in and out through pores so small they cannot be seen with the most powerful microscope. The membrane separates the cell from surrounding fluid and other cells. Under favorable conditions it heals itself rapidly if ruptured.

Cytoplasm—the colorless, transparent, sticky substance containing dissolved salts and food substances.

Nucleus—a small area within the cell with its own covering (nuclear membrane). It is filled with a substance like cytoplasm, but one important difference is that it contains *chromatin material*. This material regulates cell reproduction (division) and growth through the *genes*. Genes come from parents and are known as "hereditary units." They transmit such characteristics as color of the eyes and hair from parents to children. But they do more than that. Genes regulate the day-to-day functions of the cells by controlling what goes on within a cell and indicate if and when it should reproduce itself.

Though cell reproduction is still something of a mystery, scientists have found a few important answers during recent years. They have determined something of the physical and the chemical structure of the gene which is helping them unlock the process by which a cell reproduces and regulates itself. In the healthy body, cell reproduction is a constant and orderly process. As cells die, new ones take their place so that the body can maintain itself in the prescribed way. Cell reproduction begins in the nucleus. First, all of the genes (there are thought to be more than a million in each nucleus) and the 46 chromosomes (twenty-three pairs) duplicate themselves; then they divide and form two separate nuclei. The last step is the pulling apart or separation of the cell which produces two new daughter cells. In place of one cell, there are two cells. Cell division is called *mitosis*. Under ordinary circumstances the life cycle of a cell is from 10 to 30 hours; it takes this long from one reproduction to the next reproduction. Mitosis takes only about 30 minutes.

Some cells are mobile; they have the ability to move about freely and function where they are needed. An example is the white blood cell that moves itself through the blood vessel wall and moves on to the site where needed.

Certain cells have the ability to change their shape and according to the body's need even if they stay in place. They can shorten themselves (contract) and become stronger and thicker. Muscle cells do this. Another example of contraction is "goose flesh"; chill or fright can send a message over the nerve fibers which in turn causes them to pull up or to contract.

Water and Body Fluids

To function properly, cells need tissue fluids with right amounts of oxygen, minerals, sugar and other vital substances.

Water makes up the bulk of living matter; it is located within cells and around cells throughout the body. In addition, *all* body fluids are chiefly water; this makes it an all-important substance. Water is essential to life and accounts for more than half of the body's weight.

Tables 6–3 and 6–4 include some main functions of water and factors which influence body water balance.

Body fluids contain more than water; they also contain food nutrients, oxygen, and specific chemical substances. These chemical substances are tiny particles which are either dissolved or suspended in the water. The list of these particles is long, but some important ones are potassium, bicarbonate, phosphate, sulfate, magnesium, sodium, and chloride. They are called *electrolytes* due to their nature and work. Body fluids must contain exact amounts and strengths of these electrolytes to cause body cells to respond or behave as they should; when this is so it is called *electrolyte balance*. Electrolyte balance is essential to such vital body functions as transporting oxygen and carbon dioxide in the blood, building of bone, maintaining proper chemical balance in the blood and in the tissue fluids and permitting blood to clot.

Body fluid found within cells is called *intracellular* fluid. Body fluids found outside the cells are called *extracellular* fluids; these fluids include lymph, plasma, fluids in the digestive system, secretions of the kidneys and glands, and the fluid in the spaces between cells. When the fluid climate (intracellular and extracellular) remains in constant balance, this is called *homeostasis*.

Tissues

Tissues are groups of like cells that are joined together. Although there are trillions of cells in the body, there are only four major kinds of tissue. They are:

1. *Epithelial*. In this tissue the cells are very close together, with little space between them. This type of structure makes a good covering for surfaces either outside or inside the body (skin, nails, vessels, body cavities). Protection is one of its main functions: secretion and excretion are others.

2. *Connective*. There are many types of this tissue and it has a great variety of uses in all parts of the body. Some connective tissue is very thin and soft and tears easily. One type contains fat and is seen as fat on meat. Strong, tough, yellow and white tissues are made of

---

TABLE 6.3.   WATER—MAIN FUNCTIONS IN THE BODY

With the cell:
1. Transports materials to it.
2. Moves material through the cell wall *into* the cell itself.
3. Moves material *from* the cell through the cell wall.

With the body in general:
1. Helps regulate body temperature.
2. Assists with waste removal through the intestines, kidneys, skin, and lungs.
3. Vital to all internal transportation systems.

TABLE 6.4.   WATER BALANCE IN THE BODY

The volume of water in the body at a given time depends on a balance between the water output and the water intake; the body regulates this balance. Thirst is a signal that the body needs more water.

Factors which influence water volume and balance include:
1. The weather (hot weather contributes to greater water loss).
2. Exercise (hard exercise over a period of time contributes to a greater water loss).
3. Body temperature.
4. Water sources (liquid consumed, water in food, and water formed when food is used by the body to produce heat).

---

fibers and serve as ligaments and tendons connnected to bones. Blood is considered a connective tissue. While it is a liquid, it does contain cells (blood cells and plasma cells and others). One could say that connective tissue protects, supports, binds the body together, and nourishes it.

3. *Muscle.* This tissue helps the body move; it moves food through the digestive tract, and a special muscle tissue (cardiac) is the heart muscle. Some muscle tissue contracts because we want it to, as when we raise an arm, while other muscle tissue (heart) works automatically.

4. *Nerve.* Nerve tissue has one purpose. It conducts or carries messages or impulses. Examples are *the brain, spinal cord,* and *body nerves.*

Membranes

Membranes serve many essential functions even though they are rather thin sheets of tissue. They protect, secrete, absorb, and, in the case of the skin, help regulate body heat and serve to alert the body to sensations of heat, cold, and painful agents. They also cover or line many parts of the body. The four most common types are:

1. *Mucous.* This membrane lines passageways or cavities leading to the outside, such as the lining of the digestive tract originating in the mouth, the passageway that air follows into the lungs, and the passageway of the urinary tract. *Mucous* membrane comes from the word *mucus,* the protective, slippery, moist coating which this tissue secretes.

2. *Serous.* This membrane lines *closed* cavities, the opposite of the mucous membrane. It also covers the organs within the cavity itself. A good example is the thoracic cavity; it is lined with a serous membrane and the lungs in that cavity are covered with a serous membrane, too. A small amount of *serous* fluid (watery fluid) is between these two membranes to prevent the "rubbing" of one against the other during respiration.

3. *Synovial.* Synovial membranes line cavities between bones (joints) and the tube-like structures covering some tendons (tendon sheaths). They secrete the synovial fluid which is much like the serous fluid mentioned above.

4. *Cutaneous* (skin). The skin serves several important functions: heat regulation, sensation, protection from injury and germs, identification (finger prints).

Organs

An organ is a part of the body having a special function. Examples are: stomach, heart, intestines, lungs. Each is made up of a combination of different tissues grouped together to perform a certain task.

Glands

A gland is an organ that secretes or gives off a substance. Two main types are *exocrine* and *endocrine.* Exocrine glands secrete the substance by way of tubes or ducts, i.e., salivary glands. Endocrine glands secrete the substance directly into the blood (ductless). These substances are powerful body regulators called *hormones,* i.e., thyroid gland.

Systems

A system is a group of united organs working together to perform a major body function. For example, the digestive system (made up of several connected organs) forms the route that food follows during the digestive process. Some glands provide secretions to aid this process. The following nine systems are the more common ones. Here the discussion is brief; later chapters give more detail.

1. *Skeletal* system. Two hundred six separate bones give the body a framework and allow it to bend, twist, and turn. A joint is formed where one bone meets another.

2. *Muscular* system. More than 400 muscles (all sizes and shapes) are attached to the bony framework of the body. Some are short, others long; some are round and bulge in the middle (upper arm) while others are tough, sheathlike layers as in the abdomen. The muscular and skeletal systems working together account for man's ability to move.

3. *Circulatory* system. The major parts are: blood, blood vessels, heart, and lymph. The heart serves as a pump to move the blood through the blood vessels. Lymph (a watery liquid) circulates in the body also but without a pumping action. The lymphatic system is related to blood circulation. The main work of this entire system is transportation of food nutrients, oxygen, carbon dioxide, other cell wastes, and blood cells.

4. *Respiratory* system. This system includes the nose, pharynx, larynx, trachea, bronchi, and lungs. Its only purpose is to exchange gases (oxygen and carbon dioxide) from air to blood and from blood back to air.

5. *Digestive* system. Part of this system is called the gastrointestinal tract; this tract includes the mouth, pharynx, esophagus, stomach, small intestine, and large intestine. Salivary glands, liver, and pancreas join the gastrointestinal tract to make up the digestive system. It processes food into a liquid state so that it passes through the pores in the lining of the small intestine into the blood stream and is carried to all parts of the body.

6. *Urinary* system. It is made up of two kidneys (right and left), two ureters, a bladder, and the urethra. This system has one chief function: to collect wastes thrown off by working body cells and to expel them from the body.

7. *Nervous* system. The brain, spinal cord, and nerves make up this system. It acts as an internal messenger service — sending and receiving messages which control body activities. The nervous system reaches each of the other systems and makes it possible for the body to work as a "whole machine."

8. *Reproductive* system. The organs in this system differ in the male and in the female. The male has testes (sex glands), a series of ducts, accessory glands, and supporting structures (scrotum, penis, and spermatic cords). The female has ovaries, two fallopian tubes or oviducts, uterus, vagina, vulva, and the breasts or mammary glands. The purpose of this system is to produce the new individual.

9. *Endocrine* system. This is the name given to several essential glands located in various parts of the body. These glands pour their secretions directly into the blood stream and therefore are called *ductless glands*. There are six: pituitary, thyroid, parathyroid, adrenal, gonads (testes or ovaries), pancreas (islands of Langerhans). Hormones produced by these glands regulate many body functions such as growth and body development.

Skin and Accessory Organs

Everyone knows something about the skin, if only that it needs to be kept clean. But the skin serves several important functions including keeping a close check on the loss of water, protecting against infections, regulating body temperature (keeping us cool in summer and warm in winter), and alerting us of possible danger through its network of nerves.

The accessory organs of the skin are the following: hair, nails, small glands, and nerve receptors.

SUMMARY

The human body works as a "whole machine" even though it is made up of trillions of cells. These cells are arranged and organized to perform special functions but no cell can work alone. Each cell helps the other and together they make life possible.

Body structures include cells, water and body fluids, tissues, membranes, organs, glands, systems, skin, and accessory organs. The structural unit is the cell. It needs and gets food and oxygen; it throws off wastes which are removed and carried away. Cells make up every part of the body.

Keep in mind that a healthy human body has the ability to regulate itself—its growth, temperature, movement, nourishment of parts, and disposal of wastes; it heals and protects itself. In addition the body is capable of reproducing human life.

No machine is capable of doing all the "whole human body" can do. It is an amazing scheme of many parts working in unison quite unlike any other "machine."

GUIDES FOR STUDY AND DISCUSSION

1. Table 6–1 lists eight wonders of the body. What makes each "a wonder"?
2. What is meant by the statement "The body functions as a unified whole."?
3. What is anatomy? What is physiology?
4. Using Figure 6–1, locate the entire ventral cavity; list the three main parts. Locate the dorsal cavity; list the two main parts.
5. Think of another example for each term under the "Direction" column, Table 6–2.
6. In your opinion, what makes water an all-important body substance?
7. The cell is able to divide itself and produce two daughter cells. Of what value is this to the body?
8. Cells work. What do they do?
9. What is meant by "electrolyte balance"?
10. Study the vocabulary list at the beginning of this chapter. Can you pronounce them and define them?
11. Make a list of the nine systems in the body and state one function of each.

SUGGESTED SITUATIONS AND ACTIVITIES

1. Draw a single cell. Label the main parts and below it list as many facts as possible about the cell.
2. Watch for articles in the newspapers or magazines which tell of progress scientists are making in finding out new things about the normal human body. If one of these articles is of particular interest to you, share it with your classmates and instructor(s).

CHAPTER 7

THE SKELETAL SYSTEM

OBJECTIVES FOR THE STUDENT: Be able to:

1. State five main functions of the skeletal system.
2. Give an example of each of the five types of bones.
3. Describe the composition of bones.
4. Explain how bones grow.
5. Explain why the body has several types of joints.
6. Tell how age and sex account for differences in bone structure.

SUGGESTED STUDY VOCABULARY*

skeleton	humerus	condyle
shaft	radius	crest
articulation	ulna	foramen
ligaments	carpal	sinus
cartilage	metatarsal	spinous process
cranial	phalanges	meatus
vertebra	innominate bones	marrow
rib cage	femur	medullary cavity
sternum	patella	periosteum
clavicle	tarsal	axial skeleton
scapula	tibia	appendicular skeleton
	thorax	maturation process

*Look for any terms you already know.

INTRODUCTION

Man has need to stand erect, move about, and perform endless tasks. The *skeleton* of the body is made up of 206 separate, differently shaped bones joined together to serve in a variety of ways.

Some functions are performed solely by bones; other functions are carried out in direct cooperation between bones and muscles. Still other functions of bones are performed in concert with the body as a whole.

Use Figures 7–1 and 7–2 as often as necessary to locate bones discussed in this chapter.

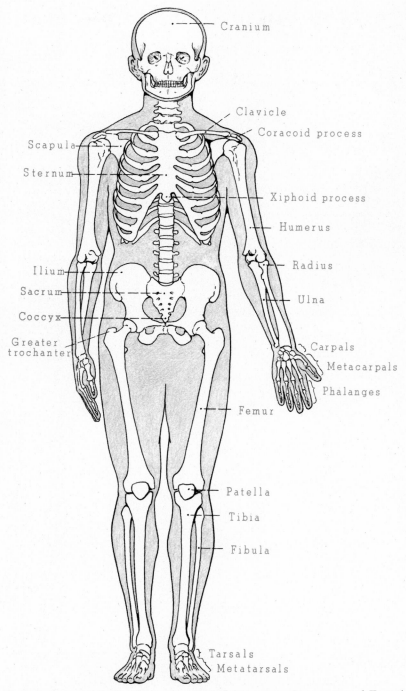

FIGURE 7–1 Anterior view of the skeleton. (Jacob and Francone: Structure and Function in Man).

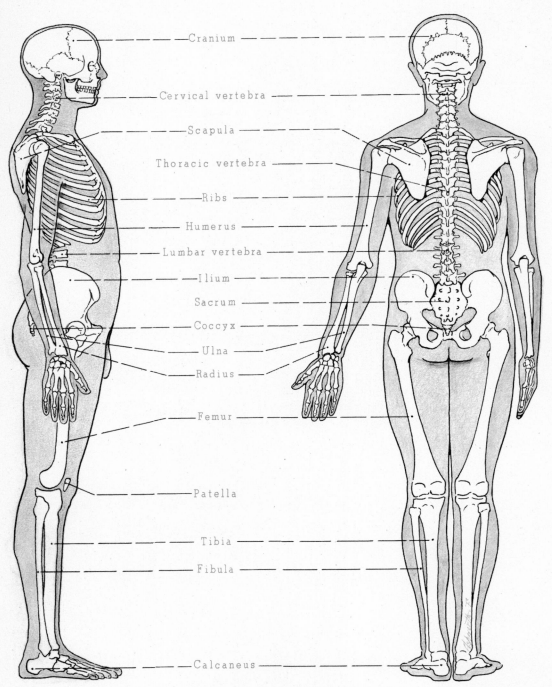

Cranium

Cervical vertebra

Scapula

Thoracic vertebra

Ribs

Humerus

Lumbar vertebra

Ilium

Sacrum

Coccyx

Ulna

Radius

Femur

Patella

Tibia

Fibula

Calcaneus

FIGURE 7–2   Lateral and posterior views of the skeleton. (Jacob and Francone: Structure and Function in Man).

FUNCTIONS OF BONES

The main functions of the skeletal system are to:

1. Give the body shape and support.

2. Assist body movement. Bones attached to muscles for "moving power" permit the body to bend, sit, turn, or stand.

3. Protect vital organs. For example, the skull protects the brain and the eye, the ribs shield the lungs and the heart.

4. Manufacture red blood cells, some types of white blood cells, and the blood platelets (see Fig. 7-3)

5. Serve as a storehouse for mineral salts such as calcium and phosphorus to be released when needed.

TYPES OF BONES

The 206 bones of the skeletal system are classified into five types according to shape: long, short, flat, irregular and sesamoid.

1. *Long bones* (examples: ulna, tibia, and femur). The long, hard portion between the two ends is called the *shaft*. It has a core (medullary canal) filled with yellow substance called marrow. The shaft is made of tightly packed cells (bone tissue) to give it strength and the capacity to take strain. Weight bearing helps keep long bones in good growth condition. The ends of long bones broaden out to provide space to articulate with the next bone (jointing) and allow space for muscle attachments.

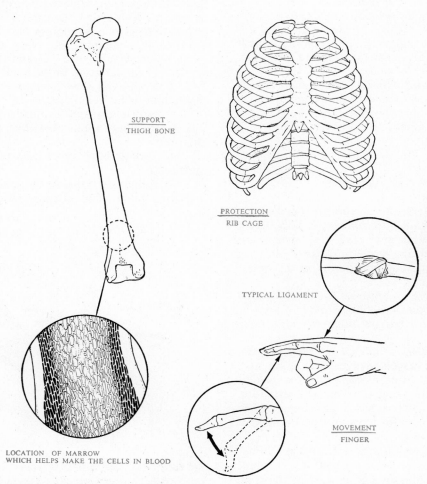

SUPPORT
THIGH BONE

PROTECTION
RIB CAGE

TYPICAL LIGAMENT

MOVEMENT
FINGER

LOCATION OF MARROW
WHICH HELPS MAKE THE CELLS IN BLOOD

FIGURE 7-3 Functions of bones. (Miller and Burt: Good Health: Personal and Community, 3rd ed.)

2. *Short bones* (examples: ankle or tarsals, wrist or carpals). These bones are not "miniature" long bones; they do not bear the same type of strain and have a thinner layer of tightly packed cells (bone tissue) covering the core. Short bones are more irregular in shape. Note the bones in the wrist (Fig. 7–1).

3. *Flat bones* (examples: ribs, scapula or shoulder blade, sternum or breast bone, frontal or forehead). These bones are protectors of soft tissues. Notice the cage formed by the ribs, the sternum, and the spinal column in Figures 7–1 and 7–2. Notice too, in Figure 7–2, how the scapula forms additional protection. The name of these bones tells their shape; being flat allows space for muscle attachments. As with other bones, there is a core space filled with spongy bone matter.

4. *Irregular bones* (examples: mandible or lower jaw, vertebra, coccyx). Bones in this group might be considered as special in a sense. They differ in shape and size to perform selected tasks. Notice in Figure 7–2 the difference in size and shape between the lumbar vertebra and the thoracic vertebra. Irregular bones have a core also.

5. *Sesamoid bones:* The name comes from their resemblance to the rounded, small sesame seed. The patella (knee cap) is the largest of the small, round bones.

MARKINGS OF BONES

There is a useful system for bone markings which relates to openings, hollows or depressions, and projections or processes; each such marking has a purpose. Following are some of the common terms in this reference system:

1. *Condyle*—a knob or rounded piece at the end of a bone. This helps make a joint.

2. *Crest*—a narrow edge or ridge on a bone.

3. *Foramen*—a hole or opening for passage of blood vessels, nerves, and ligaments.

4. *Fossa*—a depression or hollow usually to accommodate some other nearby structure.

5. *Head*—the rounded portion attached to another bone to form a joint. Notice head of femur (Fig. 7–4).

6. *Sinus*—a chamber or cavity in a bone.

7. *Spinous process* or *spine*—a pointed, slender projection on a bone. Locate these on the lumbar vertebra (Fig. 7–2).

8. *Meatus*—a long tube-like canal or passageway.

COMPOSITION AND GROWTH OF BONE

Bones need to be strong, but they must be light enough in weight to permit the body to move easily; if not, movements would be clumsy, the body would tire too easily and it would be less able to remove itself from dangerous situations.

All bones have roughly the same basic structure even though they vary in size, shape, and exact consistency (some are more compact than others). Bone is living, growing tissue needing nourishment the same as other tissues. To know how bones are nourished and grow requires some knowledge of their composition. The hard substance that gives strength to bones is calcium phosphate; hard bone looks something like ivory and is yellowish white. Use Figure 7–5 and locate:

1. Compact bone in the shaft.

2. Yellow marrow in the medullary cavity (contains fat cells).

3. Nutrient artery to furnish blood supply. Nerve fibers are located close to the blood supply.

4. Spongy bone in both extremities (end portions).

5. Epiphyses—the area toward the end of the long bone. The portion called "line of

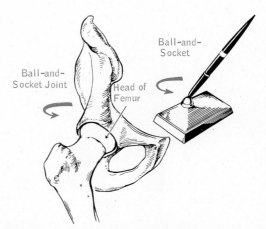

FIGURE 7–4 The ball and socket joint. (American Medical Association: The Wonderful Human Machine).

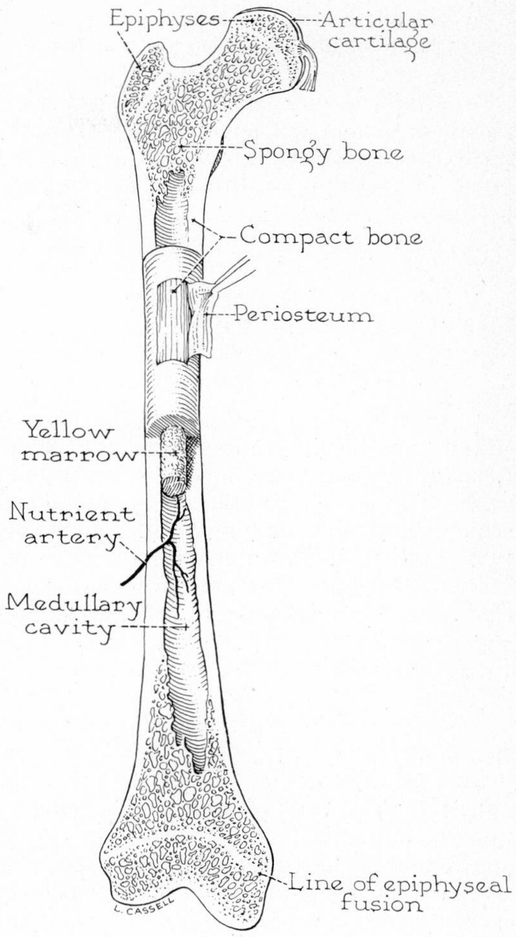

Epiphyses — Articular cartilage

Spongy bone

Compact bone

Periosteum

Yellow marrow

Nutrient artery

Medullary cavity

Line of epiphyseal fusion

L. CASSELL

FIGURE 7–5 Diagram of a structure of a long bone. (King and Showers: Human Anatomy and Physiology, 6th ed.)

epiphyseal fusion" is known as the growth plate. It is here that a bone lengthens.

6. Periosteum—the tough membrane covering the shaft but not the ends.

7. Articular cartilage—the smooth covering where joints are formed. Another substance called red marrow is present in bones, with more found in infants than in adults. It manufactures red blood cells, some white blood cells, and is found in the ends of long bones and throughout the soft tissue of irregular and flat bones.

Bones grow and they change as they grow. On the average a female needs about 20 years to attain full bone growth, while it takes the male some three years longer. At the time of birth skeletal bones are developed to the point of readiness to grow in length. They are soft and need great amounts of calcium phosphate and vitamins to grow and harden.

Noticeable growth in height takes place until puberty. With the onset of puberty, bone growth begins to slacken and, it reaches skeletal maturity at different ages for the male and for the female. From soft bone at birth, there is a gradual hardening of the bone as it grows (in length and circumference) and matures. When a bone hardens, there is a cementing together of long fibers which run in every direction. This hardening process takes place when calcium is deposited in and among these long fibers.

Nature carefully maintains a balance in bone growth. To prevent a bone from becoming solid, an orderly tearing-down process is carried on at all times in the medullary (inner) cavity as growth takes place. Every bone needs an inner space for bone marrow to make blood cells and aid in the nourishment of the bone itself. Solid bone would allow no space for marrow; it would be too heavy to carry around and would be unable to bear the strain as well.

A marked change takes place in bone between birth and old age. From soft bone at birth, bone gradually becomes hard and more brittle as years go by. Brittle bone cracks and breaks more easily.

MOVEMENT OF BONES (ARTICULATION)

Another name for articulation is joint. When two or more bones meet a joint is formed. In some joints bones are separated by cushions or by smooth, slick membranes which allow for movement. In other joints bones are bound firmly together with tough immovable fibers. The kind of tissue separating bones or binding them together depends upon the function of a joint; some need to be freely movable, and others must be fixed in position.

Where bones come together (articulate), the shape of one fits the shape of the other. They are held together by tough, fibrous bands called *ligaments* which give strength and support to the joint.

Joints are commonly classified according to the work they do. Some move freely in a wide range of motion, others twist and turn, while still others move back and forth. Some joints are immovable.

Study Figures 7–4, 7–6 and 7–7 to note three types of joint action. Self-examination of

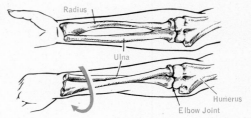

FIGURE 7–7 The wrist—condyloid. (American Medical Association: The Wonderful Human Machine).

arms, hands, and legs will help you find these types of joints and to sense their work. Table 7–1 includes some common body joints and their features. Figure 7–8 shows examples of each classification.

Movements of Joints

Certain terms describe movements of joints. See Figure 7–9.

1. *Flexion*—bending, as when the forearm bends at the elbow to bring it closer to the upper arm.

2. *Extension*—straightening, as when the forearm is straight with the upper arm.

3. *Abduction*—moving away from, as when the arm is raised.

4. *Adduction*—moving back (opposite of abduction), as when the arm is returned to the body.

5. *Rotation*—turning or revolving, as when the head is turned in one direction and then another.

TWO DIVISIONS OF THE SKELETON

The 206 bones in the body work in unison to help the body carry on its activities. However (for study purposes), the skeleton is divided into two main parts:

1. Axial skeleton (80 bones—vertebra, thorax, skull).

2. Appendicular skeleton (126 bones—upper and lower extremities, shoulder bones and pelvic bones).

Tables 7–2 (axial skeleton) and 7–3 (appendicular skeleton): name the bones in each part and include common names to help you locate them in the body.

(*Text continues on page 77.*)

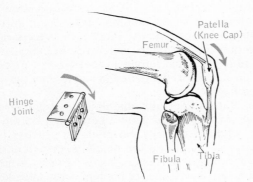

FIGURE 7–6 The hinge joint. (American Medical Association: The Wonderful Human Machine).

TABLE 7.1. JOINTS: COMMON TYPES

TYPE	MOVEMENT	FEATURES	EXAMPLE
1. Synarthrosis	No movement	No joint cavity	
a. Suture		Fibrous tissues firmly unite end margins of bones	Skull
b. Synchondroses		Cartilage unites end margins of bones	Ribs
2. Amphiarthrosis	Slight movement	May have joint cavity; fibrous, elastic tissues unite bones	Where vertebrae are joined together in spinal column
		Cartilage discs separate bones	Between vertebrae
3. Diarthroses (most joints are included in this group)	Free movement to a certain extent	Joint cavity present; cartilage covers ends of bones; cavity lined with synovial membrane and contains fluid	
a. Ball and socket (See Figure 7-6)	Free, full movement	Rounded head of bone moves in cuplike cavity (socket) of the adjoining bone	Shoulder, hip
b. Hinge (See Figure 7-8)	Forward or backward direction only		Elbow, forward only Knee, backward only
c. Condyloid (See Figure 7-9)	Forward and backward direction		Wrist
d. Pivot	Rotation	Permits turning movement	Between ulna and radius in forearm; between skull and first two vertebrae
e. Saddle	Rocking back and forth	Gets name from shape of one bone as it fits curvature of other	Thumb
f. Gliding	Chiefly back and forth	One bone glides or slides across another	In ankle In wrist

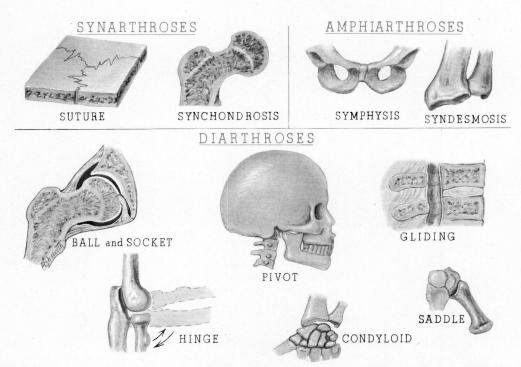

FIGURE 7–8 Joints are categorized into three groups according to the degree of movement permitted. Each of these groups is in turn subdivided with respect to the structural components of individual joints. (Jacob and Francone: Structure and Function in Man).

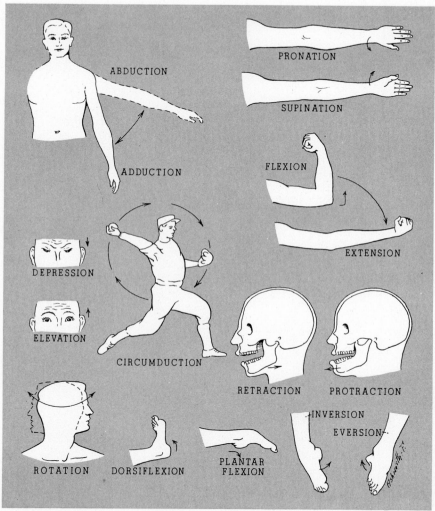

FIGURE 7–9 Types of movement permitted by diarthrodial joints. (Jacob and Francone: Structure and Function in Man).

TABLE 7.2. BONES OF AXIAL SKELETON

NAME OF BONE	LOCATION Common Term	NUMBER Single	NUMBER Paired	REMARKS
Skull (28 bones)				Contains the brain; brain and spinal cord join through the large skull opening called foramen magnum; sutures (immovable joint) located on the surface
1. *Cranium (8)*	Head			
Frontal	Forehead	1		
Parietal	Side walls of cranium		2	
Occipital	The back part of head	1		
Temporal	Pertaining to temple		2	
Sphenoid	Central part of base of cranium	1		Also closes off anterior base of the cranium
Ethmoid	Within the nose to help form passageways	1		
2. *Face (14)*				
Nasal	Bridge of nose		2	Gives shape to nose
Maxilla	Upper jaw		2	
Malar or zygoma	Cheek bone		2	Gives shape to cheek
Mandible	Lower jaw	1		Forms chin and is largest bone in the face
Lacrimal	Part of the eye socket		2	
Palatine	Hard palate		2	Roof of the mouth
Inferior nasal concha	In each nasal cavity		2	Spiral or scroll-shaped bone
Vomer	Bony nasal cavity divider	1		Shaped like a plowshare
3. *Ear (6)*				
Malleus	Hammer		2	
Incus	Anvil		2	
Stapes	Stirrup		2	
Hyoid		1		Not a part of skull; only bone in body that does not join or articulate with another bone

TABLE 7.2. (Continued)

Spinal Column (26)	Back bone		Flexible chain of bones housing the spinal cord
Vertebrae			
Cervical	In the neck	7	Below the cervical area
Thoracic	Upper back	12	Below the thoracic area
Lumbar	Mid-back	5	Below lumbar area; in the adult, 5 vertebrae fused into one bone
Sacrum	Lower back	1	Below sacrum; small triangle-shaped bone formed by 4 – 5 vertebrae fused together
Coccyx	Lower end of column	1	
Thorax (25)	Chest		Framework made up of ribs attached to sternum in front and to thoracic vertebrae in back
Ribs (24 or 12 pairs)			
True ribs	Attached to sternum and thoracic vertebrae	7	Curved, long, and slender
False ribs	Attached by cartilage to the lower edge of the rib above it (not to the sternum)	3	The term "false ribs" is sometimes used to include the floating ribs. In this case one could say there are 5 pairs of false ribs.
Floating ribs	Attached to thoracic vertebrae but not in any way attached to sternum, hence the name "floating ribs"	2	
Sternum (1)	Breast bone		Flat, tapered bone forming front piece for rib cage; at top, it articulates with collar bone (clavicle)

TABLE 7.3. BONES OF APPENDICULAR SKELETON

NAME OF BONE	LOCATION Common Term	NUMBER Single	NUMBER Paired	REMARKS
Upper Extremities (64)				
Shoulder girdle				
Clavicle	Collar bone		2	
Scapula	Shoulder bone		2	
Upper arms				
Humerus	Arm bone		2	Long shaft with 2 enlarged ends; upper end forms ball and socket joint with shoulder; lower end forms hinge joint at elbow with ulna
Forearms				
Ulna	Longer bone		2	
Radius	Shorter bone on thumb side of forearm		2	Broad lower end articulates to form wrist
Hands				
Carpals	Wrist		16	
Metacarpals	Hand		10	
Phalanges	Fingers		28	
Lower Extremities (62)				
Pelvic girdle or Innominate bone	Hip bone; forms socket for head of femur		2	3 bones fused together to form this bone (ilium, ischium, and pubic)
Upper leg				
Femur	Thigh		2	Longest, heaviest bone in body
Patella	Knee cap		2	
Lower leg				
Tibia	Shin bone		2	Larger, stronger bone of lower leg
Fibula	Located within lower leg itself; smaller than tibia		2	Not part of knee joint; articulates with tibia
Foot				
Tarsals	Ankle		14	
Metatarsals	Within foot		10	
Phalanges	Toes		28	Arch-forming bones of foot

CHANGES AND DIFFERENCES IN SKELETAL DEVELOPMENT

Two things cause skeletal changes in the normal body: age and sex.

AGE. All bones go through a "ripening" or maturing process. Cartilage and fibrous tissue are transformed into bone; this is called a maturation process. While they are "ripening" or maturing, bones likewise are growing—increasing in size; these two processes go on at the same time, the one with the other.

At the time of birth bones are ready to grow and they grow noticeably until puberty. From then until the so-called end of adolescence, growth slackens until finally the individual reaches maximum height and the bones are fully ossified (cartilage and fibrous tissue are changed to bone).

Age in years is no true index to bone maturation. Some persons develop quickly; others develop slowly. The pattern for individual development is set in the genes just as is the color of the eyes or the hair.

As stated previously, bone is living tissue. Therefore, after all cartilage and fibrous tissues (that are going to change) have become hard bone tissue, bone continues to live and change with increased age; it thickens and becomes more brittle. Adequate nourishment at any age is beneficial to bone growth, maturation, and bone maintenance.

SEX. Sex has an effect on skeletal maturation. The female matures at a faster rate than the male. On the average, the female skeleton has matured by about age 20, the male by about age 23. Other noticeable differences include a smaller, lighter skeleton in the female than in the male; a broader, more shallow and flaring pelvis in the female contrasted to the funnelshaped, deep pelvis of the male; and a wider pubic arch in the female than the male.

SUMMARY

There are 206 bones in the normal skeleton (plus three in the middle ear) making up two main skeletal systems or divisions: (1) axial skeleton, and (2) appendicular skeleton. While bones depend upon the muscles for "power," they help the body to move. In addition, bones give shape and support to the body and allow it to stand, sit, bend, and turn. Protection to vital organs is another important function. Bones manufacture red blood cells, platelets, and some types of white blood cells and serve as a storehouse for calcium.

Age and sex cause skeletal changes. Bones change throughout a lifetime, changing from soft bone at birth to hard, thick bone in later years. Noticeable skeletal differences related to sex include differing rates of maturation, as well as size and shape of some bones. Adequate nutrition at any age is essential to proper bone maturation, growth, and maintenance.

GUIDES FOR STUDY AND DISCUSSION

1. The skeleton continues to undergo change during a lifetime. Using the following headings, list some normal changes that occur during each period:
    a. infancy.
    b. adolescence.
    c. old age.
2. The skeleton serves the body in many ways. List the main functions of bones.
3. In your opinion, why is there a difference between the size and shape of the various vertebrae? between the size and shape of the bones in the feet?
4. Using Figures 7–1 and 7–2, locate examples of the five types of bones (long, short, flat, irregular, and sesamoid) found in the human body.

5. Imagine that your right femur is twice as heavy as it is. How might this fact influence your mobility?

6. Why do bones have an inner canal?

7. Bones "ripen" or mature and grow at the same time. Be ready to discuss the difference between *maturing* and *growing*.

8. In your opinion, how would it be helpful for a nurse to know that bones are soft at birth and brittle at old age?

SUGGESTED SITUATIONS AND ACTIVITIES

1. Following is a way to sense the wide range of movement in a ball and socket joint: Keeping the right arm straight and stiff at the elbow, move it into as many different positions as possible using only the shoulder joint.

2. Experience the use of other types of body joints. Identify each as to type and consider how it serves the body.

CHAPTER 8

THE MUSCULAR SYSTEM

TOPICAL HEADINGS

Introduction
Functions of Muscles
Types of Muscle Tissue
Characteristics of Muscle Tissue
General Description of Muscles

Types of Muscles
Summary
Guides for Study and Discussion
Suggested Situations and Activities

OBJECTIVES FOR THE STUDENT: Be able to:

1. Tell how muscles serve the body; give three examples.
2. Name and locate common body muscles.
3. Describe how muscles work.
4. Explain how bones, muscles, and body movement are related to each other.
5. Demonstrate four examples of proper body mechanics.

SUGGESTED STUDY VOCABULARY*

posture
body alignment
equilibrium
body mechanics
striated muscle
smooth muscle
cardiac muscle
contractility

elasticity
extensibility
irritability
tonus
muscle fatigue
flaccid
origin
insertion

tendon
abductors
adductors
levators
depressors
flexors
extensors
rotators
sphincters

---

*Look for any terms you already know.

INTRODUCTION

The power to move and to move about makes the difference between being mobile and immobile. Power gives us the ability to swallow, to move food along the food route, to move blood through its system of tubes, and to move urine along its pathway. Any body movement (even lifting a finger) requires power.

The power system of the body is its system of muscles. This system is vast. More than 400 muscles are attached to bones; others furnish power for such organs as the stomach, intestines, urinary bladder, and body openings. The heart itself is a muscle furnishing power.

Real knowledge of the structure and function of muscles began with the invention of the microscope (17th century); this instrument permitted the first close look at muscles. Today's electronic scopes and devices produce close-up pictures and graphs of muscular tissue structure and function which guide scientists in their continuing search for more information.

FUNCTIONS OF MUSCLES

Muscles serve the body in three main ways: (1) assist with movement, (2) produce heat and energy, and (3) maintain posture.

Movement

At no time is the human body without some type of movement or motion. It is easy to understand movement such as walking or jumping; but think of examples of movements which occur while sleeping or sitting. The term body movement means a variety of activities. One is *locomotion*—the power to move from one place to another. But movement also means *small* movements such as changing the size of the eye pupil to adjust to surrounding light conditions, or movement of the tongue during speech and eating. It includes internal movements where untold numbers of muscles work unnoticed, doing such things as pushing blood through blood vessels and pulling air into the lungs and forcing it out. It means controlling the entrances and exits to certain organs and forcing food through the digestive tract.

Heat and Energy

Heat and energy are the essence of life itself; in a way they represent life. It is not yet clear how the energy produced in muscle tissue is changed into movement. But it is known where the energy in a muscle comes from; it is a complicated chemical process that starts when a single muscle cell takes in food substance (sugar) and oxygen. These combine and burn. Heat (energy) and waste products are produced. Some of this energy is used for movement power, and the rest is body heat.

Chapter 12, The Process of Metabolism, discusses heat production in the body as a whole.

Posture and Body Mechanics

Posture is the alignment and position of body parts; it is the arrangement of one part in relation to another part and can be called the carriage or attitude of the body.

Muscles contribute to body posture by exerting pull to keep the body in proper position. Muscles attached to bones act as levers; some pull in one way, others pull in opposite ways. The many muscle-bone attachments and muscle to muscle attachments throughout the body make up a vast system of checks and balances to allow the body to run, lift, sit, stand, walk, and bend.

The word *mechanical* pertains to something machinelike that is power-driven. The body-machine with its movement and balance is called *body mechanics*. Bones, joints, muscles, plus nerves and the brain, work together to maintain balance and posture. Proper body posture is essential to good body mechanics (Fig. 8–1).

A person can assist the body-machine in its efforts so that it functions with the least possible effort. Following are eight rules that, when used, help conserve physical energy and reduce muscle fatigue:

1. The base of support is related to body balance. A broader base (feet slightly apart or apart with one slightly ahead of the other) provides better body balance.

2. Maintain proper alignment of body segments.

3. Proper walking habits reduce fatigue and body jar. Body weight is shifted with each forward step. Good step rhythm moves the body forward with less effort.

4. Stooping with proper body alignment and position prevents fatigue.

5. Proper body alignment in sitting reduces muscle strain and provides proper blood circulation in the thighs. Keep the trunk in the same alignment as when standing. The feet should be flat on the floor (or foot stool) to avoid pull on the muscles of the thigh and pressure on the blood vessels on the posterior surface of the thigh. Sit back in the chair to provide full back support; it is important that the depth of the chair seat (front to back) properly fits the body from hips to knees.

6. Work should be kept close to the body when performing tasks. Reaching toward the

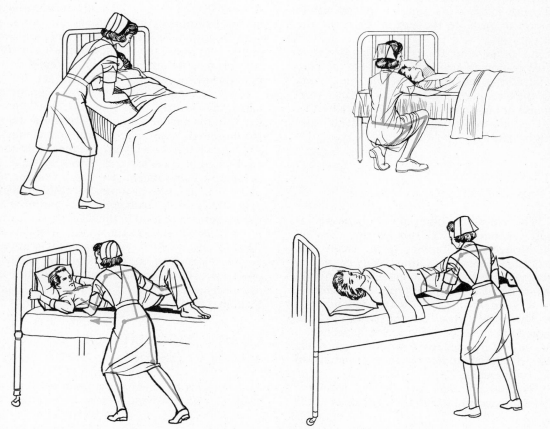

FIGURE 8–1 Body mechanics in action. Notice the position of the feet, the alignment of the back, the posture while stooping, the position of the thigh with respect to the lower part of the leg. (Kozier and DuGas: Introduction to Patient Care, 2nd ed.)

"work" from a bending or outstretched position will cause undue muscle strain and fatigue.

7. To maintain proper balance when reaching above the head, stand close to the area to be reached; keep the back in a straight line with the feet slightly spread.

8. Use as little energy as possible when moving, carrying, or lifting heavy objects. To do this, maintain proper alignment of the head and trunk, keeping the feet, knees, and legs in position to provide the power to move the body.

Keep in mind that the skeletal system shares responsibility for posture; nerves play a vital role in maintaining muscle tone, along with the circulatory system which brings oxygen and nourishment to the muscle cells. The brain is the control center for balance and equilibrium.

TYPES OF MUSCLE TISSUE

There are three types of muscle tissue: (1) *striated* (voluntary), (2) *smooth*, and (3) *cardiac.* Notice the difference in the shape and the arrangement of the three types of muscle cells in Figure 8–2. About one half of the body is made up of these three types of muscles.

Striated muscle is known as *skeletal muscle.* The word "stria" means streak or line. Striated muscle cells are long fibers, each with many nuclei encased in elastic covering. While each cell is alone in its case, it is connected to neighboring cells.

Skeletal muscles vary in size from the tiny middle ear muscle to the large ones of the thigh. The function that a muscle performs influences its size, shape, and arrangement of fibers. Each muscle has many fibers. Some have fibers that run lengthwise in bundles; others have diagonal fiber arrangements (similar to a feather); and some muscles resemble a ring-like formation with the fibers extending from the ring's edge toward the center and meeting there.

Smooth muscle (non-striated) cells are spindle-shaped (Fig. 8–2) and are controlled by the autonomic (involuntary) nervous system. Smooth muscle tissue is found in arteries, veins, arterioles, the genitourinary tract, the respiratory tract, some lymphatic vessels, and the alimentary canal or digestive tract.

For example, think of the alimentary canal as a "tube" with four different layers; the smooth muscle layer is right under (next to) the outer layer. The smooth muscle layer itself consists of two layers; the inner one contains circular muscles and the outer layer is made up of smooth muscle fibers running up and down the tube in a parallel fashion. This two-layer muscle arrangement is essential to the movement of food in the digestive process.

Cardiac muscle tissue makes up the main part of the wall of the heart; it is called *myocardium.* The myocardium and certain other specialized muscle tissue in the heart are discussed in Chapter 10, The Circulatory System.

CHARACTERISTICS OF MUSCLE TISSUE

Muscles have several unique qualities or features which provide them with the ability to

FRAMEWORK OF THE BODY

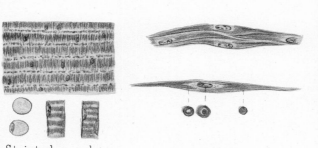
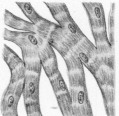

Striated or voluntary (skeletal m.)   Smooth muscle   Cardiac muscle

FIGURE 8–2   Types of muscle cells. (Jacob and Francone: Structure and Function in Man.)

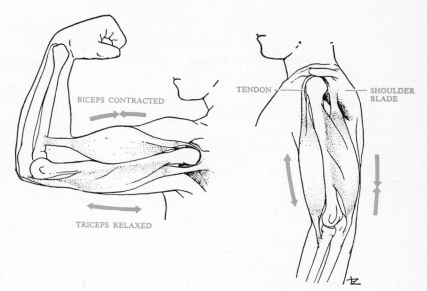

BICEPS CONTRACTED

TRICEPS RELAXED

TENDON

SHOULDER BLADE

FIGURE 8–3 Muscles almost always work in groups. (Miller and Burt: Good Health: Personal and Community, 3rd ed.)

do work; without these features they would be unable to serve the body. These unique features include:

1. *Contractility*—the ability to shorten and thicken (contract) when given the proper nervous stimulus. When a muscle shortens it exerts pull. If it is attached to a bone, the pull is exerted on the bone (Fig. 8–3).

2. *Elasticity*—the ability to return to original length after stretching.

3. *Extensibility*—the ability to stretch (Fig. 8–5).

4. *Irritability*—the ability to respond to stimulation.

5. *Tonus* (tone)—a slight tension in the muscles at all times—even when at rest. This is a state of readiness to act more easily and quickly when called upon. Without tone, muscle is flaccid (flabby). The nervous system plays a part in maintaining muscle tone.

Muscle fatigue occurs when there are prolonged periods of muscle contraction; fatigue causes the muscle to lose some of its power to contract and respond quickly to stimuli. The fibers do not continue to put out the same amount of ability to work. Sufficient rest and proper cell nourishment help restore them to a normal manner.

Continued, active use of muscle (exercise) increases its size and strength. This is why the leg muscles of the ballet dancer or the runner are large and strong. Vigorous use of muscles that have been idle for a while will

cause them to be stiff and sore. A "charley horse" comes from too much exercise of a muscle too fast (i.e., can occur during spring training for the baseball season).

Muscles lose tone and actually begin to degenerate or waste away when the nerve supply to the fibers is destroyed. This degeneration (atrophy) causes muscles to shrink in size. Disuse (or limited use) also causes muscle atrophy and it does not take too long for muscle shrinkage to occur.

GENERAL DESCRIPTION OF MUSCLES

A *muscle unit* is a muscle consisting of a framework of connective tissue with its network supply of blood, lymph, and nerves. A skeletal muscle has a *body* and *two attachments*. Within the muscle body (sometimes called muscle belly) is the bundle of tissue itself. The two attachments are made of white fibrous tissue: one is called the *origin* (more fixed); the other where movement is produced is known as the *insertion*.

When white fibrous tissue forms a direct cordlike attachment to a bone it is called a *tendon* (Fig. 8–3). If the attachment spreads out into a heavy sheet of white fibrous tissue to connect muscle to bone or muscle to muscle, this is called an *aponeurosis*.

Muscles almost always work in groups; one contracts and the other extends or relaxes, as shown in Figure 8–3. They vary in size and shape (long, short, broad, narrow, flat, bulky) depending upon their use in the body.

Names are assigned to muscles according to certain features such as origin and insertion (sternocleidomastoideus), shape (deltoid-triangular outline), number of divisions in the muscle (biceps, triceps, quadriceps), and location in the body (rectus abdominus, rectus femoris).

TYPES OF MUSCLES

Muscles are classified and labeled according to action. Following are terms which describe some common muscle action (see Fig. 7–9 for positions):

1. Abductors—draw *away* from a neighboring part or limb.
2. Adductors—draw *toward* a neighboring part or toward the midline.
3. Levators—lift up or raise a part.
4. Depressors—lower a part.
5. Flexors—bend joints.
6. Extensors—straighten joints.
7. Rotators—revolve a part on its axis.
8. Sphincters—ring-like muscles used for closing body openings.

MAIN SKELETAL MUSCLES

While it takes a good many muscles to serve the body, a practical nurse would have need to know (and use) but a select number of them—those most related to her work. Table 8–1 lists some major skeletal muscles, their general location and main functions. Locate as many as possible in Figures 8–4 and 8–5.

TABLE 8.1.   SOME MAIN SKELETAL MUSCLES

LOCATION	*MUSCLE(S)*	*MAIN FUNCTION*
Neck	Sternocleidomastoid	Rotates and flexes head
Shoulder	Deltoid	Abducts upper arm
Upper arm	Biceps brachii	Flexes and turns lower arm
	Triceps brachii	Extends lower arm
Lower arm (forearm)	Brachioradialis	Turns lower arm outward and inward
	Pronator	Turns and flexes lower arm
Back	Trapezius	Raises and lowers shoulder
	Latissimus dorsi	Extends and adducts upper arm
Chest	Pectoralis major	Flexes upper arm
	Pectoralis minor	Pulls shoulder forward and down
Abdominal wall	External oblique	Compresses abdomen, flexes trunk
	Internal oblique	Compresses abdomen
	Transversalis	Compresses abdomen
	Rectus abdominis	Compresses abdomen, aids in defecation and during childbirth
Buttocks	Gluteus maximus	Extends thigh, rotates outward
	Gluteus medius	Abducts thigh, rotates outward
	Gluteus minimus	Abducts thigh, rotates inward
Thigh	Quadriceps femoris	Extends leg
	Hamstring group	Flexes leg
Leg (lower)	Tibialis anterior	Flexes foot
	Tibialis posterior	Extends foot
	Gastrocnemius	Extends foot, flexes lower leg
Pelvic floor	Levator ani	Supports pelvic organs

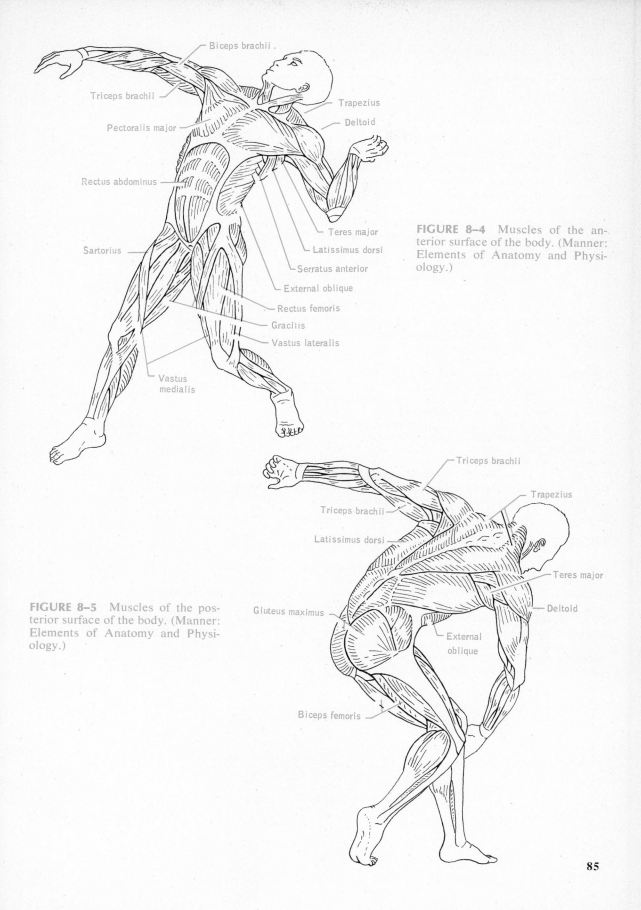

Biceps brachii

Triceps brachii

Pectoralis major

Rectus abdominus

Sartorius

Trapezius

Deltoid

Teres major

Latissimus dorsi

Serratus anterior

External oblique

Rectus femoris

Gracilis

Vastus lateralis

Vastus medialis

FIGURE 8–4 Muscles of the anterior surface of the body. (Manner: Elements of Anatomy and Physiology.)

Triceps brachii

Trapezius

Triceps brachii

Latissimus dorsi

Teres major

Deltoid

Gluteus maximus

External oblique

Biceps femoris

FIGURE 8–5 Muscles of the posterior surface of the body. (Manner: Elements of Anatomy and Physiology.)

85

SUMMARY

The muscle system is the body's power system; it produces heat and energy. Skeletal muscles furnish power for bones to move. Smooth muscles furnish power for internal organs (i.e., lungs, stomach, intestines) to function. Cardiac muscle makes up the bulk of the heart wall and has its special pumping function to perform.

Muscles serve the body in three main ways: (1) assist with movement, (2) produce heat and energy, and (3) maintain posture.

The body-machine with its movement and balance is called body mechanics. A person can benefit from body mechanics by using correct practices when standing, walking, lifting, or stooping.

Muscle tissue has such unique qualities as contractility, elasticity, extensibility, irritability, and tonus (tone).

Muscles get their names from such things as origin and insertion, shape, number of divisions, or location in the body; they are classified according to the action they perform.

GUIDES FOR STUDY AND DISCUSSION

1. As you understand it, how do muscles serve the body?
2. In what ways do muscles work with bones?
3. In general, how do skeletal muscles perform?
4. What causes muscle fatigue? What helps overcome it?
5. What is meant by the statement, "A person who practices good body mechanics tires less easily"?
6. What keeps muscles in "good muscle tone"?
7. What is the difference between muscle tone and muscle atrophy?
8. In your opinion, what are the basic requirements for healthy muscles?

SUGGESTED SITUATIONS AND ACTIVITIES

1. Assume that you have been asked to identify and make a list of the muscles you should know. While making this list, keep in mind body "landmarks" you might refer to time after time in your nursing practice. Be ready to compare your list with your classmates and with the instructor's expectations.

2. Practice standing, stooping, lifting, pushing, pulling, sitting, and walking, using the rules for proper body mechanics in carrying out your daily living activities.

3. Role play some ordinary life situation which involves the movements described in item 2. Have classmates observe and assess your actions according to the basic rules of good body mechanics.

THE RESPIRATORY SYSTEM

TOPICAL HEADINGS

OBJECTIVES FOR THE STUDENT: Be able to:

1. Describe the body's need for oxygen.
2. Trace the route oxygen takes from the lungs to the red blood cells; from the red blood cells to other body cells.
3. Trace the route carbon dioxide takes from body cells to its exit from the lungs.
4. Explain the basic functions of each organ or structure in the respiratory system.
5. Distinguish between internal respiration and external respiration.

SUGGESTED STUDY VOCABULARY*

nasal cavity	larynx	bronchial tree
septum	epiglottis	mediastinum
concha	vocal cords	pleura, parietal and visceral
ciliated	anoxia	bronchi
sinus	bronchioles	abdominal breathing
pharynx	alveoli	costal breathing
inspiration	expiration	eupnea

---

*Look for any terms you already know.

INTRODUCTION

The respiratory system has the all-important function of delivering oxygen to the circulatory system—specifically, to the red blood cells. Delivery of oxygen to the red blood cells actually involves an exchange of gases. In giving up oxygen to the blood, the lungs take out carbon dioxide as well as water. A person's breath is moist. You can witness moisture on glass as you breathe on it.

The respiratory system is responsible for moistening the inhaled air by the time it reaches the exchange area (alveoli). The moisture is picked up from the fluids on the surface (linings) of the tract.

TABLE 9.1. TYPES OF RESPIRATION

NAME	PARTS OF BODY INVOLVED	WHAT HAPPENS
1. External "lung breathing"	To inhale: nose, nasal cavity, pharynx, larynx, trachea, bronchial tubes, alveoli (lungs) To exhale: reverse route from lungs back to nose	Air is inhaled; oxygen is exchanged for carbon dioxide in air sacs of lungs; used air is exhaled This is the body's source of oxygen and a one-way route for throwing off body waste (carbon dioxide)
2. Internal "cell breathing"	Thin walls of the many alveoli and of the many capillaries in the lungs Blood and blood vessels Body cells	Through the thin walls of alveoli and capillaries, oxygen easily passes *into* red corpuscles; carbon dioxide passes *from* red corpuscle through the thin walls into air sacs Blood carries new oxygen supply through every capillary serving each body cell; in each cell there is another exchange of gases; carbon dioxide goes from cell to blood, and oxygen passes into cell to be used

Respiration is commonly called the act of breathing—drawing air into the lungs (inspiration) and expelling it (expiration). Actually, it is more complicated than that. Breathing in and breathing out is more exactly called *external* respiration (the exchange of gases in the lungs). Recalling that tissue cells need oxygen, there must be an exchange of oxygen and carbon dioxide in the tissues too. This exchange of gases between tissue cells and capillaries is called *internal* respiration. External and internal respiration represent a direct marriage or union between the respiratory and the circulatory systems. (See Table 9–1).

ORGANS

The organs of the respiratory system are shown in Figure 9–1. They are discussed in sequence beginning with the nasal cavity and moving downward into the lungs. Locate each organ and position as you proceed.

Nasal Cavity

Cavity means a hollow place. The nasal cavity starts with the nostrils (nares) and extends down into the throat or pharynx.

The nose is the port of entry for air. Part of it (external portion) protrudes from the face; a large part (internal portion) lies above the roof of the mouth. As a port of entry, it *filters, moistens,* and *warms* air as it is pulled into the body. The nose is lined with cilia (hairlike projections) on the mucous membranes, as is the rest of the respiratory tract, to aid the filtering, moistening, and warming process until the air reaches the alveoli. This lining contains the nerve (olfactory) endings for the sense of smell.

A partition called the *septum* starts in the external portion and extends inward to divide the nose into a right and a left side. This divider is made up of cartilage and several thin bones. One bone, called the palate, serves as a floor for the nasal cavity and thus becomes the roof of the mouth.

The entrance is the nostrils (nares). On each side, the nares lead into a cavity with three passageways formed by spiral-shaped bones called *concha.*

Four pairs of sinuses within the facial area empty into the nasal cavity: frontal (forehead); ethmoid (in back of nasal bones); sphenoid (in back of the ethmoid); maxillary (on either side of the nose). See Figure 9–2. The nasal cavity and facial sinuses aid in the vibration of air when a person speaks, and lack of proper vibration is noticed when normal air passages are obstructed by a head cold.

Pharynx

The nasal chambers open into the throat or pharynx, which is a sac or muscular tube-like chamber starting in the back of the mouth and extending downward about five inches. The pharynx ends below the esophagus and opens into the larynx (voice box). Two other openings into the pharynx are from the eustachian tubes. (See Middle Ear in Chapter 16.)

Larynx

Commonly called the "voice box," the larynx is located at the upper end of the trachea and serves as an entryway leading from the pharynx into the trachea. It is made of pieces of cartilage joined together to form a boxlike structure. One triangular part, the *thyroid cartilage,* commonly known as the "Adam's apple," is usually larger in men than in women.

The upper surface of the larynx has a hinged lid called the *epiglottis.* This opens for movement of air and closes when solids or liquids are swallowed. Muscles and nerves within the larynx open and close it automatically. If the epiglottis fails to close when something is swallowed, a person chokes. It is nicknamed the "Sunday throat."

Vocal cords (fibrous bands) stretch across the larynx and produce the voice. The length of the vocal cords and their tension (or lack of tension) determine the pitch (low, high) of the voice as air passes through.

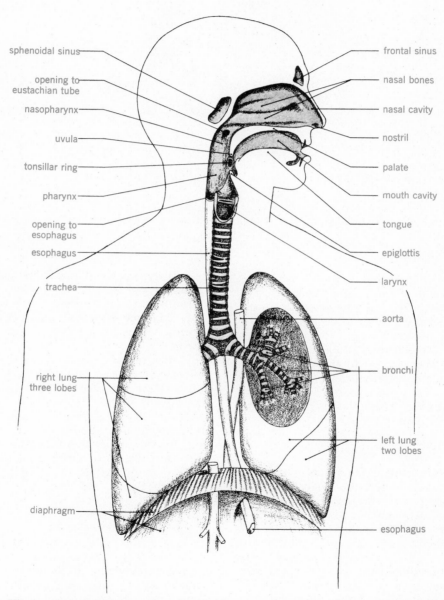

FIGURE 9-1 The human respiratory system. In this illustration the heart and most of the blood vessels have been eliminated. The left lung has been partially cut away to show the branches of the bronchi. (Schifferes: Essentials of Healthier Living. 3rd ed., John Wiley and Sons, Inc.)

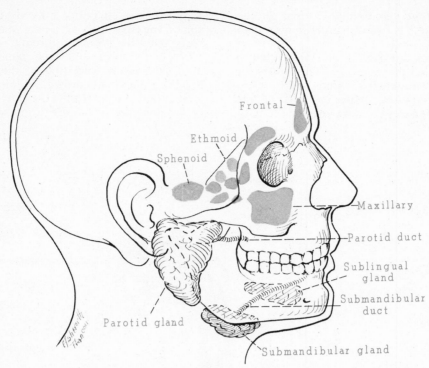

FIGURE 9-2   Lateral view of head showing sinuses and salivary glands. (Jacob and Francone: Structure and Function in Man.)

Trachea

A common name is the windpipe. The trachea is about four or five inches long and reaches from the larynx to the bronchi. Its circular wall is muscular, and at regular spaces there are C-shaped rings of cartilage open at the back. These rings hold the trachea open for movement of air at all times. The trachea serves one purpose, as a passageway for air to and from the lungs. It cannot be obstructed for very long or death occurs.

Bronchi

The lower end of the trachea branches into two tubes called the right bronchus (slightly larger and straighter) and the left bronchus. As each enters a lung it divides into numerous branches and then subdivides into small branches called *bronchioles*. Both bronchi with all their many smaller branches are called the bronchial tree, which is lined with ciliated membrane and has some cartilage rings in the walls of the larger branches.

The bronchiole tube subdivides into its smallest tubes which are called *alveolar ducts*.

At the tiny ends of the ducts are groups of small air sacs called *alveoli*. This arrangement resembles a bunch of grapes (Fig. 9–3). The bronchial tree from the trachea through to the alveoli serves one purpose, as a passageway for air.

It is in the alveoli where the actual exchange of oxygen and carbon dioxide takes place. Here the very thin membrane walls of the alveoli permit the molecules (minute particles) of oxygen to pass through into the pulmonary blood stream via tiny capillaries. Carbon dioxide molecules travel in the opposite direction. They exit through the thin capillary walls then through the thin alveolar membrane to get back into the respiratory tract to be exhaled.

At no time is blood free in the alveoli. It is contained in the smallest of capillaries which lie very close to the membranes of the alveoli. (See Fig. 9–4.) The red blood cells carry the oxygen and must rid themselves of carbon dioxide so they squeeze their way into the tiny capillaries to be as close as possible to the oxygen in the alveoli. Being close at hand speeds up the rate of exchange.

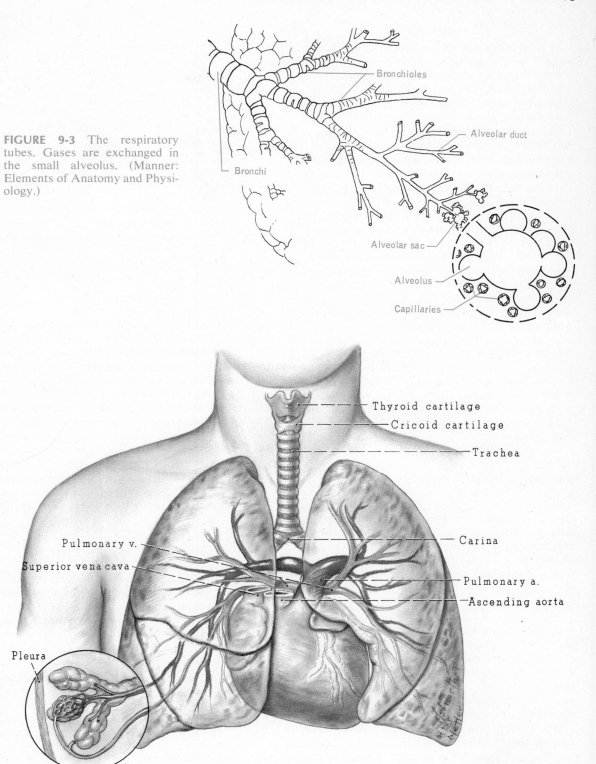

FIGURE 9-3 The respiratory tubes. Gases are exchanged in the small alveolus. (Manner: Elements of Anatomy and Physiology.)

Bronchioles

Alveolar duct

Bronchi

Alveolar sac

Alveolus

Capillaries

Thyroid cartilage

Cricoid cartilage

Trachea

Pulmonary v.

Superior vena cava

Carina

Pulmonary a.

Ascending aorta

Pleura

FIGURE 9-4 Relationships of lungs to heart and pulmonary vessels. (Jacob and Francone: Structure and Function in Man.)

Lungs

The lungs are soft, spongy, cone-shaped organs made up of multitudes of air sacs. There is one on each side of the thoracic cavity. The lungs are light in weight and elastic. The right one is larger than the left and has three lobes; the left lung has two lobes. The two lungs are separated by the heart, the large blood vessels, the esophagus, and part of the trachea and bronchi. To accommodate these other structures, the lungs are slightly concave in that area; this space is called the *mediastinum*.

Relationship of Lungs to the Heart. As previously stated the all-important function of the respiratory system is to deliver oxygen to the blood and remove carbon dioxide from it. This requires close cooperation between the lungs and the heart. The heart is the pump which keeps the blood flowing to and from the lungs, and it has a special system for this purpose called **pulmonary circulation.**

The pulmonary artery of the heart carries blood with carbon dioxide (from all parts of the body) to the alveoli of both lungs. After the exchange of carbon dioxide for oxygen is made, the pulmonary vein carries blood laden with oxygen back to the heart for more push to send it out to body tissues via the aorta. (See Fig. 9–4.)

RESPIRATION PROCESS

The respiration process involves expiration (breathing out) and inspiration (breathing in). Figure 9–5 shows what happens to the shape of the lungs, diaphragm and chest cage during expiration and during inspiration.

Thorax

This cavity (called the chest) is bounded in front by the sternum and ribs, and in back by the ribs and vertebrae. The floor is formed by the upper surface of the large muscle, the *diaphragm.*

The chest cavity contains the lungs and the mediastinum and is lined with a membrane called *parietal pleura.* Each lung is covered with a thin saclike serous membrane called *visceral pleura.* As a person breathes, the surface of one pleura comes in contact with

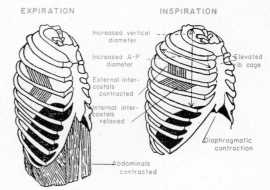

FIGURE 9-5 Expansion and contraction of the thoracic cage during expiration and inspiration, illustrating especially contraction of the diaphragm, elevation of the rib cage and function of the intercostals. (Guyton: Textbook of Medical Physiology, 4th. ed.)

the other, and a watery fluid between the two surfaces prevents friction.

The external intercostal muscles between the ribs move them to enlarge the thoracic cavity. These muscles act in cooperation with the diaphragm. When the rib muscles contract, the diaphragm contracts, becoming horizontal in shape and pulling downward. The ribs then separate, and the thoracic cavity becomes much larger, *sucking air into the lungs.* When the rib muscles relax, the ribs come together and the diaphragm relaxes and becomes dome-shaped. In this way, the chest cavity is made smaller, *pushing air out of the lungs.*

Types of Respiration

As mentioned before, two types of respiration are external and internal. When either fails to function properly *anoxia* results. This means that body cells do not have enough oxygen. Air normally contains about 20 per cent oxygen.

Table 9–1 lists the parts involved and shows what happens in the two types of respiration.

Regulation of Respiration

Breathing has depth and a rate. For example, it can be shallow and fast, or deep and slow. Depth and rate are under the control of the respiratory center in the brain (medulla). Nerves (the most important one is the phrenic nerve) send impulses to the respiratory system. For example, the intercostal muscles receive their directions for action from the intercostal nerves.

Carbon dioxide is a necessity; it acts directly on the respiratory center in the medulla. *Increased amounts of carbon dioxide in the blood step up the rate of breathing, while decreased amounts cause slower breathing.*

Under certain conditions, oxygen triggers the nerve mechanisms affecting breathing. *Lack of oxygen increases respirations.* Pain, sudden cold, exercise, fright, and anger also influence depth and rate of respiration.

Normal Respiration

Under normal conditions there are two types of breathing, *abdominal* breathing and *costal* breathing. As the diaphragm contracts and relaxes, the abdomen moves outward and inward; this deep breathing is known as abdominal breathing. *Costal* or chest breathing is shallow, the intercostal muscles moving the chest wall upward and outward. Normal breathing may be a combination of these two types. *Eupnea* is the term for quiet normal breathing. About one pint of air is expelled during a normal respiration; the average rate of breathing is about 14 to 20 respirations a minute. Babies breathe faster, while elderly persons are apt to breathe more slowly.

SUMMARY

The respiratory system is responsible for supplying oxygen to the body and for expelling carbon dioxide from it. External respiration can be called "lung breathing." Internal respiration can be called "cell breathing."

The chief functions of the nasal cavity and pharynx are to warm, moisten, filter, and guide the air on its way to the lungs. Other services include providing the body with the sense of smell (nose) and aiding in vibration of air (nasal cavity sinuses) when a person speaks.

The pharynx, with the epiglottis, serves both the respiratory system and the digestive system. The trachea is a passageway for air to and from the lungs; death occurs when it is obstructed. The "bronchial tree" consists of the two main bronchi and all their branches. At no time is the blood "free" within the alveoli in normal lung tissue. The exchange of gases is always through the very thin membranes of the air sacs and the capillaries.

The thoracic cavity houses the lungs, heart, esophagus, large blood vessels, and parts of the trachea and bronchi. The intercostal muscles and the diaphragm pull air into the lungs and push it out, in turn.

Respiration is controlled by the respiration center in the brain (medulla). Other factors which influence the rate and depth of breathing include pain, exercise, sudden cold, anger, and fright.

GUIDES FOR STUDY AND DISCUSSION

1. How many organs/structures of respiration are there? What is the function of each?

2. External respiration and internal respiration are two distinct processes. How is one related to the other?

3. What happens to the shape of the diaphragm during expiration? During inspiration?

4. Air is pushed from the lungs and in turn is sucked into the lungs. How do these two things happen?

5. Carbon dioxide acts directly on the respiratory center in the medulla. What happens when there is too little? Too much?

6. There is an exchange of gases in the lungs. Where does this exchange take place?

7. How does oxygen get from the lungs to body cells?

8. How does carbon dioxide leave body cells and then find its way back to the lungs? What happens to it in the lungs?

SUGGESTED SITUATIONS AND ACTIVITIES

1. The serious problem of air pollution is catching up with man's right to breathe clean air. Prepare an exhibit which shows the problem and which also shows some efforts being made to meet this problem.

CHAPTER 10

THE CIRCULATORY SYSTEM

TOPICAL HEADINGS

Introduction
Heart
  Coverings
  Muscle
  Chambers and Valves
  Heart at Work and at Rest
Blood Vessels
  Arteries
  Arterioles
  Capillaries
  Venules
  Veins

Blood Circulation
  Systemic
  Coronary
  Pulmonary
  Hepatic Portal
  Cerebral
  Renal
Fetal Circulation
Blood Pressure
  Meaning
  Measurement
  Pulse
Blood
  Composition

Hemostasis and
  Clotting
  Types
  Rh Factor
Lymphatic System
  Functions
  Vessels
  Nodes (Glands)
Accessory Organs
  Spleen
  Tonsils
  Thymus
Summary
Guides for Study and
  Discussion
Suggested Situations
  and Activities

OBJECTIVES FOR THE STUDENT: Be able to:

1. Explain the three general functions of the circulatory system.
2. Trace the pulmonary journey of the blood from the time it enters the heart laden with carbon dioxide until it returns with oxygen.
3. Explain the working relationship between the S-A node and the bundle of His.
4. Name the parts of the blood.
5. Describe the structure of arteries, veins and capillaries with respect to the work of each.
6. Illustrate the relationship between the circulatory system and two other systems by giving an example of each.
7. Tell how the circulatory system helps regulate body temperature.
8. Differentiate between pulse and blood pressure.
9. Explain the relationship between blood circulation and lymph circulation.
10. Tell how lymph serves the body.

SUGGESTED STUDY VOCABULARY*

apex	aortic valve	sphygmomanometer
pericardium	superior vena cava	homeostasis
epicardium	inferior vena cava	hemostasis
myocardium	pulmonary artery	agglutination
endocardium	pulmonary vein	fibrin
right atrium	arteries	cross-matching
left atrium	arterioles	lymph nodes
right ventricle	capillaries	red corpuscles
left ventricle	venules	white corpuscles
septum	veins	platelets
tricuspid valve	blood pressure	plasma
pulmonary valve	systole	lymph
mitral valve	diastole	tachycardia
		bradycardia
		arrhythmia

*Look for any terms you already know.

INTRODUCTION

This chapter includes basic information about the structure and the function of the circulatory system; it discusses the organs of circulation, defines the chief functions of the system, and attempts to point out relationships between this and other systems to reinforce the "body as a whole" concept.

The organs of the circulatory system are heart, blood, blood vessels, lymphatic vessels, and nodes.

The general functions of the system are:

1. *Transportation*—moving substances to and from body cells.

2. *Protection*—defending the body against attack by invading bacteria.

3. *Assistance*—helping to regulate body heat.

HEART

Close your hand into a fist. What you see is a shape and size somewhat like that of the heart. The human heart is a hollow, pulsating, four-chambered muscle located between the lungs, just above the diaphragm, and slightly left of the mid-line of the chest. The lower border, called the *apex*, is slightly tapered and blunt. The upper border is called the *base*; normally it lies below the second rib. The heart is a pumping station—a rhythmically pulsating muscle that keeps body fluids mixed by constantly forcing blood through the vast system of blood vessels.

Heart Coverings

Pericardium. This loose-fitting sac or jacket around the heart is a tough, fibrous covering with a smooth, moist lining.

Epicardium. This is the outside surface of the heart itself; it is a smooth, moist, and strong tissue the same as the lining of the pericardium.

Pericardial space and fluid. The slight space between the two moist surfaces described above is called the *pericardial space*. These two surfaces are moistened by a few drops of fluid, *pericardial fluid*, which lubricate and prevent friction as one surface might rub against the other. When this fluid is absent or there is more than normal the heart is in difficulty.

Heart Muscle

Myocardium is the name of the heart muscle; it is also called the cardiac muscle or the heart wall. It has an outside layer or covering (*epicardium*) and an inside lining called the *endocardium*.

The heart wall (myocardium) is made up of three interconnected types of cardiac muscle. Two types contract much like skeletal muscles, but the third type of fiber is unique; it excites or arouses the energy for the heart beat *and* transmits that charge or impulse throughout the heart itself. In a sense this special fiber system threads itself into the rest of the myocardium and prompts it to pulsate in a rhythmical manner.

Heart Chambers and Valves

There are four chambers in the heart. In Figure 10–1 locate these four chambers: *right atrium, right ventricle, left atrium, left ventricle.* The lower chambers have thicker walls than the upper chambers. As shown, the left ventricle has a thicker wall than the right one because it pushes the blood out to all parts of the body (except the lungs).

There is a wall (*septum*) down the middle of the heart that divides it into a right side and a left side. Each side has an upper and a lower chamber. Two valves serve as trapdoor gateways that permit blood to flow from the upper chamber to the lower chamber on each side. Then there are two more valves that let the blood move out of the lower chambers and continue on its way.

Locate these four valves in Figure 10–1:

right side	*left side*
tricuspid	mitral (bicuspid)
pulmonary	aortic

In the normal heart there is no way for the blood to back up; it must move on with each heart beat because the valves open only in one direction. Strong, cordlike tissues attached to the valves and anchored to the heart itself give strength and support to the valves to perform properly.

The septum or middle wall prevents blood from moving back and forth from one side to the other. You will see a specific reason for this as you trace the blood through the heart.

The Heart at Work and at Rest

As mentioned previously, the heart is a rhythmical pumping station for movement of blood to every cell in the body. The normal pumping rate of the adult heart ranges from the middle 60's to low 80's (strokes per minute). At that rate (and depending upon the size of the individual), a healthy heart pumps between five and 10 tons of blood every 24 hours. This represents a lot of work but the heart gets its rest between beats or contractions. Anything that causes the heart to beat faster (exercise, emotional strain, etc.) means that its rest periods are shortened.

The heart beats in a rhythmical way. While it might seem that all parts of the heart contract at the same time, this is not quite true. The contraction itself has its beginning in

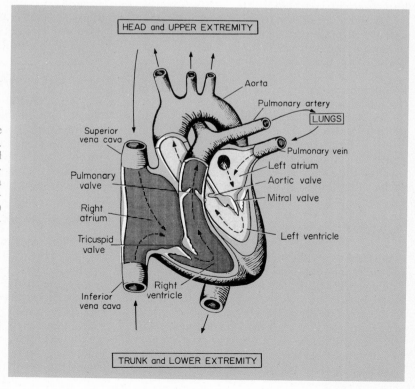

FIGURE 10-1 Details of the functional parts of the heart. (Shaded area indicates blood laden with carbon dioxide enroute to the lungs; lighter area indicates blood laden with oxygen coming from the lungs.) (Guyton: Function of the Human Body, 4th ed.)

a small mass of specialized tissue called the S-A node (sino-atrial) in the upper region of the right atrium. It begins when the S-A node gives out an impulse or signal that starts the wave of contraction. This wave spreads throughout the walls of the atria and the message travels down to the ventricles by the most direct route over a bundle of special cardiac fibers called *the bundle of His*. Then the ventricles contract.

The S-A node is called the *pacemaker* of the heart; it sends out the impulses in a certain rhythm. The atria and ventricles contract in the same well-timed rhythm to keep in step with the pacemaker. Between impulses the heart muscle relaxes and rests. Under normal conditions it rests about twice as much as it works.

A complete heart beat includes the contraction and relaxation of both atria, followed quickly by the contraction and relaxation of both ventricles. This is called a *cardiac cycle*.

Using Figure 10–1, follow the route that blood takes through the heart in this manner:

1. Locate the *superior vena cava* and the *inferior vena cava*. Blood (laden with carbon dioxide) enters the right atrium through these two veins.

2. It passes through the *tricuspid valve* into the right ventricle.

3. The blood is forced by contraction upward through the *pulmonary valve* into the *pulmonary artery* to both lungs, where the carbon dioxide is exchanged for oxygen.

4. From the lungs the (oxygen-laden) blood returns through the *pulmonary vein* to the left atrium.

5. It passes through the *mitral valve* into the left ventricle.

6. The strong muscular wall of the left ventricle contracts and forces the blood through the *aortic valve* into the aorta when it is then distributed to all parts of the body.

BLOOD VESSELS

In the body there is a "distribution route" for the blood and there is a "collection route." Each route has its own blood vessels. The "distribution route" carries blood with oxygen to all parts of the body through *arteries* into *arterioles* and then into the smallest vessels of all, the capillaries. Here there is an exchange of substances between the tiny vessels and the tissue cells. The "collection route" starts in

the capillaries: the blood, picking up carbon dioxide and other impurities, starts back toward the heart, going from the capillaries to the venules into the veins and to the right side of the heart. From there it is pumped to the lungs only to return and start the distribution route again. Other impurities are removed from the blood by the kidneys and the liver.

Figure 10–2 shows the main arteries of the body; Figure 10–3 shows the main veins. Notice that both arteries and veins are in the same general area of the body. Most large vessels are deep within the tissue for their protection.

In general, blood vessels are divided into groups according to their size, function, and characteristics. See Table 10–1.

BLOOD CIRCULATION

Blood circulates to all parts of the body. Figure 10–4 shows where the total blood volume is located in the various parts of the circulatory system.

Special names are given to blood circulation related to several parts of the body such as *systemic* circulation, *coronary* circulation, *pulmonary* circulation, *hepatic portal* circulation, *cerebral* (brain) circulation, *renal* circulation, and circulation in the body before birth called *fetal* circulation.

Systemic Circulation

This term refers to the heart pumping blood through the arteries, arterioles, and capillaries, into the venules and veins and back to the heart—and thus serving the body as a whole. Sometimes this is called the "greater circulatory system." Figure 10–5 shows this system in relation to some main body organs.

Coronary (Heart) Circulation

The heart needs and has its own blood supply (Fig. 10–6). The coronary arteries (right and left) branch off from the aorta just above the aortic valve. The left branch furnishes blood mainly to the left ventricle and the right branch furnishes blood mainly to the right ventricle. The demands made on the heart (exercise, emotional stress, sleep, etc.) influence the heart's need for oxygen; thus at times the coronary arteries bring more blood

(*Text continued on page 103.*)

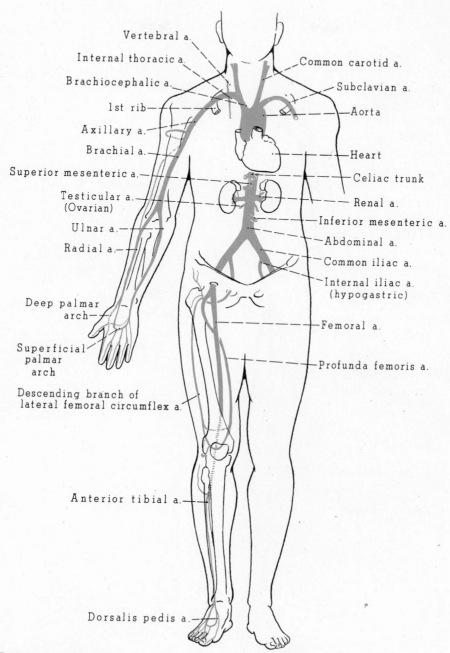

FIGURE 10-2 Major arteries of the body. (Jacob and Francone: Structure and Function in Man.)

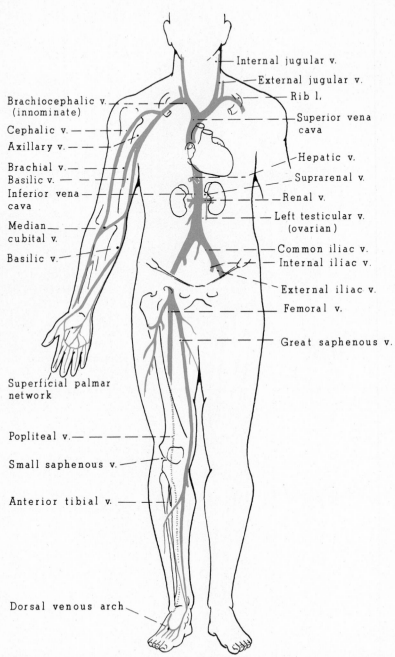

Internal jugular v.

External jugular v.

Rib 1.

Superior vena cava

Brachiocephalic v. (innominate)

Cephalic v.

Axillary v.

Hepatic v.

Brachial v.

Suprarenal v.

Basilic v.

Inferior vena cava

Renal v.

Left testicular v. (ovarian)

Median cubital v.

Common iliac v.

Internal iliac v.

Basilic v.

External iliac v.

Femoral v.

Great saphenous v.

Superficial palmar network

Popliteal v.

Small saphenous v.

Anterior tibial v.

Dorsal venous arch

FIGURE 10-3   Main veins of the body. (Jacob and Francone: Structure and Function in Man.)

TABLE 10.1. BLOOD VESSELS—TYPE, SIZE, AND WORK PERFORMED

NAME OF GROUP	SIZE	FUNCTION	CHARACTERISTICS
1. Arteries *Examples:* aorta, brachiocephalic, subclavian, common carotid, common iliac, femoral, brachial, radial.	Large and Medium (largest is aorta, about one inch in diameter)	Passageways for carrying blood from heart to body tissues (exception is the pulmonary artery leading to the lungs).	Tough, elastic vessels with smooth linings; medium size vessels have more smooth muscle tissue than larger ones which are more elastic.
2. Arterioles	Smaller branches of arteries connecting with the vast network of capillaries.	Serve as the branches (connecting links) between arteries and the capillaries carrying nourishment and oxygen.	Thin, muscular (small) vessels with smooth linings.
3. Capillaries	Smallest blood vessels forming a network among tissue cells.	The link between the arterioles and the venules which bring "on the spot" nourishment and oxygen to cells and collect wastes from them.	Smooth (one cell thickness) walls with a diameter so small blood cells barely move along; tiny pores (far apart) serve as minature passageways taking nourishment to cells and removing wastes from them.
4. Venules	Smaller branches of veins connecting with the vast network of capillaries.	Serve as branches connecting links between the capillaries and the veins carrying wastes away from cells.	Small, thin vessels with little muscle tissue.
5. Veins *Examples:* superior vena cava, brachiocephalic, internal jugular, inferior vena cava, common iliac, femoral, brachial.	Large and medium.	Passageways for blood to return to the heart; have some ability to enlarge and constrict and thus regulate blood flow, making it available as body demands it.	Thinner than arteries with much less elasticity and muscle tissue; inner lining has cuplike valves to prevent blood from flowing backward.

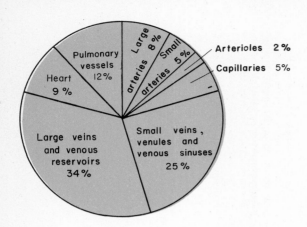

FIGURE 10-4 Percentage of the total blood volume in each portion of the circulatory system. (Guyton: Textbook of Medical Physiology, 4th ed.)

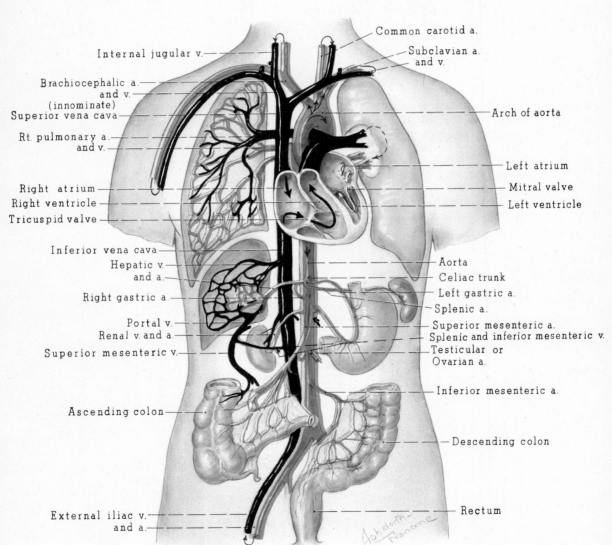

FIGURE 10-5   Arterial supply and venous drainage of organs. (Jacob and Francone: Structure and Function in Man.)

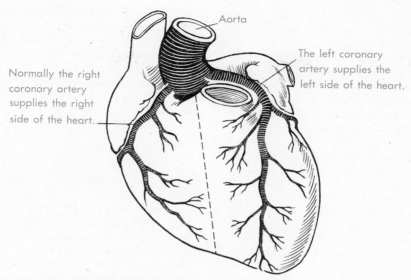

FIGURE 10-6 Coronary circulation (Miller and Burt: Good Health: Personal and Community, 2nd ed.)

to the heart muscle and at other times less blood. As the coronary arteries enter the heart wall, they become smaller and finally nourish the tissues through capillaries. In turn the venules and coronary veins carry the blood back to the right atrium of the heart (see Fig. 10–1) where it joins systemic blood on its way to the lungs.

Pulmonary Circulation

This is the name given to the flow of blood from the heart to the lungs and back to the heart. Study Figure 9–4 and trace this circular route. The purpose of this "circle" is to remove the carbon dioxide from the blood and replace it with a fresh oxygen supply. The exchange of these gases in the lungs takes place in the capillaries surrounding the small air sacs in the lung tissue (see Fig. 9–3).

Hepatic Portal Circulation

Figure 10–7 shows the extent of blood circulation in this subsystem. The stomach and the intestines require large supplies of ar-

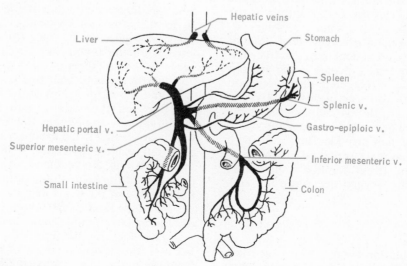

FIGURE 10-7 The major vessels of the hepatic portal circulation. (Manner: Elements of Anatomy and Physiology.)

terial blood to carry on their functions. Blood coming from these organs carries bacteria and some food nutrients, especially sugar.

The spleen serves as a blood reservoir; in particular it stores (and releases) red blood cells, plasma cells and lymphocytes. Like the liver, the spleen helps cleanse the blood.

The veins leading to the liver from these organs form the portal circulation system. The liver filters out the bacteria before the blood goes on; this serves as a built-in safety feature to prevent body infections. The liver likewise removes from the blood much of the sugar (glucose), amino acids, and some fat which were absorbed from the intestines. In due time (several hours later) the liver releases these food substances (somewhat changed) back into the systemic circulation to be used by the body.

The liver gets its blood supply through the hepatic artery. Once this blood has served the needs of the liver cells, it joins the portal supply and moves on. The liver is an organ that expands and contracts readily; thus it can handle large quantities of blood which come to it from these two sources.

The liver is essential to digestion and metabolism. (See Chapters 11 and 12.)

Cerebral (Brain) Circulation

The brain gets its blood supply through the two carotid arteries and the two vertebral arteries. They ultimately join together to form the *circle of Willis* which provides a generous blood supply to the brain. In the average adult about 15 per cent of the blood output of the heart is needed by the brain under resting conditions. Interestingly enough, this amount does not change a great deal during active conditions unless there is a change in the amount of carbon dioxide or oxygen in the blood. Too much carbon dioxide or too little oxygen causes dilation of the vessels and permits more blood to be present. This is an automatic safety feature which provides the brain with the necessary amount of blood to meet its metabolic needs. Brain damage soon occurs when brain tissue oxygen needs are not adequately met.

Renal Circulation

Renal circulation means the blood route in the kidney. The kidney is a filtering organ for the blood and this function relates to urine production which is described in Chapter 13, The Reproductive and Urinary Systems. For the present it will help to locate the *renal vein* and *renal artery* in Figure 10–5 to show you how directly they connect with the largest body blood vessels (inferior vena cava and the aorta).

Fetal Circulation

Fetal circulation is the name given to circulation in the body before birth (fetus). This circulation serves the fetus in a different way from that of the body circulation after birth. The lungs and the digestive system of the fetus do not function. Before birth the body receives oxygen through the fetal blood supply; it also receives nourishment that way. The oxygen and food are secured from the mother's blood supply. Fetal circulation is the special route blood takes to perform these two functions. In Figure 10–8, find the *umbilicus* (two umbilical arteries and one umbilical vein); follow the two umbilical arteries leading into the *placenta*. Next, locate the umbilical vein as it leaves the placenta. The placenta is a cakelike organ within the uterus which serves as a "service center" between the mother and the fetus. It puts oxygen and food into fetal blood and removes waste from it. The mother's blood and the blood of the fetus do not mix. The exchange of food, oxygen, and waste products takes place in the tiny capillaries within the placenta.

As stated, the lungs in the fetus do not function, therefore the blood does not need to go to the lungs for oxygen as it does after birth. In Figure 10–8, trace the blood in the fetus from the umbilical vein to the ductus venosus going through the liver and on through the hepatic vein to the inferior vena cava and the right atrium of the heart.

Between the right atrium and the left atrium there is an opening, the foramen ovale, which closes at birth. This opening serves as a short-cut to allow fetal blood to leave the heart without taking the regular route through the right side of the heart to the lungs and back to the left side of the heart as it does after birth.

Another fetal heart structure that is not used after birth is the *ductus arteriosus*.

The liver in the fetus is a large organ because it receives a quantity of blood directly from the placenta and from the intestine.

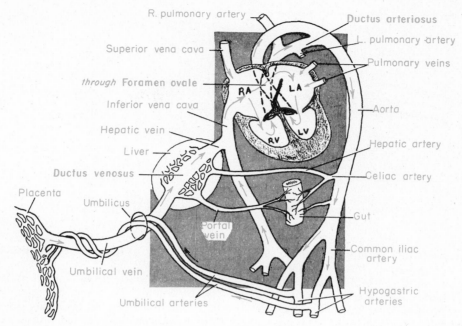

FIGURE 10-8   Fetal circulation. (Brooks: Integrated Basic Science, The C. V. Mosby Co.)

BLOOD PRESSURE

Factors Influencing Blood Pressure

By this time you are aware that the circulatory system represents a circuit—a continuous pathway where blood is on a constant journey throughout the body, sometimes moving rapidly, sometimes barely able to squeeze through tiny capillaries, sometimes moving slowly "uphill" through the veins back to the heart, and at times pooled (i.e., liver) until further notice from the body. Knowing these facts helps one understand something of the meaning of blood pressure.

As blood moves along, it presses or pushes against the walls of the vessels carrying it. This pressing action is called pressure—*blood pressure*. Some of the factors that influence blood pressure include (1) strength of heart beat, (2) elasticity of the artery wall, (3) resistance of the capillaries, (4) amount of blood present, and (5) age.

Measurement of Blood Pressure

Blood pressure has high and low points (systole—high, diastole—low). This "up" and "down" pressure corresponds to the pumping action of the heart. When the ventricles contract, it is called *systole*. When they relax, it is called *diastole*.

An instrument used to measure arterial blood pressure is called the *sphygmomanometer*. Pressure readings are recorded with two numbers, i.e., 120/80. The 120 is the systolic pressure reading; the 80 is the diastolic pressure reading. There is a difference in the blood sounds heard with the stethoscope as the sphygmomanometer is used. The systolic sound is a sharp, clear thumping sound, while the diastolic sound is faint and dull. Normal blood pressure readings vary with age (Fig. 10–9).

Pulse

The impulse felt with the expansion of an artery as the heart beats is called the *pulse*. Figure 10–10 shows several sites where it is possible to feel the pulse. One of the most common sites is the radial artery at the wrist.

Characteristics of the pulse include:

1. *Rate*—the number of beats per minute. The normal range is from middle 60's to lower 80's but some people have a normal rate in the 50's and others in the 90's. Rate can vary

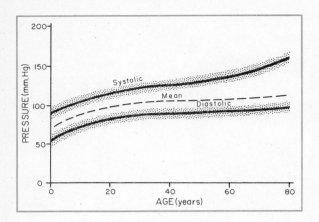

FIGURE 10-9 Changes in systolic, diastolic, and mean arterial pressure with age. The shaded areas show the normal range. (Guyton: Textbook of Medical Physiology, 4th ed.)

with: 1. Sex—slightly higher for women than for men. 2. Age—from birth to adulthood there is a gradual decrease until a person is elderly. 3. Others—size of a person, activity, body metabolism, worry, fear and pain.

Tachycardia is a term used to indicate a rapid pulse (usually over 100). Bradycardia is a term used to indicate a slow pulse (usually below 50).

2. *Rhythm*—equal time intervals between beats.

When the time intervals are not equal and beats occur at irregular intervals this is known as *arrhythmia*.

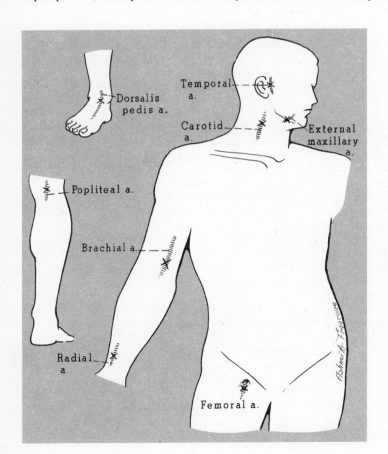

FIGURE 10-10 The pulse is readily distinguished at any of the above pressure points. (Jacob and Francone: Structure and Function in Man.)

3. *Tension*—the amount of fingertip pressure exerted to measure the strength of the pulse (can only be estimated). This pressure is related to "volume" of the pulse. If it takes considerable fingertip pressure to completely block the pulse beat, it is called a *bounding* pulse. On the other hand, if it takes light pressure to block the pulse beat, it is called *weak, thready* or *feeble.*

BLOOD

Composition of Blood

Blood is considered a tissue and it makes up about one-thirteenth (8%) of the body weight. The amount (volume) of blood in the body is influenced by sex, age, weight, and general condition of the circulatory system (adult range is about six to eight quarts, with extra body weight requiring extra blood).

Blood appears to be a simple, unmixed, liquid. This is not the case. Whole blood is a *mixture* of formed elements and plasma. Blood transports oxygen, food nutrients, water, chemical substances called hormones, and waste products, and also helps to regulate body temperature; therefore it must have parts or means for carrying out these functions. The body has an automatic means to maintain a constant, normal state of the blood (i.e., proper water, sugar, salt, protein, fat, oxygen, and calcium content; correct acid-base balance; constant temperature; proper quantities of hormones, vitamins, and other minerals). This is known as *homeostasis.*

Study Figure 10–11 to see how involved blood is. Beginning with the arrow "Blood 8 per cent," study each column, moving across the illustration from left to right. A careful look will point out how involved and intermixed blood really is. In particular notice the following:

1. *Whole blood* consists of formed elements (45 per cent) and plasma (55 per cent).

2. *Formed elements* consist of leukocytes (white cells), erythrocytes (red cells), and platelets.

3. *Plasma weight* consists of water (91.5 per cent), proteins (7 per cent), and other substances (inorganic salts, fats, enzymes, vitamins, etc.) 1.5 per cent.

The formed elements listed above and plasma deserve some basic explanation. See Table 10–2.

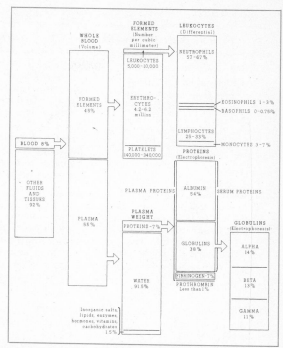

FIGURE 10-11 Composition of the blood. (Jacob and Francone: Structure and Function in Man.)

Hemostasis and Blood Clotting

Hemostasis means checking the flow of blood through any part or vessel. Means by which the body can arrest escaping blood are (1) platelet agglutination, (2) contraction of blood vessels, and (3) formation of a blood clot.

Clotting of blood is a safety feature when it prevents blood loss by sealing off or plugging an unwanted opening in a vessel. The actual details of blood coagulation and clot formation are an involved process. In general, it can be said that the platelets agglutinate or clump together (somewhat as if glued) and begin to cling to the edges of the wound. During this clumping process the platelets rupture, releasing a substance (thromboplastin) which works cooperatively with some plasma proteins to form a network of tightly woven fibers. This mass of threadlike fibers (fibrin) traps and holds blood cells, uniting them to form the clot. Platelets and plasma proteins need the help of vitamin K and calcium (among other things) to form the clot; no clot can be produced without them. Figure 10–12 shows the stages of clot development.

TABLE 10.2.   FORMED ELEMENTS AND PLASMA

FORMED ELEMENTS*	SOURCE	FUNCTION
1. Red cells (erythrocytes) (Coloring matter called *hemoglobin* comes from iron in the diet) Normal "red count" is 4.2 to 6.2 million per cubic millimeter (a million in 2 or 3 drops)	Red bone marrow (In adults less red bone marrow manufactures red cells; elderly people have the least bone marrow forming red cells) A red cell wears itself out in 3 or 4 months Red bone marrow keeps number in blood about the same at all times	Transport oxygen and carbon dioxide Oxygen-filled red cells give blood a bright red color; carbon dioxide-filled red cells give blood a dark red-brown color
2. White cells (leukocytes) Normal "white count" is 5000-10,000 per cubic millimeter of blood (during body infection this number increases)	Some types (there are several) come from red bone marrow; others from lymph nodes and spleen A white cell does not live as long as a red cell; some last a few hours, others a few days	Protect the body against microorganisms; produce antibodies White cells are able to squeeze through blood vessel wall to reach microorganisms; they kill and digest these tissue invaders; some body disorders increase the number; others decrease it
3. Platelets Average count is 140,000-340,000 per cubic millimeter of blood	Red bone marrow A platelet lives only a few days	Help blood to clot
4. Plasma* (55% of whole blood) Liquid part of the blood, chiefly water; straw colored when blood cells are absent A small part (7%) is proteins and 1.5% other substances; see Figure 10-11		Transports blood cells, mineral salts, food nutrients, hormones, antibodies, and cell wastes

* In the normal body the percentages of formed elements and plasma remain constant. When blood is lost through a wound, tissue fluid goes into the blood stream to make up the loss, if possible. Severe blood loss causes thirst.

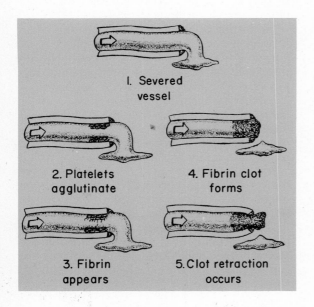

1. Severed vessel

2. Platelets agglutinate

3. Fibrin appears

4. Fibrin clot forms

5. Clot retraction occurs

FIGURE 10-12 Stages of clot development and clot retraction following injury to a blood vessel. (Redrawn from Seegers and Sharp: Hemostatic Agents. Charles C Thomas.)

TABLE 10.3.   BLOOD TYPES FOR TRANSFUSIONS

BLOOD TYPE	RECEIVE BLOOD FROM	GIVE BLOOD TO
A	A and O	A and AB
B	B and O	B and AB
AB (universal recipient)	All	AB
O (universal donor)	O	All

Simple tests are done to check clotting time; the most common is pricking the finger or ear lobe and counting the time it takes for a clot to form. Normal clotting time is three to five minutes.

Blood Types and Cross-matching

Blood from one person may be fatal to another person when transfused into his circulating blood because the blood from the two individuals may not be compatible; the two bloods may be unable to mix without clumping (agglutination) and without breaking up red cells and releasing hemoglobin (hemolysis) into the blood. The clumping can plug blood vessels. To prevent this from happening and thus ensure the safety of the person receiving the blood (the recipient), the blood of the recipient must be cross-matched with the blood of the person (donor) giving the blood. It must be determined that the two blood samples *are* compatible. Cross-matching of blood is a laboratory process.

Blood is grouped into four main types: A, B, AB, and O. Each type has its own properties. Thus each type of blood has its own uses and limitations as far as transfusions are concerned. Table 10–3 shows the uses of blood types for transfusions.

Rh Factor

There is another blood quality that needs to be determined — the Rh factor. This factor, a substance in the red blood cells, is not present in all people (85 per cent have it, 15 per cent do not). When this substance is present in the red cells, a person is said to be Rh positive; when it is absent, he is said to be Rh negative. A transfusion of Rh positive blood into Rh negative blood can cause a severe reaction (mass clumping of cells). Special care is taken when children are born to an Rh positive father and an Rh negative mother. Tests made ahead of time determine the Rh factor in case the infant needs a transfusion. (Study Fig. 10–13.) (See Rho Gam.)

LYMPHATIC SYSTEM AND ACCESSORY ORGANS

The lymphatic system is a vast network of vessels spread throughout the body (Fig. 10–14) transporting lymph without a central

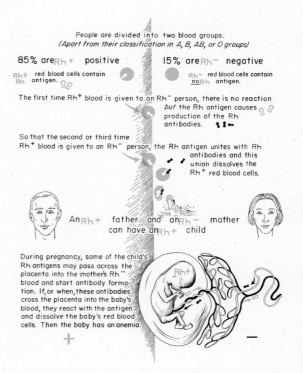

FIGURE 10-13 The Rh factor. (Dowling and Jones: That the Patient May Know.)

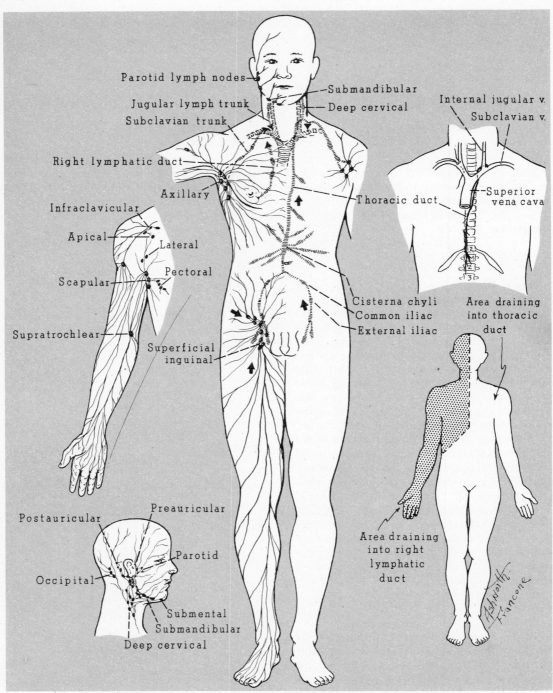

FIGURE 10-14   Plate of the lymphatic system and drainage. (Jacob and Francone: Structure and Function in Man.)

TABLE 10.4.   THE LYMPHATIC SYSTEM AND ACCESSORY ORGANS

PARTS AND FUNCTIONS	*GENERAL INFORMATION*
Functions of the System	1. Serves as a route for returning stray nutrients (especially proteins) to the blood stream that may have escaped through the blood capillaries into tissue spaces. 2. Filters out unwanted substances caused by inflammation and cancer; corners or traps such substances for disposal. 3. Aids the body in combating illness and producing immunity. 4. Aids in absorption of food during digestion.
Descriptions	A tissue fluid, generally clear in color. Contains white cells (lymphocytes) in particular. Milky color when laden with fat (chyle) after a meal. Lymph is a waterlike environment serving as a go-between substance among cells (bathes cells and removes wastes).
Types of Vessels	*Lymphatic Capillaries.* The smallest, thinwalled (single layer of cells) vessel. Dead-end tubes (with valves) reaching into all tissue spaces to carry lymph back to bigger vessels; they are in the villi (intestines) absorbing fat. Lymphatic Vessels. Threelayered vessels (varying in size much like veins) with valves to prevent "back flow" of lymph as it moves along. Note the following in Figure 10-14: 1. The extent and range of the *right lymphatic* duct drainage area. 2. The location of the *thoracic duct* (and drainage area). 3. The directions of the arrows (———▶) to denote lymph flow. 4. The lymph supply to head, arm, leg.
Lymph Nodes (Glands)	Lymph nodes are bean-shaped bodies congregated in rather widely separated areas as seen in Figure 10-14. These congregations or groups of nodes are filtering stations for lymph-removing bacteria (not viruses); they produce lymphocytes and aid the body in establishing immunity. The bacteria screened out of the lymph are sent on their way and not left to accumulate in the node(s).
Lymph Movement	With no central pump, lymph is pushed through the vessels by: 1. Increase in volume. New lymph pushes old lymph along. 2. Contraction of muscles next to vessels (squeeze, massage) and vessel walls. 3. Peristalsis of intestines. 4. Smooth muscle fibers in vessel walls rhythmically contracting. 5. Respiration which produces pressure on the thoracic duct. The rate of flow is influenced by such factors as (1) fever, (2) lack of oxygen, (3) an obstruction in a vein, and (4) exercise.
Accessory Organs *Spleen*—located on the left side of upper abdominal cavity.	Tissue structure similar to lymph node. **Functions**: 1. Filters blood to rid it of bacteria and worn out red blood cells. 2. A reservoir for blood and storehouse for red blood cells. 3. Produces lymphocytes and monocytes (white blood cells). 4. Produces red blood cells during fetal life.
Tonsils—lymphatic tissue at the entrance of the alimentary and respiratory tracts.	**Functions**: 1. Guard the entrance(s) to these tracts by "trapping" unwanted organisms and thus forming a barrier.
Thymus—(see endocrine system)	Seems to have some relation to antibody protection and immunity.

pump (such as the heart or pump for the circulatory system).

The lymphatic system is an assistant (accessory) to the blood system; it provides the means for interstitial fluids to get into the blood system. It aids in keeping a balance in the amount of interstitial fluid in the body.

Table 10–4 explains the parts and functions of this system.

SUMMARY

To know how the circulatory system serves the body will help you to understand some of the needs of patients with circulatory disorders.

Transportation, protection, and assistance in regulating body heat are three main functions of this system.

The pump is the heart; it has a saclike covering (pericardium), and the heart muscle itself is called the myocardium.

The four chambers in the heart are the right and left atria, and the right and left ventricles. The right side pumps used blood to the lungs where the carbon dioxide is replaced by oxygen. The left side receives the fresh blood with oxygen from the lungs and pumps it to all parts of the body.

Normal heart beat (pulse) ranges from middle sixties to the lower eighties per minute and the heart rests between beats. A complete heart beat is called a cardiac cycle.

The "distribution route" for the fresh blood supply is through the arteries and arterioles to the capillaries.

The "collection route" for used blood starts in the capillaries and goes on to the venules through the veins and to the right atrium of the heart.

Although the capillary is the smallest blood vessel, it serves as the bridge which takes oxygen and food substances to the cells and removes unwanted cell wastes.

The heart needs and has its own blood supply (coronary circulation). Pulmonary circulation is the flow of blood from the heart to the lungs and back to the heart. The hepatic portal circulation system is a special blood route from the intestines, stomach, and spleen to the liver. Cerebral circulation refers to the blood route through the brain. Systemic circulation is a general term referring to all of the main blood vessels in the body. Fetal circulation is circulation in the body before birth.

Blood pressure means the pressure that blood exerts on the walls of the blood vessels as the heart moves it along.

There are about six to eight quarts of blood in the body. A severe loss of blood creates thirst. Blood is a fluid made up of formed elements and plasma.

The lymphatic system aids the circulatory system in removing cell wastes and transporting food into the cell. The filtering system for lymph is the lymph node or gland.

GUIDES FOR STUDY AND DISCUSSION

1. The circulatory system has three main functions. What are they?
2. Turn to Figure 10–1 and trace the blood through the heart. Identify and learn the chambers and valves.

3. Why is it impossible for blood to back up in a normal heart?

4. The heart is a hard-working organ. List two facts which prove this.

5. What are the main differences between the "distribution route" and the "collection route" of the blood?

6. Fetal circulation serves the fetus differently from the way circulation serves the body after birth. Which main differences can you list?

7. Why does the heart have (need) a septum?

8. Name and locate the most common site to count the pulse.

9. Review Table 10–2. Be able to name the three types of blood cells, where they come from, and what they do for the body.

10. How does a blood clot form?

11. Why is it necessary to know a patient's blood type before he receives a transfusion?

12. How does lymph serve the body?

13. What is the "nickname" for the S-A node? How is it related to the bundle of His?

14. What means does the circulatory system have to help regulate body temperature?

SUGGESTED SITUATIONS AND ACTIVITIES

1. If elderly people have the least bone marrow forming red blood cells, what would this suggest to you about their "automatic" ability to make up a loss of red blood cells due to an accident?

2. Find out if there is a blood bank in your community. Visit it to determine the precautions and problems encountered in furnishing this community service.

3. Practice counting your pulse. Notice the amount of finger tension (pressure) it takes to "feel" the pulsation; notice the rhythm of the beat.

4. Complete this:

Characteristics of the Pulse	Facts to Remember
1. Rate	
2. Rhythm	
3. Tension	

CHAPTER 11

THE DIGESTIVE SYSTEM

TOPICAL HEADINGS

Introduction
Main and Accessory
  Organs
    Mouth
    Teeth
    Tongue
    Salivary Glands

Pharynx
Esophagus
Stomach
Small Intestine
Liver
Gallbladder
Pancreas

Large Intestine
Digestion
Summary
Guides for Study and
  Discussion
Suggested Situations
  and Activities

OBJECTIVES FOR THE STUDENT: Be able to:

1. Name the main organs in the digestive tract.
2. List the structures that provide accessory services to the digestive tract.
3. Trace food through the digestive tract.
4. Explain how food changes as it moves along the digestive tract.
5. Tell how and where digested food gets into the circulatory system.
6. Describe how digestion is related to proper eating habits and adequate nutrition.

SUGGESTED STUDY VOCABULARY*

esophagus
gallbladder
liver
pancreas
duodenum
jejunum
ileum
cecum
ascending colon
transverse colon
descending colon

rectum
anus
digestive process
peristalsis
incisors
canines
premolars
molars
crown of tooth
neck of tooth
root of tooth
caries

salivary glands
parotid gland
submaxillary gland
sublingual gland
enzyme
cardiac sphincter
pyloric sphincter
chyme
mesentery
sigmoid
feces
defecation

---

*Look for any terms you already know.

INTRODUCTION

No system of the body is more remarkable than the digestive system. The digestive organs have the ability to take the food we eat and prepare it for cell use. Cells require food, but they cannot use it in the form seen on the table. Food, as we know it, must be transformed into usable substance; to do this the digestive system softens, breaks up, liquefies, and chemically changes food so it can be absorbed in the circulatory system and carried to the tissues. En route, water and salts are removed as the roughage and unusable food parts are moved along and become solid wastes which are regularly eliminated from the body.

The digestive system is about 30 feet long. It is a muscular tube lined with mucous membrane which provides a smooth moist surface for easy movement of food.

Figure 11–1 shows these main parts: (1) mouth, (2) esophagus, (3) stomach, (4) duodenum, (5) jejunum, (6) ileum—nos. 4 to 6 comprise the small intestine, (7) ascending colon, (8) transverse colon, (9) descending colon, (10) sigmoid, (11) rectum—nos. 7 to 11 comprise the large intestine, and (12) anus.

In addition, the following organs (accessory or assisting) are considered a part of this system: (1) liver, (2) gallbladder, and (3) pancreas. Notice (in Fig. 11–1) that these three separate organs make their contribution through a common Y-shaped tube entering the duodenum.

Each part of the digestive tract is designed to carry out specific functions. To perform these functions automatic provisions are made for two important things—*time* and *movement*. The digestive process is automated, so to speak; it provides time enough for needed changes to take place, yet it keeps the food moving along at a rate necessary to supply body tissues and remove wastes. This fact (automatic regulation) points up a distinct "marriage" between the digestive system and the nervous system.

MAIN AND ACCESSORY ORGANS

Use Figure 11–1 to locate the main and accessory organs listed in the introduction so

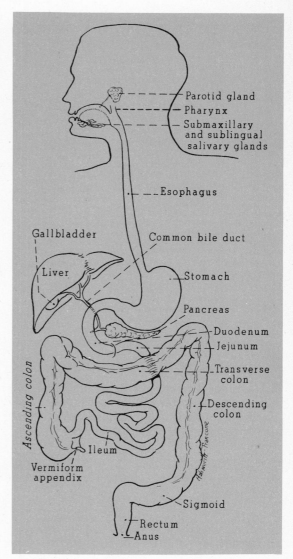

FIGURE 11-1 The digestive system and its associated structures. See Table 11-1 for digestive juices, their sources and action. (Jacob and Francone: Structure and Function in Man.)

that you become well-acquainted with the placement and arrangement of each part.

Mouth

The boundaries of the mouth include lips, cheeks, hard palate, soft palate, and pharynx. The mouth cavity contains structures (teeth, tongue, and glands) which start the process of food digestion. Here food is softened, chewed, and mixed as saliva (about 97 per cent water) sets to work to change starch to sugar. This

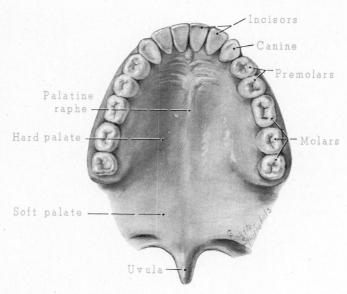

FIGURE 11–2   Roof of mouth with adult teeth. (Jacob and Francone: Structure and Function in Man.)

first chemical change is limited. Saliva does not change all starches to sugar; it merely starts the process and leaves the rest of starch digestion up to the small intestines.

Teeth
(accessory organs)

During a lifetime a person has two sets of natural teeth.

Name	Number	Comments
1. Deciduous	20	Begin to appear about six or seven months of age.
2. Permanent	32	As the deciduous teeth start to "drop out" during childhood, permanent teeth begin to replace them; this process may continue until a person is 20 or more years old.

A tooth is shaped according to the function it performs. Figure 11–2 shows *incisors* (thin edge cutters), *canines* (thin but more pointed), *premolars* (more square with irregular surfaces for chewing), and *molars* (large, grinding, chewing surfaces).

The 32 permanent teeth are equally divided between the two jaws—each has 16 teeth (see diagram below).

Study Figure 11–3 and locate the three main sections of the tooth: *crown* (portion seen above the gum), *root* (portion embedded in the jaw), and *neck* (portion connecting crown and root covered by the gum). This same figure shows blood vessels entering the root canal (for nourishment) as well as nerves.

While there is some controversy about fluoridation of drinking water in relation to health and tooth preservation, it is a rather widely accepted practice aimed at the prevention of tooth decay (caries).

Teeth in the upper jaw ⟶ 4 incisors ⟵ Teeth in the lower jaw
2 canines
4 premolars
6 molars

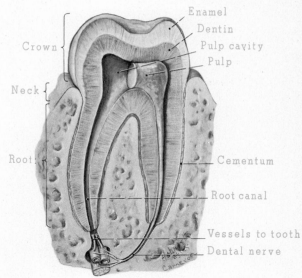

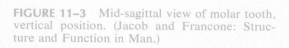

FIGURE 11–3 Mid-sagittal view of molar tooth, vertical position. (Jacob and Francone: Structure and Function in Man.)

Tongue
(accessory organ)

The tongue is a very flexible muscle on the floor of the mouth; it mixes, moves, and presses food against the teeth as saliva softens it for grinding and chewing. The tongue aids swallowing; when food is ready to move, the tongue pushes against the roof of the mouth and forces the food into the pharynx. In additon, it helps us speak and taste; taste buds are found in the nerve endings on the surface of the tongue.

Salivary Glands
(accessory organs)

These three pairs of glands empty their secretions (saliva) directly into the mouth. (See Fig. 11–1.) They are: *parotid,* located in front of and below each ear; *submaxillary,*

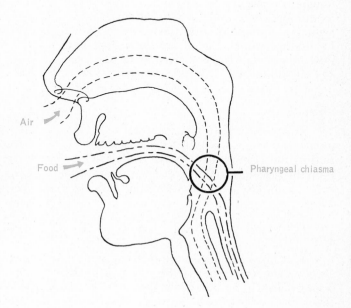

FIGURE 11–4. The air from the nose must cross the pathway of food in order to reach the larynx. (Manner: Elements of Anatomy and Physiology.)

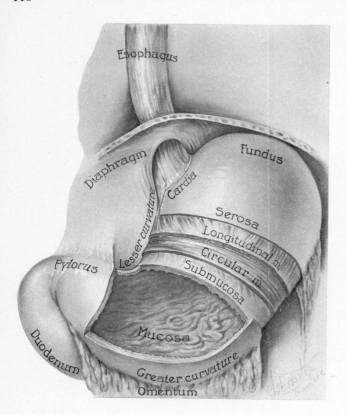

FIGURE 11–5   Anterior view of the stomach with portion of the anterior wall removed. (Note the various layers which make up the stomach wall.) (Jacob and Francone: Structure and Function in Man.)

located in back portion of mouth under the tongue; *sublingual,* located in front portion of mouth under the tongue. The presence, odor, sight, and thought of food causes these glands to produce saliva. Saliva moistens food and thus aids in chewing and swallowing. The enzyme ptyalin starts to change starch to sugar.

Pharynx

This connecting chamber between the mouth and the esophagus is discussed in relation to the respiratory system, and it serves both the digestive and the respiratory systems (Fig. 11–4). Notice that food and air pathways cross.

Esophagus

This muscular food tube is from 10 to 12 inches long and connects the pharynx to the upper (cardiac) opening into the stomach. It lies in back of the trachea and pierces the diaphragm before it joins the stomach. Swallow-

ing moves food or liquid past the pharynx into the esophagus. From here the food (aided by the moist mucous membrane lining) slips easily and quickly downward into the stomach.

Stomach

The stomach, a pouchlike enlargement of the alimentary canal, is located to the left of and just below the diaphragm. (See Fig. 11–5.) It varies in size; after a meal it is enlarged and remains that way while the food is being mixed and digested. Overeating further enlarges the stomach, and it interferes with the downward movement of the diaphragm. This can cause dyspnea (difficult breathing). An empty stomach has a wrinkled lining that stretches as food accumulates there.

The upper opening of the stomach is guarded by the *cardiac sphincter,* the lower opening by the *pyloric sphincter.* (These two muscles control the entrance and exit to the stomach.) Vomiting results when the pyloric sphincter refuses to open properly. The upper portion of the stomach is the *cardiac region;* the lower portion is the *pyloric region.* Note the area called the *fundus.* The portion marked "greater and lesser curvature" is the *body* of the stomach.

Strong muscles in the wall of the stomach are arranged in layers running in different directions, some lengthwise, others across and around. These muscles squeeze and force the food downward. The pyloric sphincter guards the lower opening, holding food back until it is properly mixed before it is released into the small intestine. The squeezing, wavelike motions of the stomach walls are called *peristaltic* waves. This movement continues until the food is thoroughly mixed with gastric juices and is in a semi-liquid form called *chyme.* Certain portions of the stomach lining secrete the gastric juices. (Study Table 11–1 for action on food.)

When food is thoroughly mixed and the gastric juices have done their work, the chyme is released by spurts through the pyloric sphincter into the duodenum of the small intestine. About four hours after a meal has been eaten, the stomach is empty and again reduced in size.

Small Intestine

Study Figure 11–6 to get an idea of the tissue structure of the small intestine. It is a tube about one inch in diameter and 20 feet long. Like other parts of the digestive system, the small intestine consists of several layers of tissue, each with its own function to perform. Notice Part C (Fig. 11–6). The inner lining or layer contains circular folds, and its surface is covered with villi. Part E (Fig. 11–6) shows the inner structure of a villus and the underlying layers of tissue. Food (chyme) is absorbed into the circulating blood through the villi. The mucous membrane layer secretes digestive juices. Lymph is present too. The muscle layers (circular and longitudinal) account for ringlike contractions and wavelike movements

TABLE 11-1. CHEMICAL DIGESTION OF CARBOHYDRATES, PROTEINS, AND FATS

SOURCE	JUICE	ACTION
Mouth Salivary glands	Saliva	Changes some starch to sugar (maltose), "Digestion begins." *Enzyme* – Ptyalin
Esophagus	None	None
Stomach Glands in lining of the stomach	Gastric	*Enzymes* Rennin – changes milk proteins to curds. Pepsin and hydrochloric acid — partially digests proteins. Lipase – changes fats to fatty acids and glycerol.*
Liver (gallbladder into duodenum)	Bile	Changes large fat droplets to small droplets.
Pancreas (into duodenum)	Pancreatic	*Enzymes* Trypsin – changes some proteins to amino acids.* Steapsin – changes small fat droplets to fatty acids and glycerol.* Amylopsin – changes starch to sugar (maltose).
Small Intestines Glands in lining of small intestines	Intestinal	*Enzymes* Erepsin – changes partially digested proteins to amino acids.* Sucrase – changes cane sugar (sucrose) to simple sugars.* Lactase – changes milk sugar (lactose) to simple sugars.* Maltase – changes malt sugar (maltose) to glucose.*
Large Intestines	None	Water and salts absorbed. Wastes stored or evacuated.

* Ready for absorption.

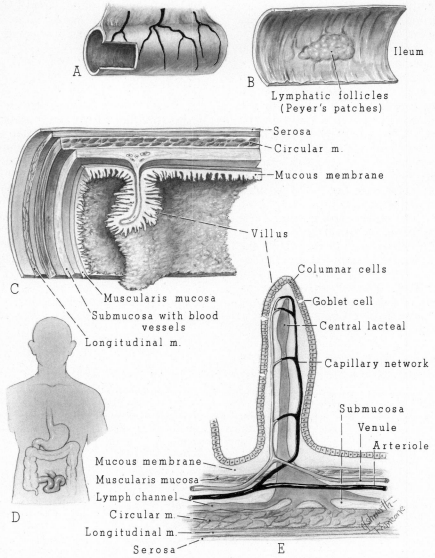

FIGURE 11–6   A, Segment of small intestine. B, Interior view of intestines with Peyer's patch. C, Layers composing intestinal wall. D, Anatomic position showing stomach and large and small intestines. E, Midsagittal section through villus. (Jacob and Francone: Structure and Function in Man.)

which squeeze and propel the chyme along at varying rates in different portions of the tube. The outer layer is attached to the posterior abdominal wall by a large fan-shaped membrane (mesentery).

In Figure 11–1, locate the following: *duodenum, jejunum,* and *ileum.* The *duodenum* is about 10 inches long. The common bile duct empties into it (Fig. 11–7). The *jejunum* is about seven feet in length. The lower portion, the *ileum* (about 14 feet long) opens into the large intestine; at this opening, there is a valve (ileocecal) to prevent substance from returning to the small intestine once it has moved on.

As stated previously, the chyme is moved along by wavelike or *peristaltic* movements, and continues to be mixed, digested, and made ready for absorption through the villi. Material that cannot be digested and passed into the blood and lymph vessels for cell use moves on through the ileocecal valve into the large intestine. Keep in mind the "automated" control of food movement. The nervous system guards the rate of movement to permit necessary chemical changes to take place.

The *liver, gallbladder,* and *pancreas* are essential accessory organs of the digestive tract. (See Figs. 11–1 and 11–7.) Locate the ducts from the gallbladder and pancreas leading into the duodenum.

Liver

This is the largest gland in the body (weighing three to four pounds) and is located in the upper right area of the abdominal cavity just below the diaphragm. The liver, a dark red gland, has a right lobe and a left lobe; each is divided into smaller compartments (lobules) by numerous small blood vessels and fibrous strands of tissue. Each such lobule has a rich blood supply (branches of hepatic artery and hepatic vein); it also has a duct for collecting *bile*. The tiny bile ducts join together in each lobe and emerge from the undersurface of the liver to form the *hepatic duct* (Fig. 11–7).

The liver has such important functions as:

1. Making bile, a yellowish green secretion. (Bile salts aid digestion.)

2. Producing plasma proteins and antibodies.

3. Destroying old red blood cells, bacteria and other debris in the blood.

4. Producing body heat from sugars and fats.

5. Changing proteins to sugars and fat for body use.

6. Storing food nutrients: sugar, amino acids (long enough to change them so that they can be used to produce energy), fats, vitamins, and minerals (especially iron).

7. Storing blood to release as needed (i.e., hemorrhage).

Gallbladder

Notice in Figure 11–7 that the gallbladder (pear-shaped pouch) is located just under the liver. It stores the bile until needed to aid the digestive process. Bile produced in the liver flows through the hepatic duct and cystic duct into the gallbladder. When needed, the bile travels through the common bile duct into the duodenum where bile salts aid digestion.

Pancreas

The pancreas is a slender fish-shaped organ lying behind the stomach. The head of the pancreas is close to the duodenum. The pancreatic duct (Fig. 11–7) runs the full length of the organ and joins the common bile duct to empty into the duodenum.

Three substances are produced in the pancreas. *Pancreatic juice* is secreted, collected in the tiny ducts, and emptied into the large pancreatic duct. Special cell clusters

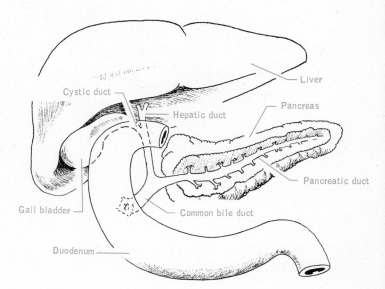

FIGURE 11–7 Accessory organs. The liver, pancreas, and gallbladder are connected to the digestive tract by the ducts shown here. (Manner: Elements of Anatomy and Physiology.)

Cystic duct

Hepatic duct

Liver

Pancreas

Pancreatic duct

Gall bladder

Common bile duct

Duodenum

scattered throughout the pancreas (islands of Langerhans) produce *insulin* and *glucagon* which pass directly into the circulating blood. Thus, one juice travels in ducts, the other two do not (ductless gland).

Large Intestine

The lower portion of the digestive tract is about five feet long and two or more inches in diameter; hence it is called the large intestine (Fig. 11–8). Its chief function is to absorb water from the material it receives, and move this material (feces) along to be eliminated from the body. The large intestine has no villi for food absorption. Glands in the wall secrete mucus, and muscle layers (circular and longitudinal) are present to control the movement of fecal material.

The large intestine has three main parts: *cecum* (first two or three inches of large intestine forming a pouch, lower part projects the

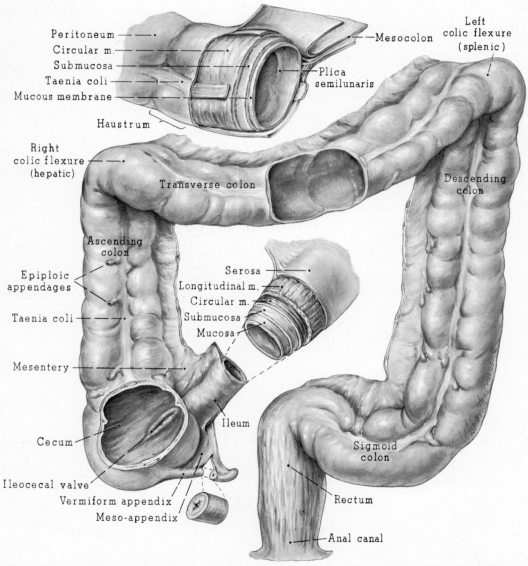

FIGURE 11–8 Position and structure of the large intestine. The walls of both large and small intestines have been enlarged and disected to show their various layers. (Jacob and Francone: Structure anf Function in Man.)

appendix); *colon* (ascending, transverse, descending, sigmoid); *rectum* (last six or seven inches of the large intestine). In Figure 11–8, follow the ascending colon upward, across the abdomen (transverse) and down the left side (descending), and note the curved portion called the sigmoid colon. The lower opening is guarded by sphincter muscles called the *anus.* Fecal material moving by peristalsis into the rectum normally stimulates that area to empty once every 24 hours (defecation).

DIGESTION

The "food route" has been outlined and the accessory organs have been noted. The preparation of food for body use involves both *mechanical* and *chemical* means. Food must be broken down to be absorbed by the circulating blood and used by the cells.

Fecal material (undigested foods, bacteria, mucus, and water) must be moved on and eliminated from the alimentary canal.

Three types of food substance are digested: carbohydrates (starches and sugars), fats, and proteins. The body also needs minerals, vitamins, water, and cellulose. Cellulose (roughage) is indigestible but adds bulk to the diet and so aids the mechanical process. Minerals, vitamins, and water are ready for body use.

Mechanical Digestion

Food must be broken into smaller pieces, moistened, and mixed with digestive juices and moved along. This action on food is called *mechanical digestion;* it starts in the mouth and continues through the entire digestive tract (chewing, swallowing, peristaltic waves in the stomach, peristalsis in both intestines). The tongue, muscles in the jaws, the pharynx, esophagus, stomach, and intestines furnish the power for mechanical digestion.

Chemical Digestion

As food is mixed with digestive juices along the way, a chemical action or change takes place. (See Table 11–1.) Digestive juices need help to perform these changes. *Enzymes,* substances that speed up the work of the digestive juices, are present.

The chief chemical changes in food are:

1. Carbohydrates (starches and sugars) are changed to *simple sugars* (mouth, stomach, small intestine).

2. Fats are turned into *fatty acids* (stomach, small intestine).

3. Proteins are changed to *amino acids* (stomach, small intestine).

These so-called *end products* of digestion are absorbed through the small intestinal villi into the blood for body use.

SUMMARY

The digestive system prepares food for body use and eliminates the unusable parts. Mucous membranes provide a smooth moist lining for the entire digestive tract. Muscles, nerves, and glandular secretions are essential to the digestive process.

Digestion of food begins in the mouth, continues in the stomach, and is completed in the small intestine. Peristaltic waves move food along. In each of the three organs digestive juices act on the food to help change it for body use. The absorption of chyme through the villi in the small intestine puts the digested food directly into the circulating blood. The large intestine absorbs water from indigestible materials as they move along the tract to be eliminated from the body.

Six accessory organs are teeth, tongue, salivary glands, liver, gallbladder, and pancreas. The function(s) of each should be understood.

Mechanical and chemical means are used to digest food. They work together, yet act upon food in different ways.

GUIDES FOR STUDY AND DISCUSSION

1. Use Figure 11–1 to help you complete the following chart. Use an asterisk (*) to indicate accessory organs.

The Journey of Food

Organs Involved	Function of Each

2. What is meant by the statement, "The liver is an accessory organ"? How many accessory organs can you name?

3. In your own words, explain the difference between mechanical and chemical digestion.

4. The body has need for seven dietary substances. What does each one do for the body?

5. As you understand it, what relation(s) do you see between good food habits and the digestive system?

6. The pancreas could be nicknamed a "duct-ductless" gland. Why?

7. Villi play an important role in the digestive process. What is that role?

SUGGESTED SITUATIONS AND ACTIVITIES

1. Select one food you have eaten during the last 24 hours and try to trace it through the digestive process.

2. During the study of the digestive system, pay particular attention to your eating habits. Decide on two things you could do to improve them.

3. Prepare an exhibit of news items about food fads and dieting.

THE PROCESS OF METABOLISM

OBJECTIVES FOR THE STUDENT: Be able to:

1. Tell where body heat comes from.
2. Describe the process of metabolism in general terms.
3. Explain how heat production is influenced in the body.
4. Tell how the healthy body maintains a constant temperature range.

SUGGESTED STUDY VOCABULARY*

metabolism
anabolism
catabolism

metabolic rate
basal metabolic rate
calorie

"normal" body temperature
oxidize
absolute rest

*Look for any terms you already know.

INTRODUCTION

A living cell is a working cell; it is a receiving, using, and storing unit of living matter. You will recall (Chapter 6) the cell could be nicknamed a "mini-factory" because it takes in food substance and oxygen, produces heat-energy, and has waste by-products. The food is the fuel; the oxygen makes it burn.

Producing heat-energy and making it available from food keep body cells busy because body activities constantly make various demands upon the body's energy supply. The muscles need energy; the absorption of chyme through the small intestine wall requires it. Energy is used by glands and nerves; the cell itself uses energy as it does work.

Cells must continue to live and work if the whole body is to live and have heat-energy to perform its functions.

METABOLISM—WHAT IS IT?

Metabolism is a complicated chemical process in cells whereby energy is released to tissues in such manner that they can perform their selective functions. This process includes using food substances, storing these substances until needed, and ridding the cells of waste. So it can be said that metabolism is the sum or total of all chemical reactions in all body cells. This total chemical reaction has two distinct phases—a constructive process dealing with the use of food by cells (anabo-

125

TABLE 12-1. FOOD AT WORK

ESSENTIAL DIETARY SUBSTANCE	WHAT EACH DOES FOR THE BODY
CARBOHYDRATES	
Starch Examples: wheat, corn, rice, macaroni, bread, crackers, potatoes	Furnish heat energy for body work (digestion, work of muscles, etc.) and to keep it warm (body temperature)
Sugar Examples: table sugar, honey, jam, syrup, candy	
One gram furnishes 4 calories of heat. In our country more than one-half of daily calories in diet are carbohydrates.	
FATS	
Fats and Oils Examples: butter, cream, bacon, vegetable oils	1. Furnish heat energy for body work and warmth 2. Help some vitamins do their work better
One gram furnishes 9 calories of heat (over twice as much as carbohydrates and proteins).	
PROTEINS	
Proteins Examples: meat, eggs, milk, cheese, poultry, nuts	1. Build and repair body tissues (muscles, blood, glands, etc.); no other dietary substance can take its place for this function 2. Furnish body energy 3. Regulate body processes (water balance in body tissues)
One gram furnishes 4 calories of heat. Not quite one-half of protein eaten is changed to fatty acid, the rest is changed to glucose (sugar).	

(Table 12–1 continues on opposite page.)

TABLE 12-1. (Continued)

ESSENTIAL DIETARY SUBSTANCE	WHAT EACH DOES FOR THE BODY
MINERALS	
Sodium While food contains some salt, chief source is that added to food in preparation	Necessary for proper water balance in body; aids body chemical control scheme
Iron Good sources: liver, oysters, turkey, beef hamburger, shrimp, cooked peas, raisins	Makes hemoglobin (coloring matter in red blood cells) to carry oxygen in blood
Calcium Good sources: skim milk, cheddar cheese, raw cabbage, orange, spinach	1. Makes up part of nerve and muscle tissue and of body fluids 2. Builds teeth and bones
Iodine Good sources: sea foods, water and milk under certain conditions.	Makes up part of thyroid gland (regulates the rate energy is used by body)
Other essential minerals include: phosphorus, magnesium, potassium, manganese; they help maintain the body's chemical control scheme and proper water balance.	
VITAMINS	
Vitamins (2 groups) 1. Fat soluble (A, D, E, and K) (See Chapter 25 for examples) 2. Water soluble (B complex and C) (See Chapter 25 for examples)	1. Necessary to proper growth because they serve as "helpers," to carbohydrates, fats, proteins, minerals in their functions 2. Do not furnish any calories 3. Help regulate metabolism 4. Appears there is much yet to be discovered about vitamins and their role in proper body functioning

lism) and a destructive process within cells to release energy (catabolism).

While cells are at work chemically releasing energy for tissue use, they produce heat too. It has been determined that more than half the energy in food becomes heat.

METABOLIC RATE

The rate at which heat is produced in the body is called the *metabolic rate*. The unit for measuring this heat is called a *calorie*.

Carbohydrates, proteins, and fats all can be turned into body heat-energy. Study Table 12–1. Notice that one gram of carbohydrate produces 4 calories of heat, one gram of fat 9 calories of heat, and one gram of protein 4 calories of heat. Factors which influence the rate of heat production in the body are amount of exercise, age and size, amount of thyroid hormone, abnormal fever, drugs taken, emotions experienced, state of pregnancy, external climate, sleep, and presence of malnutrition.

The daily calorie requirements for individuals vary. A person doing hard physical labor uses more heat energy than a secretary. Daily activities influence calorie requirements. Some days a secretary may use more calories than others and the laborer use fewer. When an individual ingests more calories than he uses, the remainder is stored as body fat; when he uses more than he ingests, the stored fat is changed into simple sugars and the body uses them. When this happens a person loses weight.

BASAL METABOLIC RATE

Basal metabolic rate (BMR) represents the total number of calories used by a person awake but at absolute rest. To say it another way, it is the lowest rate of metabolism a person can get along with. The minimum heat energy requirements of the body at rest are measured by a test called a basal metabolic test; it measures the oxygen intake and the carbon dioxide output. This shows the oxidation that has taken place and the calories used to expend the energy. Food is withheld from the person for 12 hours or more prior to the test.

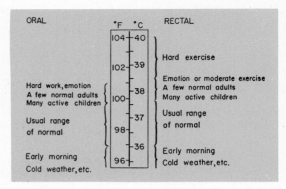

FIGURE 12–1   Estimated range of body temperature in normal persons. (From DuBois: Fever. Charles C Thomas.)

BODY TEMPERATURE

Tissue and organ temperature within the body *(core temperature)* remain almost constant. Temperature of the skin varies with surrounding conditions *(skin temperature)*. However, there is a range of average body temperatures influenced by climate, age, time of day, and activity. In Figure 12–1 notice the usual range of normal temperature. Under ordinary circumstances mouth temperature is about 98.6 F., or 37° C.; it may well vary a degree or more either way. During illness this variation may be several degrees.

Cells at work produce heat as they "burn" food substance. Some tissues produce more heat than others—namely, the more active parts of the body (i.e., muscles and liver). They oxidize more food substances and thus they produce more heat.

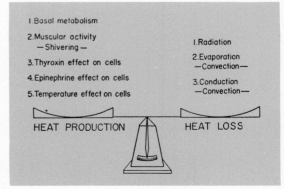

FIGURE 12–2   Balance of heat production versus heat loss. (Guyton: Textbook of Medical Physiology, 4th Ed.)

The amount of heat produced depends upon body activity. Hard work and exercise (and shivering) produce more heat. Other factors influencing heat production are low environmental temperatures and intake of food. To maintain an even body temperature, body heat production and heat loss must be equal (heat balance). (See Fig. 12–2.)

Heat is lost in several ways:

1. From the skin—over 80 per cent of all body heat loss is through evaporation of sweat, radiation (transfer of heat from one object to another without touching it), and conduction (transfer of heat from one object to another by touching it, hence the wrist watch you wear feels warm).

2. From the lungs—a small amount lost through carbon dioxide.

3. Cold food and drink require body heat to warm them.

Heat is regulated in a region of the brain called the hypothalamus. It is stimulated by nerve impulses from the skin and the temperature of the blood circulating through it. The heat-regulating center in the newborn does not work well for a while. The infant needs to be kept warm because of this; the premature infant has even greater need for additional warmth.

SUMMARY

Metabolism is a complicated chemical process in cells where food substances are turned into heat-energy for body use. The sum total of all body cells producing heat-energy is called metabolism. The rate of heat production is called metabolic rate; basal metabolic rate (BMR) is the number of calories used by a person who is awake but at absolute rest.

Factors which influence normal temperature range include climate, age, time of day, and activity. Core temperatures remain almost constant while skin temperatures vary with surrounding conditions. When the amount of body heat produced is equal to the amount of heat lost, this is known as heat balance.

GUIDES FOR STUDY AND DISCUSSION

1. What is metabolism? Where does it take place?
2. Using Table 12–1, determine which essential dietary substances furnish body heat energy.
3. In your opinion, what would you need to know about the process of body heat production to nurse a patient?
4. Why is body core temperature more constant than body skin temperature?
5. Where is the body's heat regulating center? Why are people especially careful to see that a newborn baby is kept warm?
6. How is body heat lost?
7. What factors influence the amount of heat produced?

SUGGESTED SITUATION AND ACTIVITY

1. For a period of one week take and record your temperature by mouth under a variety of circumstances. Use the same thermometer; position it in the same way in your mouth and leave it in position the same length of time each time. See if you can prove or disprove any statements in this chapter about range of body temperature.

THE REPRODUCTIVE AND URINARY SYSTEMS

OBJECTIVES FOR THE STUDENT: Be able to:

1. Name the main structures and functions of the female reproductive system.
2. Name the main structures and functions of the male reproductive system.
3. Explain the meaning of conception and how it takes place.
4. Describe the need for good hygiene habits with respect to these two systems.
5. Compare the structures of the female and the male urinary systems pointing out the similarities and the differences.
6. Describe the menstrual cycle.
7. Name the male and the female hormones.
8. List the functions of the urinary system.
9. Describe the characteristics of normal urine.

SUGGESTED STUDY VOCABULARY*

orifice	epididymis	labia majora
semen	vas deferens	labia minora
urine	vagina	vulva
puberty	enzyme	estrogen
conception	follicles (graafian)	progesterone
reproduction	hormones	testosterone
sperm	uterine or fallopian tube	menopause
ovum	cervix	seminal vesicle
embryo	uterus	prostate gland
penis	fundus	Cowper's gland
testes	ovary	urethra
		ureter

*Look for any terms you already know.

INTRODUCTION

The reproductive system and the urinary system overlap in some respects. For instance, in the male, the same tract is used to discharge both semen and urine from the body. While the same statement is not true of the female, the very close proximity of the urethral orifice to the vaginal orifice makes it clearly necessary to understand the location of each. This knowledge directly relates to safe nursing practice. A nursing measure ordered for the urinary bladder could be a serious error if mistakenly performed in the vaginal tract. This understanding also relates to proper personal hygiene habits.

For these and other reasons the two systems are discussed side by side, so to speak. While they may well be taught as separate units, you will be helped to more easily transfer what you learn about one system to the other system if you come to understand the overlapping anatomical structures and pay particular attention to the close proximity of one system to the other. Use the illustrations interchangeably as you study each system to help you see these relationships.

PART I—REPRODUCTIVE SYSTEM

Man instinctively desires to and does continue himself through reproduction. In fact, all living things have this built-in purpose and capability. Reproduction, a powerful drive among all living things, is controlled in different ways among different creatures and plants.

In the human, the female after reaching puberty and until menopause is capable of conception at any time except during certain portions of each month; this fact is directly related to the performance of certain endocrine glands. This is another example of system to system relationships in the "body as a whole."

REPRODUCTION: HOW IS IT INITIATED?

At the moment of conception, reproduction starts. The moment of conception is when one mature sperm (male germ cell) penetrates one ripe ovum (female egg). From that moment on there is an orderly procession of developments as the new "individual" (embryo) grows and matures in preparation for separation from the mother nine months later. Conception requires the union of a live sperm and a mature ovum. A chain of events leads to this union. The live sperm must be present at the right time—namely, when the mature ovum is available and in the right place.

Sperm are *very* minute germ cells, each with a spear-shaped head, neck, and a long tail. The wiggling tail propels the cell; it causes it to "swim" or move along about an inch every 20 minutes. Billions of sperm are produced in the testes of the male during a lifetime and are transported out of the male in a white, semi-liquid fluid called *semen*. The amount of semen introduced into the vagina (female) via the penis (male) during copulation or sexual union actually is very small (normally about 2 to 5 cc.), but this small amount of semen contains literally several hundred million sperm (1 cc. contains about 100 million sperm).

Ordinarily, it takes live sperm about four to six hours to move along the female tract to the uterus. The exact cause of sperm movement is not clear; some believe the long tail propels it along, others feel that muscular contractions of the uterus are responsible. In any event, as the sperm does move along, it "prepares" itself to fertilize the ovum. This means that when the sperm encounters the mature ovum, it has developed an enzyme strength sufficient to penetrate the ovum with its spear-like head. Once the head is within the egg and the egg is fertilized, the sperm sheds its tail. Only *one* sperm head penetrates and fertilizes the ovum. When this happens, the ovum is somehow able to ward off all other sperm cells.

Sperm cells have a short life span. Some die in the vagina and get no further; all unused sperm cells that do reach the uterus may live a day or even longer, but within about 72 hours they too have died.

What about the ovum, the other "half" of conception? You will recall that the ovum must be mature; it must be ripe to be able to join with the sperm and be fertilized. A ripe ovum has a short life span also; it is thought to be about 48 hours. Considering the approximate life span of each—the sperm and the ovum—one can readily see why timing is such an important factor in conception.

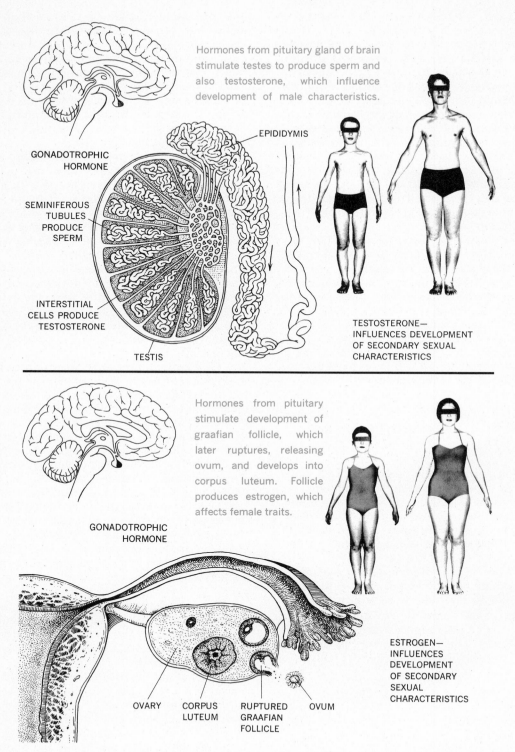

Hormones from pituitary gland of brain stimulate testes to produce sperm and also testosterone, which influence development of male characteristics.

EPIDIDYMIS

GONADOTROPHIC HORMONE

SEMINIFEROUS TUBULES PRODUCE SPERM

INTERSTITIAL CELLS PRODUCE TESTOSTERONE

TESTIS

TESTOSTERONE—INFLUENCES DEVELOPMENT OF SECONDARY SEXUAL CHARACTERISTICS

Hormones from pituitary stimulate development of graafian follicle, which later ruptures, releasing ovum, and develops into corpus luteum. Follicle produces estrogen, which affects female traits.

GONADOTROPHIC HORMONE

OVARY   CORPUS LUTEUM   RUPTURED GRAAFIAN FOLLICLE   OVUM

ESTROGEN—INFLUENCES DEVELOPMENT OF SECONDARY SEXUAL CHARACTERISTICS

FIGURE 13–1 Primary reproductive organs of the male and female. (Courtesy of Western Publishing Company.)

An ovum comes from an ovary; it is about the size of a dot made by a pencil on paper and is barely noticeable to the naked eye. The ovum contains a nucleus which is surrounded by cytoplasm and some food nutrients. The ovary (there are two) has the built-in capacity ordinarily to release one ovum at one time. This means that from puberty to menopause, the well-regulated process of egg maturation goes on continuously and involves both ovaries. It has been estimated that at birth, each ovary has the potential for producing some 200,000 graafian follicles (each potentially can produce an ovum). Hormones control this well-regulated process, namely the maturing of the follicle and its rupture to release the mature egg. This process follows a regular cycle.

Following the rupture of the graafian follicle (there is uncertainty about what triggers this rupture), the ovum is free in the abdomen. Study Figure 13–1 and locate the "free" egg. The ovum is close to the fringed end of the uterine or fallopian tube, but it has no self-power to move toward the tube. Movement of the fringed ends, the cilia, and the muscular contractions of the tube and the uterus are responsible for capturing the ovum and directing it toward the uterus. The trip takes from six to eight days. Fertilization (if it is to take place) usually occurs when the ovum is about one-third of the way through the uterine tube. If there is no fertilization, the egg moves into the uterus and soon breaks up and is expelled.

Multiple Births

On occasion, the ovaries release more than one mature ovum at or about the same time. When the ova are fertilized, multiple births occur. In the case of twins, each ovum is fertilized separately from the other; such twins are called *fraternal twins*. *Identical* twins result from *one* fertilized ovum that subdivides after it is fertilized; these two embryos come from the same egg.

THE FEMALE REPRODUCTIVE SYSTEM

The internal and the external parts of the female reproductive system are listed first; a description of the structure and function of each follows.

Reproductive Organs of the Female

Internal	*External* (Vulva)*
vagina	
cervix	mons pubis
uterus	labia majora
uterine or fallopian	labia minora
tubes (2)	clitoris
ovaries (2), "primary	vaginal orifice
reproductive organs"	glands
	perineum
	breasts (mammary
	glands)

Locate each organ, opening, or part in Figures 13–2 and 13–3 as it is discussed. This will help you become familiar with the structures and to notice the close proximity of some of the body orifices.

Internal Organs

Vagina. The vagina, located between bladder and rectum, is an expandable, muscular tube about three to five inches long; it extends from the uterus to the *vulva*. The outer opening called *vaginal orifice* is partially closed by a ring-shaped fold of mucous membrane called the *hymen*.

The vagina serves three functions: (1) forms the lower part of the birth canal; (2) receives semen from the male; and (3) serves as exit duct for menstrual flow and uterine secretions.

Cervix. The cervix is the lower, tapered part of the uterus that projects into the vagina.

Uterus. The uterus is a pear-shaped hollow organ which lies between the bladder and the rectum. Its thick muscular walls (three layers) are capable of great expansion during pregnancy; otherwise, the approximate size is three inches long, two inches wide (widest part), and an inch thick. The rounded portion above the cervix is called the *body* of the uterus and the dome-shaped portion between the uterine tubes is known as the *fundus*. The uterus has a rich blood supply and is held in place by several strong ligaments. The main function of the uterus is to provide an abode for and protect and nourish the embryo.

Uterine or fallopian tubes. The two

---

*Urethral orifice (urinary system) and anus (digestive system). Note the close proximity of these openings to the vaginal orifice.

uterine tubes extend slightly upward and away from each side of the dome-shaped portion of the uterus; they then arch downward ending very close to the ovary. These slender, muscular tubes (about four inches long) have fringe-like ends and serve as pathways for the ovum to reach the uterus. Fertilization of the ovum by the sperm normally takes place in the first one-third of the tube.

Ovaries (primary sex organs). The two ovaries are almond-shaped structures (about one and one-half inches long) located on each side of the uterus and attached by a long stem or (ovarian) ligament; they also are suspended from the broad ligament of the uterus by a fold of peritoneum. Each ovary has a store of tiny follicles (graafian) in varying stages of devel-

opment; each follicle produces a germ cell or ovum. Ordinarily, one mature ovum is released about every 28 days. This supply of follicles lasts about 35 years; when exhausted, menopause (cessation of menstruation) occurs and the body adjusts to a changed body chemistry (see menopause).

From puberty to menopause the ovary produces two types of hormones: (1) *Estrogen:* responsible for growth and development of reproductive organs during puberty, for development of other sex characteristics, for thickening the lining of the uterus prior to ovulation and repairing it after menstruation. (2) *Progesterone*—further prepares the lining of the uterus to receive the fertilized ovum and aids its implantation in the uterine lining. It

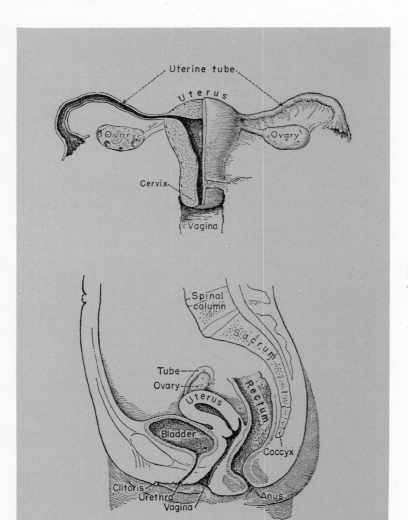

FIGURE 13–2 The female reproductive system. (Dowling and Jones: That the Patient May Know.)

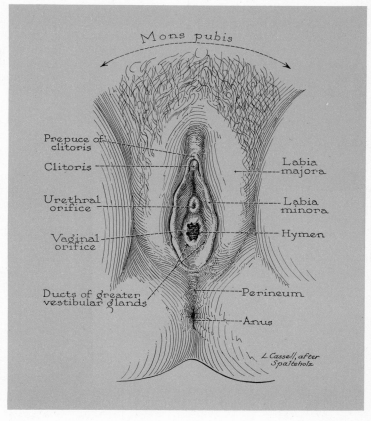

FIGURE 13–3 The vulva. (King and Showers: Human Anatomy and Physiology, 6th ed.)

promotes the development of the placenta and prevents the production of more ova during pregnancy. Progesterone causes breast enlargement during pregnancy.

Study Figure 13–4 to notice when, during the month, these hormones perform; note also the presence of progesterone during pregnancy.

External Organs

The term *vulva* refers to *all* of the external genitals.

Mons pubis.   This is the rounded, fatty, fibrous tissue which crowns the vulva; from puberty it is covered with hair.

Labia majora.   The labia majora consist of a pair of elongated folds of membrane which extend downward from the mons pubis toward the perineum surrounding the labia minora.

Labia minora.   The labia minora are two thinner, highly sensitive folds under the labia majora. They extend from the clitoris to the hymen.

Clitoris.   Where the labia majora and the labia minora meet at the top, there is a very sensitive tissue called the clitoris which becomes erect during sexual excitation.

Vaginal Orifice.   This is the opening to the vagina.

Glands.   During sexual stimulation two sets of glands (Bartholin's and Skene's) secrete lubricating fluids; they are situated near the vaginal orifice.

Perineum.   The term perineum is clinically used to mean the area between the vaginal orifice and the anus. However, the full use of the term means the area (including all structures) between the pubic symphysis and the coccyx; used in this context, it includes the entire pelvic outlet.

Breasts (mammary glands)

The breasts secrete milk for the newborn. Clusters of glands with ducts, each resembling a bunch of grapes with a stem, make up a lobe; there are about 20 such lobes in each breast cushioned in fat and connective tissue. They radiate from the nipple similarly to spokes in a wheel, and each opens separately on the tip of the nipple. About three days after delivery of the newborn, the mammary glands begin to secrete milk and continue to do so for several months. Progesterone promotes the development of the milk-secreting cells of the breast.

Puberty

Many changes occur among normal children between the ages of 10 and 14 years. Puberty is the age at which secondary sex characteristics develop and the reproductive organs become workable or operative. Exact ages for the onset of puberty in girls and in boys vary a great deal. (See Fig. 19–4). Physical changes occurring in the female are breast enlargement, appearance of pubic and axillary hair, menstruation, and increased body growth

with body contour changes; girls grow faster during this period than boys. Puberty in the male marks the time when sperm are produced in sufficient quantity to effect reproduction. There is the development of such secondary sex characteristics as full growth of the penis, body hair growth (pubic, axilla, face, chest, etc.), and lower pitching of the voice due to increased size of larynx.

Menstruation

When the menstrual flow first occurs, generally at 12 or 13 years of age, the reproductive organs are able to function. (See Fig. 13–4.) Menstruation is the body's means for periodically discharging extra blood and tissue it has prepared for an ovum in case it is fertilized, but which has not been used. Although menstrual cycles vary, usually there is about a 28-day interval from one menstrual

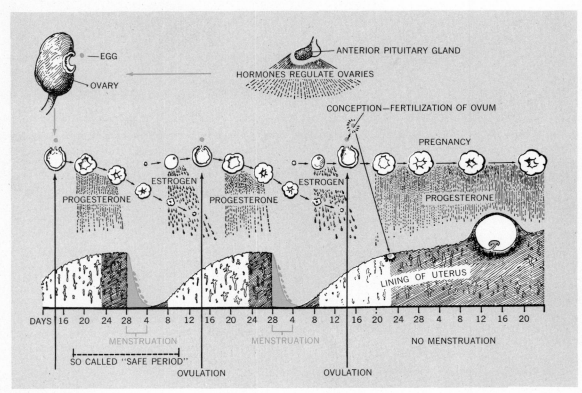

FIGURE 13–4 Diagram shows the chain of events that occurs during the average 28-day menstrual cycle. The cycle begins when hormones from the pituitary gland stimulate the development of an egg in a follicle inside one of the ovaries. About the 14th day ovulation occurs. The follicle bursts, and an egg is discharged from the ovary. Three successive ovulations are shown here. After the first two, the egg is not fertilized, and the cycles end in menstruation on the 28th day. After the third ovulation, the egg is fertilized and pregnancy begins. (Dowling and Jones: That the Patient May Know.)

period to the next. On the average, the flow lasts from three to five days.

During each 28-day cycle, certain things occur on a regular basis. Beginning with the first day of menstrual flow, one (seldom more than one) of the many ova in the ovary begins to mature. It is enclosed in a small sac (graafian follicle) which fills with fluid and causes the follicle to swell until it reaches the periphery of the ovary. By the fourteenth day it has swelled to such a size that it ruptures and the ovum is released into the abdominal cavity (ovulation). During this time the follicle has been producing *estrogen* and has been under the control of the pituitary gland. Shortly after ovulation, the fringed end of the fallopian tube sweeps the ovum into the tube and the ovum is slowly propelled through the tube by the waving motion of hairlike projections of its lining. Midway through the tube the ovum has matured and, if met and joined there by a sperm cell from the male, it is fertilized; if not, it passes on into the uterus and is expelled from the body.

The ruptured follicle fills with lipoid or golden-colored substance and is called the corpus luteum. While it grows (six or seven days) it secretes greater amounts of progesterone and estrogens but after that, if the ovum has not been fertilized, the corpus luteum and its secretions diminish. By the end of the 28-day cycle very little estrogen is secreted, and no progesterone.

Meanwhile, what is happening within the uterus? Changes in the uterine lining are directly related to the work of the ovaries. About every 28 days, part of the epithelial lining is sloughed off and blood and tissue are released for several days. Following that (as the ovarian follicle increases in size) this lining starts to rebuild itself and continues to do so until the ovarian follicle ruptures. Then the progesterone from the corpus luteum causes the mucous membrane of the uterus to increase in thickness. The glands begin to secrete a mucoid substance, arteriole coils tighten, and the venous capillaries fill with blood. The uterus now is ready to receive and nourish the fertilized ovum. If the ovum is not fertilized, the uterus has no need for the extra blood, and menstrual flow begins. This starts a new cycle.

The matter of meticulous personal hygiene, essential at all times, requires extra attention during menstruation. Good personal hygiene habits are essential and not harmful; exercise and ordinary pursuit of living without going to excess can be and should be carried on. Many myths from the ancient Hebrews, early Christians, Greeks and Romans are just that—something handed down from early imagination with no basis in fact.

The Menopause

Menopause is a normal happening in the life of the female; it is the cessation of menstruation and signals the end of reproductive power. It usually occurs between 45 and 50 years of age, but it may occur earlier or later. Prior to the last menstrual flow (premenopausal years), a woman may experience mood swings, irregular menstrual cycles, hot flushes, and cold sweats. Many factors influence the beginning and ending of menstruation but one of the best indicators of duration is the familial history. Overwork, ill health, and poor nourishment can interfere with normal ovarian function and thus contribute to an early menopause. Obesity is thought also to have its effects upon early menopause.

THE MALE REPRODUCTIVE SYSTEM

The internal and external parts of the male reproductive system are listed first; a description of the structure and function of each follows.

Reproductive Organs of the Male

Internal	*External*
seminal vesicle (2)	penis
prostate gland	urethra
Cowper's gland (2)	erectile tissue
spermatic cord or vas deferens (2)	glands
bladder*	scrotum
	testes (2)
	epididymis
	vas deferens (2)

Locate each organ, gland, or part in Figure 13–5 as it is discussed; this will help you visualize location(s) and appearance(s).

---

*Note the common pathway used by urine and semen from the prostate gland through the penis.

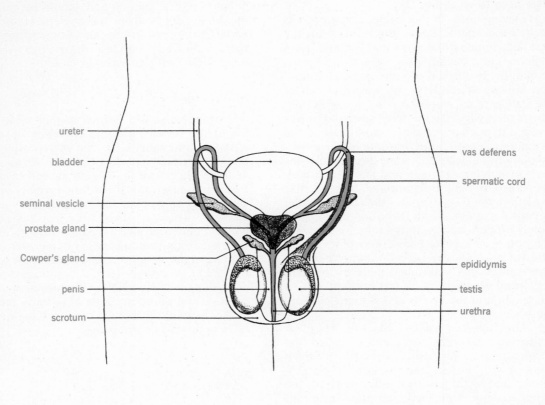

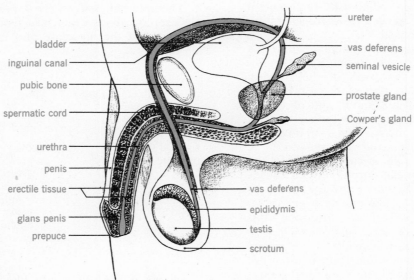

FIGURE 13–5 The male reproductive system. The upper diagram is a straight front view. The lower diagram is a side view shown as if a section had been made a little to one side of the center of the body from the front to back. (Schifferes: Essentials of Healthier Living, 3rd. ed., John Wiley and Sons, Inc.)

Internal Organs

Seminal vesicles. These two structures add essential components to the semen in the vas deferens.

Prostate gland. This gland likewise adds essential components to the semen in the vas deferens.

Cowper's gland. This gland also adds essential components to the semen in the vas deferens.

Vas deferens (spermatic cord). This is a duct or tube (one attached to each testis) for transporting sperm from the testes. In this duct the sperm follow a devious or crooked route upon leaving the scrotum. The duct enters the lower abdomen and loops around picking up needed contributions from the three glandular structures previously listed to form semen.

External Organs

Scrotum. This saclike structure (posterior to the penis) serves as a protection for the testes. One of its most important functions is to regulate and maintain a proper temperature for the sperm produced in the testes.

Testes. (See Fig. 13–1.) The two testes are primary sex glands (compared with ovaries in the female) located in the scrotum and capable of producing billions of germ cells or sperm in a lifetime. Sperm production lasts from puberty to old age. The activity, size and purpose of the sperm is discussed elsewhere in this chapter (Reproduction – How Is It Initiated?).

Another function of the testes is to produce the male sex hormone testosterone; this hormone influences body metabolism in a general way and is responsible for producing secondary sex characteristics (see Fig. 13–6). Small amounts of estrogen are produced in the male but their function is not known.

Epididymis. (See Fig. 13–1.) The epididymis is a hoodlike structure over the testes; it is a coiled-up tube that collects and stores sperm while they mature.

Vas deferens or spermatic cord. Both internal and external.

Penis. The penis, the male organ for copulation, is suspended from the pubic arch, anterior to the scrotum; it carries semen into the vagina (through the urethra) during copulation. Erectile tissue surrounding the urethra is capable of erection during sexual excitation. Under these circumstances this tissue holds

Testes and penis	Increase in size begins, 10–12 years. Rapid growth, 12–15 years.
Pubic hair	Initial appearance, 12–14 years. Abundant and curly, 13–16 years.
Axillary hair	Initial appearance, 13–16 years.
Facial and body hair	Initial appearance, 13–16 years.
Mature sperm	Average, about 14–16 years.
Breasts	Some hypertrophy, often assuming a firm nodularity, 12–14 years. Disappearance of hypertrophy, 14–17 years.

FIGURE 13–6 Time of appearance of sexual characteristics in American boys. (Watson and Lowrey: Growth and Development, Year Book Publishers)

large amounts of arteriolar blood, causing the penis to become firm rather than flaccid as under ordinary circumstances.

Glands. The bulbo-urethral glands add a secretion that lubricates the urethra.

PART II – URINARY SYSTEM

The body machine cannot operate long without a coordinated means for waste disposal and regulation. While other structures (large intestine, lungs, skin, lymphatics) do their part and play unique roles in waste disposal, the urinary system plays a singular role in this respect. It could be called the role of "body regulator" because, in the main, the urinary system (1) filters liquid metabolic wastes from the circulation and eliminates them from the body, and (2) helps regulate the water balance in the body and the acid-base balance in the blood.

Organs of the urinary system include:
Kidneys (2)
Ureters (2)
Bladder
Urethra
(Adrenal glands atop the kidneys are a part of the endocrine system)

Locate each organ, gland, or part (Figs. 13–7 and 13–8) as it is discussed; this will help you realize the positions of these main structures and to visualize their appearance.

The four parts to the urinary system work with a united purpose in a "1–2–3–4" order – urine formed in the kidneys is carried through the ureters to the bladder and discharged from there through the urethra.

Kidneys

These two bean-shaped organs lie behind the peritoneum, one on either side of the spine and just back of the lower five ribs. The left kidney is a little higher than the right because the liver is to the right of the abdominal cavity. They are held in place by adipose tissue and fascia which bind them to muscles in that area.

The smooth outer covering of the kidney is a thin membrane called the *capsule*. The interior portion known as the *medulla* is made up of triangular units (from eight to 12) called *renal pyramids*. Within each pyramid, large tubes collect the liquid wastes filtered out of the blood by more than a million minute filtering units called *nephrons*. Figure 13–9 shows the arteriole (blood supply) within the renal corpuscle. Here the blood flows slowly through the glomerulus to permit filtration; it is under pressure within the corpuscle and

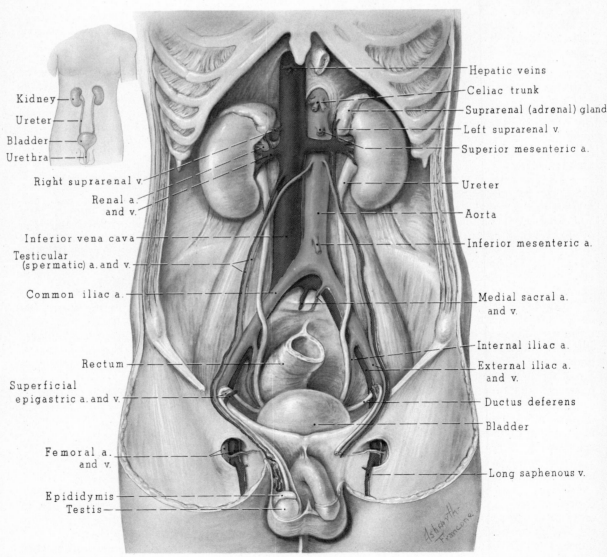

Kidney
Ureter
Bladder
Urethra

Right suprarenal v.
Renal a. and v.

Inferior vena cava
Testicular (spermatic) a. and v.

Common iliac a.

Rectum

Superficial epigastric a. and v.

Femoral a. and v.

Epididymis
Testis

Hepatic veins
Celiac trunk
Suprarenal (adrenal) gland
Left suprarenal v.
Superior mesenteric a.

Ureter

Aorta

Inferior mesenteric a.

Medial sacral a. and v.

Internal iliac a.
External iliac a. and v.

Ductus deferens

Bladder

Long saphenous v.

FIGURE 13–7   Posterior abdominal wall, showing relationship of urinary system, genital system, and great vessels. (Jacob and Francone: Structure and Function in Man.)

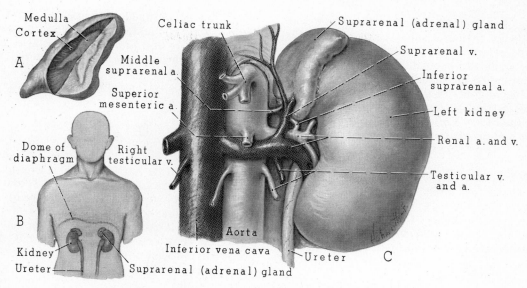

FIGURE 13–8 A, Suprarenal gland sectioned to show the medulla. B, Anatomic position of kidney and suprarenal glands. C, Anterior aspect of left kidney, showing adrenal gland and vascular supply. (Jacob and Francone: Structure and Function in Man.)

this, too, aids the filtering process. With so many filtering units at work in the kidneys, the blood is relieved of liquid wastes.

Liquid waste removal is the beginning of the formation of urine. Water and solutes forced through the membranes travel through the irregularly looped tubule on their way to the collecting tubule. While traveling this route, about 98 per cent of the water and some

of the solutes filter back into the circulating blood. During this winding journey, most mineral salts and all glucose are reabsorbed; this is a selective reabsorption process. When glucose is not filtered out, but remains in the urine, it produces a condition called *renal glycosuria.* Filtration of water, mineral salts, and sugar back into the blood is essential to proper electrolyte balance in the body. Tests

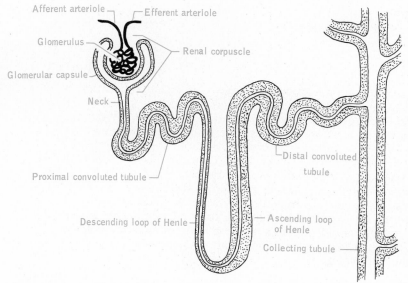

FIGURE 13–9   The nephron—the renal unit. (Manner: Elements of Anatomy and Physiology.)

are used to show the concentration power of the kidney. Mineral salts removed from the blood combine with water to form urine that is collected in the tubules and passed through the ureters to the bladder.

The quantity of urine secreted in a day is influenced by the amount of water removed from the blood; normally it is from one to one and a half quarts (see urine).

Ureters

These two tubes, 10 to 12 inches long, connect the kidneys with the bladder and serve as passageways for urine. Contraction of the middle (muscular) layer creates peristaltic waves from the upper funnel-shaped end to the bladder; here the opening is controlled by valves (Fig. 13–7).

Bladder

The urinary bladder is a storehouse or reservoir for urine. It is a hollow muscle somewhat triangular-shaped at the bottom and its activity is controlled by the para-sympathetic nervous system. As the bladder becomes moderately filled, there is a desire to void (micturate). Ordinarily it holds about one pint; as the urine volume increases, pressure within the bladder increases. Voluntary control can be exerted up to a point of extreme pressure, but involuntary micturition occurs in time if pressure is not released. The elasticity of the bladder wall permits expansion and contraction.

The bladder is located in front of the rectum in the male and in front of the uterus and the vagina in the female. It has three controlled openings, two where the ureters join it and one where it opens into the urethra. The latter opening is controlled by a sphincter.

Urethra

This tube extends from the bladder to the outside of the body (Fig. 13–5). It differs in the sexes. In the female the tube, one to one and one-half inches long, has two sphincters (internal and external). The female urethral orifice is so close to the vaginal orifice and the rectum that it can easily become irritated and infected. The urethra of the male has three parts: the prostatic (in the prostate); the membranous, extending from the prostate to the urethra; and the cavernous, extending to the external opening. Altogether it is about eight inches long.

Urine

Normal urine has the following characteristics: The amount (in 24 hours) varies according to fluid intake, perspiration, and other factors, but usually it is about three pints (1500 ml.). It is a clear straw-colored liquid, becoming cloudy upon standing. The usual urine odor takes on a smell of ammonia when it stands. Its specific gravity varies from 1.015 to 1.025 (highest in the morning), and it is slightly acid. Vegetables in the diet can make urine alkaline, and so can staleness.

SUMMARY

The male and female reproductive organs are equally important in the start of reproduction and in influencing hereditary factors. The female produces the ovum which is fertilized by the sperm of the male. Growth of the embryo takes place in the uterus of the female, and birth takes place after nine months. Hormones in both the male and the female influence reproductive power. Puberty occurs in both sexes. In the female, reproductive power ceases when menstruation ceases.

The urinary system produces urine, ridding the body of liquid metabolism wastes, and helps to regulate body water balance and the acid-base balance in the blood. The filtering unit of the kidney is the nephron; there are untold numbers of these units in each pyramid of the kidney. Together they serve a vital purpose, that of removing waste materials from the blood.

GUIDES FOR STUDY AND DISCUSSION

1. Prepare a chart as follows and complete the information

Female Reproductive System

Structure(s)   Function of

Hormone

Male Reproductive System

Structure(s)   Function of

Hormone

2. By the fourteenth day of the menstrual cycle, a graafian follicle ruptures, releasing an ovum. Assume the ovum is to be fertilized. What happens to it once it is released?

3. What, if anything, is the relationship between ovulation and conception?

4. What causes menstrual flow? Why does it cease during pregnancy?

5. Why should a nurse know the length of the female urethra and the male urethra? When would this knowledge be useful?

6. What is the relationship of good personal hygiene habits to these two systems?

7. Puberty occurs in both sexes. What are the differences? The similarities?

8. Where is urine formed? What are its characteristics?

9. Prepare a chart as follows and complete the information:

Female Urinary System

Structure(s)   Functions of

Male Urinary System

Structure(s)   Functions of

SUGGESTED SITUATIONS AND ACTIVITIES

1. The urinary system is a body regulator. Prepare a visual aid that shows the various ways it regulates the body.

2. Use the index and locate information elsewhere in the text about puberty and adolescence. Using the new knowledge you have gained studying the reproductive system, see in how many ways you can relate it to puberty and adolescence.

CHAPTER 14

THE ENDOCRINE SYSTEM

TOPICAL HEADINGS

Introduction	Adrenal Glands	Summary
Pituitary Gland	Pancreas	Guides for Study and
Thyroid Gland	Ovary	Discussion
Parathyroid Glands	Testis	Suggested Situation
Thymus Gland	Pineal Gland	and Activity

OBJECTIVES FOR THE STUDENT: Be able to:

1. Given a list of nine endocrine glands,
   a. Locate each one.
   b. Tell how each serves the body.
2. Explain the anatomical difference between "duct" and "ductless" glands.
3. Describe the two general ways hormones influence cell metabolism.
4. Give an example of a man-made medicine prescribed to assist a faulty endocrine gland.

SUGGESTED STUDY VOCABULARY*

hormone	parathyroid	insulin
endocrine	thymus	estrogen
pituitary	adrenal	progesterone
thyroid	epinephrine (adrenaline)	testosterone
thyroxine	islet cells (Langerhans)	pineal

*Look for any terms you already know.

INTRODUCTION

One could argue that the nervous system is the central seat of power when it comes to coordinating body functions, but it would be more logical to say that such power is shared with the endocrine system.

The endocrine system is made up of a series of "ductless" glands, scattered throughout the body, that wield great chemical power in promoting or impeding all body processes.

There is a distinct "marriage" between the nervous and endocrine systems; some glands require direct "stimuli" from the brain to produce secretions. But the hormones secreted by the endocrine glands, moving directly into the circulating blood and other body fluids, reach all cells and "orchestrate" an untold number of cell tissue and organ activities throughout the entire body. The rate of secretion is controlled by the needs of the body.

The secretions (hormones) of the endocrine glands seem to have a great deal of influence in regulating cell metabolism. This influence has: 1. An all-at-once effect in some instances (i.e., insulin in response to hyperglycemia). 2. A slow, steady effect in other instances (i.e., growth hormone; thyroxine on regular normal growth).

A hormone is a chemical substance secreted chiefly by the endocrine glands. Some other body tissues and organs contribute as well (i.e., adrenaline, long thought of as produced in the adrenal gland is also produced at nerve endings throughout the body).

The knowledge about hormones is incomplete in many respects such as the exact number produced in the human body or *how* hormones (chemically) function in cellular metabolism. What is known is the chemical make-up of many of the known hormones. This makes it possible to duplicate them in the laboratory so they may be used as medicine (i.e., insulin, thyroxine, ACTH, epinephrine).

Several other facts about hormones include:

1. They are *very powerful* chemical substances.

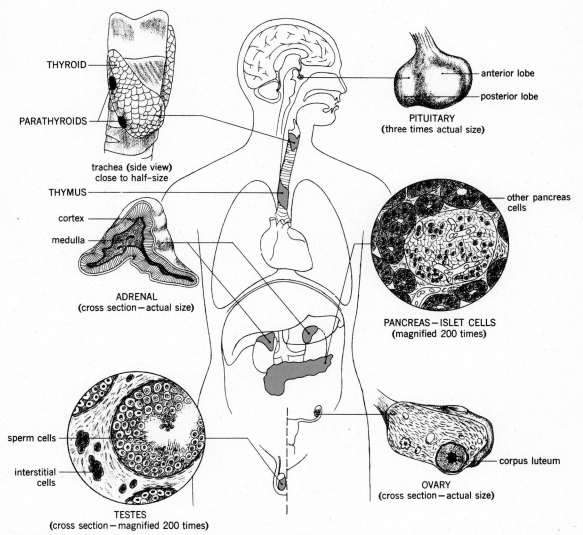

FIGURE 14–1 Endocrine glands. Reading from top to bottom, the endocrine glands of the human body are pituitary, thyroid, parathyroid, thymus (its endocrine status is questionable), adrenals, pancreas (the islet cells only), and ovaries or testes. (Schifferes: Essentials of Healthier Living, 3rd Ed. John Wiley and Sons, Inc.)

2. It seems to take such a *very* small amount of a hormone to do the work.

3. The amounts are so small that a new system of measurement had to be developed to name the amounts (billionths and trillionths of a gram).

4. They have their own "targets"; they know where to go. The target may be a single cell (or cluster) close by or one far away. In either event, their speed of travel is lightning quick. It is unknown how a particular hormone knows where to go and how it gets there so fast.

Use Figure 14–1 to locate the glands discussed in this chapter.

THE PITUITARY GLAND

For years the pituitary gland has been thought of as the "master gland" which served as a master control station for stimulating, coordinating, and regulating other endocrine glands. But scientists are finding that it is an "errand boy" carrying out commands from the brain. These are thought to be chemical commands coming by way of the blood stream from the brain to the gland.

The pituitary gland is a small piece of tissue about the size of a pea which hangs from the base of the brain just behind the eyes. It consists of two lobes (anterior and posterior)

and a very small central area. The work of the anterior lobe and of the posterior lobe is described in Table 14–1. Notice how often the pituitary hormones assist other endocrine glands.

Oversecretion or undersecretion of this powerful little gland directly alters body growth and development. If a malfunction occurs during childhood, giantism or dwarfism may result. In adult life, oversecretion and undersecretion cause changes in appearance and sometimes general ill health.

THE THYROID GLAND

Attached to the trachea, this gland is located beneath the larynx and above the sternum; it is U-shaped (two lobes connected by an isthmus) and secretes a hormone called *thyroxine*. The thyroid gland *regulates body metabolism* and *influences growth and temperature sensitivity*. The pituitary gland stimulates the thyroid gland to produce thyroxine which is formed in part from iodine.

Thyroxine is released, as needed, into the blood stream where it immediately is combined with several plasma proteins. This holds the thyroxine captive so to speak; it is then released very slowly to the cells even though the blood itself moves rapidly through the body. It is estimated that about one half of the

TABLE 14.1. PITUITARY GLAND HORMONES

Anterior Lobe	
HORMONE	FUNCTIONS
1. Growth	Promotes steady growth; affects metabolism
2. Prolactin	Works with other hormones on mammary (breast) tissue.
3. Follicle-stimulating	Necessary for normal cyclic growth of ovarian follicle.
4. Luteinizing	Essential for ovulation and forming of corpus luteum.
5. Thyrotrophin	Directly related to work (secretion) of the thyroid.
6. Adrenocorticotrophin (ACTH)	Influences the work of the adrenal cortex; stimulates production and release of cortisol, androgen and corticosterone; is related to metabolism of fats, glucose and proteins.
7. Melanocyte	A stimulating hormone but little is known about its functional role.

Posterior Lobe	
HORMONE	FUNCTIONS
1. Antidiuretic (Stored until needed)	Acts upon kidney tissue to save body water; reduces urine volume and increases its concentration. Hemorrhage can trigger the release of this hormone, so can some drugs (i.e., morphine).
2. Oxytocin (Pitocin)	Plays a part in getting breast milk from gland to the nipple; acts on human uterine muscle.

"captive" thyroxine in the blood is released to body cells every eight days. The supply is slow, steady and constant.

THE PARATHYROID GLANDS

This cluster of tiny pea-sized glands (usually four) is attached to the posterior base of the thyroid. The parathyroid hormone controls *the level of calcium in the blood* and *the metabolism of calcium and phosphorus*. In this way, it is related to the development of teeth and bone and to proper nerve and muscle tissue functions (Table 12–1).

THE THYMUS GLAND

The thymus gland is located beneath the sternum and in front of (anterior to) the trachea. Locate its position, Figure 14–1.

The thymus grows from birth to puberty and then it starts to get smaller, changing some of its tissue to fat and fiber. Some thymic tissue remains. It has been determined that the thymus gland serves the fetus and newborn by somehow influencing the formation of antibody cells for immunity purposes. Likewise it has something to do with the establishment of the lymphoid system. There is a question about a hormone from this gland.

THE ADRENAL GLANDS

Locate the adrenal glands attached to the top of each kidney (Fig. 14–1). Each gland has an outer portion called the *cortex* and an inner portion called the *medulla*. Each produces its own hormones. The cortex secretes *corticoids* which influence metabolism of fats, carbohydrates, and proteins, and body fluids and electrolytes. It also secretes some sex hormones. The medulla secretes *epinephrine* or *adrenaline* in response to excitement or stress; this secretion increases heart rate; blood supply to the heart, smooth muscles, and the nervous system; and the amount of glucose poured into the circulating blood from the liver. The cooperation between the medulla and the sympathetic nervous system in stress situations serves as an emergency system for the body. Adrenaline is also produced at nerve endings throughout the body.

PANCREAS—ISLET CELLS (LANGERHANS)

The organ, the pancreas, is discussed as an accessory organ in The Digestive System, Chapter 11. Our concern here is only with the special cell clusters scattered throughout the organ, known as islets of Langerhans. These special cells secrete two hormones: *insulin* and *glucagon*. The first hormone, insulin, is well-known for its relationship(s) to regulation of metabolism (carbohydrates in particular and, to a lesser extent, the body's use of protein for growth purposes). Insulin has been found to influence the transportation of phosphate and potassium into cells. Glucagon, the second hormone, indirectly helps regulate blood glucose. Insulin and glucagon are not emptied into ducts and carried away, but pass directly into the blood stream—thus, the islets are "ductless."

OVARY

The ovary is the primary sex organ of the female. See Chapter 13, The Reproductive System, to review the functions of the hormones *estrogen* and *progesterone*.

TESTIS

The testis is the primary sex organ of the male. See Chapter 13, The Reproductive System, to review the functions of the hormone *testosterone*.

PINEAL GLAND

The pineal "body," located at about the middle of the brain (not shown in Fig. 14–1), is sometimes included as an endocrine gland. It is a very small, gray-colored organ and little is known about its function. There is no concrete evidence that it produces a hormone. It is known that the pineal gland often becomes calcified in adults.

SUMMARY

No body system carries more responsibility for normal growth and function than that of the several endocrine (ductless) glands located in various parts of the body. The "master gland," the pituitary, stimulates and coordinates the work of other glands so that all work together to regulate the body. Some general knowledge of these glands is necessary for effective patient care.

GUIDES FOR STUDY AND DISCUSSION

1. There are eight, possibly nine, endocrine glands. Why is there a question about the exact number? Make a list of the endocrine glands; tell the known or suspected function of each. Notice how many seem to help each other. Can you tell where each is located?

2. Sometimes this system is called "the gland orchestra." Why might this be an appropriate nickname?

3. Why can one say that the endocrine system shares regulating power with the nervous system?

4. Using Figure 13–1 to help you, try to explain to yourself the relationship of the pituitary gland to growth and development (male and female).

5. In your opinion, what is the most interesting fact you learned about this system?

SUGGESTED SITUATION AND ACTIVITY

1. The endocrine gland system seems to influence many aspects of body processes as well as its growth and development. Use your imagination and create some type of visual aid which points out the relationship of one (or more) endocrine gland to a body function or process. Be ready to explain that relationship to a classmate or the instructor.

CHAPTER 15

THE NERVOUS SYSTEM

TOPICAL HEADINGS

Introduction
  Two Functions of the
    Nervous System
Sensory Division
Motor Division
Levels of Functions

"Systems" Within the
  Nervous System
    Central Nervous
      System
    Peripheral
      Nervous System
    Autonomic Nervous
      System

The Nerve Cell
  (The Neuron)
Summary
Guides for Study
  and Discussion
Suggested Situations
  and Activities

OBJECTIVES FOR THE STUDENT: Be able to:

1. Explain the two functions of the nervous system.
2. Give three examples of ways in which man has contact with his external environment.
3. Give four examples of the body regulating its internal environment.
4. Describe the difference between the work of the sensory nerves and the motor nerves.
5. Given a list of the three general levels of function in the nervous system, describe an activity carried on in each level.
6. Defend the statement "The body is controlled by the nervous and the endocrine systems" by giving one example.
7. Describe the functions of the three parts of a nerve cell.
8. State reasons why the nervous system is known as the "control system" of the body as a whole.

SUGGESTED STUDY VOCABULARY*

sensory—afferent
motor—efferent
cerebrum
cerebral cortex
memory
cerebellum
medulla
pons

midbrain
hypothalamus
thalamus
basal ganglia
reflex
reflex arc
peripheral
autonomic

end-plate
neuron
cell body (cyton)
dendrite
axon
ganglion
myelin sheath

---

*Look for any terms you already know.

INTRODUCTION

The nervous system reaches all parts of the body; all living tissues are served by its nerve fibers. Together with the endocrine system it controls body functions.

The purpose of this chapter is to acquaint you with the work of the nervous system and the structures which carry it out.

The nervous system is complicated and perhaps the most difficult body system to understand. So many of its functions are difficult to perceive and the structures make up a complex network of interrelated pathways. Then, too, the system has some parts and features with vague qualities and locations such as "the mind," "feelings" and "thinking."

Content in this chapter is arranged from general purposes of the nervous system, to levels of function for handling nerve impulses and the various sub-systems for transmitting nerve impulses within the body. The nerve cell, its structure and function, is discussed last, with the thought that it will be more meaningful once you have some notion how the entire system functions to serve the body as a whole; however, there is nothing to prevent reading about the nerve cell first *and* last if you wish.

TWO FUNCTIONS OF THE NERVOUS SYSTEM

The nervous system is commonly thought of as a communication system with two main functions:

1. It maintains man's contact with his *external environment*. It alerts him to what is happening around him so he can respond accordingly.

2. It controls and coordinates man's *internal environment*. Action within the body is constant; sometimes more rapid than others. Examples of internal environmental controls include: peristaltic action in the small intestine, releasing proper amounts of digestive juices as needed; and contracting and relaxing muscles of every description.

The word "communication" implies an exchange of information (messages) going on in this system; there is such an exchange. It takes one set of nerves, the *Sensory Division,* to pick up and transmit messages to the brain; it takes another set of nerves, the *Motor Divi-*

sion, to return the message from the brain to control body functions. The work of each division is described below.

SENSORY DIVISION (AFFERENT NERVES → INPUT)

The sensory division of the nervous system picks up all manner of impulses by way of its many sensory receptors located in all parts of the body. For instance, things seen, heard, touched and otherwise experienced by the body including stimuli from internal structures. The nerves of the sensory division are called *afferent nerves*.

A sensory receptor actually is the supersensitive nerve end of the afferent nerve equipped to pick up "local messages" and send them on their way. Where are these messages sent? To the appropriate *level of function* in the central nervous system. For example, notice in Table 15–1, **Lower Brain Level**, that "balance and equilibrium" sensory impulses come here.

It should be remembered that while a person is conscious of some of these stimuli, many of them are relayed to some part of the brain without person-awareness because they do not call attention to themselves. The brain sorts them out for "no action now" and codes them in such a manner as to retrieve or call them up later, sometimes even months and years later.

Body unawareness may readily turn into body awareness if the stimuli persist long or strongly enough. For example, sitting in a chair may evoke no conscious body response at first even though receptors in the thighs pick up the touch sensation of the body against the chair; however, prolonged sitting ultimately calls attention to itself and the body shifts around to a "more comfortable position." If sitting continues, one becomes quite aware of the need to stand, stretch, and move about.

Some stimuli evoke body reactions automatically and completely without body awareness. Functions of internal structures proceed in an automatic, orderly, on-time basis (i.e., bile released from the gallbladder into the duodenum, gastric juice released into the stomach, progesterone produced for the

TABLE 15-1. NERVOUS SYSTEM—LEVELS OF FUNCTION

STRUCTURES INVOLVED	GENERAL INFORMATION
Higher Brain Level *Cortex of the Cerebrum* (the grey, irregular folded outer layer of the cerebrum) This layer contains approximately 3/4 of all neurons (nerve cell bodies) in the entire nervous system. This layer has direct connections with lower brain levels which in turn connect with the spinal cord and peripheral nerves. This layer has designated areas for particular functions. Figure 15-1 shows some of the areas.	The cortex stores information. With 3/4 of all body nerve cells located in the cortex, it has an information storage capacity to more than equal an electronic computer tube as tall as a skyscraper. A capacity such as this makes it possible for the cortex to carry on a vast number of independent and interrelated functions. Local nerve cells handle specific functions in a cortex area but inter-connecting pathways between and among areas make it possible to relate the functions of one area to another as the need may be. Certain cortex areas have been designated as having definite functions. Note (Fig. 15-1) the motor-sensory activities related to the leg(s), chest, arm(s), hand(s), face and tongue. Notice also designated areas for memory, vision, personality, and character; there are many more designations. Some lobes or sections of the cerebral cortex (prefrontal and parts of parietal and temporal) are not directly connected to the motor-sensory area. These areas are the "thought" areas; some locations deal with simple thought processes and others deal with deeper thought processes. When some part of the cortex is destroyed (by whatever means), some information is lost; some pathways for processing information are lost as well. Knowing this, one realizes that every portion of the cerebral cortex has its own and related functions to perform.
Lower Brain Level *cerebellum, medulla, pons, midbrain, hypothalmus, thalmus, basal ganglia.*	Some of these structures (medulla, pons) are the sites of origin for many of the 12 cranial nerves. This level of nervous system function controls the subconscious and coordinated activities essential to life processes: i.e., arterial blood pressure control, breathing, coordination of turning movements of the body (e.g., eye ball movements), balance and equilibrium. This level has structures to relay impulses to the higher brain level; one activation from this level to the higher brain level has to do with sleep and wakefulness.
Spinal Cord Level *spinal cord, spinal nerves* and their many branches and sub-branches.	The spinal cord can process a local reaction. A simple reflex can occur (see Fig. 15-2). A complex reflex can occur – there is a dividing of the sensory impulse (within the spinal cord) sending one part of it up the spinal cord to the cerebral cortex and sending the other part through the bow-like curve (arc) out of the cord via a motor neuron to the effector muscle. A reflex is a "patterned" response and serves as safety and regulating mechanism for the body; it provides immediate and automatic reaction. One commonly thinks of it in terms of burning a finger and the fast action of the body in withdrawing it from the source of heat. Other reflexes commonly handled (chiefly) at the spinal cord level are emptying the urinary bladder, bowel evacuation, and local heating and cooling of the skin. The spinal cord is a main impulse pathway between the brain and other parts of the body. Destruction of part(s) of this pathway produces disuse of body parts and can lead to death if destruction is sufficiently extensive.

uterus, peristalsis of the intestines) in a healthy body.

Ordinarily, walking is an automatically controlled body response and little thought is given to putting one foot ahead of the other except under unusual conditions (e.g., when walking on slippery surfaces, having a sprained ankle, or wearing ill-fitting shoes).

Most sensory stimuli are stored because the body is not capable of effectively responding to every bit of stimulus that comes its way. In fact, it is felt that 99 stimuli out of every 100 are coded as "no action needed now" and stored for recall. The stimuli needing "attention now" are relayed to the motor division of the brain and action results.

Under circumstances calling for immediate response, the nervous system has a built-in mechanism (reflex) to short-circuit the sensory-motor pathways to produce immediate action. The reflex arc (impulse pathway) is discussed in Table 15–1 under **spinal cord level of function.**

Memory is the term given to stored information (Fig. 15–1). Experiments continue to produce new facts about how the brain stores and retrieves information, but there is much more to be determined about memory. For instance, why is some information lost from memory after a short time while other information lasts and lasts? What triggers the brain to recall long since "forgotten" information and have it for reuse? Questions about memory and retrieving stored information have many uncertain answers.

MOTOR DIVISION (EFFERENT NERVES → OUTPUT)

The motor division of the nervous system controls body reactions (automatic or otherwise) by carrying impulses from the brain to a "function" area. The nerves of the motor division are called *efferent nerves.*

This statement is an oversimplification of a very complex process as is true of the general description of the sensory division. However, keep in mind that many rapid and continuing internal body processes must be regulated and controlled, some at the conscious level and many at the subconscious level. Likewise, remember that some reactions need to be immediate while others occur in a regulated, orderly manner.

LEVELS OF FUNCTIONS

All incoming and all outgoing stimuli are not handled in the same way or in the same location of the central nervous system. To simplify, let us divide the receiving and sending centers into three "levels of function." (1) The higher brain level, (2) the lower brain level, and (3) the spinal cord level. The work of each level of function is described in Table 15–1 in general, simplified terms; no attempt is made to deal with the complexity of the structures and the functions of these three levels.

"SYSTEMS" WITHIN THE NERVOUS SYSTEM

According to purposes served, the nervous system is divided into parts (also called "systems"). Each of these "systems is interconnected with every other "system" to make up the total nervous system. To say it another way, the nervous system is made up of separate but interconnected systems.

Three such separate yet interconnected systems are: (1) *central,* (2) *peripheral,* and (3)

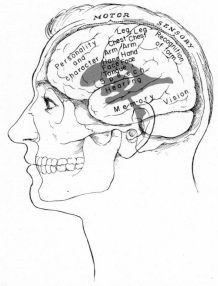

FIGURE 15–1   The brain showing functional areas. (Dowling and Jones: That the Patient May Know.)

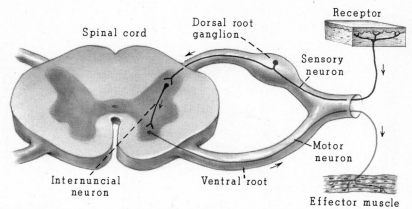

FIGURE 15–2   Simple reflex arc. (Jacob and Francone: Structure and Function in Man.)

autonomic. Each system is briefly described and Figure 15–3 shows their locations.

THE CENTRAL NERVOUS SYSTEM (CEREBROSPINAL OR VOLUNTARY)

This system includes the *brain* and the *spinal cord.*

Brain

The brain weighs about three pounds at full growth. Rapid growth takes place during the first four or five years of life and reaches full growth in about 20 years; by this time it fills the skull. The power of the brain reaches its peak much later. Figure 17–2 shows how reasoning and judgment continue to mount through the middle adult years and continue at a high level into advancing age.

While the previous information about the "levels of functions" has included names of various parts of the brain, the following subdivisions (and their general functions) are included for reference:

1. *Cerebrum*—Largest area of the brain and divided into right and left hemispheres. Has cortex centers for speech, hearing, vision, personality, character, motor and sensory areas, recognition of form, etc. Has capacity for reasoning, memory, learning, and will. Outer surface, the cortex, is gray matter about one-eighth inch in thickness.

2. *Cerebellum*—Divided into right and left hemispheres. Mainly serves as a reflex center for muscle coordination, posture, and equilibrium (walking, playing active games, dancing, etc.).

3. *Midbrain*—Third and fourth cranial nerve nuclei located here. Important cerebrospinal canal (aqueduct of Sylvius) passes through it lengthwise.

4. *Pons*—Fifth, sixth, seventh, and eighth cranial nerve nuclei located here. Chiefly a vital pathway of fibers connecting the cerebrum and cerebellum.

5. *Medulla*—All ascending and descending nerve pathways pass through it; some end here, others cross from one side to the other. Cranial nerves 9 through 12 have their nuclei in this section. It is the center for such vital body functions as temperature, breathing, heart rate, swallowing, and control of the size of blood vessel openings.

The gray matter surface of the brain is grooved or furrowed in an unordered way. It is infolded upon itself with furrows going in many directions, causing curved surfaces between the furrows called *convolutions.* By infolding the surface, more brain area is provided than if it were without furrows and simply lay flat and smooth. These furrows divide the cerebrum into special areas of function.

Two essential fluids circulate in the brain. One is the clear, slightly sticky cerebrospinal fluid that circulates in the subarachnoid spaces about the brain and spinal column to cushion and protect these organs; the other is blood. The brain cells cannot long survive without oxygen from the blood. The rich blood supply at the base of the brain comes through a network of large arteries which form the *arterial circle;* from here vessels fan out into smaller blood tubes and penetrate brain tissue to nourish it and remove wastes. Other large vessels located at the side of the head pass over the upper and outer surfaces.

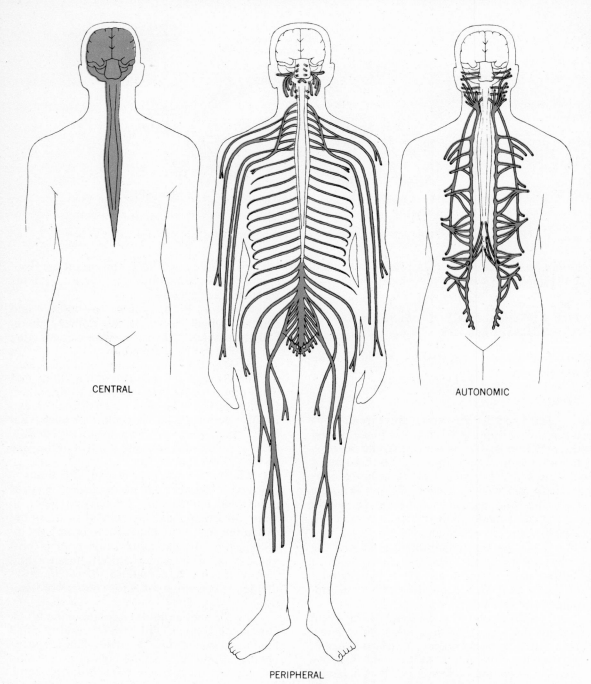

CENTRAL

PERIPHERAL

AUTONOMIC

FIGURE 15–3 The human nervous systems are pictured here in highly simplified fashion. Actually they are all interconnected and integrated with each other.

The central nervous system includes the brain and spinal cord. The peripheral nervous system reaches out to end organs, such as the retina of the eye and nerve endings on the surface of the skin. As shown in the simplified picture above, the nerve trunks originating from the central nervous system have been cut off before branching out and reaching the end organs. Many fine, complex branches are not shown.

The autonomic nervous system which parallels but lies outside the spinal cord, includes both sympathetic and parasympathetic nerves and their junctions (ganglia). The system "automatically" controls many body functions, such as breathing and digestion. (Schifferes: Essentials of Healthier Living, 3rd ed., John Wiley and Sons, Inc.)

The Spinal Cord

The spinal cord is an oval-shaped bundle of nerve pathways that extends from the medulla of the brain through the spinal cavity about 18 inches; it then begins to taper into a "horse tail" of fibers that finally ends in the coccyx area. The outer covering consists of white matter, and the center is an H-shaped core of gray matter. The cord is protected by the spinal column.

The spinal cord serves two main functions:

1. Is a pathway for nerve impulses between the peripheral nerves and the brain.

2. Has many reflex centers that serve as message switchboards (Table 15–1).

The white matter is composed of bundles of long nerve fibers (both sensory and motor) that connect with the brain, and each serves a specific function. The center core of gray matter consists of nerve cell bodies and fibers. Impulses come to the spinal cord from all body areas.

The vital importance of the spinal cord to all parts of the body is seen when it is injured, and main body functions are impaired or death results.

THE PERIPHERAL NERVOUS SYSTEM

This system is a vast network of nerve fibers consisting of the cranial nerves (12 pairs) and the spinal nerves (31 pairs). Table 15–2 shows that all but two cranial nerves (I and II) originate in some part of the brain. The spinal nerves are attached to either side of the

TABLE 15.2. THE 12 CRANIAL NERVES

NUMBER, NAME	ORIGIN	PURPOSE SERVED
I. Olfactory (sensory)	Nasal chamber	Sense of smell
II. Optic (sensory)	Retina	Sense of sight
III. Oculomotor (motor)	Midbrain	Controls eyeball muscles
IV. Trochlear (motor)	Midbrain	Controls eyeball muscles
V. Trigeminal (sensory and mixed)	Pons	Three branches: serve eye, upper portion of face, ear, lower lip, teeth, gums, muscles for chewing
VI. Abducens (motor)	Pons	Controls eyeball muscles
VII. Facial (mixed)	Pons	Facial muscles, middle ear, taste
VIII. Auditory (sensory)	Pons	Sense of hearing and balance
IX. Glossopharyngeal (mixed)	Medulla	Taste, swallowing
X. Vagus (mixed)	Medulla	Swallowing, hunger, speech muscles, breathing, heart rate, peristalsis, control of glands in stomach and pancreas
XI. Spinal accessory (motor)	Medulla	Controls muscles of neck and upper back
XII. Hypoglossal (motor)	Medulla	Controls muscles of tongue

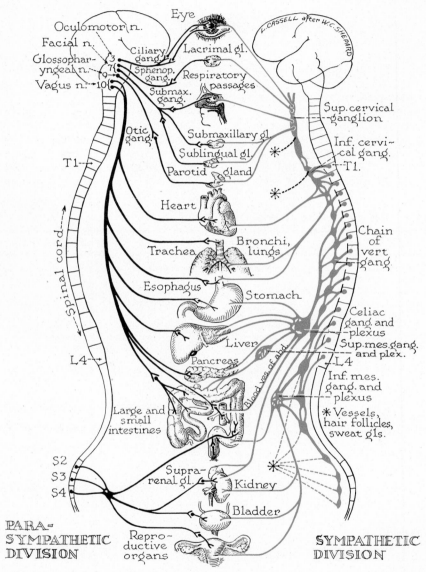

FIGURE 15–4 Diagram of the autonomic nervous system. The craniosacral division is shown in black, the thoracolumbar division in green. (King and Showers: Human Anatomy and Physiology, 6th ed.)

spinal cord in an orderly fashion serving the body from the neck down to the coccygeal area of the cord.

The work of this widespread system is to carry messages to and from the central nervous system. Some carry impulses from skeletal muscles, joints, skin, and large internal organs to the central nervous system; some carry messages back for function/action.

These nerves receive impulses or pick up their messages through *receptors* (end organs) and transmit them over sensory (afferent) nerves to the central nervous system. The return message comes back via the motor (efferent) nerves. Examples of end organs which pick up stimuli through receptors are located in the ear, in the eye, and in the nose. Receptors in various parts of the body to sense heat, cold, pain, pressure, thirst or tickling sensations are other examples.

THE AUTONOMIC NERVOUS SYSTEM (INVOLUNTARY)

The term autonomic indicates that this system acts independently of a person's will and carries on certain body functions without our control. While these nerves are sometimes considered a sub-system of the peripheral nervous system, they are very much a part of the total nervous system.

They have specific functions in governing activities of the heart, glands, lungs, digestive tract, urinary bladder, body temperature control, sweating, and arterial blood pressure (Fig. 15–4).

The autonomic nervous system has two divisions with one counteracting the actions of the other: they are the *sympathetic* division (thoracolumbar) and the *parasympathetic* division (craniosacral).

THE NERVE CELL (THE NEURON)

The nerve cell (Fig. 15–5) is the smallest functioning unit in the nervous system. It has three parts; each part performs its own unique functions. The three parts, their functions and characteristics are as follows:

1. The *cell body* (cyton) acts as a receiv-

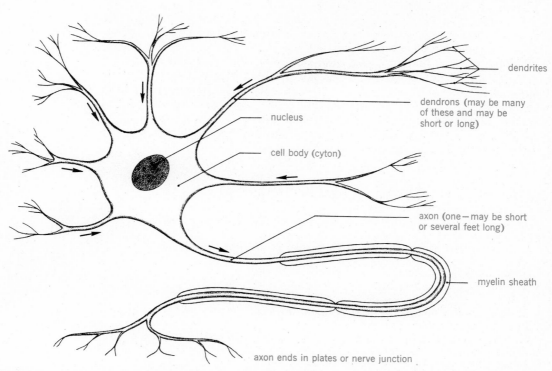

FIGURE 15–5 Nerve cell. A typical nerve cell (neuron). Arrows show the direction of nerve impulses within the nerve cell to and from the cell body (cyton). (Schifferes: Essentials of Healthier Living, 3rd ed., John Wiley and Sons, Inc.)

ing and sending center, carries on metabolism, stores energy, and contains a nucleus.

2. The *dendrite,* a branching, tree-like figure, carries impulses to the cell body via short fibers of nervous tissue. A neuron may have several dendrites.

3. The *axon* conducts impulses away from the cell body to an end-plate or to junction (synapse) with the dendrites of another neuron. A neuron has *one* axon (may be short or long) which is covered by a protective coating called the *myelin sheath.*

Due to functions in various parts of the body, neurons differ according to the size of the cell body; length, number, and size of dendrites; size and length of axon; and according to whether or not they synapse with other neurons or terminate in an end-plate. A com-

ing together or collection of nerve cells is called a *ganglion.*

Nerve tissue, unlike other tissue, has two unique characteristics: (1) *irritability,* meaning it can be stimulated, and (2) *conductivity,* meaning it can carry impulses.

A nerve, as we think of it, is actually a bundle of nerve fibers (both dendrites and axons from one or more cell bodies) with a flexible covering; the fibers themselves are separated from each other by myelin sheaths. However, nerves within the central nervous system have no protective sheath and do not have the ability to repair themselves. Neither the optic nerve nor the auditory nerve can repair itself. The ability of a nerve to repair itself depends upon which nerves are involved and the extent and location of damage.

SUMMARY

The nervous system is a communication system that connects man to his external environment and regulates his internal body activities. Information is transmitted as impulses moving along nerve cells from one to the other. While much is known about the structures and functions of the nervous system, the brain seems to provoke more questions for scientists than other structures do.

The nervous system (along with the endocrine system) controls and promotes body actions and reactions. It is a highly complicated network of special tissues reaching all parts of the body for the purpose of picking up all sorts of stimuli, relaying them to appropriate levels for sorting, and producing proper body responses.

Under certain circumstances some damaged nerve tissue can repair itself and some cannot.

GUIDES FOR STUDY AND DISCUSSION

1. The nervous system connects man to his external environment. What means are provided for this?

2. The nervous system regulates man's internal environment. How does this occur?

3. Where is the cerebral cortex? What happens there?

4. How does the spinal cord serve the body?

5. What is the work of the sensory nerves? Of the motor nerves?

6. The nervous system operates on three levels of function. What are they? What occurs in each level?

7. In your opinion, why is it said that the nervous system and the endocrine system control body functions?

8. How is nerve tissue unlike other body tissues?

9. What are the three parts of a nerve cell? What is the work of each? What does a receptor look like?

SUGGESTED SITUATIONS AND ACTIVITIES

1. The nervous system is subjected to all manner and type of stimuli during waking hours. Some stimuli require body awareness; others do not. Using your day yesterday, list in a column called "A" as many stimuli as you can that required immediate body reaction. In column "B" (to the left of column "A") assign *one* of the following terms to each stimulus you listed: (a) aware, (b) unaware, or (c) uncertain.

2. Your brain has vast storage capacity. As a student you are putting in endless amounts of bits and pieces of new information. How can you aid your brain in changing these bits and pieces into a meaningful something called "understanding"? What things can you do (or stop doing) that will help you *understand rather than merely memorize?*

CHAPTER 16

SOMATIC AND SPECIAL SENSE MECHANISMS

TOPICAL HEADINGS

Introduction
Somatic Senses
Special Senses
  Seeing

Hearing and Equi-
  librium
  Smelling and Tasting
Skin

Summary
Guides for Study and
  Discussion
Suggested Situation
  and Activity

OBJECTIVES FOR THE STUDENT: Be able to:

1. Name some of the ways the body has for receiving sensory information.
2. Explain how sensory information is useful to the body.
3. List the basic parts of the eye, ear, nose, and tongue.
4. List the basic function(s) of each of these sense organs.
5. Describe the structure of the skin.
6. Explain how the skin serves the body.

SUGGESTED STUDY VOCABULARY*

somatic	lens	anvil
auditory nerve	iris	stirrup
optic nerve	focus	eustachian tube
olfactory nerve	aqueous humor	cochlea
glossopharyngeal nerve	vitreous humor	semicircular canals
receptors	equilibrium	taste buds
retina	outer ear	epidermis
rods and cones	middle ear	dermis
cerebral cortex	inner ear	sebaceous glands
pupil	hammer	sweat glands

*Look for any terms you already know.

INTRODUCTION

Sensory information is collected from two main sources:
  1. Somatic senses.
  2. Special senses.

While this chapter is primarily concerned with the special senses and the purposes of the skin, brief mention is made of somatic senses to help you understand the wide somatic sensory capability of the human body which can be useful in giving patient care.

SOMATIC SENSES

The word *somatic* means something which pertains to the body. Somatic senses are related to special nerve tissue mechanisms that gather stimuli from all parts of the body to guide it in its minute to minute pursuits and activities. These mechanisms do *not* include the eye, ear, nose, and tongue, which are called "special sense organs" and are discussed separately in this chapter.

Somatic senses are classified and described in great detail for students of medicine; but for purposes here, a few of the more common somatic senses are listed for general information which can be extended into nursing care practices as you go along. *Such a list could include* touch, pressure, kinesthetic sensations (recognizing the position of one part of the body with relation to another, body movements, and the rate of such movements), and muscular sensations (sensing weight of objects, amount of push or pull felt). The list could also include the sensing of vibrations, tingling, pain, heat, cold, tickling and itching.

The nervous system is capable of receiving somatic sensory stimuli through a wide variety of receptors (some near the surface, others in deep tissue) and transmitting the information to various levels of function for body reaction, protection, and safety. Somatic sensations are difficult to describe in exact or precise terms, thus often making it necessary for the doctor or the nurse to ask more informational questions than the patient may think necessary.

THE SPECIAL SENSES

The body is equipped with several receptor organs which provide direct communication with the outside world. These receptor organs are commonly called the "special senses"; they include the eyes, ears, nose, and tongue. In the case of each, there is direct nerve contact with particular levels of function in the brain (by way of certain cranial nerves).

1. The eye—*the optic nerve for seeing.*
2. The ear—*the auditory nerve for hearing and balance.*
3. The nose—*the olfactory nerve for smelling.*
4. The tongue—*the glossopharyngeal nerve for tasting.*

Use Table 15–2 to locate and trace these nerves.

Seeing

The sight mechanism includes the eye, the optic nerve, and the vision area of the brain where impulses are translated (Fig. 16–1).

The eye has three layers or coats: outer, middle, and inner. As the *outer coat* reaches the front of the eyeball, it is called the *cornea* and is a clear, transparent covering over the front, forming a "picture window." The *middle coat* attaches to the eye muscles in the front and controls the movements of the *iris* and the *lens;* it contains blood vessels to nourish the eye. The *inner coat*, the *retina*, contains over a million light receptors and is made up of eight layers of nerve tissue.

Special light sensitive nerve cells called *rods and cones* are most directly related to vision. The rods pick up the light rays and send them via the optic nerve to the brain; the cones do the same task with color stimuli. The image is formed in the vision area of the cerebral cortex.

Light rays enter the eye through the pupil. The size of this opening is adjusted by the iris, which accommodates itself according to the amount of light present. The light rays are adjusted as they then pass through the lens to focus the image on the retina. The eye muscles adjust the shape of the lens to permit the proper focus. Notice in Figure 16–1 a front chamber filled with *aqueous humor* and a large rear chamber filled with *vitreous humor;* they prevent the eyeball from collapsing.

Eyes are delicate organs, but they have the protection of the bony sockets in the skull, as well as eyelids, lashes, and eyebrows. They are kept moist and continue to cleanse themselves under ordinary conditions.

Hearing and Equilibrium

Sound causes air to vibrate, and hearing results when these air vibrations are carried across the hearing mechanism to the hearing area of the cerebral cortex. The mechanism consists of the outer, middle, and inner ears, and the auditory nerve pathway to the cortex. Balance or equilibrium is controlled by this mechanism also.

Figure 16–2 shows a sectional diagram of the structure of the ear (outer, middle, and

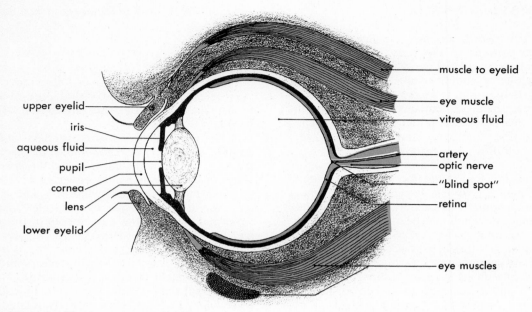

FIGURE 16-1   The human eye. (Schifferes: Essentials of Healthier Living, 3rd ed., John Wiley and Sons, Inc.)

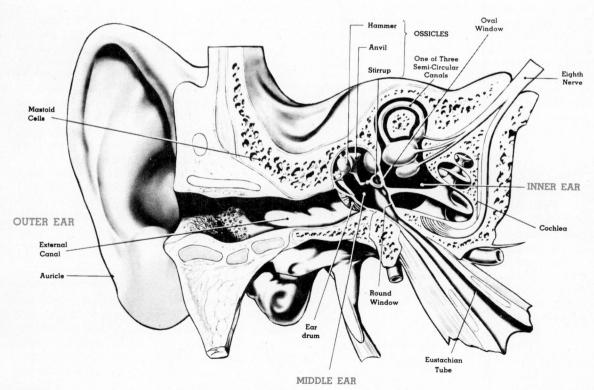

FIGURE 16-2   Sectional diagram of the human ear. (Courtesy of Sonotone Corporation, Elmsford, New York. Falkner: Human Development.)

inner portions). The *outer ear* (visible outside portion) catches air vibrations and the *external canal* guides the vibrations to the *ear drum* which vibrates as the air waves strike it. The *middle ear* starts with the ear drum and ends at the membranes stretched across the *oval and the round windows*. Within this chamber the following occurs: As the ear drum vibrates, it sets into motion a chain of three small bones (hammer, anvil, stirrup) which transmit the vibrations to the oval window membrane and the round window membrane.

Within the middle ear chamber is a safety device to maintain equal pressure on the ear drum. In Figure 16–2, locate the eustachian tube passageway; it leads from the middle ear to the pharynx. A sudden pressure change—as when one rides into higher or lower altitudes—will cause the ears to feel full and ear drums will crackle or pop. Once the tube has equalized the middle ear pressure with the outside pressure, the discomfort is gone.

The *inner ear* starts at the membrane of the round window and includes an irregular bony structure made up of three areas: cochlea (snail-shaped), semicircular canals (three), and vestibule (area between). This set of bony passageways contains membranes and fluids. As the *stapes* vibrates the oval window membrane, the fluid on the other side is set into motion. Hair cells on some membranes vibrate and touch other membranes to stimulate them. The pitch of the sound determines which hair cells and membranes will be set into motion; this is the way we can distinguish different pitches. Figure 16–2 shows that the

eighth nerve (auditory) branches and attaches to the cochlea and to the semicircular canals and the vestibule.

Equilibrium or balance is controlled by the inner ear. For example, when the head is tilted to one side, the receptors in the semicircular canals feel the fluid move and are thus alerted to a changed position of the head. Another equilibrium control area (two small sacs) is located next to the cochlea.

Smelling and Tasting

Smelling and tasting sensations are related. To smell something being chewed influences one's taste of it. In reverse, recall how tasteless food seems when nasal passages are closed due to a head cold.

The structures of the smelling mechanism and the tasting mechanism are much easier to locate and describe than are their functions (Figs. 16–3 and 16–4). Tasting and smelling are believed to be reactions to chemical processes.

The olfactory nerve is the receptor for odors; it is a small bulb of nerve tissue with dendrites very close to the surface of the mucosa and it is generally thought (though there are some differences of opinion) that these dendrites select different smells by first dissolving the odor in the mucus secreted by the mucosa (Fig. 16–4). This would make it a chemical process. Once the receptor(s) sorts out the odor, the stimulus is relayed to the appropriate area of the cerebral cortex.

The tongue as it relates to digestion is dis-

FIGURE 16-3 Taste bud and section from tongue showing where it is found. (Jacob and Francone: Structure and Function in Man.)

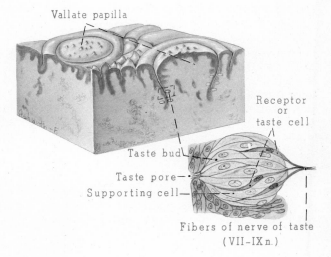

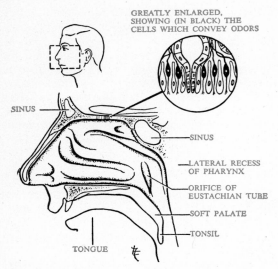

GREATLY ENLARGED, SHOWING (IN BLACK) THE CELLS WHICH CONVEY ODORS

SINUS

SINUS

LATERAL RECESS OF PHARYNX

ORIFICE OF EUSTACHIAN TUBE

SOFT PALATE

TONSIL

TONGUE

FIGURE 16-4   The nose. (Miller and Burt: Good Health, 2nd ed.)

cussed in Chapter 11, The Digestive System. Mention is made there of the nerve endings in the tongue called *taste buds*. Figure 16–3 shows a taste bud and its related nerve fibers. Notice the tiny opening called the *taste pore;* to pass through this small opening, substances must be in solution. The solution entering the pore sets up the chemical reaction which relays the stimulus to the appropriate area of the cerebral cortex.

Various parts of the surface of the tongue are known as "taste centers"—the front tip is the "salt and sugar" area, the sides are the "sour" area, while the back portion of the tongue is the "bitter" area. Yet there seem to be taste relationships among all areas.

The sense of taste has much to do with a person's appetite. If fatigue of the olfactory nerve and the taste buds occurs (this happens, though the reasons for it are not clear) or the odor is unappealing, a person is not interested in food. If this is prolonged, malnutrition can result.

THE SKIN

The skin serves the body in several essential ways. While this chapter shows the rela-

tionship of the skin to somatic senses, other functions are included.

Functions of the skin (other than sensory) include:

1. *Protection.* The entire body is covered to prevent invasion by microorganisms and to protect deeper tissues from drying out and being injured.

2. *Excretion.* The sweat glands throw off some moisture and salts.

3. *Absorption.* The skin has limited ability to absorb anything. Lotions and ointments made of certain compounds can penetrate the skin barrier. Basically, however, under normal conditions the skin remains a stopping place for most substances.

4. *Regulation of body temperature.* This is a major role of the skin and is closely associated with body metabolism, the circulatory system, and climatic conditions.

Sensory function of the skin is one of its most important purposes even though receptors are scattered over the body in a somewhat uneven manner. As a body covering, it provides a vast source of somatic sensations ranging from the slightest tickling sensation to severe pain depending upon the intensity of the stimulation. The greater the stimulation, the more receptors involved and the greater the pain. Other sensations include warmth, cold, and touch.

Figure 16–5 shows the two main layers of the skin: the *epidermis* and the *dermis*. You will notice nerve receptors for *warmth, pain, cold,* and *touch* in the corium portion of the dermis while the receptor for *deep pressure* is embedded in a deeper layer of fatty tissue. All of the sensory nerve sensations in the skin travel to the spinal cord and ultimately to the cerebral cortex where they are consciously experienced if the stimuli are strong enough to call attention to themselves.

There are several other facts about the skin worth remembering. It has great ability to reconstruct and renew itself. It resists outside interference such as bumps and bruises, thus offering protection for underlying tissues. Sebaceous glands produce oil to lubricate the skin, and sweat glands help regulate body temperature by the evaporation of perspiration. Accessory features of the skin are hair and nails. Figure 16–6 illustrates the structural relationships of hair follicles, oil glands, sweat glands, and the structure of the finger nail.

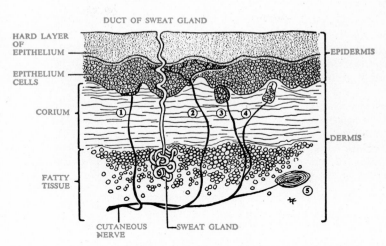

FIGURE 16-5   Structure of the skin. The numbers indicate the sensory nerve endings: 1, warmth; 2, pain; 3, cold; 4, touch; and 5, deep pressure. (Miller and Burt: Good Health, 2nd ed.)

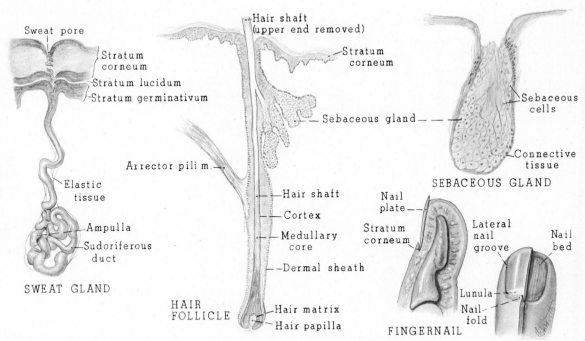

FIGURE 16-6   The appendages associated with the skin. (Jacob and Francone. Structure and Function in Man.)

SUMMARY

Body activities are guided by sensory information collected by the somatic senses and by the special senses.

Somatic sense receptors are located in a wide variety of places. Some are near the body surface, others in deep body tissues. These receptors gather stimuli which guide the body's minute to minute activities.

The special senses provide direct communication with the outside world through receptor organs: the eye, the ear, the nose and the tongue. Each receptor organ has a direct nerve pathway to the brain.

The close relationship of the sensory mechanisms to the brain is a unique communication system which guides man in relation to his external and internal environment.

GUIDES FOR STUDY AND DISCUSSION

1. Why does the body need both somatic and special senses?
2. Why is it that somatic sensations are sometimes hard to describe?
3. How many special senses are there? What is meant by saying each one has a receptor organ?
4. Thinking of the skin as an envelope for the body, what purposes does it serve?

SUGGESTED SITUATION AND ACTIVITY

1. Sensory information, whether somatic or special, is related to other body systems. Make a list from your present knowledge of these various system relationships. Be ready to explain any one of the relationships you include in your list. Your explanation might even include how you feel this information could be useful to you as you care for patients.

HUMAN DEVELOPMENT: THE LIFE SPAN

The purpose of this unit is to help you understand that during a lifetime, a human being undergoes many changes. Man matures slowly, and his body functions decline slowly. All this time the human is learning how to live with others and adjust to circumstances.

The newborn comes from his fluid environment, within the uterus, equipped with some survival mechanisms to start the long process of humanization. The culture or society he enters begins immediately to make its particular demands and exert its influences. Cultural patterns and the expectations of society surround its members from birth on. Even after death, the body is disposed of in a manner prescribed by that culture.

Man develops (grows, matures, ages) according to his gene-code and the influences of his environment. It is difficult, in many instances, to say whether it is heredity or environment that causes a person to develop the way he does. Often it is a combination of both working together or against each other.

The word development, as used in this unit, includes both physical growth and all maturing processes because the two words *growth* and *development* overlap and are difficult to separate.

As a practical nurse, you will use knowledge of normal development to help you understand why patients of different ages and at different stages of life behave as they do. You will also use knowledge of changing body structure and function to make sounder judgments in providing nursing care.

CHAPTER 17

THE NATURE OF
HUMAN DEVELOPMENT

TOPICAL HEADINGS

Introduction
The Journey of a
   Lifetime
What Influences Hu-
   man Development?

The Several "Faces"
   of Human Develop-
   ment
Summary

Guides for Study and
   Discussion
Suggested Situations
   and Activities

OBJECTIVES FOR THE STUDENT: Be able to:

1. Describe each of the various periods of human development from conception through old age.
2. State five reasons why the life span is lengthening.
3. Describe the relationship between "genes in the chromosomes" and "heredity."
4. Restate this definition in your own words, "personality is selfhood."
5. Explain the meaning of the terms physical, mental, social and emotional development.
6. Compare the terms in the preceding item to show if and how they are related.

SUGGESTED STUDY VOCABULARY*

maturation	childhood	environment
conception	puberty	personality
prenatal	adolescence	emotions
neonatal	adulthood	social relations
infant	chromosome	memory
toddler	gene	reasoning
preschooler	heredity	judgment

*Look for any terms you already know.

INTRODUCTION

You might ask, "Why study the nature or the distinguishing qualities of human development?" To side-step the long and involved answer, some understanding of the factors which "shape" a person within and without helps

one accept other people better. A little insight into what one might expect from a newborn infant, an elderly neighbor, an adolescent, or a preschooler helps a practical nurse provide more intelligent nursing care.

It would be much easier to learn about the nature of human development and maturity if humans were more alike and more predictable — more like "peas in a pod" — but they are not. In the past, it has been common practice to set up averages for people in different age groups and compare individuals against these averages. Now we realize that this is a little risky because too many things can and do influence individual size, features, intellect, temperament, actions, and maturation. Thus, if any such comparison is made, it must be very general and not specific.

This chapter is designed to furnish some general information about the factors which influence human development and maturation. Keep these factors in mind as you study the other chapters in this unit; they will help you understand what "shapes" people in the various stages in life.

THE JOURNEY OF A LIFETIME

At the turn of this century, a lifetime journey was not as long as it is now in this country. People died much earlier. Today, reaching the age of 100 is not a rarity. It is thought by some that people will live 125 years or more in the future and that this will not be a rarity either.

There are many reasons for the lengthening span of life. Among them are concern for better and proper nutrition; the means to prevent certain diseases from spreading; the means to cure certain diseases once they have started; the means to arrest disastrous results from some diseases that cannot be cured but can be halted; and the means to remove, repair and replace defective body parts.

Reference Points

While the journey is a continuous one from conception to the last moment of life, man has given labels to various groups or "like clusters" of people along the span for purposes of study and identification.

The following list of life span reference points includes commonly used labels:

Conception — "the beginning"; when the ovum is fertilized.

Prenatal — existing before birth.

Neonatal — pertaining to the first four weeks after birth.

Infant — designates the young child from birth or from the neonatal period until he assumes the upright position (12 to 14 months).

Toddler — pertains to getting around, though clumsily (12 to 14 months).

Preschooler — the very active period prior to starting school when the human is filled with questions (three to five years).

Childhood — actually means from infancy to puberty, but commonly means the period when the child starts school until puberty (6 to 11 or 12 years).

Puberty — the state of first being able to bear offspring; sexual maturity is reached (marked by menstruation in female).

Adolescence — sometimes called "that part of life's journey when a human is crossing over from childhood to adulthood" (12 to 20 years).

Adulthood — the state of being grown to full size and strength; coming to full development (maturation). This period is usually subdivided into the *young adult, middle-aged adult,* and the *elderly adult.* The human undergoes a pattern of changes once full size, strength and maturation have been reached. So marked are the differences between the young adult and the elderly adult that the oldest humans are often referred to as "senior citizen," in the "golden years," "elderly," or "aged."

WHAT INFLUENCES HUMAN DEVELOPMENT?

As you know, human development starts at "the beginning" when the ovum of the female is fertilized by the sperm of the male. At that point a few decisions concerning the offspring have already been made. For example, the sex of the child is determined; the sperm carries "the code" (in a gene) as to whether the offspring will be male or female. Blood type has been determined and so have the color of the eyes and the hair. "The code" in the genes can get mixed up causing "inborn errors."

Heredity

Particular qualities or traits are handed down from parents to offspring through the genes in the chromosomes. This transmission is called *heredity.* Figure 17–1 gives you

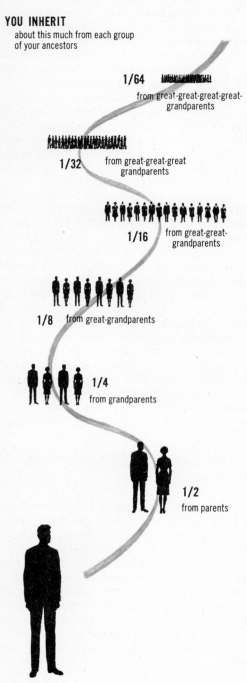

YOU INHERIT
about this much from each group
of your ancestors

1/64 from great-great-great-great-
grandparents

1/32 from great-great-great
grandparents

1/16 from great-great-
grandparents

1/8 from great-grandparents

1/4 from grandparents

1/2 from parents

FIGURE 17-1 Galton's law (Sir Francis Galton worked out this scheme of ancestral heredity) indicates where the individual's traits come from. (Schifferes: Essentials of Healthier Living, 3rd Ed. John Wiley and Sons, Inc.)

an idea of how far back your ancestors have influenced your qualities and traits.

There is a gap in knowledge today; it is difficult to determine what is actually handed down from ancestors and what is the result of environment. For the most part, however, it is felt that heredity has much to do with the structure of the body and its physical form (e.g., features, stature or natural height). This is why physicians pay attention to the size, build, and so forth, of parents when assessing the growth of an offspring. If he discovers a faulty metabolism, for instance, he looks back to the parents; did one parent have an "inborn error" in metabolism?

Environment

The term environment, as used here, is the sum total of all external conditions (e.g., climate, housing, food, air, health and living practices, interaction with people — the family, at school, at work, at play, "on the street") and influences affecting the life and development of the offspring. When you pause to think about this definition you can begin to see why it is not easy to neatly separate heredity and environment. In fact, they are all but inseparable in many instances when trying to determine what actually was responsible for a certain growth pattern. For example, when an abnormality appears, the physician needs to consider if this is something that has been inherited, if it is the result of environmental causes, or if it is a mixture of both.

Criminal behavior is one type of development that puzzles those who study it. What traits are inherited? Can internal instability be passed along through the genes? What part do outside (environmental) influences play in the criminal's development? These questions are raised merely to give you an idea of just how inseparable heredity and environment can be.

Personality and Behavior

The word "person" within the term personality means individual identity. Personality means the qualities the individual possesses, his identifying characteristics which set him apart from all others. The term "personality" is used loosely when someone says, "She has a good personality" or "He has personality plus." They mean that the person they are talking about is pleasant to be with or that he radiates more than the "usual" amount of self to others. Actually, it is more nearly correct to think of personality as selfhood or inner man. Inside qualities constitute one's personality; they have a way of showing through in behavior and it is this behavior (reflection of inner self) that others see and respond to.

Heredity plays a part in personality and behavior. Many studies have been done to show that the body's metabolic functioning affects behavior. If "the code" in the genes established the body chemistry process to begin with, then one sees a direct line between heredity and behavior (personality). Couple this inner chemical activity (e.g., it may cause irritability, ability or inability to stand up under stress, dullness, boredom, alertness, sadness, happiness, fatigue, extra energy, etc.) with what is happening environmentally and you can begin to understand why some people seem to "come through" as they do. It should be mentioned, however, that all personality traits are not clearly influenced by environment. It has been found that despite changes in the environment certain qualities or traits do not seem to change much, if any. So far one might conclude that, generally speaking, personality is influenced by heredity, environment, and social culture in varying degrees and extents.

Disorder and Disease

It is easy to understand that if some part of the body malfunctions, the rest of it may not develop as it should. Of course it depends upon where the malfunction was located as to how extensively the body would be harmed or its normal growth pattern blocked. For example, let us assume that the malfunction had to do with the body's inability to use calcium correctly, and the bones did not develop as they should. This situation could rather drastically influence physical development. Or, in the instance of a disease that infects the brain tissue of a five-year-old and destroys part of its usefulness, this child would live without full use of the part(s) of the brain that controlled speech and thought processes.

The lack of proper nourishment influences human development. This lack may be due to not eating (or being unable to eat) an adequate diet or it may be due to the body's inability to properly use the diet even if it is adequate. In either case, the cells suffer from malnourishment and are unable to perform as they should. Growth can be stunted, energy can be limited, and a person's mentality and outlook on life can be affected.

Mention should be made of the fact that the mother's state of health during pregnancy can influence the growth and development of the embryo and fetus. Her lack of a proper diet, insufficient oxygen supply, having infectious diseases (e.g., German measles), and taking certain drugs during pregnancy are some examples of mother factors which can influence the development of the offspring.

THE SEVERAL "FACES" OF HUMAN DEVELOPMENT

While it is impossible to actually separate a person into physical, emotional, mental, and social parts, it is possible to discuss them, remembering that in "real life" these several "faces" of development are occurring together and are companion developments.

Physical Development

Growing takes place in a pretty orderly fashion from conception to maturity, but it is by no means at the same rate among people, even among children of the same family. The pattern is an individual affair; this makes it a little misleading to say that a "normal" time for such and such to occur is at such and such an age. Each individual has his own "genecode" which makes up his inheritance, his own set of environmental factors, his own selfhood and his own chances for disease or disorder to alter his growth pattern.

During the journey of a lifetime, the human grows from one cell to a "full-term" baby in nine months, to a fast-growing young child, to a fast-growing older child, to a developing adolescent who matures and arrives at adulthood at full size and full strength. Adulthood is the longest span of the journey. During this period the body continues to alter with the passing of time until in the elderly adult one sees certain marked changes in physical appearance and endurance. No place along this span is there a point where physical development is the same for everyone. There are several landmarks, however.

Emotional Development and Social Relations

Emotions are feeling tones that well up inside as a response to someone, something, or some experience and they prompt the individual to behave in certain ways. An inner adjustment is made in the feeling tones as the autonomic nervous system responds by adjusting blood pressure, heart beat, and so forth, and the individual demonstrates his feelings through his behavior. For example, notice the behavior of a person meeting an old and dear friend unexpectedly. There is warmth in the voice and facial expression; there are smiles, laughter, and maybe even tears. Or observe the person who flies off the handle; his feeling tones have welled up within him to the point where he lashes out with a verbal blast. Silence and a blank stare may accompany the hearing of a "shocking" incident. Some people "keep their feelings to themselves" and show few, if any, outward signs of emotional reaction.

Only a few built-in feeling tones are present at birth. Excitability is a major one. The newborn is quiet or restless, calm or agitated, but he soon begins to respond to hunger, love, and affection and develops different types of crying patterns to communicate his needs.

Some emotional responses come from happenings. For example, a person is not born afraid of dogs; if he has such a fear, he has learned it through some type of experience.

As the human grows and matures in physical stature, he likewise grows and matures emotionally. When a person behaves like someone much younger, demonstrating "inappropriate" behavior, a common remark is, "He's never grown up" or "He's emotionally immature." Emotional stability is demonstrated when a person is able to cope with stress in a manner that does not upset his "balance" and perspective.

Social relations are the ways humans behave in their physical encounters with each other. Social behavior, itself, has many "faces" that change as the person changes physically, emotionally, and mentally.

When a person is said to be *sociable*, what is meant is that by his nature he is inclined to be friendly, cordial, and companionable. The term *unsociable* means the opposite; the person does not seek companionship and is apt to avoid physical encounters unless necessary. Such words as inhospitable, self-sufficient, unfriendly, withdrawn, hermit are examples of terms others use in describing the person who seems to prefer his own company. Many times such labels are unfairly used through ignorance. A snap judgment is made on the basis of too little information or insight. It is fair to say that many people are both sociable and unsociable, meaning that at times they seek companionship and at times they seek their own company according to their particular needs.

During the journey of a lifetime, a person develops as a "social creature" going through all manner of changes in his mode(s) of interacting with and encountering others. These

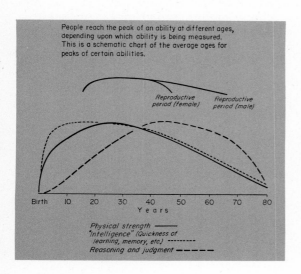

FIGURE 17-2   Mental and physical faculties at different ages. (Dowling and Jones: That the Patient May Know.)

changes are perhaps most noticeable during the early years of life but, for each person, a social pattern emerges over a lifetime that is uniquely his.

Mental Development

This important aspect of human development has been studied for many years; often the study of intellectual development has been viewed along with the physical-emotional-social aspects of development even though scientists have sought to separate it.

Today, the search is even more direct. Efforts are being made to gain more specific knowledge about thought processes, to see how they relate to understanding and to the ability to call up one's understanding in order to solve problems in new situations.

It is a known fact that the first few years of life are filled with finding out what words are for. The world around the child fills him with questions that he continues to ask. But mental growth (memory, quickness of learning, reasoning, and judgment) continues for years; reasoning and judgment "ripen" well along in the span of life. Study Figure 17–2 and notice the differences and similarities among the various curves representing mental and physical faculties at different ages.

SUMMARY

Human development has been likened to a journey stretching over the span from conception through old age. This span is lengthening for good reasons and with this gradual change one can expect that we will continue to learn and know more about what happens to a person—all aspects of him—as he lives and lives on.

The development of an individual is a very gradual process. Months and years bring changes; some are easy to detect and others are not. These changes occur in anatomical structures, physiological processes, mental powers, and emotional capacities in an individual way for each person. Heredity and environment influence how a person develops and matures.

GUIDES FOR STUDY AND DISCUSSION

1. In your opinion, what are the most important factors contributing to an increased life span?
2. Why do you suppose there are "reference points" across the life span?
3. Give an illustration of one environmental factor which can influence development and be ready to explain why.
4. What is heredity? What does it influence?
5. What is personality? What things can influence an individual's personality?
6. Disease and disorder can influence development. Think of some instance of this that you know about. Be ready to share it with your classmates.

SUGGESTED SITUATIONS AND ACTIVITIES

1. Prepare some visual aid (poster, drawings, etc.):
   a. showing as many types of emotional responses of the human face as you can.
   b. showing a variety of human social relation situations.
In each case use all age groups.

2. Prepare a chart you can use to keep track of the *main* ideas you gather (from reading, discussing, listening, and thinking) about human development and changes across the span of life. Here is a sample:

Life Span Changes

Life Span Reference Points	Physical	Emotional	Social	Mental
1.				
2.				
3.				

CHAPTER 18

LIFE BEFORE BIRTH AND DURING THE FIRST YEAR

TOPICAL HEADINGS

Introduction	The Newborn	Guides for Study and Discussion
The Beginning of Life	The Infant	Suggested Situations and
Growth Follows a Plan	Summary	Activities

OBJECTIVES FOR THE STUDENT: Be able to:

1. Tell how the ovum is fertilized.
2. Trace the journey of the fertilized ovum to its implantation.
3. Explain what mitosis has to do with the beginning of life.
4. Describe the environment of the embryo-fetus by telling what it provides.
5. Describe, in general terms, the orderly way in which a normal offspring develops to full term.
6. Show by giving examples the meaning of the phrase "growth follows a plan."
7. Name the inborn abilities of the newborn.
8. Describe how the human begins to socialize and become a family member.
9. Describe how the human begins to verbalize and communicate with others.
10. Compare the abilities of the infant during the neonatal period with those of the infant at 12 months.

SUGGESTED STUDY VOCABULARY*

ovum	sperm	chromosome
gene	heredity	implantation
embryo	fetus	vernix caseosa
amniotic sac	amniotic fluid	cell differentiation
prenatal	neonatal	infant
mitosis	fontanel	reflexes

*Look for any terms you already know.

INTRODUCTION

Life begins when the single sperm cell fertilizes the ovum. Mitosis starts at once but it takes "nine months" of dividing and subdividing of cells to bring the offspring to full-term.

As this process goes on, cells become specialized; some become muscle, some bone, some blood, and so forth. Science does not yet know what controls cells to make them change in substance and structure so that specialization can take place. This is called *cell differentia-*

tion; when it becomes known what controls it, medical science will know a great deal more about body functions than is known presently.

As pointed out in the preceding chapter, parents and ancestors contribute to certain traits and characteristics of the offspring through the genes in the chromosomes. Normal conditions in the uterine environment also contribute to normal growth of the fetus, while "abnormal" conditions in that environment may contribute to "abnormal" fetal development.

The focus here is normal, not abnormal, fetal development, except to say that when the "gene-code" gets mixed up or when the environment in the uterus is not what it needs to be, "inborn errors" can result.

The purpose of this chapter is to help you gain some general understanding of the beginning of life and of the fact that a newborn is actually nine months old at birth. Review Chapter 13, The Reproductive System and the Urinary System, to help you recall how reproduction is initiated, what sperm is, and under what circumstances an ovum becomes fertilized.

THE BEGINNING OF LIFE

You will recall that each male germ cell contains 23 chromosomes and so does each female egg (ovum); therefore, when brought together at the time of fertilization, the newly fertilized ovum has a total of 46 chromosomes when it starts to subdivide; this makes it a normal cell. If for some reason the number of chromosomes is not 46, the orderliness of cell division and cell differentiation is disrupted. At the present time little is known about the structure of chromosomes except that they have two parts: genes and protein.

The genes control heredity; they carry the "coded" information that determines sex, features, color of eyes and hair, structural form, and inborn strengths and weaknesses. Aside from controlling heredity, genes also control the work and the reproduction of all body cells *before birth and after*. One is apt to overlook the fact that the work of genes is ongoing throughout life. The normal body stays in cell balance (new cells replace missing cells) with the assistance of genes in the chromosomes.

The gene has to be very small because it is estimated that more than a million reside in a nucleus of a human cell. The electronic microscope has made it possible to study the structure of the gene and some of its functions within the cell. This helps scientists to understand more about how we inherit characteristics and qualities from our parents (strengths and weaknesses) and what goes wrong when people fail to develop in a normal way. Such information may some day help prevent mental and physical deficiencies.

Implantation

Embryo means the earliest stage of development; in the human this stage lasts seven to nine weeks. After a single sperm penetrates and fertilizes an ovum, cell growth and reproduction (cleavage) begin in a rapid and orderly fashion. What regulates this orderliness (some cells having one kind of structure and function and other cells other kinds of structure and function) is still a mystery. From the time of fertilization, the human embryo takes about 72 hours to reach the uterus (Fig. 18–1). During this time the first cell has redivided many times until it is a solid mulberry-like mass of cells.

Within three or four days after the fertilized ovum has reached the uterus, *implantation* takes place. This means that the fertilized ovum is embedded in the inner wall of the uterus. It has become a small bladder-like structure with fluid between the inner cell mass and the outer layer of cells. The outer layer of cells produces fingers of tissue (villi) which attach themselves to the inner uterine wall where they make contact with the rich supply of uterine blood vessels. It is sometimes called the "feeding" layer because it provides the means for getting nourishment and oxygen to the embryo. Gradually the structure becomes embedded in its own nest in the uterine wall.

The bladder-like structure and fluid represent the beginning of the amniotic sac and the amniotic fluid which house the embryo-fetus until birth. The amniotic sac with the amniotic fluid is often called "the bag of waters." It is within this sac that the embryo-fetus lives and moves about. The fluid provides protection and an even temperature for the embryo-fetus. It is thought that the fetus drinks the amniotic fluid.

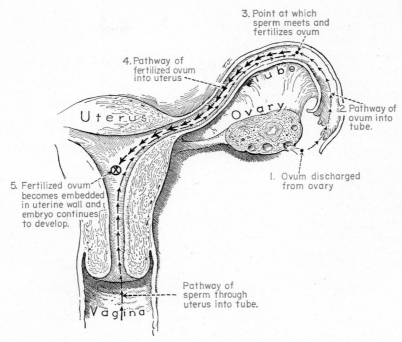

3. Point at which sperm meets and fertilizes ovum

4. Pathway of fertilized ovum into uterus

2. Pathway of ovum into tube.

Uterus

Ovary

5. Fertilized ovum becomes embedded in uterine wall and embryo continues to develop.

1. Ovum discharged from ovary

Pathway of sperm through uterus into tube.

Vagina

FIGURE 18-1   Fertilization of the ovum. (Dowling and Jones: That the Patient May Know.)

The outer cells multiply quickly to form a stalk or means by which the young embryo is nourished.

1. *First Month.* Within a month, the cell mass has developed into a minute embryo, but this body form has little resemblance to the body of the newborn, even though there is early evidence of eyes, ears, and extremities. The placenta begins to form. It is a nearly round flat cake about eight inches across when fully developed in three months. The placenta is firmly attached to the inner wall of the uterus where it serves as a connection between the mother and the fetus via the umbilical cord. It is a "service center" providing the fetus with nourishment, oxygen, antibodies, hormones and removal of wastes.

2. *Second Month.* By eight weeks, body form is becoming human. Eyes and ears are beginning to show definite positions, the face is forming, and so are extremities. The head is disproportionately large for the rest of the body. The placenta is well established.

3. *Third Month.* The embryo is now called a *fetus;* all organs and major structures have been formed. The head (though still large) is erect; nasal bones are forming, and so is the palate. Fingers and toes show beginning

nail formations, and external genitalia reveal the sex. The placenta attains full growth.

4. *Fourth Month.* Fetal movements are active by the end of this month; heart beat can be heard with a stethoscope, and the face looks distinctly human. Hair has appeared on the scalp and the body.

5. *Fifth Month.* By this time the skin is less transparent. Nails are evident, as are eyebrows and eyelashes. A cheesy protective substance called *vernix caseosa* covers the body.

6. *Sixth Month.* The fetus weighs more than a pound and is long and thin, with wrinkled (little fatty padding) red skin. The nostrils are open, but the eyes are not.

7. *Seventh Month.* Fine hair covers the thin, red body. Movements are fairly strong. If delivered prematurely, the fetus has a weak cry. Weight is little more than two pounds.

8. *Eighth Month.* From the seventh month through the eighth month the fetus gains in size and all but doubles its weight, but because there is little fatty padding, the skin is somewhat wrinkled.

9. *Ninth Month.* The fetus weighs about five pounds, and the skin, though red, begins to lose the wrinkled appearance as subcutan-

eous fat develops. The body resembles that of a full-term fetus as it continues to round itself out, creating folds in the skin, and as it becomes pink in color. The fine body hair has disappeared, but hair growth tends to be heavy. By the end of intrauterine life, the fetus weights about seven and a half pounds.

Twins and Multiple Pregnancy

Identical twins result when a single fertilized ovum divides into two cell masses and each becomes a separate embryo. *Fraternal* twins result when two separate ova are fertilized. Each embryo has its own membranes and placenta. Multiple births, other than twins, are thought to develop from either multiple ova or a single fertilized ovum subdividing itself into several cell masses.

Prenatal Period

The development of the embryo-fetus within the uterus is called the *prenatal period*. The mother's needs are influenced during pregnancy; these adjustments are discussed in Chapter 52, Nursing the Mother.

GROWTH FOLLOWS A PLAN

Growth before and following birth proceeds according to a plan. Figure 18–2 is a good "12-month yardstick" for behavioral development the first year and the following laws of growth give you some notion of how the growth plan proceeds.

1. *Growth is orderly and continuous.* The body develops according to its "gene-code" messages. Pairs, such as arms or legs, grow at the same rate; while there are periods of faster and of slower growth, all parts of the body grow in proportion to all other parts.

2. *Growth starts with simple actions and continues to complicated actions.* The newborn does little except eat and sleep. He cannot move around on his own; he stays put. From being picked up and fed, he grows up and can walk to a table and feed himself with utensils.

3. *Growth* (development of muscular control) *proceeds from head to foot* and from near to far (see Fig. 18–3).

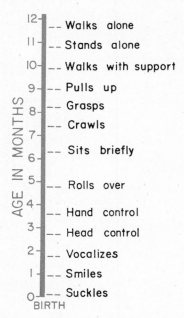

FIGURE 18-2   Behavioral development of the infant during the first year of life. (Guyton: Textbook of Medical Physiology, 4th ed.)

4. *Each individual has his own development pattern.* Comparison at a given age can be general, but not specific.

5. *Growth means over-all development.* This includes all parts of the humanizing process (physical, emotional, mental, and social).

THE NEWBORN

The first four weeks after birth are known as the *neonatal period* — a time when the body begins to work as a whole. The word *infant* refers to the young child either from birth or from the neonatal period until he assumes an upright position which is about 12 to 14 months. During this time remarkable changes occur in his appearance, his personality, and his social development.

Physical Appearance of the Newborn

The newborn's skin is wrinkled and red and may be partially covered with *vernix caseosa*, the cheesy substance that covered the fetus in the uterus. His head seems too large for the rest of him and his eyes are closed most of the time. The neck is only a fold of skin. The newborn's flat and stubby nose and his receding chin make it easy for him to get his mouth next to the nipple to suck.

Skeletal bones are soft, and the "soft spot" (fontanel) on the head is visible. The body soon begins to round out and birth wrinkles disappear as the newborn begins to gain weight.

Activities and Abilities of the Newborn

Two main "diversions" of the newborn are sleeping and eating. Born with the ability to suck, the newborn (with nose and chin out of the way) "roots" about with his lips and tongue in search of the nipple.

Science is showing us that the newborn can do more than was thought possible. For example, studies show that even the fetus responds (with faster heart beat) to musical

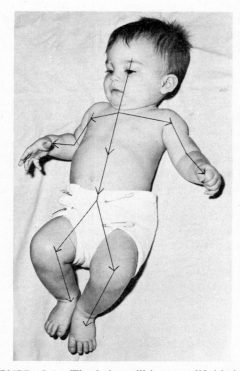

FIGURE 18-3 The baby will learn to lift his head and do "push ups" to look around before he learns to scoot around on his buttocks and then walk. (Marlow: Textbook of Pediatric Nursing, 4th ed.)

sounds; shortly after birth (within minutes to hours) the newborn "follows" sound by turning his head. He is found capable of certain eye movements, even though the eyes do not seem to focus well at first.

The newborn has built-in mechanisms called *reflexes* which help him get started as safely as possible. For instance, he can sneeze and yawn (increases oxygen supply), and hiccup and vomit. He has a sense of balance and responds to sudden position changes by pulling up his legs and extending his arms. Loud, sudden noises cause him to jerk and cry.

It does not take the newborn long to turn and lift his head and to use his arms to try and lift himself when he is lying on his stomach. In addition to his ability to suck, he can swallow and breathe while sucking. He cries when hungry, sighs and grunts, and smiles after a fashion. He responds to love and body contact.

From the standpoint of "what he knows," he has everything to learn; but he soon starts. Very quickly he knows his mother's voice, and responds to her presence and to being picked up and held. He comes to like and want this person to be near and pay attention to him.

THE INFANT

When one thinks about a person's life spanning sixty, seventy, and eighty years, it is easy to imagine that there must be periods of significant growth and developmental changes. The first year is one of these periods. The infant undergoes tremendous changes in size, habits, personality, and abilities. The brain grows very fast. Keep in mind that each individual grows at his own rate; there is no set time for things to happen.

Race makes a difference in infant maturity. For instance, it is known that the American black infant is more advanced in physical development than the white infant (e.g., sitting up, tooth development).

Some of the significant changes in the infant during the first year include:

1. *Physical size.* The body length increases 50 per cent; the weight triples.

2. *Ability to move about.* Getting on one's feet for the first time is a slow, gradual

process for the human. Earlier in this chapter it was pointed out that the development of muscular control proceeds from head to foot; this is why, almost from the start, the infant begins to lift his head while in a prone position. Then, in about three or four months, he sits with support; in another eight or ten weeks he sits alone and begins to move himself about on his hands and knees and on his buttocks. By the time he is about ten or eleven months old (some sooner, some later) he stands up with support. The infant gradually learns to stand alone, takes the first faltering steps, and proceeds to walk in an unsteady manner with help. By the time he is twelve months old, he is usually on his feet with the assistance of furniture or a helping hand. He can sit down by himself from a standing position.

3. *Other signs of physical development.* Somewhere between the fifth and eighth months teeth begin to erupt so that the "one-year-old" has several teeth (usually six). During the latter months of the first year, the infant is using his hands to hold and transport bits of food to his mouth; he enjoys helping to hold the cup or the spoon but would just as soon eat everything with his fingers and is not at all particular whether all the food gets into his mouth. He uses his hands to hold and manipulate (move, poke, squeeze, throw) objects.

4. *Nourishment.* The infant grows very rapidly during the first year of life because he is catching up with body development. Thus his caloric intake is high considering his size. In the beginning the human digestive tract handles liquids only—in small amounts and frequently. Then strained foods are introduced in the diet. Sometime between three and six months, solid foods are added and by the end of the first year the infant is eating three meals a day and having nourishing snacks between.

5. *Bowel control.* This comes earlier than bladder control; it can be started as early as the eighth month but some authorities agree that it is perhaps better to wait until after the first year. Bladder control takes much longer, two years or more to be reliable.

6. *Behavior undergoes noticeable changes.* The infant has to find his niche or place in the family. Remember that his mind is a clean slate at the beginning. This means that he begins with the sights and sounds around

him and proceeds to absorb them and make some meaning out of them. The mother in his life, at this point, is the center of his world; her voice and presence are reassuring. She comes to represent coddling, affection, security, and such other "creature comforts" as cleanliness, dry diapers, and a full stomach.

The infant can vocalize from the beginning with his grunts, squeaks, and cries. But it is not long before he extends these abilities and adds to them. By the second or third month he has "classified" his crying so that others can tell whether he is hungry, has pain, or wants attention.

For the first month or two, the infant is not too sociable; he is chiefly interested in his needs (as he feels them) for food and for sleeping in comfort. Gradually he comes around and starts (by the second or third month) to smile when coaxed and when another person smiles. This soon leads to laughing aloud and cooing in his own language.

During the fourth and fifth months he begins to show definite signs of sociability. He initiates the smile and "talks" his own babbling language and begins to want people around. In fact, he wants and demands attention. Smiling and crying are not too far apart now and for some time to come.

Along about the fifth or sixth month the infant really begins to know who is his family and who is a stranger and shows some concern in the presence of strangers (e.g., he might be afraid, shy, refuse to have anything to do with them, and even cry or scream) which continues for some months.

By the eighth or ninth month vocalizing moves from babbling to some distinct sounds such as "ma, ma, da, da" as he tries to imitate others. He soon outgrows these sounds and replaces them with "Mama and Dada." By the time he is busy learning to walk he may know a few other words including his name, but at this point he is usually much more interested in getting around than in learning new words. Figure 18–4 shows four types of abilities the infant possesses at 12 months.

The human is capable of showing anger, love, frustration, jealousy, and other emotions including concern for himself by the time he has lived one year. He is completely dependent upon others to help him meet all his daily living needs; high on this list is the need for love and attention.

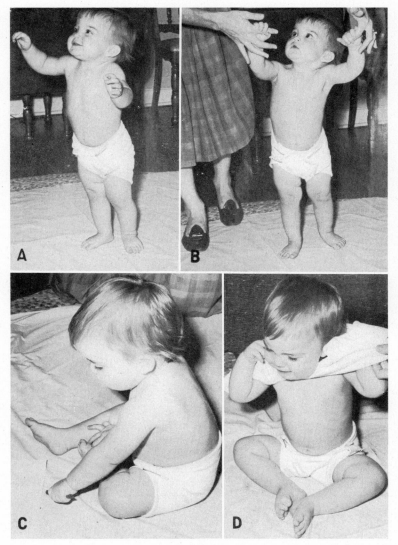

FIGURE 18–4   The 12-month-old infant. A, stands alone for a moment or possibly longer; B, walks with help; C, holds a crayon adaptively to make a stroke, and can mark on a piece of paper; D, cooperates in dressing, puts arm through sleeve. (Marlow: Textbook of Pediatric Nursing, 4th ed.)

SUMMARY

Growth and development from conception to an infant's first birthday is an amazing process, individualized for each offspring. Cell differentiation is cell specialization which is responsible for the various types of body tissue. The embryo grows to become a fetus. The fetus matures to full term in nine calendar months (prenatal period); therefore, one could say an offspring is nine months old at birth, but age is counted from the time of birth on.

Growth and development follow a plan: they are orderly and continuous; they start with simple actions and proceed to complicated actions; development of muscular control proceeds from head to foot and from near to far.

The neonatal period is the first four weeks after birth and represents a time when the body begins to work as a whole.

Each day in the life of the infant creates change (growth and development); however, one has to observe the infant in periods of time to see noticeable differences. Growth and development of the infant is generally discussed in terms of what happens month by month during the first year after birth. While the practical nurse does not use the details of this developmental growth in carrying out her responsibilities in Roles I and II, she does need a general understanding of what occurs.

GUIDES FOR STUDY AND DISCUSSION

1. Cell division and cell reproduction start with fertilization of the ovum. Describe the appearance and location of the cell mass approximately 72 hours after fertilization. When does implantation take place?

2. The embryo becomes a fetus when all organs and major structures have been formed. When does this occur? What might the mother begin to experience soon after?

3. The fetus is suspended in amniotic fluid in the sac. How does it meet its needs for nourishment and air? How does the fluid protect the fetus?

4. Imagine yourself helping to care for a newborn. Knowing his state of complete dependency upon others, what would be his first needs?

5. When does an infant begin to be sociable? How does he show his sociability?

6. In your opinion, what are the most remarkable signs of human development during the first year after birth? How will this knowledge help you as a practical nurse?

SUGGESTED SITUATIONS AND ACTIVITIES

1. Prepare a two minute talk on one of the following topics:
   a. The infant finding his niche in the family.
   b. The infant's struggle to get on his feet.
   c. How the infant's diet changes from birth to his first birthday.
   d. Progress in vocalizing the first year.

2. Make a poster showing how eating and food requirements change during the first year.

3. Write a meaningful sentence or two for each of the nine daily living needs of the one-year-old infant.

CHAPTER 19

CHILDHOOD

TOPICAL HEADINGS

Introduction
The Toddler—Years
   Two and Three

The Preschool Child—
   Years Four and Five
The School Child—Age
   Six to Puberty
Summary

Guides for Study and
   Discussion
Suggested Situations and
   Activities

OBJECTIVES FOR THE STUDENT: Be able to:

1. Give three reasons why growth and development may vary from one toddler to another.
2. Describe the general physical developments during the life of the toddler, the preschool child, the young school child and the "middle-aged" school child.
3. Compare the socializing traits among the four groups of children listed in objective 2.
4. Predict how these traits might influence behavior when hospitalized.
5. Predict how these traits might influence your nursing actions when these children are your patients.

SUGGESTED STUDY VOCABULARY*

heredity
environment
toddler
enuresis

defecation
attention span
mimicking
muscle coordination

prepuberty
puberty
irritability
solitude

*Look for any terms you already know.

INTRODUCTION

The term *childhood* covers the period between infancy and puberty. While the number of years is inexact because each person develops at his own rate, childhood generally includes the span from two to eleven or twelve when puberty is usually underway. During these nine or ten years there are some distinct time clusters when the human develops in certain ways and to certain extents; this is why childhood is artificially divided into parts, each with a label.

For purposes of learning about the various growth changes during childhood, the content in this chapter is divided into three parts: the toddler, the preschool child, and the school child to puberty. As you study the childhood years, notice what happens to physical, mental, emotional, and social develop-

183

ment patterns. It will help to compare one age cluster with the next to see what happens to the human as he moves along.

Keep in mind that descriptions of behavior and other developments associated with a certain year(s) are inexact because growth, by nature, is not the same from one person to another; therefore, what is "normal" for one may not be normal for another at the same age. Too many factors (heredity, environment, disease, etc.) influence human development to give it any more than a general likeness from one individual to another.

THE TODDLER—YEARS TWO AND THREE

To toddle is to walk with short uncertain steps. The term *toddler* covers the period from the first birthday to the third one when the human is learning how to remain steady on his feet and walk without falling. The period starts at about 12 to 14 months; by the third birthday the toddler is most capable of getting where he wants to be. Very often it is where he should *not* be. He explores everything he can in his quest to find out "what" and "why." A safe environment is essential because the toddler needs to explore and does so constantly. (See Fig. 19–1.)

Physical Development and Appearance

During years two and three, physical growth is about half as fast as it was during the first year. The round chubbiness of infancy gradually disappears as the body shows some changes in posture and proportion (the back is straighter, the chest and shoulders are broader, and the abdomen protrudes less).

About midway or so in this period, the toddler has a full set (20) of temporary teeth.

Eating and Sleeping Habits

With teeth for chewing and with muscle coordination developing, the toddler becomes more independent at the table. By the age of two he holds his spoon and manages fairly well to get food into his mouth. The toddler also learns to hold a glass and drink by himself.

Getting ready for bed begins to be a

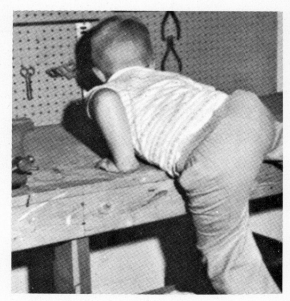

FIGURE 19-1 The aggressive toddler goes after what he wants. (Brisbane: The Developing Child. Charles A. Bennett Co.)

chore; the toddler makes all types of demands in the process. He takes regular naps or rest periods and sleeps about 12 hours at night.

Toilet Training

Toilet training is related to muscle development. Usually it is started about the end of the first year; an anxious mother might try to start it earlier. The control of defecation (bowel movement) usually comes sooner than bladder control (urination). The attitude of the mother can play a part in how soon a child is toilet trained. If she is severe and anxious, the child senses this and often is slower in his training. By the time a child is four to four and one half years old he has learned both bowel and bladder control.

Behavior and Socialization

"Getting on one's feet" represents a move toward independence and individuality. The toddler wants to do things for himself; often this means mimicking his parents or others about him. He has much to find out and busies himself doing just that—exploring all manner of things and places. In the process of finding out, he does not appreciate being stopped or told "no." He is negative at this period and uses the word "no" himself but does not know its real meaning. Trying to be independent, the toddler becomes very upset when he is blocked in his efforts. But he is not quite sure about his dependence and independence since very often he says "no" but proceeds to do as asked, thinking no more about it. His attention span is short.

Parents need to remember that a toddler does not know right from wrong and can let him help do things to fulfill a request. For example, if toys are to be put away at bedtime and not all kept in the crib with the child, he can help put them away.

Years two and three are vocabulary building years. You recall the "clean slated mind" at birth and what a vast amount of things there are for the child to learn and learn about. As soon as the human begins to ambulate, he expands his "world." Everything within reach needs to be touched, examined, and inquired about. The toddler has an endless list of questions and is always asking, "What?" "Why?" One of the things that provokes him (and causes him to cry) is that he does not have enough words at his command and cannot always get his point across. This fact forces him to put words into sentences—awkward sentences sometimes at first—but nonetheless, as he continues to try, his vocabulary grows. By this time the brain is almost adult size.

The toddler begins to relate to members of his family. He likes to do it on his own terms, as a rule, but learning how to conform and meet others half way is part of the discipline that goes along with being a toddler. By mimicking, he learns how to go about washing his face, cleaning his teeth, and so forth; grooming can become a messy pursuit, especially if explored on his own. Mimicking is very much a part of the toddler's activity (see Fig. 19-2).

A CAPSULE VIEW OF THE TODDLER

Physical Development

Growth is slower than during infancy.
Height (two years) about 32 to 33 inches.
Weight (two years) about 26 to 28 pounds.

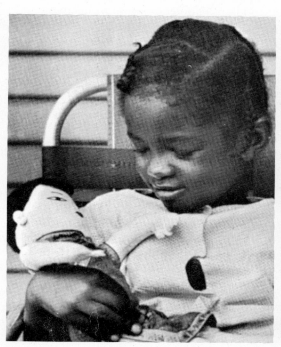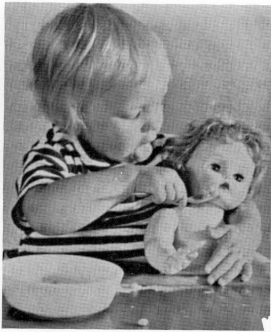

FIGURE 19-2   The toddler is a mimicker. This habit develops imagination and should be encouraged. (Brisbane: The Developing Child. Charles A. Bennett Co. Courtesy Jean Garner, Photographer.)

Pulse (two years) range 90 to 120 per minute.

Respiration (two years) range 20 to 35 per minute.

Has a full set (20) of temporary teeth.

Body changes from a round, chubby appearance to having a "growing up" look. Back is straighter, chest and shoulders proportionately larger, abdomen protrudes less. Brain all but reaches adult size.

Muscle Control

Large body muscles coordinate fairly well.

Small muscle coordination just beginning: scribbles, turns pages, stacks up blocks, etc.

Becomes more sure-footed; runs, jumps, climbs, falls easily.

Climbs stairs up and down by holding onto something; turns door knobs, light switches; pulls cabinet doors open; holds spoon.

Toilet training is progressing.

Eating is a messy experience but the toddler does not mind; he mixes play and exercise with getting food into his mouth.

Behavior and Socialization

Interest span is short.

Becomes negative as independence is sought.

Does not know right from wrong.

Does not have enough words to express himself.

Constantly exploring "his world."

Begins to relate to family; mimics parents, brothers and sisters.

Does not particularly like to share what he thinks is his; therefore, does not get along too well in a group with the same ideas; prefers one playmate at a time.

Enjoys games with action: peekaboo, jack-in-the-box, etc.

Finds excuses for delay at bedtime.

THE PRESCHOOL CHILD—YEARS FOUR AND FIVE

From the third through the fifth year, the human perhaps learns as much as he does in any other two-year-period in his life span. While physical development proceeds and there are some noticeable changes in the child, his mental, emotional, and social development are even more pronounced.

Life for the preschooler is filled with "learning." He has ways of learning that make sense to him; perhaps this is why he learns so fast and so much. He learns by doing—for himself and by himself; he tries to find out where he came from and what his body is like. The preschooler is a great imitator; this improves his imagination, creativity, and intellect.

Physical Development and Appearance

By the time a child is around five, he is about twice as long and about five times as heavy as he was at birth. Boys are somewhat taller and heavier than girls, but there are no set standards for either sex. This is apparent when you see a group of four- or five-year-olds together; they vary considerably in height and weight regardless of sex.

The body is now slimmer and straighter; the chest is flatter and the shoulders are wider. Legs are straight now, having lost the bowed shape or the knock-kneed appearance of the toddler. The neck begins to lengthen and the head no longer seems to rest atop the shoulders.

Eating and Sleeping Habits

The preschooler may or may not have a "good" appetite; a lot depends upon how busy he is at mealtime or how much he is imitating other family members at the table. He does have food preferences which may make it difficult to maintain a balanced diet.

Muscle coordination has developed so that he can handle a spoon very well and begins to use a fork to advantage. His eating habits are neater than the toddler's, but he does not pay too much attention to table niceties unless he is reminded or is imitating someone who does.

Because the preschooler is so active and uses his body energy in so many ways, it is not uncommon for him to need a midday nap besides 11 or 12 hours of sleep at night. Delaying tactics at bedtime diminish during this period. The preschooler comes to know the meaning of bedtime and enjoys a "goodnight story."

Behavior and Socialization

Play, imitation of others, and freedom fill the life of the preschooler. In the main, small groups get along fairly well together and even though anger and frustration surface easily, all is soon forgotten and play continues.

It should be mentioned that the four-year-old generally has more difficulty getting along than he does later because he is bossy, likes to argue, is more selfish, and tells tall tales. But he just as quickly seeks approval and love from his parents and is himself loving and affectionate. He changes "best friends" often.

By the age of five, the preschooler is more settled and has a noticeably longer attention span which keeps him occupied with one thing for long spells, instead of flitting from one thing to another and another. He is more realistic and tells things as they are rather than "making believe" as does the younger preschooler. In the main the five-year-old seems

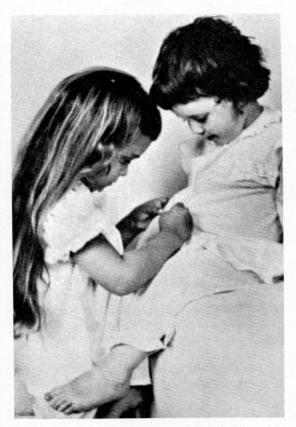

FIGURE 19-3 The five-year-old is helpful and is even protective of younger brothers and sisters. (Brisbane: The Developing Child. Charles A. Bennett Co. Courtesy of Jean Garner, Photographer.)

to get along fairly well by himself and with others, follows directions, is friendly, helpful, and looks to adults for approval (see Fig. 19-3).

Toilet training is completed during this period, usually by age four. Enuresis (bed wetting) may occur if boisterous play precedes going to bed.

The child's ability to use words and express himself improves tremendously as he explores his "bigger world" asking "what" and "why", and finds things out for himself through pictures, television, stories, conversation, and participation in all types of activities inside the home and out.

A CAPSULE VIEW OF THE PRESCHOOLER

Physical Development:

The body grows to become twice its length at birth.

Body weight increases to about five times that of birth weight.

Boys are somewhat taller and heavier than girls.

Body is straighter and slimmer; abdomen less pronounced and the neck begins to lengthen.

Legs are straight and stance is firm.

Muscle Control:

Play activity develops large and small muscle control.

Learns to help with his personal hygiene, dressing, and undressing.

Rides a tricycle, climbs, jumps, runs, dances, moves forward and backward.

Uses a scissors; draws "after a fashion" trying to copy pictures, figures, numbers; laces shoes; buttons and unbuttons clothing; pulls a zipper.

Feeds himself using a spoon and starts using a fork and a knife (to spread with but not to cut).

Toilet training completed.

Behavior and Socialization

Three-year-old
Plays simple games; gets along with others.

Imitates family living habits and activities.

Speaks in short sentences to himself and others.

Feels secure in the family.

Has a good memory.

Has a vocabulary of about 900 words.

Inquires about everything; tries to keep track of days, events, i.e., "Is this tomorrow?"

Is affectionate and loving.

Four-year-old

Tattles, is bossy, quarrelsome, argues, is selfish, loving, and affectionate.

Fickle to friends and has "new ones" every little while.

Tells imaginary tales to make-believe companions or to others.

Likes to talk things over.

Likes to run away.

Does not like restrictions.

Has a vocabulary of about 1500 words.

Is toilet trained.

Five-year-old

More settled and quiet.

Interest span is longer; stays with a project and/or goes back to it.

Has less fantasy; tells things as they are.

Follows directions; is reliable and wants approval.

Friendly; makes friends easily, trusts others.

Sensitive about criticism and not getting approval.

Has a vocabulary of about 2100 words (notice what has happened since age three).

Talks a great deal.

Counts; knows coins and days of the week.

Is a good errand-runner.

THE SCHOOL CHILD—AGE SIX TO PUBERTY

The cluster of years from age six to puberty is (1) period of many changes in human development, and (2) period that cannot be boxed in with exactness because puberty is an individual experience, coming at different times for different people.

To help understand the gradual phasing-in of sexual maturity, study Figure 19–4. This information helps account for many physical changes, certain emotional developments, and changing social patterns common to this period of life.

To further understand this period, the term *prepuberty,* meaning the few years leading up to puberty, could be substituted for the term *childhood* in Figure 19–4. *Puberty* means the period marked by the beginning of secondary sex characteristics (distribution of hair, breast size changes, voice changes, hip contour changes, beginning of menstruation). Puberty leads into the adolescent period discussed in the following chapter.

No doubt, you can already predict that "the school child" undergoes considerable development from the age of six to puberty. This fact makes it necessary to describe him at various stages after we look at this period in general.

It is a period of discovery; of finding out about people outside the family (up to now family has been the child's world, so to speak); of exploring things beyond home; and of beginning to compete with others (in school and out) and get along with them (surviving the process in good shape).

The "six to puberty" child moves considerably toward independence; but he alternates between wanting independence and not wanting it. As new things happen and he has decisions to make, he gradually learns to cope with people and events, although it is still a common practice to turn to family and home for sympathy and understanding. This aspect of behavior changes somewhat during prepuberty and puberty, as pointed out later.

Physical growth meanders along for awhile and then takes a rapid spurt. Appetites follow suit. The endocrine glands account for this stepped-up change in size and appearance. All traces of babyhood disappear, including the beginning replacement of temporary teeth. Children undergo stress, at times, especially if teased about their appearance. The child-body begins to resemble the adult-body.

A CAPSULE VIEW OF THE YOUNG SCHOOL CHILD (YEARS SIX TO EIGHT)

The young school child is a *busy* person.

Physical Development

Uneven growth of body parts begins.

Growth is slow and gradual (only four or

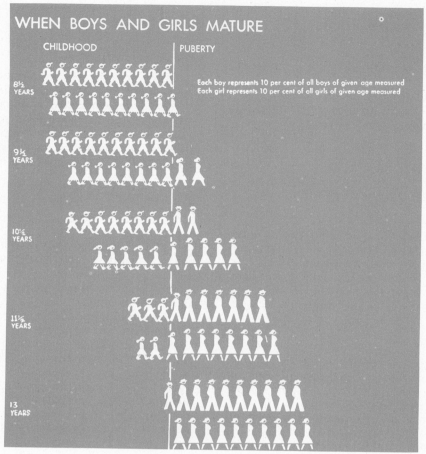

FIGURE 19-4 Notice how early in childhood sexual maturation starts, how long it takes, and the difference in rate between boys and girls. (Breckenridge and Vincent: Child Development, 5th Ed.)

five pounds and two or three inches per year) until prepuberty.

Body develops a gangly, awkward appearance; legs and arms seem too long and hands grow bigger.

Large muscles better developed than small ones.

Permanent teeth start replacing "the temporary twenty"; incisors are replaced first.

Facial features (nose, chin, mouth) begin to lose their "small child" appearance.

Muscle Control

Constant physical activity (running, climbing, jumping) develops the large muscles.

Boys pay close attention to "how strong" they are.

School and hobby work improve small muscle control.

Sense of balance improves with fence walking, bicycle riding, hop scotch, etc.

Behavior and Socialization

Companionship of children his own age is sought.

Both sexes share in group activities, but generally prefer their own sex for play.

Enjoys his own company now and then.

Curiosity is high about everything.

Wants to learn to do things well; is able to stay with and return to a project.

Enjoys mystery and high adventure in play and in stories.

Wants to measure up to competition and expectations.

Is helpful at home and at school.

Begins to take care of own grooming; girls are better about this than boys.

A CAPSULE VIEW OF THE MIDDLE-AGED CHILD (PREPUBERTY TO PUBERTY)

Being a middle-aged child has its problems as well as pleasures. Everything points toward growing up; experiences occur fast and seem to be endless. Changing body chemistry accounts for much of the up and down mood swing common during puberty.

Physical Growth

Body growth speeds up faster for girls than boys; period for out-growing clothes.

Sex organs begin to mature; girls mature about two years ahead of boys.

Secondary sex characteristics begin to appear.

Adult look continues to erase more childhood characteristics. Boys have broader shoulders (still lanky) and a flat abdomen; girls beginning to develop roundness in the hips and breasts.

Permanent teeth complete except for wisdom teeth.

Muscle Control

Boys are especially interested in developing athletic skills and building muscles.

Small muscle control is refined; mechanical skills such as assembling models (cars, planes, boats) and sewing, knitting, painting, drawing, and playing musical instruments develop small muscle control and intellect, too.

Behavior and Socialization

The move is toward assertive independence.

The "telling-all" to parents tends to change; loyalty is to the "club" or "clan" until a situation becomes overwhelming and then there is a retreat to parents for security, love, and understanding.

Selecting friends is a definite trait now.

Interest in the opposite sex begins; shyness, self-consciousness, and boisterous activity are all ingredients in mixed groups.

Frustration, anger, wonderment, irritability, solitude, happiness and unhappiness take turns in the behavior pattern.

Concern for personal appearance heightens; much time is spent in "getting ready."

Daydreaming and goal-setting are common.

The prepuberty child seeks companionship with older children.

SUMMARY

No other part of the life span provides the opportunity for freedom, inquiry, wonderment, and whole person involvement that childhood does. Each segment of it has its own type of physical development, explorations, frustrations, learning challenges, and humanizing processes; each makes its contribution toward an individual's growing up physically, emotionally, and mentally.

What is important for the practical nurse in childhood development is to have general ideas of the gradualness of the development and how the child reacts to himself, his family, and others as he joins society. These general ideas will serve you well when helping the sick child to meet his needs.

GUIDES FOR STUDY AND DISCUSSION

1. What are the chief differences between the toddler and the preschool child? The similarities?

2. What are the chief differences between the preschool child and the child who has been in school a year or two? The similarities?

3. When is the trait of *stubbornness* quite pronounced in childhood?

4. What are the most noticeable differences between a four-year-old and a five-year-old?

5. What is meant by the terms prepuberty and puberty?

6. Why does the 11- or 12-year-old girl seem to have her ups and downs?

7. What are the characteristics of boys around the ages of nine and ten?

8. In your opinion, what is the most interesting thing about human development during childhood?

9. When does the search for independence start in childhood? How is it demonstrated?

SUGGESTED SITUATIONS AND ACTIVITIES

1. Visit a nursery school. Observe children in organized and free play activities, and during nourishment and rest periods. While observing, raise in your own mind a question or two that you would like to discuss later with classmates. See what information you can gather ahead of time to help in the discussion.

2. Select a child (any age) and prepare some type of poster or chart to show how his particular daily needs are met.

CHAPTER 20

ADOLESCENCE

OBJECTIVES FOR THE STUDENT: Be able to:

1. Defend this statement: "Adolescence is that part of life's journey when a person is crossing over from childhood to adulthood," by giving one example.
2. Explain, in general terms, the main physical, mental, emotional, and social developments during adolescence.
3. Give five examples which show that males and females mature at different rates during adolescence.
4. Identify several adolescent traits which influence daily living needs.
5. Compare the physical development of an adolescent with that of a child during prepuberty.
6. Predict how the traits of adolescence might influence behavior during hospitalization by giving two examples.

SUGGESTED STUDY VOCABULARY*

adolescence	behavior	menarche
frustration	endocrine forces	scrotum
stress	self-conscious	testes
values	testosterone	penis
beliefs	estrogens	larynx
development	progesterone	peer group
maturation	embryonic development	conformity

*Look for any terms you already know.

INTRODUCTION

Life never stops changing people. Some periods bring tremendous developments as during the first year of life, while other periods seem to bring little change. During the entire life span there seems to be no period when the person experiences more physical and emotional changes than during adolescence.

Adolescence has been called "that part of life's journey when a person is crossing over from childhood to adulthood"—a journey of

192

several years which is noted for steady physical development and emotional see-sawing, leading to maturity. During this time the human is trying to find his place in society, square away his beliefs and values, and declare his independence while reaching for adulthood. This is a frustrating and stressful period for offspring and parent alike. It has not always received the attention it does at present; in fact, child development as a whole is a fairly new concern of society, a concern that has arisen since the century started.

This chapter is designed to help you understand what are some of the traits of the adolescent so that your nursing action in assisting him might be more realistic for you and the patient.

WHO IS THE ADOLESCENT?

Popular use of the term *adolescent* refers to the person taking the journey from childhood to adulthood. Specifically, it refers to the individual from his development of secondary sex characteristics to full body development and personal maturity (ability to assume responsibility in society). The starting and the completion ages are inexact due to individual differences. The cause of the onset of puberty is still a mystery to medical science, but it does come to each human. Generally speaking, by age 12 or 13 adolescence is underway and ends in the late teens or early twenties when full body development is reached.

Development is a process and no period presents the individual with more "process perplexities" than adolescence. Humans develop and mature slowly; the process ebbs and flows throughout life. Adolescence is marked by a see-sawing of feelings and actions as the body advances toward full development. During this period it is almost impossible to separate what is a physical development and what is an emotional-social development since one so much affects the other.

This period has many common labels, i.e., teen years, growing-up period, coming of age, years of decision, the difficult years, and so forth. Regardless of the label, it brings about many physical, emotional, and social changes that result in a certain amount of confusion and frustration for the offspring and the parents. As a developmental period, it is a dif-

ficult one to experience and to understand, but as stages go in life, it is one of the most important of human experiences.

Review the developments of the prepuberty period and compare what happens then to what occurs during adolescence. Notice the changes that occur and how they influence behavior.

DEVELOPMENT DURING ADOLESCENCE

Boys and girls share many of the same feelings and reactions during adolescence. While the rate of maturation differs between the sexes, as pointed out later, endocrine forces (notably sex hormones) within the body prompt it to develop physically and mature emotionally. Keep in mind that endocrine forces also call a halt to physical growth and help the body adjust to its new plateau of maturation. The "gene-code" predetermines some factors about the individual's size and build. Environment, nutrition, and disease or disorder influence development in great measure also.

Rapid and Uneven Physical Growth

A boy is apt to be wearing adult-sized shoes before wearing adult-sized trousers. This is to say that feet grow faster (in proportion) than the body frame. In fact adolescence is a time of uneven growth; a time for the body to "catch up with itself" and become well-proportioned. Body appearance is lanky as arms (and hands) and legs (and feet) take on new size, often leaving the owner with a feeling of awkwardness. Large muscles develop better and faster than small ones.

The rate of growth is noticeable, but may not be as fast as the spurt of growth during prepuberty and early puberty. The adolescent is quite aware of his growth and appearance, often feeling self-conscious and clumsy during this "catching up" period.

Production of the male sex hormone, *testosterone*, increases rapidly as puberty starts and continues throughout life but at a diminishing rate after about age 35 to 40. Testosterone is often called the "youth hormone" because it is so essential to body growth and particularly muscle development. It is vital to male development from the embryonic period to the end of life. It accounts for the rapid enlargement of the scrotum, penis, and testes during adolescence as well as other male secondary sex characteristics; for growth of the larynx (change in pitch of voice); and for increased thickness of the skin, secretions of the sweat and sebaceous glands and increased metabolic rate. Muscle and bone development likewise are related directly to this hormone.

Of the two female hormones, *estrogens* and *progesterone,* estrogens influence the growth of sex organs and many of the secondary sex characteristics. During puberty the production of estrogens in the female increases greatly (the amount is 20 times as much as during childhood) and estrogens are responsible for the increased size of external and internal sex organs. They also influence the growth of the lining of the uterus and the fallopian tubes. Bone growth is controlled by estrogens; they are responsible for causing bones to cease growing sooner in females than testosterone does in males. Thus, the male continues to grow a couple of years after the female has stopped growing. Estrogens do not seem to influence hair growth (except pubic) the way testosterone does in the male, nor to thicken the skin of the female to any great extent. They do make the skin more vascular, causing the female to bleed more readily than the male. Estrogens are related to metabolism (slight increase), fat deposits in breasts and other tissue, and somehow control the change of the pelvis from a narrow funnel shape to a broad oval shape. Why this change occurs is not clear at present.

Progesterone promotes the functions of the lining of the uterus, especially as these functions relate to the implantation of the fertilized ovum; it readies the lining to receive the ovum and nourish it. Progesterone also influences the lining of the fallopian tubes by promoting secretions which nourish the ovum en route to the uterus. It helps the breasts develop so they can secrete milk, but is not directly responsible for milk secretion.

As you can see, sex hormones are very necessary factors in both male and female development. The changes they bring about (in fairly rapid order) often make the adolescent self-conscious. To avoid embarrassment and to handle his or her sensitivity, the adolescent seeks privacy during personal hygiene routines, often asserting independence about this in the family situation.

Rate of Maturation Differs Between Sexes

To *mature* is to come to fullness of development: *maturation* is the process of coming to fullness of development or the continuous change leading to full development.

The male and the female do not develop at quite the same rate during prepuberty and adolescence. Figure 19–4 shows the girl starting to move ahead of the boy as early as ages eight to nine. She continues this "front" position until about age 16 to 18 when the boy overtakes and surpasses her. During this time, certain female characteristics appear, as do certain male characteristics.

The Female Reproductive System: Signs of Maturation

Process takes about five years.

Menarche appears first.

Ovum production begins about one year later.

Uterine maturity follows ovum production.

Distribution of hair: pubic hair begins to appear as breasts enlarge and axillary hair follows.

External and internal sex organs increase in size.

Contour of breasts, hips, pelvis: breast development is one of the first signs of sexual maturation; hips widen as pelvis broadens and becomes rounded.

Height increase levels off as sexual-maturity is reached; consequently the female (usually) reaches maximum height sooner than the male because sexual maturity occurs a year or two sooner.

The Male Reproductive System: Signs of Maturation

Process takes about seven years.

Sperm production at about age 15 or 16.

Distribution of hair: pubic hair growth accompanies testicular growth or follows it; axillary hair growth is followed by facial hair; abdominal hair extending up from pubic area (diamond-shaped pattern) generally occurs in late adolescence.

Growth of scrotum, testes, penis: growth (sometimes rapid) of male sex organs starts early in puberty and continues until late teens or early twenties; height increases accompany these changes.

Contour of breasts, hips, pelvis: breast changes occur; enlargement may be temporary (lasting a year or so) or permanent; hips are narrow in contrast to shoulders; pelvis is narrow and funnel-shaped.

Voice deepens as the larynx grows, most noticeably after about age 15.

Behavior and Socialization

Friendship is a key word in describing one of the emotional needs of the adolescent (Fig. 20–1). From puberty through adolescence, peer (own group) relationships see-saw back and forth but always are present.

Early in puberty the "clan or club" drive is apparent; groups form easily. Boys join with boys and girls with girls. Best-friend relationships are present too, but they can change fairly fast; this is apt to occur more among girls than boys. Girls have more noticeable ups and downs during this period.

Interest in the opposite sex makes itself known early. At first it is apt to be a boisterous, show-off time for boys when they openly

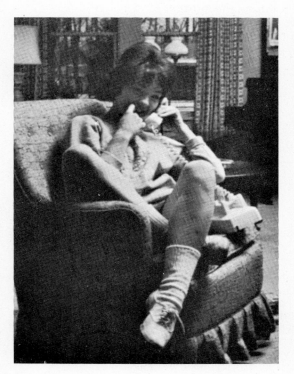

FIGURE 20-1 Friendships are a way of life for the teenager. (Brisbane: The Developing Child. Charles A. Bennett Co. Courtesy of Honeywell.)

socialize with girls. This is replaced (at about age 15 or 16) by interest in particular individuals on a more serious basis. There is concern for the future and a shaping of values.

Conformity is another key word. The adolescent wants to be "in"; he seeks group approval and wants their good opinion of him. This need on the part of the adolescent influences his manner, speech, dress, and his behavior in general, be it good or bad.

The Need for Independence

There is a strong drive for independence during adolescence. The person wants freedom in action and in decision making; he declares this need for independence in all aspects of behavior (deed and word) because he is trying to find his place among others. At the same time modesty and sensitivity overtake the individual. Adolescents like to have their own room and be able to take their own time with grooming, because looking "just right" becomes increasingly important as interest in the opposite sex heightens.

Concern for appearance, along with trying to look and act mature, causes some anxious moments. Feelings of awkwardness or self-consciousness about looks, mannerisms, and social efforts are normal. No one likes to be laughed at, teased, or ridiculed—least of all adolescents—so they strive to be like their peers in dress, mannerisms, and language usage. In seeking independence they use the comparison technique with parents: "Why can't I do so and so; all the other kids do," or "I'd drop dead before I'd wear that; nobody else does."

Through all of the striving for independence to make decisions and to be liked (accepted) by his own group, the adolescent still likes to know his parents will help him. Such help and support should have flexible and reasonable limits.

Life is Ahead

For adolescents, life is ahead. The future captures their daydreams as they think about what they want to do, where they want to go, and how they plan to get there. Plans for earning money, going to school, finding employment, and getting married are discussed among themselves. They think about the future and like to discuss serious problems confronting people, nations and the world, as they move toward adulthood.

Immediate needs are met for many by part-time employment. Adolescents want to have their own money and to decide how to spend it.

Knowing the adolescent's need to be independent, and his feelings of insecurity, sensitivity, and occasional confusion make it easier to understand why this person's emotions can change readily. There are "see-saw" feelings with flares of emotion which puzzle others who do not stop to think that any individual must gradually learn to control and handle himself. This control, for the human being, is a slow process.

SUMMARY

Adolescence has been called "that part of life's journey when a person is crossing over from childhood to adulthood." This part of the journey is one of development leading to maturity. The offspring finds himself frustrated by his growth pattern, serious in his efforts to reach independence, and puzzling to adults.

Sex hormones play important roles in the development of both sexes. Girls reach maturity in physical stature earlier than boys; this fact may account, in some ways, for their more noticeable mood swings.

The behavior of the adolescent is more understandable when one stops to consider how many things within him or her change in a few short years. Knowing in general what to expect during this portion of the life span can be useful to the practical nurse. Nursing actions, communications, relationships, and judgment, can be more sensible when viewed in the light of the unique needs of this person.

GUIDES FOR STUDY AND DISCUSSION

1. Adolescence is a period of great change. Complete the following by listing the changes under each heading:

	Physical	Mental	Emotional	Social
Male				
Female				

2. Study Figure 19–4. Notice which sex is more highly developed at age 13. Why is this so? When does the male catch up and pass the female? Why is this so?

3. Values change during adolescence. Think of some things adolescents question and hold opinions on. Who and what helps shape these values?

4. Adolescence influences daily living needs. In what way(s) is this true?

5. In comparing the prepuberty period with adolescence, what are the most noticeable developmental changes?

6. Knowing that the adolescent seeks and appreciates privacy, how will this knowledge influence your actions when you are providing nursing care?

SUGGESTED SITUATIONS AND ACTIVITIES

1. If you are an adolescent, try this: Use the daily living needs of the individual outlined in Chapter 22 and describe your own reactions. Be as forthright as possible in your self-assessment.

2. If you are an adult, use the daily living needs of the individual outlined in Chapter 22 to describe an adolescent you know well.

3. Prepare a piece of visual material which will show how the traits of the adolescent might influence a practical nurse's common sense in providing nursing care.

4. Visit a community agency (church, social, official) which you think is trying to work with young people. Find out what activities they offer, how they are funded and how many young people are involved. Ask if the agency has a stated purpose and how well they think they are meeting this purpose. Prepare a written outline of the information you gathered. Be ready to discuss it in class.

CHAPTER 21

ADULTHOOD

TOPICAL HEADINGS

Introduction
Who is the Adult?
The Young Adult
The Middle Aged
    Adult

The Years Ahead: The
    Older Adult and the
    Elderly Adult
Summary

Guides for Study and
    Discussion
Suggested Situations and
    Activities

OBJECTIVES FOR THE STUDENT: Be able to:

1. Name the four terms used to identify general divisions of adulthood.
2. Describe the main body changes taking place during each division of adulthood.
3. Compare the emotional characteristics of the young adult with the adolescent.
4. Give two examples which show that the decline of vitality is slow during adulthood.
5. Distinguish between the activities of the middle-aged adult and the older adult.
6. Describe three problems of "old age" in this society.
7. Differentiate between Medicare and Medicaid.
8. Tell how a local community shows concern for the elderly; how the national community shows concern.

SUGGESTED STUDY VOCABULARY*

vitality
vigor
wisdom
climacteric
aging

identity
dignity
senile
chronic

boredom
purposeful living
reminisce
geriatrics
gerontology

---

*Look for any terms you already know.

INTRODUCTION

This chapter concludes the journey of a lifetime. As mentioned previously, life never stops changing people. Adulthood is no exception; humans change slowly but surely after adolescence.

It is difficult to say when a person slips into the role of a mature adult; it has to be a gradual process. Knowing that each person's development pattern is unique to him, one could never say, with exactness, when young adulthood leaves adolescence behind. One could presume that "old adolescence" overlaps young adulthood; the overlapping would be a "gray area" between the two, difficult to define as one or the other.

The aging process starts with conception and continues throughout life. The word aging is commonly used in terms of someone who is well along in years, but actually this is a misuse of the word. Aging has some distinct landmarks; at first these landmarks are called "growth and development"; after that one thinks of the body as declining in many respects. When the body reaches full development and all body systems are fully active, there is a period of years when a person is vigorous and active. This period gradually fades across another stretch of years when a person is less vigorous and his activity is less strenuous. As body tissues continue to age, there is a gradual coming of signs of older age and then of elderliness.

This chapter discusses adulthood in four parts: The Young, The Middle-aged, The Older and the Elderly Adult. This does not mean that one period abruptly ends and the next begins, but when you compare the appearance of persons at ages 25, 50, and 75, it is very apparent that the body does undergo considerable change. These changes influence how one's daily living needs are met, and thus they are related to how his nursing care is adjusted in patient-centered nursing care.

WHO IS THE ADULT?

The word *adult* means grown to full size and strength. *Adulthood* represents the period in life described by such terms as full age, full bloom, ripe age, grown up, and oldness. If you stop to rethink these terms, it is plain to see that adulthood represents a long period of time. In fact, it is the longest segment of the life span and during the course of these years, the body and mind continue to change.

The society in which the adult lives and works has a lot to do with his efforts and his well-being. If the society puts a premium on youth and the young adult, those who slip toward the middle age and into elderliness can easily find themselves in a bind when it comes to work and purposeful living. For example, business, industry, government all might be promoting early retirement if they think in terms of "Putting people out to pasture after such and such an age," "Making room for the young, the vigorous," and "Permitting those who have worked thirty or forty years to stop and enjoy life." If the adult is ready to cease functioning in his life-long work role and has the means to provide for purposeful retirement, he no doubt welcomes this change. If

he is not ready to step aside, he is apt to be unhappy and frustrated whether or not he has the means to retire.

The number of elderly adults in this country is increasing and their unique needs are beginning to command the attention of society; this attention is long overdue.

THE YOUNG ADULT

As the journey from childhood to adulthood draws to an end, the body reaches full physical maturity and capacities are there waiting to be developed or extended. One begins to see more stable emotions, less frustration in making decisions, and an emerging set of values which guide behavior. In other words, a person is showing some ability to function independently in a grown-up way — in a grown-up world. He is an adult, a young adult with a "lifetime" of work and responsibility ahead of him.

Concerns of the Young Adult

The young adults (in their early twenties to late thirties) are busy establishing homes of their own and finding places in the world of work. Young adulthood represents the first years (in the development process) of true independence and full responsibility. These years bring more stable behavior, a settling down, so to speak, and new interests. By comparison, many things that seemed important at age 16 or 17 no longer hold the same interest — at least not in the same way. Along with this turn toward a more mature outlook, a person's values change. The things he sets store by, believes in, and practices are related to his new goals, expectations, and plans for the future. The individual is apt to accept change and necessary adjustments without the same type of emotional upset as in earlier years because his judgment improves as he lives through one experience after another.

Two things are particularly important to the young adult group: establishing a home and a family (Fig. 21–1), and finding a place in the world of work that is satisfying and challenging.

Establishing a home makes new demands on the young adult; he or she is required to share with the others the good and the bad, the frustrating and the pleasant, and to make ad-

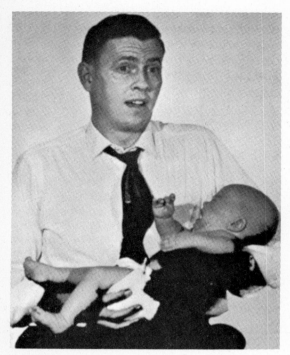

FIGURE 21-1   Another home responsibility. (Brisbane: The Developing Child)

justments which may not always give the person "his own way". The clamor of earlier years to make one's own decisions is replaced by necessity, with making joint decisions and, perhaps more importantly, accepting the consequences of those decisions. Such behavior indicates a forward step in the maturing process.

The young male adult is aware of the need to find his place in the world of work. His goals are achievement, advancement, and success in what he does. He is a newcomer to the adult world of work, often rubbing elbows with people who have achieved and have learned through experience what it means to share and to carry responsibility. Vitality, interest in getting ahead, and being in the prime of physical life are plus factors the young adult brings to his work. The process of working with others begins to shape and mold his judgment, his capacity to share, to give and to take, to stand up to the consequences of his own actions and develop wisdom.

The young adult female in our culture also enters the world of work (in increasing numbers) carrying home-family responsibilities. Her needs as an individual are served; she wants to be a part of community effort. In addition, her income helps to provide for home and family needs. The activities of the "working mother" have made it necessary for the "working father" to take a more active role in the home and family rearing responsibilities — something that was almost unheard of a generation or two ago.

Physical Changes Taking Place

The how and why of the aging process still baffles medical science. Much is known about what the signs of maturation are (early-life changes, middle-life changes, and late-life changes), but answers are being sought as to how and why these gradual, continuous changes occur. The journey of life from conception through adolescence is filled with examples of physical growth, mental and emotional development, and things that humanize the offspring as he learns to live with and get along with others. From that point on, the adult continues to mature in many aspects of his being (judgment, mental powers, socialization, etc.) but some aspects of the physical being begin to show signs of change. Some might call it "decline."

What happens when the body reaches full physical maturity? Does it remain in that vigorous state very long? What are some of the signs that indicate gradual body change even at the "prime of life"? These questions bring us to the young adult who remains one for 15 or twenty years. The healthy body continues to be vigorous and full of energy during this prime of life period. While exercise is not as strenuous nor carried on for as long periods as before, it includes all manner of energy-consuming activities and the body remains able to restore itself promptly after adequate rest. As middle age approaches, one might notice that it seems to take a little less strenuous exercise and a little more rest to maintain full energy, but the "decline" of vitality is slow.

Perhaps the most noticeable beginning signs of aging are a change in skin texture and in color, texture, and amount of hair (particularly in the male when thin or bald areas appear). Skin begins to lose some of its elasticity as indicated by traces of furrows or wrinkles across the brow and around the eyes and mouth. Because the "look of youth" is sought in our culture, both the male and the female often take whatever cosmetic steps they feel necessary to cover up the balding spots, the receding hairline, or the graying hair. The female has long been concerned about tell-tale signs of aging and tries to remedy them; the male, up to this time, has not been nearly as openly determined to conceal skin changes which occur.

Less noticeable signs of aging (alteration of structures and functions of body tissues) might be thought of as a type of petty larceny. This is to say that age robs the body of its youth, a little bit at a time, causing its tissues to change and later their functions (e.g., metabolism, blood pressure, circulation, digestion, elimination, respiration, bones, muscles, vision, hearing). These changes often are ever so slight that they go unnoticed until they call attention to themselves.

A person's social environment, his demands on himself, and his emotional make-up (where and how he works, his goals, what he gives to living, how he reacts) go hand in hand with time and alteration of body tissues. A young, eager-to-get ahead male may age himself faster by the pace he sets for himself and the goals he seeks than if he were less eager or in a different social environment.

Young adulthood could be summarized by stating that it is a period of some 15 to 20 years when the body-mind experiences vigorous productivity. The decline, if any, goes almost undetected, but body tissues are changing and altering their functions with the passing of each year. Consequently, the person at age 39 is quite different from the person he was at 21.

THE MIDDLE-AGED ADULT

Many important things happen during this part of the journey of life commonly called middle age. The label "middle-aged" is quite an inexact and difficult term to define. For one thing, it covers some 20 years (from the forties to the late fifties or early sixties) when the body and mind both change considerably. Study Figure 17–2 and notice what happens to physical strength, intelligence, reasoning ability, and judgment from about age 40 to 60. Notice too that the reproductive period for the female ends about midway while the male reproductive period continues for several more years. You can easily see, in many instances, that these 20 years bring some marked changes when you compare a male or

female at age 40 with a male or female at age 60. Keep in mind that development is an individual matter and a person of 40 may look much older than his years and a person of 60 look much younger. A person in the forties perhaps resents the label middle-aged while another in the late fifties enjoys this reference to himself and hangs onto it as long as possible.

Concerns of the Middle-Aged Adult

Despite the fact that this 20-year period (more or less) produces many changes, it has several things in common with the young adult period. In fact, these things are simply continuations: family rearing, homemaking, and success in the world of work. These three concerns do change considerably during this period, as pointed out in the following discussion.

Children Grow Up and Leave Home. They start new homes and the middle-aged parents become grandparents. Or the children finish school and leave home to continue their education or seek employment. In any event, sooner or later, middle-aged parents find themselves "homemaking" alone. Adjustment to this is often more difficult for the mother than for the father; her home activities change while he continues his work. The mother has time for other things and may go back to work or become more active in community efforts (Fig. 21–2). Some middle-aged adults manage

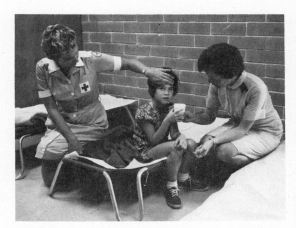

FIGURE 21-2 A Gray Lady (a volunteer) and a public health nurse look after a sick child in the health room of the S. Bryan Jennings Elementary School, Orange Park, Florida. (Florida Health Notes, Division of Health of the Florida Department of Health and Rehabilitative Services.)

to adjust to this change in the home better than others.

Community Activity is Common. Many middle-aged adults are active community supporters. They are interested in and actively support such community endeavors as public school efforts, fund drives for worthy causes (health, safety, recreation, etc.), better government, boys' or girls' club sponsorship, and church-related activities.

Job or Position Advancement Commonly Occurs. As might be expected (and predicted) from studying Figure 17–2, this is a period of high productivity for the adult. Reasoning and judgment are at their peak; experience has improved skills and understanding along the way. Many continue to study and take advantage of special training or continue to study and broaden their educational background to cope with present job needs and competition. The middle-aged adult realizes he is living the most productive portion of his life and seeks job or position advancement to increase his earning power and enjoy the satisfaction of moving up in his work.

Physical Changes are Noticeable

As the body ages, there is increasing evidence that tissues are altering their structure and function; this evidence, of course, is more noticeable in some than in others. One noticeable addition is eyeglasses. The middle-aged person hesitates to buy glasses and postpones this purchase as long as he can because it tells others his eyes are not as good as they were. Vision does become less sharp; eye muscles (the same as any other body muscles) are less elastic and adjust or focus more slowly. In time, glasses with two-level vision (bifocals) are required to accommodate sluggish vision and eye focus.

Another evidence of middle age is the tendency toward being overweight. As the metabolic rate decreases, tissues seem not to require the amount of fuel they once did; but food intake is not adjusted accordingly. When you combine less physical exercise and a continuing good appetite with a decreased metabolic rate and a body that has attained full development, you begin to understand why the middle-aged person tends to gain weight.

The lack of exercise causes changes in blood circulation. The cells are denied adequate oxygen and with exertion there is shortness of breath. Today there is a renewed interest in walking, jogging, bicycle riding, swimming, and so forth to improve muscle and body vigor. People are not physically active enough today. They ride instead of walk; they are sport spectators instead of participants. Medical science is concerned that the human body be exercised to help it maintain a lively, adequate circulatory system and good muscle tone. Scientists are especially looking at the middle-aged group. You will come to find that many in this age group have cardiovascular disorders. This is also a time when gastrointestinal disorders begin to make their appearance.

Changes in hair texture, color, and amount are now quite apparent. Graying continues and there is a pronounced thinning of the male's hair. At present these signs (both male and female) are not as noticeable as they would be due to the social acceptance of color rinses and hair pieces.

Another bit of evidence that tissues alter their structure and function is found in the skin and nails. Skin texture changes; it is drier and less elastic. Facial wrinkles and furrows begin to appear around the eyes and mouth and across the forehead. Fingernails tend to be more brittle.

During this age span, body posture begins to shift position; it is not apt to be as erect. One notices a slight sloping of the shoulders, a pouching of the abdomen and a general slumping down as muscles become less firm. This type of posture actually begins to reduce a person's height. In addition, the waistline and the hips increase.

Much Lies Ahead

The middle-aged individual has more years ahead of him than ever before since people are living longer. (See Table 21–1). These can be years of opportunity and fulfillment because judgment and reasoning powers are high. One could think of it as "contribution time"—a period when a person should be able to contribute his best in work and social effort. There are fewer financial obligations when the children leave home; there is new time found as the family pace changes. These things provide opportunity for new types of challenges, service, recreation, and plans for the future.

TABLE 21–1. AVERAGE REMAINING YEARS OF LIFE AT AGES 45, 65, AND 75. BY SEX AND COLOR: UNITED STATES, 1968

SEX AND COLOR	AVERAGE REMAINING YEARS OF LIFE		
	At age 45	At age 65	At age 75
SEX			
Men	26.8	12.8	8.2
Women	32.5	16.3	9.9
COLOR			
White	30.0	14.7	9.0
All other	26.2	13.7	10.8

SOURCE: U.S. Department of Health, Education and Welfare, Public Health Service, Health Services and Mental Health Administration. Adapted from: *Health in the Later Years*, October, 1971.

THE YEARS AHEAD: THE OLDER ADULT AND THE ELDERLY ADULT

Since 1900 more than 20 years have been added to the average life span. Today the expectation of life is more than 71 years; in 1900 it was 47 years. The more that is known about how to maintain health and restore it, the longer people will live. Presently the group of people over 70 years of age in this country is growing faster than the population as a whole. This means there is an increasing number of older persons in our society.

When is a person considered to be an older adult? He is not middle-aged one day and older the next. As with any stage of life, middle age blends into older age in a gradual way. Actually, the older middle-aged person can be considered in the "youth of old age."

Older adult is a label which means the next general stage of development following the middle adult years.

The *elderly adult* is the person who is living additional or bonus years; marked changes appear in body tissue structure and function as these years go on.

THE OLDER ADULT

Who is the Older Adult?

People just entering this general category do not usually consider themselves old; they find it easy to refer to other persons who may be just a few years older than they as "old folks." Age is as much a point of view as it is the number of years involved.

The older adult is a blend of the changes which have occurred in the body to date; he is also a blend of the experiences of living—those things which have shaped his attitudes, socializing habits, reasoning, and judgment.

The mind has continued to grow; it now shows maturity in such things as reasoning, judgment, and insight because it is schooled in experience. The reproductive power of the female ceased earlier and now the male experiences *climacteric*.

For purposes of discussion, let us consider the label "older adult" to include persons in the late fifties to the mid sixties.

Characteristics of the Older Adult

Financial Security. Family responsibilities have decreased, making it a time when less money is needed to run the home and educate the children. A husband and wife will have more financial security because earning power is still high and they can pursue their retirement plans in earnest. On the other hand, if the older adult should happen to be replaced by a younger worker or a machine, it can be a very discouraging period since the working years ahead are few and plans for retirement may be hampered.

Increased Leisure. Noticeable also is the increased amount of leisure time; this is especially true for the wife if she is not employed. It is not uncommon, however, for the mother and wife to find some type of part or full-time employment. She has the time and may need the income to help provide for the future.

Climacteric. The reproductive power of the female has ceased and the body is adjusting to hormone changes. This is known as the climacteric (menopause); during this time it is not uncommon for the female to experience up-and-down emotions. With the family gone and more leisure time at hand, it suggests the need for new interests and activities, such as helping in community efforts, pursuing learning (courses of special interest to the person), part- or full-time employment, or pursuing hobbies. In the male, the climacteric generally occurs some 10 to 15 years later (late fifties to middle or late sixties).

The Prospect of Retirement. People approaching retirement view it in different ways. Some plan for years ahead of time; others do not. In fact, some people do not want to retire while others look forward to it.

The word *retire* has many shades of meaning (depart, disappear, seclude onself, retreat, shrink). Retirement somehow means withdrawing. In the case of the person and his work, it means withdrawing from the work, the active duty, or the business which has produced a living. Many times (and for many reasons) people resist retirement; they feel they are not ready to withdraw.

In our society age 65 has come to mean the time to stop the familiar means of making a living if one is working for a business firm, government, and the like. There is some talk and effort to make it earlier than age 65. Some agencies retire workers after 20, 25, or 30 years of employment which means a person starting at a young age may be retired from this work during his middle years.

The prospect of retirement can cause some emotional stress too if there seems little likelihood of enough money to live on. Financial retirement plans are a way of life in this society. Social security, pensions or payments from the employer and employee, and private plans for income are some examples of retirement income sources. To retire happily and successfully requires planning. Actually, this planning should start when the young adult starts working. Definite plans should be taking from for that "new design for living" well ahead of actual retirement.

Noticeable Physical Changes

Noticeable changes occur in appearance and in body function during this period:

Vision is decidedly less sharp.

Hair is grayer and thinner (especially in men).

Body weight increases with little or no effort.

Skin is more wrinkled as underlying tissues lose firmness and elasticity.

Posture changes to accommodate weight and skeletal changes.

Walking gait may change to accommodate postural changes.

Digestive tract is less tolerant of food variety and sudden change.

Circulatory system produces blood pressure changes.

Hearing may be less sharp.

Opportunity Ahead. By the time the adult becomes "older," many body-mind changes have occurred; many things are behind and newer things are taking their place. These can be choice, productive years in the life span for the individual who welcomes and lives them with understanding.

THE ELDERLY ADULT

Who can say when one becomes elderly? Actually no one can because the blending of change is so gradual and so different from one individual to another that a number of years have to slip by before the label *elderly* is attached to a person. The act of retiring at age 65 does not automatically make a person elderly. In fact retirement may make him feel freer and younger than he did. Adequate and proper exercise keeps him vigorous and active for some time to come.

The aging process is still a mystery when it comes to such questions as: What causes cells to change in structure and function? Why does one person show signs of elderliness so much earlier in life than another person?

For our purposes, let us consider the elderly person as one who lives well beyond the compulsory retirement age of 65. While this is an inexact way to group people during the later years of life, it may help you think in terms of a definite part of the span of life.

In our society the elderly person is one who has lived beyond the labor market. In other words, he or she has lived beyond the years which demand high productivity, strenuous exercise, and shouldering responsibility for others. In these respects there is a noticeable tapering-off of activity. On the other hand, getting older does not necessarily mean a decline in one's interest in life and and in learning, nor in activity within physical means. The individual experiences a change of pace in keeping with his own body-mind capacities to learn, work, play, and relax. It should be stated that as elderliness proceeds into advanced years certain characteristics do become apparent; these are discussed later.

The Elderly Group Grows

In this country more than 3700 people celebrate their 65th birthday every day. Both the United States and Canada are experiencing a rapid rate of growth in the elderly group. It may surprise you to know that as a group, people living 85 years or more represent the fastest growing group in our society. The number to reach 100 years is over 12,000 at present.

It is projected that by the year 2000 there will be over 28 million Americans aged 65 and over.[1] Some predict it will be possible to live to the ripe old age of 125 years in due time.

Living longer is the result of better means for maintaining health, preventing illness, detecting illness early, restoring the body and assisting it while it is being restored, and providing good nourishment.

The Meaning of Aging

One could say that aging has many "faces" because when the term aging is defined, mention is made of years (chronological aging), physical appearance changes, body function changes, psychological changes, and neurological changes.

There is common misinformation about the elderly person which tends to influence how he is treated by others (younger). For one thing, old age does not decrease intelligence; there are many living examples of people who, though old in years, have full power to understand and to meet a situation successfully. Another point to remember is that senility is a feebleness of body and mind but it is not common to all elderly people. Then, too, elderliness is not second childhood.

The study of man's problems as he ages, how aging affects different parts of the body, and what are solutions to needs (social, economic, cultural) of older people is called *gerontology.*

The care of people in later years dealing with both health and sickness is called *geriatrics;* it is a practice of medicine that crosses all branches of medical care (i.e., an elderly patient may have more than one health problem) to help older people recover or maintain their health.

The Elderly Person has Identity

Many elderly people resent being treated different from others; they resent the "senior

citizen" title or being reminded that theirs are the "sunset years." Nor are they impressed with homey titles of "gramps" or "granny" attached to them by other than family members. They do appreciate and are entitled to the same titles (Mr., Mrs., or Miss) they have been called for years.

Some nationalities or societies show noticeable respect for their elderly; they are looked to as the wisest and as the head of the family. Younger family members recognize the eldest by using proper titles and considering them the head of the group.

Elderly people have the same rights they have always had; age has nothing to do with their being treated differently from others. Living has provided them with a storehouse of experience and understanding. Your relationships should take this into account. At no time should an elderly person feel he is a member of the queer, end-of-the-line group that somehow makes him child-like and he should not be treated accordingly.

Like people of another age group, the elderly have the same daily living needs. They have special need for identity, dignity, self-importance, independence, and meaningful living. As a practical nurse, you should keep these special needs in mind because while most elderly people get around, about eight out of 10 have one or more chronic health problems and they spend more time in clinics and hospitals than do other age groups. Medicare and Medicaid are making it possible for increasing numbers of elderly people to receive medical attention.

The Retirement Revolution

The retirement picture in our society is changing. Increased numbers of retirees alone would force some changes, but there is more to the problem than that. A human needs a purpose for living. Putting him on the shelf hastens physical decline (Fig. 21-3).

Up to now, a person reaching retirement age has been expected to sit back and rock and be satisfied with his leisure of nothing special to do—a sort of putting a person on the shelf and leaving him there. Our society is beginning to awaken to the fact that this is not what retirees need. They need an interest and a purpose in life, and they need this as much as they need an adequate income.

The federal government is beginning to study the problem of meaningful activity in

1. U. S. Administration on Aging, Facts About Older Americans, Publication No. 410 (Washington, D.C.: U. S. Government Printing Office, May, 1966).

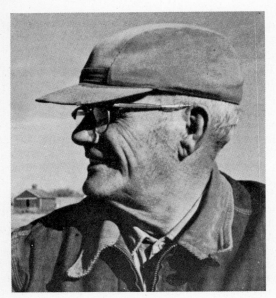

FIGURE 21-3   Ready for work and happy about it. (On Growing Older. President's Council on Aging, Washington, D.C., 1964.)

retirement; this problem (challenge) increases with time. It is projected that by the year 2000, one out of every three Americans living today will reach retirement age. People will come to live 20 and 25 years or more in retirement. Think for a moment of the vast numbers of people who will be living beyond the labor market. How can they make their lives purposeful for 20 or 25 years? What will they be doing with their time? It is a known fact that a person needs a purpose for living. Being isolated does not satisfy that need. Studies show that the people who reach the upper age limits are busy people; they are not do-nothing retirees. Is it possible to die from boredom? Some think so.

Purposeful activity is essential to purposeful living. Man has the capacity for creativity and imagination. The human body and mind thrive on use and wither without it. It has been proved that mind power does not decline with age up to 50 and that purposeful, mind-stretching activity keeps it going many years beyond that. Why not have retirees busy using their minds and bodies purposefully (Figs. 21–4 and 21–5)?

Medical science will soon make possible a 100-year-old body-mind. Automation is reducing physical work and body muscles are not getting the exercise they once did. For young and old alike, emphasis is being placed on exercise to keep the body in good working order. Considering that people will be living many years after retirement, the challenge of what to do about active, purposeful living is a serious challenge facing everyone.

Efforts to understand this challenge are now underway with people in their adolescence. If attitudes are to change, the young must be informed.

A Change in Attitude is Needed

The public needs to change its attitude toward the elderly. And the elderly person needs to change his attitude toward himself. A change in one will promote a change in the other.

The elderly person likes his independence, in fact, he fights to keep it. If he is physically fit, he can preserve his independence. Efforts (meetings, classes) are now underway to help the elderly person understand what the aging process is and how he can live with it to the best advantage. Hopefully if he understands what the body-mind needs as it ages, the elderly person's attitude toward himself and his role in society will change.

The public (since all are headed toward

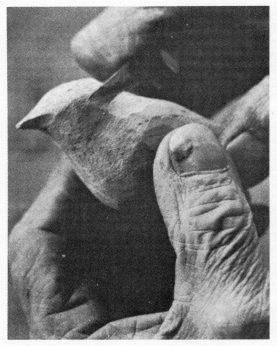

FIGURE 21-4   Creativity at work. (On Growing Older. President's Council on Aging, Washington, D.C., 1964.)

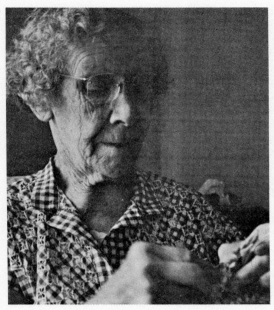

FIGURE 21-5 "A hobby should be a wing instead of a crutch." Notice her interest in what she is doing. (On Growing Older. President's Council on Aging, Washington, D.C., 1964.)

retirement) needs to recognize that *advanced age is a natural part of the life span.* Humans who reach the upper years need the same basic things to keep on living as do the younger members of society. Our emphasis on youth, vigor, and vitality has left too little room for meeting many of these needs. The older person can and should be making his contribution and should be experiencing a purposeful life.

Two words which too often color a person's viewpoint when he thinks about the elderly person are *senile* and *chronic.* Neither word is appropriate for the healthy elderly adult. Senile pertains to a progressive feebleness of body and mind which may show up in various ways when a person ages. But to be elderly does not automatically mean a person is senile. Chronic does not refer to age at all, but to the duration of an illness; it means lasting or persisting over a long period of time.

Who Assumes Responsibility?

The person who has retired from regular earning activities and lives for years beyond runs the chance of having one or more major problems (reduced income, housing problems, malnutrition, health expenses, inactivity, loneliness, and a feeling of uselessness).

Who is responsible to help the elderly? As mentioned previously, the challenge is great, and attitudes of society are important in meeting this challenge. As a practical nurse and a citizen your attitude is part of society's attitude. You will have opportunity in caring for the sick and feeble elderly to show your understanding of their needs. As a citizen you have an opportunity to help shape the attitudes of others by your willingness to help the community better its life for elderly people.

SOCIETY. Governments (local and federal) can and do pass laws related to housing and health facilities, medical assistance, Medicare, fraud and quackery, and income (social security, tax exemptions, etc.). They study the problems and provide safeguards for welfare and health. It is now apparent that more must be done to make life more purposeful for the retiree.

Coordinated federal concern for the elderly first made its appearance in August, 1950, when President Truman called some 800 delegates together in Washington, D.C. for the first National Conference on Aging.

1959—The Senate Subcommittee on Problems of the Aging and the Aged was formed to study their problems and needs, and how the various federal agencies were meeting or failing to meet them.

1961—The Special Senate Committee on Aging replaced the above subcommittee and at present is one of the largest committees in the U.S. Senate. Their work includes gathering information (they held 36 "grass roots" hearings throughout the country), and holding special Washington hearings on housing, income, and health matters including cost of medical care and drugs, nursing homes, frauds, quackery, and other ways the elderly might be cheated.

1961—The first White House Conference on Aging was held at the request of President Eisenhower. This conference brought together over 300 national organizations as well as representatives from all levels of government. The theme was "Aging With a Future—Every Citizen's Concern."

1962—The President's Council on Aging was created by order of President Kennedy. The Council membership included cabinet members (Secretary of Health, Education, and Welfare, Secretaries of Agriculture, Commerce, Labor, and Treasury), chairman of the Civil Service Commission, and administrators of Veteran Affairs, Housing and Home Financing Agency. This group made recommendations to the President concerning federal responsibilities to the aging members in society.

1965 — The Health Insurance for the Aged Act (Medicare) was passed and became effective in 1966. *Medicare* (health insurance) is a means to *help* persons 65 years or older pay for health services (inpatient hospital services, skilled nursing homes, outpatient diagnostic services, home health services). While there are limits and requirements attached to these services, Medicare is making it possible for many older people to receive health care that would otherwise be out of their financial reach.

1971 — White House Conference on Aging called by President Nixon. More than 3500 delegates came prepared to push for more federal action on issues concerned with income, health, nutrition, housing, property taxes, transportation, employment and retirement, among other concerns. Discussion helped point the way for all branches of federal government to act in the 1970's.

Medicaid is not the same as Medicare. Medicaid is an assistance program for certain kinds of needy and low-income people (i.e., 65 and older, blind, disabled, members of families with dependent children, some other children). This program is financed by federal, state and local tax monies — thus it is a financial partnership. Medicaid can pay what Medicare does not pay for people who are eligible for both programs.[1]

Community agencies promote a variety of programs that provide recreation and productive activity to help the elderly adult feel a part of the community and maintain his self-respect.

Organizations such as the American Association of Retired Persons (AARP) and the National Association of Retired Teachers (NART) not only bring people together for recreation, study and companionship, but to have a voice in the well-being of elderly people.

The elderly adult group represents a vast and almost untapped source of brain power and manpower. Some of the great contributions to music, art, literature, and teaching have been made by mature older minds with the capacity and time to express themselves. Some are asking — why not have a choice between continuing employment as long as possible or retiring on adequate income?

THE INDIVIDUAL AND THE FAMILY. While society has a responsibility for meeting certain needs of the elderly, the individual carries some also. He has no right to automatically expect others to do for him what he should have begun to plan early in life for himself. Much (not all) depends upon financial security in the advanced years; plans for adequate income should start years ahead of retirement. Other forms of security relate to physical and emotional health, comfort, usefulness, safety, and companionship.

The individual can provide some of these things for himself especially if he sees the importance of them. Public and private agencies can help him understand the meaning of aging and the needs of older people. Consider the matters of usefulness and companionship. Elderly people can become involved with helping each other. They can be trained to advise others approaching retirement (or even the adolescent and young adult) on how to plan for the changes one faces in retirement.

Family members can promote or smother the independence of an elderly patient. Preserving independence and doing their own decision-making are typical desires of older people. Who is to say when a person is unable to make decisions for himself? Sometimes the courts have to decide. One concern of the family should be to help older family members retain their independence, dignity, self-determination, and feeling of usefulness.

Concerns of the Elderly Person

One important concern was discussed earlier in this chapter — having a purpose for living. Boredom, loneliness, and a feeling of uselessness can rob this adult of vitality and innermost joy in living. Boredom withers a person on the inside, and this shriveling of the spirit shows on the outside (see section entitled The Retirment Revolution).

Adequate financial security and income are big concerns of many elderly people. Incomes for this group, as a whole, are low or moderate. Less money means less of something else. The three things first affected by this decrease are usually food, housing, and medical care.

Food does not have to be expensive to be nourishing but food does cost money. If a person needs to scrimp to get by, the food bill is one of the first things the retiree thinks of. His

---

1. *Medicaid and Medicare: Which is which?* U.S. Government Printing Office, Washington, D.C.

lack of understanding of what is an adequate diet for an elderly person often hampers him. Poor nourishment directly influences his state of health.

Many elderly live alone so getting adequate food and preparing it is often a problem—sometimes because of lack of transportation, limited mobility, lack of interest in eating and little or no money to purchase it.

The federal government is attempting to locate elderly persons who qualify for food stamps and commodities through an effort called *Project Find*. This nationwide effort involves both federal and voluntary agencies.

Housing has a lot to do with the elderly adult's frame of mind as well as his safety and general well-being. It takes a sizable amount of his income to house himself. If the individual needs help with diet problems, general health habits, and some degree of protection for his safety, these things somewhat dictate a type of place to live. If he is capable of taking care of himself, he has many other alternatives; if he is sick, this means being where he can receive medical and nursing care.

Medical care can be costly and the elderly worry about not having enough money to "take care of themselves." Medicare and Medicaid provide limited means to many who otherwise would go without medical assistance or postpone it.

The elderly person (eight of 10) is apt to have one or more chronic disorders. This means that often there is a continuing need to take medicine and have regular medical checkups. It often means periodic hospitalization to correct or to regulate some malfunction. All these things cost money. Social security income, and pensions, and life savings can dwindle quickly in the face of constant medical payments. This is why the elderly adult worries about having enough to take care of him. He wants to be independent and pay his way, if at all possible. These factors have meaning for the nurse who recognizes the need of a patient to sense independence, dignity, and self-esteem.

A nurse, as much as or perhaps more than anyone else, should acquaint herself with new efforts to help the elderly adult. It is through knowing the problems and frustrations of this patient and knowing what are the changes which come with normal aging that she can help this patient retain his identity and find some purpose in living. You will find no "procedures" for bringing this needed quality to the nursing care you give. You will need to use

"you"—your insight, imagination, fellow-feeling, and willingness to help.

Changes in Body Structure and Function, Appearance and Behavior

TISSUE CHANGES

Changes in body tissues continue to occur throughout the journey of a lifetime. Bones, muscles, fatty tissue, nerve and brain cells, blood vessel tissue, skin, nails, hair, etc., all undergo gradual change. But the normal aging process produces some definite changes by the time a person is elderly. Following are some of the changes.

The amount of cellular fluid is reduced.

The metabolic rate is slower and some cell products (normally used up) seem to accumulate there.

There is steady increase in the amount of fatty tissue (even though weight remains the same).

Less kidney tissue (nephron) provides less kidney power.

Less plasma filters through the kidneys.

Less oxygen is used during rest.

Breathing capacity is considerably reduced.

Lymphoid tissue decreases steadily.

Connective tissue is less pliable.

Blood vessels thicken.

The brain decreases in size.

Sight and hearing are less sharp.

The senses of smell and taste decline.

CHANGES IN PHYSICAL APPEARANCE

The skin becomes loose, flabby, dry, and wrinkled; the texture and color change.

Hair on the head thins (men are often bald); facial hair increases on women (upper lip and chin).

Fingernails become thin and brittle; toenails thicken.

Eyeballs seem deep set and eyelids turn outward as they lose their elasticity.

Ear lobes seem to lengthen.

The torso gradually shortens and thickens; abdominal muscles sag.

The neck is shorter.

The walking gait changes to accommodate posture changes; often there is need to hold onto someone's arm to steady the gait.

Movements are slower.

CHANGES IN BEHAVIOR

Attitudes are less flexible.

There is a tendency to reminisce.

Recent memory is reduced.

A tendency of doing things in a certain

way or at a certain time (going to bed, eating, dressing, etc.).

A tendency to want to be alone or not engage in relationships with others; a detachment from others.

Each of these clusters of change (tissue, physical appearance, behavior) has meaning for the practical nurse in giving safe, effective nursing care. To know something of how the body-mind of an elderly person functions helps you to use good judgment in doing things for and with this patient.

SUMMARY

Adulthood is a period of development too. After reaching full maturity with all body systems functioning, the human continues to learn and to adjust to people and situations. During adulthood body tissues gradually change and the body is less able to stand vigorous exertion; more time is needed to restore it. The metabolic rate declines and cells seem to be less and less able to fully use cellular substances. Body fluid movement is changed; there is less fluid within cells, less kidney function, and less lymphoid tissue and lymph.

One segment of the adult population needing more attention is the fast growing group, the elderly. Their problems are many and include such essentials as proper nutrition, an income on which they can live rather than just exist, adequate health care and adequate housing. Other needs are solutions to the problems of loneliness, boredom and isolation.

GUIDES FOR STUDY AND DISCUSSION

1. Adulthood is the longest part of the life span. Many changes take place in the body during this time. Under each of the following headings, list as many such changes as you can.
   Young Adult   Middle-aged Adult   Older Adult   Elderly Adult
2. What are the chief differences between adolescence and young adulthood?
3. How does the behavior of the elderly person differ from that of the middle-aged person?
4. Body vitality slows down after adolescence. Why is this so? Be ready to give some examples which show this is a gradual process.
5. What does it mean to say, "People should start to plan for retirement when they are young"?
6. Why is boredom such an "enemy" of the elderly?
7. Why do people move from one type of living arrangement to another and perhaps another as they become older?
8. If you were 80 years of age, where would you like to live? Why?
9. From what you know about middle-aged adults, how might you expect them to act when they are hospitalized? List as many things as you can.
10. Independence, dignity and self-esteem are needs of the elderly—sick or well. What can you do to help meet these three needs when you are nursing elderly patients?
11. Who is eligible for Medicare? Medicaid?

SUGGESTED SITUATIONS AND ACTIVITIES

1. Use the nine essential daily living needs and prepare a chart or poster that shows what these mean in the life of the young adult.
2. Think up some type of purposeful diversion for an elderly person who lives in a retirement home with other elderly people. Be ready to describe it.
3. See if you can find out what your community does for its elderly residents. Prepare a brief report on your findings.
4. Prepare a display of information showing what the government provides in the way of official health insurance and assistance for older adults.

HEALTH: INDIVIDUAL, FAMILY, AND COMMUNITY

CHAPTER 22. **HEALTH OF THE INDIVIDUAL**

CHAPTER 23. **THE FAMILY UNIT AND HEALTH**

CHAPTER 24. **THE COMMUNITY AND HEALTH**

Unit V consists of three chapters; the first one is a stepping stone to the next one, and it in turn leads to the third chapter. Chapter 22 begins by defining health in general terms and pointing out what are the health problems facing our society. This will give you a beginning understanding of the health of an individual like yourself. One of the most important features of Chapter 22 is a set of *nine essential daily living needs* of people when they are well. To learn these needs for health (your health) will give you the basis for learning the ten essential daily needs common to all patients found in Chapter 32. These two lists are very similar; compare them as you study Chapter 22. In this way you can build your own structure for learning "individual-centered" nursing care, and at the same time you will be learning the essential things related to your own healthful living.

Chapter 23 focuses on the family as the basic social unit in our culture and the role it plays in the health and well-being of family members. General knowledge of the family will help in understanding the importance of family members when illness occurs.

Chapter 24, The Community and Health, is designed to help you understand how our society is organized to meet the health needs of its citizens. Meeting health needs is among the largest industries in our country, and the practical nurse should have a general idea of what is involved in this large and growing community responsibility.

HEALTH OF THE INDIVIDUAL

OBJECTIVES FOR THE STUDENT: Be able to:

1. Define the word "health" in meaningful, useful terms.
2. Explain why people are living longer.
3. List the leading causes of death in this country.
4. Given a list of nine basic daily needs of the individual, describe the relationship of each to good health.
5. Evaluate your personal health habits according to the nine basic daily needs.
6. Name the factors influencing health.

SUGGESTED STUDY VOCABULARY*

mortality	suicide	axilla
heredity	homicide	meticulous hygiene habits
environment	predispose	life expectancy
fatigue	rehabilitate	diversion
halitosis	optimum	body alignment
congenital malformation	deodorant	posture
		self-medication

*Look for any terms you already know.

INTRODUCTION

It would be easier to describe the condition *health* if it had a common meaning for every person, but it does not. Health is not easy to measure because it is a state that varies from person to person. A narrow description might label it "the absence of disease"; an elaborate definition (such as the one developed by the World Health Organization quoted later in this chapter) takes in far more than absence of disease. As a practical nurse, you will need to have a reasonable understanding of what health is so that you can use it as a basis for understanding disabilities, disorders, rehabilitation, and prevention.

This chapter can help you now and will continue to serve you throughout the program by:

1. Furnishing you with a baseline for defining and understanding the term health.

2. Showing that all people (yourself included) *regardless of age,* have certain needs to be met every day; these are called *essential daily living needs* and are grouped into nine categories.

3. Providing a structure or foundation of needs which will help you understand how you can assist people when they become ill. People continue to have the same basic needs when they are sick, but because they are sick they need help to meet these needs (see Chapter 32).

THE MEANING OF HEALTH

What we think of today as health is something quite different from its earliest meanings. The word health comes from the Old English *hoelth* meaning a state of being safe and sound.

Table 2–1 points out ancient man's ideas about sickness and health. Since then the concept of health has broadened so that today man's interest has come to include more than the *cure of sickness;* it also includes *prevention* and *rehabilitation* as well as *research* to find answers to old questions while raising new ones.

A state of health is actually a constant adjustment process. Health is a state in which the body is functioning comfortably without especially calling attention to itself because of its ability to adjust to the environment, and to renew and restore itself physically and mentally. Such a definition allows for individual differences (within a normal range) in making such adjustments.

Health care is a vast group of measures used to cure illness, to prevent it in the first place, and to rehabilitate or restore people to their fullest capacity to function.

Health care has come to include the work going on in research laboratories where scientists are seeking new knowledge about housing, food, air, water, accidents, disease, equipment, drugs, the aging process, cure, prevention, and rehabilitation. Emotional as well as physical aspects of life and living are being studied.

Health care requires the skills of persons like yourself who prepare for work in the health industry. There are about 375 different job *titles* of health careers; this means about 375 different types of health care workers. Some spend years training for specialized types of work; others take short, intensive courses such as a course in practical nursing. All are valuable, essential workers in this growing, complex service industry.

Health Definition of the World Health Organization

While the World Health Organization (WHO) is discussed in more detail in Chapter 24, this special agency of the United Nations works toward the following purpose: "The attainment of all peoples of the highest possible level of health." Here is the WHO definition of health:

Health is a state of complete physical, mental and social well-being and not merely the absence of disease or infirmity.

The enjoyment of the highest attainable standard of health is one of the fundamental rights of every human being without distinction of race, religion, political belief, economic or social condition.

The health of all people is fundamental to the attainment of peace and security and is dependent upon the fullest cooperation of individuals and states.

Thus health is "well-being"—a basic right of every human being wherever he may be found.

STATUS OF HEALTH IN OUR COUNTRY

Much has been learned about health and illness in the last 50 years. Medical and related health sciences have learned not only how to cure many diseases, but how to prevent many diseases, and how to restore people to usefulness (rehabilitate). Such progress has been made in the last 25 years that many diseases are no longer a serious health problem. Scientists have provided vaccines, medicines, equipment, and instruments to help prevent, control, diagnose, treat, and/or cure such dreaded and once-prevalent diseases as pneumonia, tuberculosis, poliomyelitis, smallpox, scarlet fever, diphtheria, typhoid fever, and measles. Progress has also been made in dealing with congenital defects, chronic physical and mental illness, and mental retardation. Many more answers are needed.

People in our country receive reasonably good health care due to the active part local, state, and federal governments play in our daily lives; to improved hospital and clinic facilities; and to a knowledgeable public aware of the values of good health habits and practices (good daily habits, regular medical examinations, proper diets, etc.) and having a higher living standard than most countries of the world. However, the United States does not do as well as some countries in meeting the health needs of its people. Much research goes on and answers are found but there is often a lag between getting the answers and putting them to work. Air pollution and water pollution problems are two examples of the lag between what we know should be done and what is being done.

Today people live longer. There has been a remarkable and steady increase in the life span. The National Center for Health Statistics of the United States Public Health Service (Department of Health, Education, and Welfare) records the *vital statistics* of our population. These data include number and rate of deaths, births, infant mortality, maternal mortality, average expectancy of life, death by causes, and other information which shows the changes and trends in the population and the general status of health in this country.

Life expectancy is the average number of years in the lifetime. Since 1900 life expectancy in the U. S. has increased by more than 23 years. Table 22–1, *Expectation of Life,*

TABLE 22–1.　EXPECTATION OF LIFE

YEAR	AVERAGE LENGTH OF LIFE IN YEARS
1971 (Est.)	71.1
1970 (Est.)	70.8
1969	70.4
1968	70.2
1967	70.5
1966	70.1
1965	70.2
1925	59.0
1900	47.3

Source: U.S. Department of Health, Education, and Welfare, Public Health Service, National Center for Health Statistics.

Adapted from: Annual Summary for the United States, 1971. Vol. 20, No. 13, August 30, 1972.

shows remarkable progress since the turn of the century.

The year 1971 showed an estimated life expectancy of 71.1 years (highest ever reached). This means that a baby born in this country in 1971 could be expected to live 71.1 years. Canada has a life expectancy of 72 years.

The United States is capable of having healthier citizens than it presently does. Many countries have made more progress and, in some instances, faster progress in health care than we have. For example, in 1969, twelve countries had lower death rates among newborns than did the United States. These countries were Sweden, the Netherlands, Finland, Norway, Japan, Denmark, Switzerland, Australia, New Zealand, United Kingdom, East Germany and France. Canada rated 14th, just below the United States. Studies show that poor nutrition, lack of prenatal care, immaturity, birth injuries, and congenital malformations are some of the main causes of our high mortality rate.

Many citizens neglect their health due to lack of money, lack of interest, fear of what may be wrong, carelessness, and lack of information (understanding) about what is available to prevent disease and treat it.

This does not mean that no progress has been made. Immunization now prevents many diseases that used to kill endless numbers of people and leave scores of others imparied (e.g., smallpox, diphtheria, polio, whooping cough, measles, and tetanus). Equipment of all kinds (e.g., respirator) keeps vital body processes going while artificial parts (e.g., artificial kidney) replace defective body parts and organs from one body are being transplanted to another.

The leading causes of death in a country (see Table 22–2) are an index to its health problems. The list changes as the years go by because habits change, new discoveries are made, and new knowledge helps solve old problems. A disease common twenty years ago may be curable or controllable now. A vaccine used to immunize against a disease may all but wipe it out, as in the case of smallpox and polio, if people use it properly.

For many years tuberculosis ranked among the top ten causes of death; however, it has not been in the list since 1959. Two drugs, streptomycin and isoniazid, changed the course of this disease.

Accidents have been one of the first 10

TABLE 22–2. TEN LEADING CAUSES OF DEATH: UNITED STATES, 1971

RANK	CAUSE OF DEATH	PER CENT OF TOTAL DEATHS
1.	Heart Diseases	38.6
2.	Cancer	17.3
3.	Stroke	10.8
4.	Accidents	5.8
5.	Influenza and Pneumonia	2.9
6.	Diseases of Early Infancy	2.1
7.	Diabetes Mellitus	2.0
8.	Cirrhosis of Liver	1.7
9.	Arteriosclerosis	1.7
10.	Bronchitis, Emphysema and Asthma	1.6
11.	All Other Causes	15.6

Source: U.S. Department of Health, Education, and Welfare, Public Health Service, National Center for Health Statistics.

Adapted from: Annual Summary for the United States, 1971. Vol. 20, No. 13, August 30, 1972.

causes of death for some years. Fatal motor vehicle accidents outrank any other cause of accidental deaths the year around. Falls rank second, with little variance as to season. In the United States there are more deaths from accidents in the summer (June to August) than in any other season of the year, the main causes being drownings, boat and motor accidents, and lightning bolts. Other accidents occur from fires and explosions, firearms, poisoning, and railway and aircraft accidents.

In recent years suicides, homicides, and motor vehicle accidents have increased the death rates among adolescents, especially boys.

Because of the health improvement in our country, changes in the numbers of a particular segment or age group in our population have resulted. These can produce problems, and sometimes solutions come slowly. Today we face adjustments owing to the increased numbers in our aging population.

FACTORS INVOLVED IN HEALTH

How many people enjoy *health?* Certainly not everyone who is not on the "sick list." Possibly one out of every 10 is physically and mentally fit and free from defects, and about one out of every 10 persons is ill or incapacitated and cannot work. Between the fit and unfit, there are the eight out of every 10 (80 per cent) who vary in their states of health. Consideration of some of the factors which influence health should help one to understand why these conditions can exist.

Heredity is one such factor; it is the passing of physical and mental traits from one generation to another. Most persons inherit physical and mental traits within a normal range, but some are born with physical or mental deformities. Such weaknesses or variations do not necessarily render a person unfit for work, or useless. Heredity can predispose some toward certain diseases such as diabetes and some eye or nervous conditions.

Environment is another factor affecting health. Some environmental conditions are direct and others are indirect. For example, the conditions under which a person lives and works contribute to or predispose him to some illnesses or to a state of good health.

Care received during infancy and childhood influences the state of health for a lifetime. Adequate and safe environment, proper nutrition, proper health habits for cleanliness and rest, and a secure home life all help to develop a healthy body and mind.

Nutrition has a greater influence on health than is generally known. Proper diet is essential to good health. Improper diet can lead to overweight or underweight; prevent normal development of teeth, bones, muscles; cause limited functioning of some body parts; and can encourage development of certain diseases.

Another common factor influencing health is *accidents.* Accidents in the home, at work, or on the highway not only take many lives annually but leave far more injured or crippled. Accidents in the home rank especially high for the younger and older age groups, falls, burns, and poisons being the most frequent causes. The kitchen and the bathroom are the two most hazard-filled rooms.

Increased travel can transfer disease and health problems from one area or country to another very quickly and easily if strict controls and precautions are not enforced.

Lack of medical attention or refusal to go to a hospital for treatment when one is ill can sometimes do untold harm to one's health. Modern hospitals have laboratories equipped to help the physician make the earliest possible correct diagnosis and they have equipment to aid in medical care.

The health of a nation (or the world) actually means the health of the individuals who make up that nation. The right to experience optimum health belongs to each person. A country has a responsibility to protect and preserve the health of its people. This responsibility includes efforts to cure and prevent illness, rehabilitate persons to optimum capacities, and continue to search for solutions to and new knowledge about health problems so that all people are healthier people. Massive health education is needed in this country and is carried on to a certain extent; some citizens "listen and learn"; some do not. There are countries in the world where even the simplest health care is nonexistent. This is one of the biggest problems facing mankind today.

THE HEALTH OF THE INDIVIDUAL

A person's health is the total of his *physical, mental,* and *social* well-being. These three ingredients cannot be separated because an individual cannot be separated into parts. He responds as a whole unit; he is made up of a physical body, he has a mind, and he is influenced by his surroundings. The healthy individual experiences a reasonable balance among these three ingredients within his being. To help you understand physical, mental, and social well-being in relation to health, nine essential daily living needs are listed and discussed (see Fig. 22–1). They apply to you. As a practical nurse you will want and need to practice effective health habits for your own sake and for the sake of the people with whom you work (patients included). In a sense, you become an example-setter for patients and their families; but perhaps more importantly, how you look, how you feel about yourself and others, and how you conduct yourself very definitely influence the way others respond and react to you. Do not underestimate the impact that your health habits have on others.

Every person, regardless of age, has the same basic daily living needs.

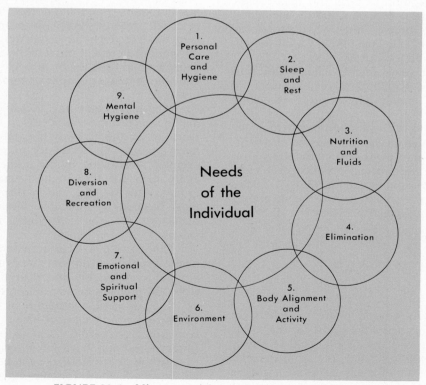

FIGURE 22-1   Nine essential daily living needs for health.

When a person is well, he takes care of his own needs (if he is old enough to do so); when he is ill, he needs assistance to help him meet these daily living needs. Nursing is the process of helping him or giving him this assistance. The amount and kind of assistance he requires depends upon his state of dependency at the time. If you learn what are *your* basic daily living needs, this will give you a head start for knowing the patient's daily needs. They are very similar.

Study the following list of the essential needs for health. Chapter 32 discusses each need relative to the patient and introduces a tenth need of the patient — medical treatment and care.

ESSENTIAL DAILY NEEDS

1. Personal care and hygiene.
2. Sleep and rest.
3. Nutrition and fluids.
4. Elimination.
5. Body alignment and activity.
6. Environment.
7. Emotional and spiritual support.
8. Diversion and recreation.
9. Mental hygiene.

THE MEANING OF EACH ESSENTIAL NEED

Each of the nine essential daily living needs is discussed to help you (1) assess your own health habits and practices, and (2) to help you assist patients in meeting their daily living needs.

Personal Care and Hygiene

Cleanliness promotes a feeling of well-being and self-respect. Clean skin, hands, nails, teeth, hair, and clothing contribute to physical, mental, and social well-being, as well as give protection against infection and illness.

Daily and regular habits of *bathing* and wearing *clean clothes* are basic to good personal hygiene. The skin constantly gives off oily substances and perspiration. If these become dry and accumulate, an odor soon results. This odor often increases when temperatures rise, physical activity increases and certain emotions are felt. The daily bath (tub or shower) with the generous use of soap and water removes perspiration and most bacteria. Everyone needs to use an effective deodorant (and antiperspirant) regularly each day or more often. The armpits (axilla) should be kept free of hair. Body cleanliness and freshness are a "must" for good grooming, especially for a nurse.

Hands and nails are never free of bacteria. Frequent washing with soap and water and scrubbing with a stiff brush are necessary to keep the hands and nails as free as possible of bacteria. Putting the hands to the face or rubbing the eyes should be avoided. Care is needed for the nails and cuticles to prevent infection and to provide a well-groomed appearance. Hand lotion will help keep the hands smooth and chap-free.

Hair needs regular attention. It should be shampooed at least once a week to give it a clean, well-groomed appearance. Dirt and dust harbor microorganisms which collect easily and quickly on hair. This is why care should be taken to avoid touching the hair or having loose and falling hair touch the face, clothing, food, etc. Clean, attractive hair adds to a person's sense of well-being.

Clean *teeth and mouth* are essential to good health and well-being. Brushing the teeth at least twice a day or after each meal is recommended for proper mouth hygiene. Well-brushed, clean teeth help prevent tooth decay and an unpleasant breath; the use of a mouthwash helps control unpleasant breath (halitosis) which can be offensive to others.

Personal hygiene during menstruation should be meticulous. Many mistaken ideas about bathing and physical activities at time of menstruation have developed through the years. Medical advice continues to point out the need for regular, daily practices of cleanliness and exercise during menstruation. Extraordinary care in controlling body odors must be used; it means more frequent bathing and regular use of deodorants.

Sleep and Rest

The age and size of the individual, his activities, and physical and mental condition help to determine the amount of sleep and rest needed. Sleep comes naturally to a healthy person. The average healthy adult needs about eight hours of sleep and 16 hours of activity for every 24-hour period. The body requires regular sleep because there is no way it can be "stored."

Activity causes fatigue; to tire is normal. Proper amounts of sleep and rest will restore the healthy body in cases of average fatigue. Fatigue may result from a state of mind rather than a physical need. Periodic relaxation during the day helps the body restore itself. Prolonged or continuous sleeplessness is not normal, and a physician's help should be sought to determine the cause.

Nutrition and Fluids

It is known that there is a direct relationship between nutrition and health. A faulty diet and poor eating habits all too often result in problems of health. (See Chapter 25 for normal, daily nutritional needs of the body.)

Many people in this country, though surrounded by good nourishing food, have very poor eating habits. The lack of money is not always the cause of these poor habits. Sometimes it is ignorance, and often it is carelessness. Good eating and food habits include a balanced diet, regularity of meals, adequate time to eat, and conditions for an enjoyable experience at mealtime.

Water is an essential requirement for life but it does not nourish the body. Drinking six to eight glasses of water a day, in addition to the intake in food and beverages, is recommended for proper body processes, and thus is a good health practice.

Elimination

Proper elimination of wastes from the body by the skin, kidneys, and intestines is essential to health. Body wastes (perspiration, urine, feces) are affected by diet, fluids, temperatures, exercise, posture, and habits, but emotions often have an effect on the amount and regularity of elimination too. Excitement, fear, anger, lack of privacy, pain, unpleasant sights and sounds, and other factors may increase or decrease the normal or regular elimination of wastes. Normal elimination, especially of the bowel, is misunderstood by many, and poor habits and practices have resulted. The healthy person has no need to resort to the regular or frequent use of medication or enema. Elimination is a regular and automatic function of the healthy body.

Body Alignment and Activity

Body alignment means that the parts of the body are in position to allow for maximum, comfortable, and graceful use. Posture is an individual matter affected by one's bone and muscle structure and habits. Working against gravity, as the body always does, the parts of the body should be so aligned as to allow maximum comfort in standing, sitting, or walking and at the same time aid body respiration, digestion, elimination, and circulation. Natural alignment helps prevent fatigue.

An individual needs to find his natural posture and maintain it, taking care not to fall into careless sitting or slouching habits which result in stooped shoulders, protruding abdomen, or unsightly walking gait.

A well-aligned, naturally postured body can be graceful in movement — walking, sitting, bending, lifting, and standing — and make a person feel better because he looks better.

Exercise is necessary for proper muscle tone and body function. Many persons do not obtain proper and sufficient physical exercise each day. Experts agree that some type of exercise is beneficial if it is within the individual's physical capacity and affords him opportunity to use muscles not ordinarily used in his work activity.

Work affords activity for almost all people throughout the greatest part of their lives; for some work may be physical rather than mental, for others the opposite is true. In addition to providing one's livelihood, work is important to one's mental well-being if it affords self-respect, dignity, and a feeling of satisfaction and worth. And, indeed, success in work may depend to a great degree on good physical and mental health.

Environment

Environment surrounds and influences a person internally and externally; man responds to his immediate surroundings and he can usually do something about it, however so slightly, to better meet his needs. Environment directly and indirectly affects health. When it is clean, safe, and comfortable as well as attractive it has a direct bearing on one's mental and physical health regardless of age.

Today there is increasing concern about environmental pollution — air, water, odor, noise, etc. (See Chapter 24). Steps are being taken to try and control these man-made problems. Control helps prevent disease, infections and accidents.

Distressful environment factors interrupt work, sleep, relaxation, one's right to privacy and the ability to relax, and often lead to occupational accidents, disabilities and unhappy living situations. Oxygen is one essential part of environment. Man's need for it is basic to life itself; each living cell must have oxygen on a regular and a sustained basis. Clean air is essential to man's oxygen requirements and, as such, he is entitled to have it.

Emotional and Spiritual Support

Emotions influence health. The mind and body work together as one. The body reacts upon the mind and the mind upon the body; they are inseparable.

Everyone has emotions and need for emotions. And they can act for us in favorable or unfavorable ways. Emotions influence body functions and bring about bodily changes, desirable or otherwise. Excitement, fear, anger, and worry are some of the emotions all of us have experienced, some more often than others and in varying degrees. For example, no doubt many have noted that the hands perspire or the heart pounds when they are excited, angry, or afraid. Grief, joy, surprise, and disgust are other well-known emotions which cause body reactions.

Emotions, in and of themselves, do not cause emotional problems; it is the *way* we handle our emotions that causes problems. Everyone needs to have some understanding of emotions in order to understand himself and others with whom he lives and works, because it is in everyday situations when we are tired, under stress, nervous, or physically ill that our emotional conflicts are difficult for us and others to accept. Early in life we need to learn to use our emotions constructively, as our emotional well-being influences our health in general and our outlook on life in particular.

One's emotional and spiritual needs are often closely related. People seek to meet their spiritual and religious needs in many ways. Many follow religious practices established early in life. Regardless of our own needs and beliefs, it is important that we respect the habits and practices of others as they meet their spiritual needs. Each person is unique in his feelings and beliefs. Prejudices and bigotry find no place in the mind of the mature, emotionally stable person who wants

to enjoy real health; such should be the case of the nurse who works with all types of individuals.

Diversion and Recreation

Diversion means to turn aside or away from one's usual pursuits. Recreation is the refreshment of body and mind; the activity and time needed for refreshment vary from one person to another. To some recreation means entertainment and to others it means a change of pace — doing something different. Leisure time is abundant in our society, and this makes diversion and recreation a vital part of our lives. Attention should be given to using this time in activities which will help us to re-create our minds and bodies; we need some purposeful physical and mental diversion from work or full-time activity.

It is a known fact that in the years just ahead people are going to have more leisure time than they do now; people need to learn how to put leisure time to beneficial use. Society is beginning to concern itself with this challenge.

While one's main interest, joy, and greatest satisfactions may come from his work, his level of work performance is better if some time and attention are given to different activities. Some recreational pursuits, with a little imagination, effort, and time, often bring stimulating and worthwhile returns. Everyone should have fun, but not all recreation or leisure can be spent at having fun, because this soon becomes tiresome. Man is creative and a balance between work and recreation can help to promote a happy, healthy person. Established habits of diversion during the working years stand one in good stead for the retirement years ahead. Retirement should be a boon to man's well-being and not a bore.

Mental Hygiene

If we remember that the body and mind work together harmoniously for good health, it becomes apparent that desirable mental health habits are as necessary as good physical health habits.

Mental hygiene is the practice of good habits of the mind. To understand how and why mental hygiene is important, one needs to know what is considered a healthy mind. Qualities of a mentally healthy adult include:

1. Being happy and enjoying life for self and others.

2. Working well with others and realizing satisfaction from doing work to the best of one's ability.

3. Taking criticism with understanding; taking disappointments and difficulties in stride; seeking help when needed.

4. Knowing one's abilities and inabilities and making good use of capacities to serve well.

5. Trusting people and expecting them to trust one.

6. Respecting the rights of others to their beliefs and opinions.

Everyone has certain basic needs throughout life. They include the need to love and be loved; to be wanted, useful, and needed; to feel secure and to belong; to have respect and acceptance of self and others.

Each person has many experiences during a lifetime, and the reactions to these experiences and the adjustments made to satisfy inner needs influence the *personality*. Each one has certain traits, ways of thinking, acting, and feeling, and the way one uses these traits affects the people around him. Personality is difficult to measure, but the person with a so-called "good" personality has qualities which others seem to find agreeable. He accepts himself as a person and is able to make needed adjustments and decisions with reasonable ease; he likes and respects the needs of other people and has the ability to get along with them; he accepts and carries responsibilities according to his abilities and has a healthy respect for work as a necessity. No individual lives without worry, anxiety, doubt, discontent, discouragement, disappointment, defeat, unpleasantness, or anxious moments or times; these cannot be avoided. *It is how we are able to handle these problems in one situation after another that makes for good or poor mental health.*

People use *mental devices* to "protect" themselves. Two of the more convenient and commonly used ones are *forgetting* and *rationalization*. Forgetting is a subconscious protection against the unwanted or unpleasant, and when properly used, it can be an acceptable mental hygiene habit. Rationalization is a process of unconscious self-deception. It is a way of fooling ourselves by the manufacturing of a plausible reason for behavior for which we would rather not acknowledge the real reason. It is used quite often, as when we failed in some undertaking, wanted something, or did or did not want to do something. Recognizing when such devices are honestly used helps one in the practice of good mental hygiene. Such self-understanding promotes good mental health.

SUMMARY

The term health has many descriptions and definitions. From early times to the present, its meaning has grown and changed from a narrow base—being "safe and sound"—to a lengthy description by WHO declaring it a state of ". . . complete physical, mental and social well-being and not merely the absence of disease. . . ." WHO further states that it is a fundamental right of every person to enjoy the highest possible standard of health. To make it possible for the people of the world to enjoy higher health standards, governments must be concerned with such things as improved housing, food and water supplies, immunization programs, and medical services which reach people.

While health is the total of a person's physical, mental, and social well-being, it is an individual matter. So-called healthy people vary in body structure; perhaps one out of ten has an anatomically "perfect" body or a body that performs its functions accordingly. Yet, the other nine are not sick. This means there is a *range* within the "physical, mental and social well-being" description, and most well people are *within the range* but are not necessarily "perfect."

People need to learn how to *stay* well (practice health habits which prevent illness). This is as important as, or even more important than, getting well once illness strikes.

Massive world-wide education must continue and increase if all peoples are to enjoy longer, more healthy lives.

An individual has basic needs to meet every day. They are present when he is well; they are present when he is ill. Practicing good health habits in relation to these basic needs will help you as a person and as a practical nurse. In turn, you will understand how to assist the patient when he needs your help.

GUIDES FOR STUDY AND DISCUSSION

1. Health does not have a clear-cut definition. What makes this a true statement?

2. What are some of the major health problems facing the world today?

3. Some countries do better in meeting the health needs of their people than this country. In your opinion, what could be the reason for this?

4. Why must research keep on asking new questions?

5. If you were 100% healthy, how would you feel?

6. Using the nine essential daily living needs as a guide, list under each the changes you could make in your daily health habits which would be an improvement for you.

7. How do you account for the tremendous increase in the life span since 1900?

SUGGESTED SITUATIONS AND ACTIVITIES

1. Using any common news media (newpapers, magazines, radio, television), discover some health problem in another country. Find out if it is a problem in this country also.

2. Identify two or three health problems in your area.

3. Locate a definition of health from another source. Compare it with definitions in this chapter. Then, write your own definition of health telling what it means to you.

4. List under each heading the items you believe improve health:

Physical Well-Being   *Mental Well-Being*   *Social Well-Being*

THE FAMILY UNIT AND HEALTH

OBJECTIVES FOR THE STUDENT: Be able to:

1. Explain the difference between "nuclear" family and "extended" family.
2. Describe the functions of the nuclear family.
3. Name four ways the family serves itself.
4. Name three ways the family serves others.
5. Explain how the shift from rural to urban living is affecting the family unit.
6. Compare family responsibilities for health care today with those of fifty years ago.
7. Describe some of the main changes which have taken place in family living in the past generation or two.

SUGGESTED STUDY VOCABULARY*

primitive peoples	extended family	code
generation	longevity	indigent
progenitor	code of conduct	universal
kindred	procreation	beliefs
nuclear family	urbanization	values

*Look for any terms you already know.

INTRODUCTION

This chapter is designed to help you look rather closely at *the family as a unit* having certain and definite responsibilities for the health of its members. This information will deepen your understanding of people as it relates to human growth and development. Likewise, it will be useful to help you to appreciate a family's concern when one of its members is ill.

The previous chapter, Health of the Individual, is a stepping stone to understanding the family because a family is made up of individuals. Attempt to see the family as a most influential group of people who relate and belong to each other; these relationships influence the way each family member meets his daily living needs.

MEANINGS OF THE TERM FAMILY

Looking across the long stretch of history, the institution we think of as *the family* is older and more universal than just about anything one could name. Authorities have long studied (and not always agreed about) the origins of family life; the fact that a human is dependent for years upon his family for just about everything related to his basic needs makes the family an essential, ongoing concern of society.

The family in our culture is but one of many patterns of family life around the world. The patterns are especially different among primitive peoples. Despite the differences, in each culture the young are cared for and instructed; but there is no guarantee that a certain people or tribe or nationality will carry out these responsibilities in the same way even from family to family or generation to generation. In fact, the contrary is true within the family culture we know best—namely our own.

Down through the ages, groups of people descending from a common, direct ancestry have been labeled a race, clan, tribe, nationality, group of descendants, breed, kindred, and family. The term *family* includes such definitions as a group formed by parents and children, a body of individuals who live in one house under "one head," one's children, immediate kindred, or those descended from a common progenitor.

The word "family" in our culture commonly refers to a group formed by parents and children. However, it is interesting to note that this term broadens to include others at certain times. For instance, it is common to hear a remark such as, "Our whole family will be together for Christmas dinner." In this case grandparents, aunts, uncles, cousins, brothers, sisters, and in-laws are present and are considered *family*. As another example, consider those who come to a family reunion. To distinguish between these two meanings of "family," sociologists refer to the parents-children unit as the *nuclear* family; this family unit plus relatives is called the *extended* family.

In discussing family responsibilities for health care, we are concerned with the nuclear family. This is not to say that other kindred (grandparents, for example) might not be living in the home; they may well be. However, this practice is not as common as it used to be,

and some of the reasons for the noticeable change are included in this chapter.

FUNCTIONS OF THE FAMILY UNIT

It is fair to say the family is a unit (something put together to make "one") which serves many intermixed functions. These functions serve the members of the household and, in turn, the society of which the family is a part. The term "society" includes local, regional, national, and world-wide communities as they relate one to the other.

Because of its many functions, the family unit can be viewed from many directions. For instance, the family is a consuming group; it uses all manner of food, clothing, equipment, and supplies. Because it is a consumer of supplies, industry and business view it from the standpoint of how much of what kinds of things will family units need and purchase. Other aspects of society view the family from their standpoint, e.g., medical science, government.

Table 23–1 shows several ways the family serves itself and society. This information will help you understand why the family is viewed (studied) from many directions, all of which have some bearing on family responsibilities for health and health care.

TODAY'S FAMILY IN A CHANGING SOCIETY

Families make up a society. When time brings about changes in the ways society does things and takes action (by voting, passing laws, setting standards of conduct, etc.) to provide for the well-being of all, the family unit is involved in these changes. This has been true in the past and will be true in the future. Beginning with the earliest families and through the ages, family life has felt the impact of such things as discoveries, inventions, wars, famines, widespread diseases, natural disasters, and man's imagination and need to explore. Consider what families have inherited over the years due to man's ability to make possible such things as the wheel, gunpowder, the printing press, steel, the steam engine, automobiles, aircraft, atomic power,

TABLE 23-1. FUNCTION OF THE FAMILY UNIT

HOW IT SERVES ITSELF

1. To continue the race by having children and providing for them until the children are able to do this for themselves.	The human needs protection and help for years before he is able to go out on his own and start his family. Marriage is the social means of perpetuating or continuing a people While satisfying sexual drives, marriage has a much broader purpose — that of extending love, care, protection, and security to its members Population "explosions" are causing societies to study the problem of birth control; it involves great differences of opinion and basic beliefs among people.
2. To provide a way of living which in turn influences beliefs, values, attitudes, and goals.	Children are influenced by what the family stands for. Early in life the things the parents stand for begin to influence the ways children respond. Parental actions have an impact on the lives of each individual in the family
3. To serve as the first instructional source for the human.	The child finds the ways he can depend upon his family and experiences a period filled with learning; it is believed to be the most rapid period of learning in the life span (see Fig. 23-1).
4. To provide love, care, and protection among its members and to promote security and a sense of well-being.	In this respect, the family unit functions in a way closely intermixed with its other functions. It is not easy to describe "caring" and "security" apart from helping a child meet his daily living needs, or apart from his feelings and beliefs about his family.

HOW IT SERVES OTHERS

1. A consuming and producing unit.	The family has many needs related to food, shelter, clothing, health, transportation, recreation, etc. It purchases services and supplies of every description, and therefore supports many aspects of society. Family members work to help produce for others. Thus, being a consuming-producing unit, it is an essential feature of all business and industry.
2. A biological unit.	The family unit is studied for purposes of statistics — births, deaths, illnesses, ages — to provide information about health, illness, and longevity.
3. A social unit.	The family unit is also studied for its patterns of conduct as they relate to crime, social welfare, education, marriage, divorce, and general living patterns.

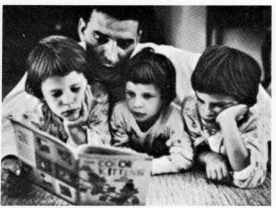

FIGURE 23-1   A bedtime story — a time to share and to learn. (Brisbane: The Developing Child, Charles A. Bennett Co. (Courtesy of the Hoover Co.)

and space travel. The future holds much change and rapid change; man will continue to imagine, explore, invent, and discover, and families will continue to be influenced by his efforts.

To deserve the title "society" a people must gauge its conduct by certain codes or standards for itself. These standards serve as an adhesive which holds the social structure together. When a society loses its commitment to acceptable conduct and allows "the code" to fall by the wayside, it loses its adhesiveness. It is then that unlikely and unacceptable things occur which jar its stability.

Family stability is directly influenced by what the surrounding society permits, encourages, discourages, and condemns. Therefore, if society's commitment to standards is firm, the family unit inherits the benefits; if such commitment is lacking, the family is likewise involved in the "fall-out."

From a Rural to an Urban Society

In this country the shift from a rural to an urban way of life has changed and is continuing to change many aspects of family life. These changes affect where and how people are housed, how they make a living, how they acquire food and clothing, and how they get an education. Urbanization creates health problems dealing with sanitation, water and air pollution, and overcrowding, all of which in turn contribute to the spread of disease, lack of space for recreation, and lack of purposeful use of leisure time. Huge concentrations of people overtax hospital and health clinic facilities, schools, streets, and highways as families try to live, work, play, travel, and receive care when they are sick.

Changes in Family Life

Two or three generations ago, all family members were involved in the activities which produced much of what the family needed. At that time the family often included grandparents who had raised their family on "the home place" and stayed on to live with a son or daughter and their family. Family ties were close and when something happened to one member, the others were immediately involved because they were close at hand.

Neighbors knew neighbors; they helped each other in all kinds of situations. There was much face to face contact among the same people year after year which influenced relationships and how people felt about each other. A neighborhood had its own qualities and "flavor" which generated from its people, their beliefs and values, and the way they conducted their lives. While remnants of such a society still exist in parts of the country, an increasing majority of people today live in quite another way; the importance of one family to another has diminished.

Today's Family

Parents and children make up this unit. As a rule the household does not include grandparents or other kindred. They live apart from their children, often for good reasons. Chapter 21 discusses the elderly adult and his needs in our society.

Providing for the needs of today's family

and the "extras" it feels are needed is directly related (or should be) to the family's ability to purchase these things. With increasing frequency, this means that both the father and the mother are wage-earners and away from the household, often at the same time.

The necessity for both parents to work is bringing about another noticeable change in family life: *increasing numbers of small children are being cared for by other than family members,* often in facilities outside the home. Day care centers and "nursery" schools are common sights in almost every community.

One-parent Households

Family life is altered when a mother or father is left to manage the household and support the family. Here again, the children may be under the charge of a non-family member. The lone parent wears two hats, so to speak, in fulfilling obligations of providing love, security, protection, early instruction, and a worthy system of values for the children.

Restudy Table 23–1 and notice that a family serves itself by its value system or what it believes in, lives by, and works toward; it serves as the first instructional source for the offspring and provides love, care, protection, and security. When a society substitutes the natural home environment with such agencies as day care centers to take care of its young for about one-third of their lives, until they are old enough to be turned over to a school system, it must concern itself with the importance of setting standards to see that these substitute "homes" go as far as possible to realistically provide a safe, clean, child-worthy environment which helps promote basic family functions.

Time has not altered the basic functions of the family (procreation, value-setting, goal-setting, early instruction, providing love, security and protection) but time does alter *how* and *how well* the family unit fulfills these basic functions.

Concern for One Another

Family members have less face to face contact with each other than in the past and very much less contact with their neighbors. In fact, next door neighbors are apt to be strangers to each other in every respect. The most they have in common is the fact they are busy, working human beings who nod to each other in passing. Less face to face contact between and among family members (and neighbors) can lead to a feeling of individual independence and less accountability to others; this in turn can result in less concern for other persons and their well-being.

Independence is a characteristic of children today. As family members, they share in planning activities and feel free to make their wishes known. Many families arrive at decisions by democratic means where all points of view are considered and the final decision is one that seems to be the best for the family unit. It is understandable that not every family member is happy with every decision, but each learns to live by the rules and decisions of the home just as a citizen must abide by standards set by government whether he likes them or not because ours is a government of laws created by a democracy.

Independence during childhood can lead to more rapid maturation. Early maturity is noticeable in our society; some family situations force it more than others by what is permitted, promoted, and encouraged in the way of social goals for the children. While children or youth marry at an earlier age in some other societies, youthful marriages today are more common in our society than in past generations.

In short, today's family unit is quite different from earlier units. It lives, works, plays, and carries on its basic functions amidst more crowded living conditions; less open space for recreation; more laws to control safety, health and welfare; less face to face contact with one another on a long term basis; and less apparent sense of concern for the other individual, especially if he is a "stranger." The costs of meeting family goals is forcing changes in the pattern of day to day living which have an immediate influence upon the lives of each family member.

FAMILY HEALTH CARE

Family health care is really a two-way situation. The family influences health care and health care influences the family. The family is responsible for providing health care (medical, dental, hospital, preventive measures, etc.) for its members. Sometimes the family is able to pay for this care and sometimes it is not. However, in either instance, the parents are responsible to see that care is provided by one means or another. This often means that help is sought from some government agencies and/or voluntary organizations. Thus the family affects the extent of health measures provided—adequate or inadequate.

In turn, health problems influence the family. The extent and seriousness of health problems often make extraordinary demands upon the family and result in restructuring the family unit: For instance, the child who needs care in a special hospital for long periods of time or even for life; or the family member who is being cared for in the home.

People are more health-conscious today because they are aware of the benefits of proper nutrition and adequate housing, the worth of immunization programs, safe water, clean air, and the need to practice safety in the home, on the job, and during travel.

State and federal governments are deeply involved in family health through their efforts to help the family meet its obligations to get well and stay well. While our society expects the family to be responsible for meeting its individual health needs if it is able, laws are passed to insure the proper production of food, drugs, and water supplies, and to insure housing standards through building codes and zoning regulations. Governments likewise provide direct health care services to the indigent family unable to provide for its members; the question of the quality of this care must continue to be a concern of society.

The Cost of Health Care

The family health dollar is spread in several directions, generally in this order of cost: hospital, physician, drugs, dentist, health insurance, appliances and other incidental health expenses. Here again, government concerns itself with the rising costs and the quality as well as the quantity of health care available to the family. Families experiencing frequent illness, long term illness, or unemployment are faced with serious financial difficulties. Families without health insurance ("sickness" insurance, "sickness" benefits) may soon use up their savings and be forced to turn to others for necessary health care.

Communities have agencies and organizations to help needy families in some circumstances, but often the family is hesitant to seek help. The community, not the neighbor, extends help to the family. But security and a sense of belonging cannot be provided by an agency or organization in the same effective way that home and family can.

Regardless of who is ill in the family,

sickness can cause concern and hardships. Health insurance helps meet financial costs but often these costs exceed the insurance coverage. It is doubly hard if the ill member is the family "breadwinner." Worry, anxiety and fear often take over within the family unit and feelings are sometimes expressed in unusual ways. An acceptance of this fact will help you understand how to better relate to the family as well as to the patient.

SUMMARY

The family is the basic unit of society. It serves itself and it serves others; therefore, what the family is (or is not) affects society. The reverse is also true—what society stands for or fails to stand for influences the family unit.

The basic functions of the family—to continue the human race and provide for its young—remain the same; the manner in which the family meets its obligations alters as time and circumstances change.

Shifting from a rural to an urban society brings about changes which often result in problems for the family and for society in general. However, urban living has many advantages as well.

Health care is costly, whether it is money paid to get well or to stay well. The trend in this country toward more families being protected by prepaid health insurance plans is an indication that people recognize they have responsibilities to meet their sickness needs. Not all people can afford prepaid insurance plans and often turn to the government for assistance.

GUIDES FOR STUDY AND DISCUSSION

1. Why is it necessary to specify who is part of the family unit? Who makes up the "nuclear" family? The "extended" family?
2. How have relationships among family members changed as society moves toward urbanization?
3. A family is made up of individuals, each with basic daily living needs. What are some things parents need to provide, or be aware of, in seeing that family members' needs are met?
4. What is meant by—*family influences health and health influences family?*
5. A neighbor is a person who lives near another. To be a neighbor today is apt to be different from being a neighbor in 1900. Why is this so?
6. The family is the first source of instruction for the child. What does the child learn from his parents?
7. Table 23–1 indicates that the family is a "social unit" (among other things). Why would a society study the family as "a social unit"? How can such information be useful?
8. Taking care of family health needs has changed a great deal in the past thirty to forty years. List as many of these changes as you can think of. What changes do you see ahead?
9. When illness strikes a family it can disrupt the family unit. Why is this so?

SUGGESTED SITUATIONS AND ACTIVITIES

1. Communities help promote family health. Find out what agencies in your community are available to families who have health problems.
2. News media are often accused of pointing out the "care less" attitudes among people rather than their "care more" attitudes. For several days, follow your usual news sources closely while keeping this accusation in mind. Estimate whether it is true or not as you observe.
3. If there were an *ideal family,* what would it be like?

CHAPTER 24

THE COMMUNITY AND HEALTH

TOPICAL HEADINGS

Introduction
Meaning of Community
The Work of Health Agencies

Health Problems Facing the Nation
Health Facilities in the Community
Community Responsibilities in a Disaster

Summary
Guides for Study and Discussion
Suggested Situation and Activity

OBJECTIVES FOR THE STUDENT: Be able to:

1. Give examples of various sizes of communities.
2. List some world-wide health problems facing humanity.
3. Explain how health problems in one part of the world can be of direct concern to people living elsewhere.
4. Give one example of a health agency under: a. international control; b. national control; c. state/province control; d. local control.
5. Differentiate between official and nonofficial health agencies by giving two examples of each.
6. Describe the general functions of the local health agency.
7. Describe the role of the community before, during and following a disaster.
8. Use two examples which show why people need survival training.
9. Explain how any of your daily living needs are influenced by public health activities in *your* community.

SUGGESTED STUDY VOCABULARY*

community	rehabilitation	health education
behavior	quackery	immunization
rural	fraud	civil defense
urban	congenital malformation	progressive patient care
welfare	official	disaster
humanity	nonofficial	emergency

*Look for any terms you already know.

INTRODUCTION

This chapter rounds out the so-called "health picture." You are already aware of the daily living needs of the individual and how they can be best practiced to promote health. You are likewise aware of the functions of the family and its responsibilities to itself and so-ciety. Next comes a look at the functions of "society" and its responsibilities to the people. This chapter is concerned with community (from the largest to the smallest) efforts to promote health and the things that are being done on a world-wide, nation-wide, and local community level to help improve health and to safeguard the lives of people. Keep in mind the basic needs of all people as you learn about the community, because people *make* the community; remember also that the number of people in the world is increasing at an alarming rate and this awesome fact has a vital relationship to health and health care.

MEANING OF COMMUNITY

A *community* is a body of people living in the same place under the same laws and regulations. It is made up of individuals and families in a particular place, and includes all phases of their lives. On first thought one is apt to think "small" in terms of size when the term community is used because one definition of the word is "people living in the same place." However, the term is also used to refer to society in general and this can mean people on a large, even world-wide, basis.

Communities have their own characteristics and may differ widely as to rules, customs, and behavior. A nation has its language or languages, its customs and its habits. There are remarkable differences in the diet and eating practices among the peoples of the world; customs related to religious practices, marriage, divorce, the role of women, dress, work, and education likewise show great variations around the globe.

Individuals reflect the influences of the family and the community in their behavior. Thus, it is important for you to know about the patient as an individual so your behavior will show regard for him as a person first and a patient second.

Levels of Communities

Communities vary according to size. They are sometimes known as rural or urban. Generally speaking, the rural community includes farms and villages of fewer than 2500 people, and the urban community includes the nonfarm areas with towns and cities of populations over 2500.

Life in one community affects life in other communities, and each is a part of a larger community. The larger the community, the larger and more varied are its responsibilities toward its citizens. As pointed out in Chapter 23, the demands of living in the large urban communities are complex, and there must be planning and direction for the good of all.

The growing trend toward urbanization in this country is rapidly making each urban center take needed steps to provide such vital things as adequate water supplies, sewage disposal, decent housing, control of vermin, more effective garbage and trash collection, improved schools, noise control, crime control, fire protection, traffic congestion, and air pollution, as well as facilities for recreation and adequate health care services. These mounting problems are related to the health and welfare of people. Today a city, facing these and related problems, often turns to the federal government for financial help because costs involved overburden the local community.

In order to make provisions for community welfare (including services, laws, regulations, and personnel) a community must have some type of organization or governing body. This may be a district organized for school purposes, or fire protection, or the incorporated village, the township, or the county. Counties make up the state, and the states the national or federal government. Canada is made up of ten provinces and two territories.

National health and welfare programs, regulations, and laws are instituted with the needs of people in mind; such efforts generally flow through state government channels to reach the individual citizen (see Fig. 24–1).

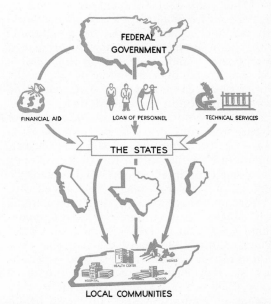

FIGURE 24-1 Federal health aid to states and local communities. (*Guide to Health Organization in the United States*, U. S. Government Printing Office.)

THE WORK OF HEALTH AGENCIES

Health programs and activities are carried out by two types of organizations, the *official* and the *nonofficial*. Health organizations supported by tax money and organized on an international, federal, state, or local basis are known as official agencies, while health organizations supported by gifts and fund-raising drives are known as nonofficial or voluntary agencies and are run by groups of interested citizens.

OFFICIAL HEALTH AGENCIES

International

Health problems in one section of the world can fast become the problems of other sections due to rapid travel and instant communication. These two things, among others, make the world very much smaller. A person can spread a disease from one continent to another in a matter of hours. The ravages of a typhoon in the southwest Pacific are known here while it is happening. Calls for help for food, clothing, and medical supplies bring fast results.

The health needs of mankind are becoming the concern of all. People around the world are healthier. The life span is lengthening while the infant mortality rate is lowering, and this means rapid increases in population. There are well over 3 billion people in the world; some 21 million live in Canada and over 203 million in the United States.

Earliest efforts to control the spread of disease from country to country go back many years to the detention of shipping vessels (quarantine) in the harbor for 40 days if they had come from infected ports. To control the spread of cholera, plague, yellow fever, typhus, and smallpox, the first international conferences (International Sanitary Conventions) were held in 1897 (Venice) and 1903 (Paris). Until 1938 these conventions were held to modernize the controls. The Americas had the Pan American Sanitary Bureau to serve their needs. Other organizations, e.g., League of Nations, worked on world health problems too.

WORLD HEALTH ORGANIZATION. *"The attainment of all peoples of the highest possible level of health" is its main objective.* In 1946, under the parent organization, the United Nations, efforts started which led to the formation of the World Health Organization (WHO) in 1948. Dr. Brock Chrisholm, a Canadian psychiatrist, was its first director. Today well over one hundred nations are members in this organization which actually serves a public health role around the world.

WHO headquarters are in Geneva, Switzerland, while several regional offices in various parts of the world bring the public health programs closer to peoples and their needs. These programs include attention to tuberculosis, malaria, maternal and child health, venereal disease, nutrition, mental health, and environmental hygiene (see Figs. 24–2 and 24–3).

National

The federal government plays a responsible and expanding role in the health of all citizens through the United States Public Health Service (USPHS). It was organized in 1798 to render care to merchant seamen (Marine Hospital Service). Its responsibilities multiplied as the nation grew, and in 1912 the organization

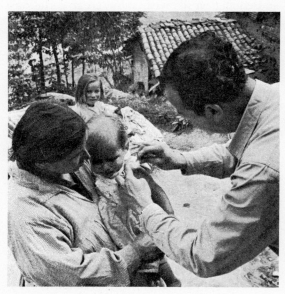

FIGURE 24-2 Colombia: A worried mother brings her child for examination by a World Health Organization doctor. (Schifferes: Essentials of Healthier Living, 3rd Ed. John Wiley and Sons, Inc.)

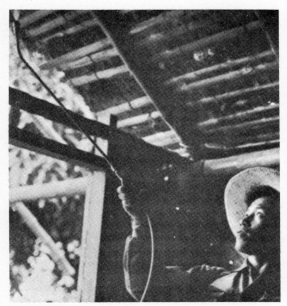

FIGURE 24-3 Philippines: Spraying to control malaria. The local government carries on a regular spraying program with the help of WHO. (Schifferes: Essentials of Healthier Living, 3rd Ed. John Wiley and Sons, Inc.)

was renamed the United States Public Health Service. Today it reaches people through regional offices and services as shown in Figure 24–4.

Since 1953 the USPHS has been a vital section of the Department of Health, Education and Welfare (HEW) which has subdivisions to carry out a wide variety of related functions, as shown in Table 24–1.

Other departments of the federal government carrying responsibility for health include the Department of Agriculture (e.g., meat inspection), the Armed Services health care programs in the Defense Department, and the Veteran's Administration services to veterans.

Figure 24–1 illustrates the three ways (money, personnel, and services) the federal government helps a state meet its health needs.

State

Each state is responsible for providing its own laws and regulations to protect the health and welfare of its people; however, a state law

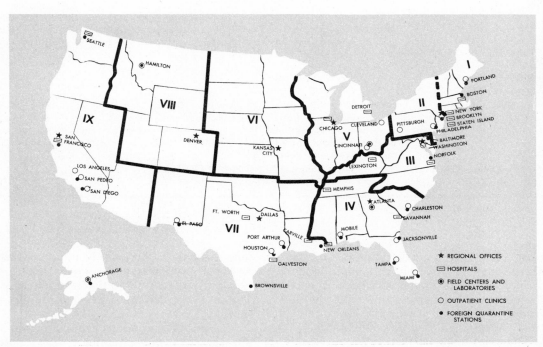

FIGURE 24-4 Public Health Service offices in the United States. Regional offices have since been established in Anchorage, Alaska, and Honolulu, Hawaii. (From Public Health Service Today, U. S. Government Printing Office.)

TABLE 24–1. DEPARTMENT OF HEALTH, EDUCATION AND WELFARE

SUBDIVISION	FUNCTIONS *
1. Public Health Service *Office of the Surgeon General*	
National Institute of Health	Investigates illnesses and conducts research. Grants money to others to carry on teaching and research programs.
Bureau of State Services	As the name implies, it serves state (and local) communities by providing assistance (money, consultation, etc.) to cope with such health problems as cancer, heart disease, venereal disease, mental illness, and tuberculosis. It concerns itself with air and water pollution, sewage control, adequate hospital construction, collecting vital statistics (deaths, births, etc.). accident prevention, food sanitation, public health education, and renders aid during and following disasters.
Bureau of Medical Services	Enforces quarantine regulations related to all types of incoming personnel; operates hospitals (which are important to research efforts) for PHS, Coast Guard, and civil service employees; responsible for health services to the American Indian, Eskimos, federal prisoners. Conducts research on food and water contamination, noise hazards, mental illness, cancer, and vaccines. Prisoners in the federal prisons may (and do) volunteer to be used in many research projects.
2. Office of Education	
3. Office of Vocational Rehabilitation	Provides programs for and assistance (money, consultation) to states to carry on efforts to rehabilitate handicapped persons including amputees, emotionally disturbed persons, the blind, people afflicted with epilepsy and cerebral palsy.
4. Food and Drug Administration	Responsible for setting standards concerning food, drugs, and cosmetics. A watchdog protecting consumers against dangerous and contaminated foods, dangerous drugs, "unproven" drugs, quackery with respect to medical devices and medicines, and fraudulent claims for cosmetics. (See Chapters 25 (Nutrition) and 29 (Drugs) for further discussion of this service.)
5. Social Security Administration *Office of Commissioner, Bureau of Federal Credit Unions, Bureau of Old Age and Survivors' Assistance*	This administration handles *Medicare,* hospital insurance to help pay for hospital care, out-patient services, and, if elected, medical insurance to help pay for physicians' services for persons over 65 who receive monthly social security benefits.
Children's Bureau	Since 1912 this bureau has been guarding the well-being of children through its assistance to states. It is concerned with maternal and child well-being, long-term disabling conditions, congenital malformation, and is now looking at the problems of children (delinquency, crime, battered or neglected child, migrant workers' families).
6. St. Elizabeth's Hospital	Psychiatric hospital in District of Columbia.
7. Welfare Administration	

* Only health-related functions discussed.

cannot contradict the Constitution of the United States, or any law, regulation, or enforcement of the federal government. In each state there is a department of health, the official agency concerned with the health interests of the people within its boundaries.

The chief responsibility of a state health department is to study the health needs of the people and to provide ways to protect and meet these needs, as well as serve in an advisory capacity to the local health department. Although programs and services may differ widely from one state to the next, all carry on certain basic activities which generally include:

1. Inspection and licensure of certain businesses, i.e., public eating places, hotels, motels, dairies, bakeries, canning factories, hospitals, and nursing homes.

2. Collection of data and keeping of

records (vital statistics) of births, deaths, marriages, population, incidence of diseases, etc.

3. Prevention and control of communicable diseases through health education, immunization, x-ray programs, and hospitals or clinics for treatment and cure.

4. Prevention, control, treatment, and rehabilitation related to chronic diseases and illnesses, disabilities, and handicaps.

5. Health education and welfare of mothers, infants, and children.

6. Provision for adequate and safe measures covering water supply, sewage disposal, milk, food and food handlers, rodent and insect control; disposal of industrial wastes; contamination of air, soil, and water; and housing.

7. Health education of the public in all phases of health work with printed materials, radio and television programs, teaching, and training.

8. Provision for safety and accident prevention.

9. Public health nursing to provide consultation, education, services, assistance with setting up programs and clinics, its main purpose being that of health counseling and supervision.

The state department of health helps to set the pattern for public health care in the local units.

Local

Local health departments work very closely with the state department in carrying out their health programs. The local unit may be the county, city, or a combination city-county unit depending upon the population, health needs and services, and money available. It is at the local level that the individual receives direct help with health problems. The immediate and direct responsibility for carrying out the health laws, regulations, and programs is generally that of the local health department. Some of its activities include:

1. Immunization against smallpox, diphtheria, polio, whooping cough, tetanus. Many states require a health record showing that children attending public schools have been immunized against certain communicable diseases.

2. Tuberculin testing and chest x-rays to detect and control tuberculosis.

3. Physical examinations and chest x-rays for food handlers.

4. Laboratory tests to detect and control venereal diseases. Most states require a premarital examination of both parties for venereal disease before a marriage license will be issued.

5. Clinics for pre- and postnatal care, care of infants, dental, mental, eye, diabetic, and many other health problems.

6. Health education, counseling, and supervision for the family and the follow-up of a patient who has returned home from the hospital.

7. Work with other health agencies to find needed help for the patient, i.e., referral for rehabilitation, child guidance, or aid to dependent children.

These are only examples of how the local health department works and serves in meeting the responsibility delegated to it by the state.

NONOFFICIAL OR VOLUNTARY HEALTH AGENCIES

Official and nonofficial health organizations and agencies often work very closely together on national, state, and local levels to meet health problems.

There are many hundreds of voluntary (nonprofit, nontax supported) health agencies, and over the years many have made valuable contributions to the health of this country. Some are large organizations and are nationally organized, while others are local. Large or small, all concern themselves with health needs and problems. Very often through the efforts of a voluntary health agency come the solutions to serious health problems (e.g., "The March of Dimes" and the control of polio).

Voluntary health agencies may be managed and staffed by professional or nonprofessional personnel, or by both; some are paid and others serve as volunteers.

The functions of the voluntary health agencies vary; most provide for research and education while some provide services. Education is through printed materials, programs, conferences, teaching, and scholarships. News releases, radio and television programs, films, and exhibits are furnished to educate the general public, school children, and special groups. Funds are furnished for research in the prevention, treatment, or cure of some disease or health problem. Some agencies

WHICH OF THESE HEALTH-AGENCY SYMBOLS DO YOU RECOGNIZE?

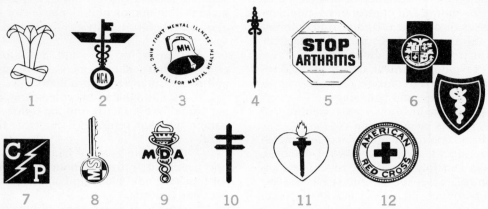

FIGURE 24-5 Health agency symbols: 1, National Society for Crippled Children (Easter Seal Society). 2, The National Council on Alcoholism, Inc. 3, National Association for Mental Health. 4, American Cancer Society. 5, Arthritis Foundation. 6, Blue Cross and Blue Shield. 7, United Cerebral Palsy Association. 8, National Multiple Sclerosis Society. 9, Muscular Dystrophy Association of America. 10, National Tuberculosis Association. 11, American Heart Association. 12, American Red Cross. (Schifferes: Essentials of Healthier Living, 3rd Ed. John Wiley and Sons, Inc.)

serve patients by providing equipment and personnel for use on loan, e.g., the respirator, recreation.

Figure 24–5 includes symbols for only twelve agencies from a list that could cover several pages. You no doubt have had some first-hand experience or have information about these and others in your community. Figure 21–2 is a familiar scene in our country; it represents a way of life, that of giving volunteer health service.

HEALTH PROBLEMS FACING THE NATION

The limits placed on the term "health problems" help determine what would be included in the list. One could make such a list by naming the major causes of death and stop there; it would (and does) represent some serious problems calling for solutions and right answers. However, this approach limits the scope of the matter. A society has all kinds of factors which relate to each other in a chain-like fashion when it comes to health. One has only to think of housing, sanitation, safe water, and proper garbage disposal to disclose a nest of contributing factors. But any list could (and should) be lengthened to include such vital things as available hospital beds, outpatient clinic facilities, public health

programs in disease prevention, mental health programs, school health efforts, and programs to rehabilitate persons with crippling conditions. Add the problems of air and water pollution, noise control, poisoning, malnutrition, drug addiction, abortion, misuse of pesticides and the list becomes increasingly more complex and awesome. And yet this list still does not exhaust the problems related to health by any means.

The United States, a changing, mobile, health-conscious nation of more than two hundred million, where three out of four families carry some type of health insurance, is finding that it may outrun its ability to provide quality and quantity health care if it does not keep pace with needed changes. What was needed in the 1950's and used in the 1960's will not suit the needs of the 1970's or the 1980's.

The importance of this challenge has the attention of concerned segments of society as well as state and federal governments. The rising costs of health care and the gaps appearing in the quality and distribution of health services call for new answers.

Shortages of trained people at all levels of health care are serious. The need to keep abreast of new knowledge and be flexible in accepting change stares all personnel in the face.

Physical facilities need to reflect more imagination, variety, and flexibility. The "traditional" hospital plan hampers the effective use of many technical lifesaving devices today; it influences how personnel are used—often to the disadvantage of patient and worker alike.

One of the greatest challenges to providing health care is the quality and quantity of health personnel themselves; they have much to do with the quality and the quantity of service rendered. A person trained ten years ago, who has not made it his business to keep up to date, is out of date. As a licensed practical nurse you will be one of these people working in situations calling for change. Your attitude and your willingness (or unwillingness) to participate in change are part of this challenge.

It is fair to say that the immediate future will require the very best efforts of all (federal government down to the individual) if health needs are to be safely met. Billions of dollars are spent on health care; it must be the goal of all involved to provide the quality as well as quantity of care needed by our citizens. Answers to health care problems facing us today and tomorrow will not be met by yesterday's solutions. New answers must come from the minds of visionary, flexible people.

HEALTH FACILITIES IN THE COMMUNITY

The Hospital

A country faced with a growing population and ever-new types of technical devices to save and prolong life, needs to design its hospital facilities to meet the demands and needs for health care. Many hospitals have been built or expanded in this country since 1946 when Congress passed the Hill-Burton Act (Hospital Survey and Construction Act), yet there are serious gaps in the services available to people.

Hospitals may be classified in several ways, according to financial support, ownership, management, purpose, type of patient, or illness. When hospitals are built and operated by the city, county, state, or federal government, they are known as public or nonprofit hospitals and may be general or special. Hospitals built, owned, and operated by private individuals or by religious or fraternal organizations are generally known as private, but also may be general or special.

A general hospital is usually able to provide care for patients of any age and with any health or illness need. A hospital that cares for patients in a certain age group or with a certain disease or health need is commonly called *special.* For example, there are hospitals that care for children or the aged; others that care for patients with mental illness, cancer, alcoholism, chronic diseases, orthopedic, and eye, ear, nose, and throat conditions; while others care for certain groups (maternity) or those in need of a certain therapy or rehabilitation. State and federal hospitals are usually for patients with certain long-term disorders such as mental retardation and mental illness, or they accommodate a specific group such as ex-servicemen in the Veteran's Administration Hospital. Organizations often support hospitals for their members (railroads, miners) or for special groups (crippled children).

The local general hospital is an important facility for health care in a community. A hospital must meet certain standards for approval by the Joint Commission on Accreditation of Hospitals to become an *accredited hospital.* A hospital must have a license which is granted by some state agency and renewed at regular intervals; to keep a license, a hospital must maintain its facilities and services according to the state agency's regulations.

Increased numbers of people use the hospital each year because people have learned that the hospital is the best place to receive proper care when one is ill. They have not always held this faith; some years ago the general public held that only the very poor or the dying were taken to the hospital. People were cared for in the home until advances in medical science and treatment made it almost necessary for them to be in the hospital. Soon after the turn of the century, the physician and the patient looked to the hospital as the place for the safe and best treatment of diseases, for surgery, for mothers and newborns, and for emergencies.

Today, the physician heads a team of personnel and uses a vast array of technical equipment in making a more accurate and quick diagnosis to assure better treatment and recovery. Many devices and supportive services (computerized record keeping, inhalation therapy, x-ray facilities, blood and other fluid therapies, etc.) are available to the physician and members of the health team.

Larger hospitals and those in teaching centers frequently have other responsibilities;

they provide the clinical environment for research and the education of personnel in the health professions. Research into the prevention and cure of illness, rehabilitation, and all phases of patient care is carried out by medical, nursing, dietary, social science, and other personnel. These same groups and others use the hospital for learning purposes; thus it serves to educate many.

Progressive patient care (PPC) refers to patients being assigned to specific service units equipped and staffed according to the needs of the patients in that unit. This concept of patient care, dating from about 1955, has not taken hold as a "whole package" idea. However, the trend seems to be in that direction. One part of the "package" that has been widely adopted is the *intensive care unit*.

Other Health Facilities

Many communities are finding a need for other facilities and services to help meet the health and welfare needs of their people. With increasing emphasis on prevention and rehabilitation, these facilities and services may or may not be connected with the hospital, depending upon the interest, support, and resources in the community.

Clinics are often established for a specific purpose (condition or illness) with public or private support. Most clinics have a program of prevention, rehabilitation, patient and family teaching, and follow-up. Examples of the more commonly found clinics include those for mental hygiene, diabetes, crippling conditions of children, and other chronic and long-term illnesses including disabilities of eye, ear, or speech.

Intermediate care facilities (a facet of the PPC concept), sometimes called *extended care facilities* are beginning to come into the facilities picture. They are emerging as a facility to render service between the hospital and home or the hospital and the *nursing home*. There have been justified objections to the use of the word "home" in the title of any institution or agency, and it is interesting to note the omission of this word in the name of many long-term care facilities. When the patient does not need the type of care the hospital is equipped to furnish it is often more satisfactory, convenient, and economical for him to use some other type of facility, especially if the patient is ambulatory, can care for himself,

is recovering from an acute illness, is receiving some specific therapy, or needs this type of care as a part of his therapy.

Another facet of the PPC concept that is slowly emerging is the *Home Care Program*. "For the patient who can be treated at home, this is often the best place for him to be. It is the physical and emotional environment with which he is most familiar."* Public health departments or Visiting Nurse Association provide home visits. Home health aids or assistants are being trained to help with some aspects of home care programs.

Even though the total PPC concept has been slowly adopted in established hospitals, it will be interesting to see if communities move more rapidly in the direction of specific service facilities as health care demands increase.

COMMUNITY RESPONSIBILITIES IN A DISASTER

A *disaster* is a situation in which many people are killed or injured, and even larger numbers made homeless and suddenly deprived of property and possessions. Disasters are sudden accidents on a large scale. The number of people involved in a disaster, the extent and severity of destruction, the area covered, and the size and resources of the community where it occurs are factors which may label an accident a disaster.

Severe windstorms, tornadoes, hurricanes, earthquakes, floods, and explosions often cause disasters. Other causes are fires in a hotel, hospital, school, or other building or an area where a large number of people are found; epidemics of disease causing death and illness to many; and the wreck or crash of a bus, train, plane, or boat. Then, of course, the result of nuclear warfare, with its devastation, is a disaster of such proportions as are hard to imagine (see Civil Defense).

Relief After Disaster

A congressional charter authorizes the American Red Cross to act to relieve suffering

---

*Griffin, John R.: *Taking the Hospital to the Patient*, W. K. Kellogg Foundation, Battle Creek, Michigan, p. 9.

and to provide material assistance and funds in the event of a major emergency or disaster. The relief which the American Red Cross offers is based on need and is extended without regard to race, creed, color, or to political, religious, or financial status. Local chapters give aid to people and not to commercial, industrial, educational, or religious organizations.

The assistance given in times of emergencies is cooperative, local and state chapters of the American Red Cross being joined by the national organization. Funds raised yearly by public subscription are supplemented by the federal government. In addition to providing medical and nursing care for the injured, food, clothing, and shelter are supplied.

The people of the community who are not injured but who have lost homes and means of taking care of themselves will be provided with the necessities of living. Food and shelter will be provided at some central place, and water and milk will be made safe. Lost persons will be located, if possible, and families brought together. Well persons should be provided with work to do so that they may be useful and regain their composure. Gradually, the community life will return to more normal patterns and reconstruction will be started. As long as there is need for help from outside the community, the American Red Cross assists. The federal government furnishes financial aid to communities declared disaster communities.

Community Planning

Each local community should have a plan of action which is coordinated with the national and state plans for disaster relief. This plan permits the local organization to move into action at home or in a neighboring area with medical and nursing personnel, supplies, food, and funds so that lives may be saved and a degree of order restored. This can be accomplished only if enough trained workers volunteer or are available locally to form efficient teams of doctors, nurses, volunteers, and workers to carry out the basic plan for assistance. Every able-bodied person should be ready to care for the injured and the homeless and to restore order in the community.

The local chapters of the American Red Cross work constantly to be ready to serve in the event of an emergency or a disaster. Special committees are active in each of the following areas: to survey the local resources available for emergencies and disasters; to warn the community in the event of a disaster; to rescue people and to evacuate them; to supply food to injured and homeless; to supply clothing and provide shelter; to provide transportation and communication; to inform the public of the situation; and to provide a central purchase and supply department.

Types of Injuries Involved

Disaster victims are exposed to cold, hunger, water hazards, injury, and fright. Homes are destroyed, families are separated, and some members are lost. Disaster injuries include all degrees of burns; shock, fractures, open wounds, hemorrhage; foreign bodies in the eye or fleshy parts of the body; immersion; and exposure. Mothers must be delivered and patients with contagious diseases must be isolated. Some people will die from drowning, shock, and severe injury. Care will be given in shelters, emergency stations, and hospitals.

Preparation for Nursing in Disasters

The extent of the disaster determines who will be available to aid the injured. In some cases people aid each other without the benefit of trained health workers. They do what they know how to do or think they should do. Such measures can be safe or hazardous depending upon the knowledge of the person giving assistance (see Civil Defense).

Nurses usually represent the largest group of health workers in a community. During a disaster, they are called upon to render immediate life-saving measures in keeping with their ability to do so. If medical direction is available, leadership rests with that group; if not, the next best prepared person takes such measures as he is prepared to give. He may have to direct the activities of others less prepared who are assisting. This is why as many people as possible should enroll in a course (see Medical Self-Help) for training in first aid and survival in disasters; in fact, some states require all of their employees to attend such a course.

Fear, anxiety, and confusion beset many victims who have suffered no physical disability, and they too require attention and understanding. Nurses are prepared to understand the needs of people during emergency situations and to render specific measures to save lives. See Chapter 51 for specific emergency care measures.

Civil Defense

The Office of Civil Defense, part of the U.S. Department of Defense, receives its authority from Congress. Its function is to plan and carry out steps to protect the citizens of this country from major disaster and to help them as well as possible to meet their essential needs following such destruction. Each state and local community, indeed the general public, has clear-cut responsibilities according to the National Plan for Civil Defense.

Civil defense and defense mobilization is the concern of every citizen. The individual must be capable in the event of an attack of caring for himself and of contributing to the organized community effort. The family must be trained and prepared to solve its own emergency problems as well as to assist others in need. Survival could be a starkly personal matter.*

---

*Office of Civil and Defense Mobilization: What You Should Know about the National Plan for Civil Defense and Defense Mobilization. U.S. Government Printing Office, Washington, D.C., 1958.

The Department of Health, Education, and Welfare with its United States Public Health Service has the responsibility for directing the health and medical care of all who survive a thermonuclear attack. Such a plan involves all health workers and an informed people as well.

To help inform the general public, the Office of Civil Defense and the U.S. Public Health Service have taken steps to prepare people for survival in a disaster when no health personnel or services are available through a program called *Medical Self-Help*. The goal is to train at least one member of each household in this country in Medical Self-Help. The course consists of 16 hours of instruction covering information vital to survival in a disaster when the family is without assistance and helpful, too, during lesser emergencies, when relieving suffering and saving lives—important at all times (see Table 24–2).

As a licensed practical nurse, you will know many of the measures covered in the Medical Self-Help course; however, there is something in it for every citizen (regardless of preparation) to learn because it is a "what-to-do" and "how-to-do" under circumstances

TABLE 24–2. "KNOWLEDGE REPLACES FEAR"—THE MEDICAL SELF-HELP TRAINING PROGRAM**

TITLE OF LESSON	CONTENT
Radioactive Fallout and Shelter	Meaning of "radioactive fallout," the dangers involved and protective measures to use.
Healthful Living in Emergencies	Public Fallout Shelters and supplies available; private shelter information concerning water, food, emergency sanitation, leaving the shelter.
Emergency Measures:	
Artificial Respiration	Mouth-to-mouth and back-pressure arm-lift methods.
Bleeding and Bandaging	What to do and how to carry out measures.
Fractures and Splinting	What to do and how to carry out measures.
Transportation of Injured	What to do and how to carry out measures.
Burns	What to do and what *not* to do.
Shock	What to do and how to carry out measures.
Nursing Care of Sick and Injured	General measures for caring for people who are suffering from some common disorders (e.g., chills, toothache, fever, common cold, convulsions, headache, nosebleed, insect bites, poisoning, etc.).
Infant and Child Care	Care of the new baby, feeding the infant, and attention to his body and safety. Precautions for the premature infant.
Emergency Childbirth	What to do and how to carry out measures.

*Source: Family Guide Emergency Health Care. U. S. Department of Defense,
* Office of Civil Defense and U. S. Department of Health, Education, and Welfare, Public Health Service. Revised 1965.

foreign to everyone. Thus, it would seem important that you participate in this course at some time. As the *Introduction** states: "Individuals and families have an essential role in

*Family Guide Emergency Health Care. U.S. Department of Defense, Office of Civil Defense and U.S. Department of Health, Education, and Welfare, Public Health Service, Revised 1965.

national defense—a role that is both simple and complex: simple because it requires rather elementary preparedness measures on the part of every person and complex because it demands that each person be ready to *live on his own* for 2 weeks—the period following a nuclear attack when outside assistance might not be available."

SUMMARY

The term "community" includes people at large as well as those living in the same place. Health problems of the world community have more meaning today for the local community due to rapid travel and instant communication.

International health efforts are promoted by WHO through its several regional facilities located in various parts of the world. Over 100 countries hold membership in this organization.

The life of every U.S. citizen is affected in many ways by community health agencies and services. National, state, and local levels of both official and nonofficial health agencies often work together to provide the most effective means of serving health needs in communities. The local community retains the main responsibility for meeting its health needs and problems, and, to a great extent, it is the local community health agency which directly serves the individual.

The community is responsible for the safety, survival, and welfare and its citizens in times of disasters. Planned programs with action at the local, state, and national levels are necessary to permit immediate action in sudden and unexpected disasters. The role of the nurse is most essential in any disaster and she should be prepared and ready to assume responsibilities that will be hers during any natural or manmade disaster. She has a responsibility to be informed and to promote community interests toward its welfare.

GUIDES FOR STUDY AND DISCUSSION

1. When you read or hear the word "community" what do you think of? In its broadest sense what does it mean?

2. What are the main differences between official and nonofficial health agencies?

3. This country no longer has certain health problems. Why is this so? What health problems seem to be under control? What does it take to keep them under control?

4. What health agencies are located or are active in your immediate community? How is each supported? What are the main types of work done by each?

5. How does a state board of health work with a county board of health?

6. Many people in this country have unmet health needs. How many reasons can you give for this situation? In your opinion, what should be done?

7. What is the value of a hospital license to: (a) the hospital itself? (b) the individual? (c) the community? (d) the state?

8. Does your community have a plan for meeting disasters? If so, what part does your hospital play in this plan?

9. Find out if your hospital has any type of disaster plan of its own.

10. Why are nurses so valuable to a community during and after a widespread disaster?

SUGGESTED SITUATION AND ACTIVITY

1. From the list of nine topics given below, select one (or supply another of your choice) and watch for it in the news. Prepare some means for informing your classmates about it. You may prefer to work in small groups.

Suggested Topics:
1. Child abuse or "the battered child."
2. Congenital malformation among newborns.
3. The food needs of some nation.
4. A local community health problem.
5. A contribution to health care made by some individual.
6. Food poisoning.
7. The migrant worker and a health problem he faces.
8. Lead poisoning in children.
9. A disaster.

NUTRITION: ITS RELATION TO HEALTH AND ILLNESS

CHAPTER 25. **NUTRITIONAL NEEDS IN HEALTH**

CHAPTER 26. **NUTRITIONAL NEEDS DURING ILLNESS**

This unit covers two large topics: *Nutritional Needs in Health* and *Nutritional Needs During Illness*. The first topic is foundation information useful in understanding the second topic. It stands to reason, if one can become acquainted with food requirements necessary to maintain health, it will be easier to understand why diet adjustments are so often necessary during illness.

Throughout this unit frequent reference is made to new discoveries about the use of food in the body and the continuing search for further information. No period in history has studied normal and abnormal nutrition and body metabolism as much as the present one nor has any period produced as much evidence to show that the food we eat *does* make a difference. The electron microscope is making it possible to study how the individual cell works to produce heat and energy from food nutrients. This scientific search for new truths will continue to bring changes in the use of foods during health and during illness.

As a practical nurse, you need a general understanding of body food requirements for three main reasons: (1) to maintain personal health, (2) to give more understanding care to patients, and (3) to assist with community understanding of problems related to proper nourishment.

NUTRITIONAL NEEDS IN HEALTH

OBJECTIVES FOR THE STUDENT: Be able to:

1. Explain the difference(s) between a good state of nourishment and a poor state of nourishment.
2. Describe five ways good nutritional condition serves the body.
3. Name seven basic food substances needed by the body.
4. Explain how the seven basic food substances jointly serve the body by naming four things they provide together.
5. Differentiate between carbohydrates, fats, and proteins by telling how each serves the body and naming three sources of each food substance.
6. Name seven ways vitamins promote health.
7. Identify five places in the body where minerals are found.
8. Using the "Essential 4," describe an adequate daily diet for a teenager; for a preschool child.
9. Explain how *age* makes a difference in the makeup of an adequate diet.
10. Using the four age groups in *growth and development factors related to nutrition*, identify two factors which influence an adequate diet for each group.
11. Describe, in general, the role of the federal government in food protection.

SUGGESTED STUDY VOCABULARY*

nutrition	enzymes	controversy
nutrient	proteins	toxicity
nourishment	fats	therapeutic
research	minerals	prophylactic
vitality	vitamins	optimum weight
carbohydrates	cellulose	pesticides
		amino acids

*Look for any terms you already know.

INTRODUCTION

The well-established fact that proper nourishment is vital to good health makes food, diet habits, food fads, and food protection all popular topics in today's news. Research continues to tell us new things about food *nutrients* and how the body uses them. It is possible for people to be healthier today than ever before. However, the matter is not that simple for a number of reasons: diet habits are hard to break, ignorance sometimes prevails, food is scarce (some kinds in some places), and family income must be considered. In addition, careless or excessive eating, bizarre food habits, hurried living practices, and pet notions (fads) about body nourishment make up another cluster of factors which undermine attempts to promote good *nutrition.* Thus, despite the new knowledge about bodily needs and uses of food, adequate nutrition for all peoples is far from a reality today. In fact, in some countries, such as India, it is a pressing problem.

The purpose of this chapter is to help you understand some basic facts about nutritional needs in health prior to learning facts about nutritional needs during illness.

One of the nine essential daily living needs is nutrition and fluids (see Chapter 22). You will learn (in Chapter 32) that both are daily needs when people are disabled, too. The physician writes the "order" for the patient's diet; this diet may be as important to the patient's well-being as any other therapy the physician uses or orders. In other words, *consider nutrition a vital human need.* Find out as much as you can about its relationship to good health; in this way you will be better equipped to understand and sense the vital role nutrition and fluids play during illness. To view nutrition and fluids in this light may help you understand your own food habits and sense the excitement of learning about normal body requirements.

THE SEVEN BASIC FOOD SUBSTANCES

While you have some knowledge of food and good eating habits, you may have some good and perhaps some poor eating habits of your own. You also have certain attitudes—likes and dislikes—toward food.

Nutrition is the study of foods and their relation to health; it is a science. Through study and experimentation, man is finding out *what* foods should be eaten, *how much* food a person needs, and perhaps most importantly, scientists are beginning to find out *how body cells utilize* food substances. The more we can know about how the body uses food *nutrients* (growth and repair substances) the better we will be able to provide the body with *what it needs to preserve health.* A licensed practical nurse is expected to possess acceptable food habits to indicate that she knows what to eat, and how much to eat, in order to *maintain proper body weight and proper body function.*

In meeting one's daily living needs, *adequate diet* (nutrition and fluids) *is as essential as any one of the other eight basic needs.* In fact, it can have a direct influence on one's state of mental health, elimination, and energy supply to carry out needed activities. When you look at adequate diet in this way it could actually head the list of daily living needs.

Good State of Nourishment

What is a good state of nourishment for any person? A good state of nourishment is present when a person profits from eating a balanced diet. In this case, the body not only *gets the proper amounts and kinds of food nutrients,* but it *uses them to advantage.* A poor state of nourishment would mean that one or more of the preceding facts would not be true.

Scientists know from study what foods should be eaten to maintain good nutritional condition. They also know that they contain certain substances the body needs to function properly. More recently, scientists have concentrated on how the human body uses food substances within the cell, from cell to cell, and in the production of body heat and energy. In short, metabolism is as much the concern of food scientists as any other health workers. To know what goes on in a healthy body is most helpful when treating the sick body. This is a good reason for you to know some of the "why's" of proper nourishment.

Let us go back to the matter of good nutritional condition of the body. How does a person profit from this condition? In the main, good nutrition helps to do the following:

1. Promotes a healthier body and mind.

2. Provides greater personal energy and vitality.

3. Resists illness.

4. Speeds up repairs.

5. Produces bones regular in size and shape and builds firm muscles.

6. Promotes good posture.

7. Helps the owner feel better, sleep better, and possess a general sense of well-being.

Seven basic food substances are needed by the body. They are *carbohydrates, fats, proteins, minerals, vitamins, cellulose* (roughage), and *water*. While each performs its own function(s), *together they supply heat and energy, promote growth, repair tissues, and regulate body processes*. Return to Chapter 6 and restudy water and body fluids.

Carbohydrates

Carbohydrates (also called starches and sugars) produce body heat and energy. (See Figs. 25–1 and 25–2.) One gram furnishes four calories. The chief sources are: fruits, vegetables, honey, corn syrup, sugars, breads, and cereals. Some meats (luncheon cold cuts), sea foods (oysters), milk, and milk products also provide carbohydrates.

People eat an abundance of carbohydrates. One reason is that they usually cost less. In America they make up more than one-half of all food eaten. In some other countries the amount is even higher. Normally, between 40 and 50 per cent of daily calorie requirements should come from carbohydrates. Excess is stored as fat and may cause obesity.

Not all carbohydrates serve the body best. Syrups and sugars do not nourish as well as do cereals, flour, vegetables, and fruits. While carbohydrates are the most easily obtained and least costly of the food substances, overuse of them can impair good nutritional status. The following paragraph will help you understand why overuse of carbohydrates can be harmful to health.

Return to Table 11–1. Starting with the mouth and saliva, follow the digestion of carbohydrates along the food route. Notice where and what things happen to prepare carbohydrates for body use. This journey changes carbohydrates into simple sugars because simple sugar is the only form the body can use. The simple sugars are absorbed into the blood stream through the villi in the small intestines and are (1) used by cells to produce heat and energy, (2) stored in the liver and muscles, (3) changed to body fat, and (4) retained in body fluids, e.g., sugar in the blood (normal level 70 to 100 mg. per 100 cc.).

Fats

Fats are concentrated sources of heat and energy. (See Figs. 25–3 and 25–4.) Gram for gram, fats furnish two and one quarter times more heat and energy than do carbohydrates or proteins. Thus, fats reduce the amount of food needed because they produce more calories.

Food fats in the diet come from *visible* and *invisible sources*. The "visible" sources of

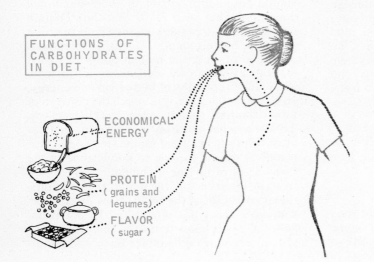

FUNCTIONS OF CARBOHYDRATES IN DIET

ECONOMICAL ENERGY

PROTEIN (grains and legumes)

FLAVOR (sugar)

FIGURE 25-1 Functions of carbohydrates in diet. (Bogert, Briggs and Calloway: Nutrition and Physical Fitness, 8th. ed.)

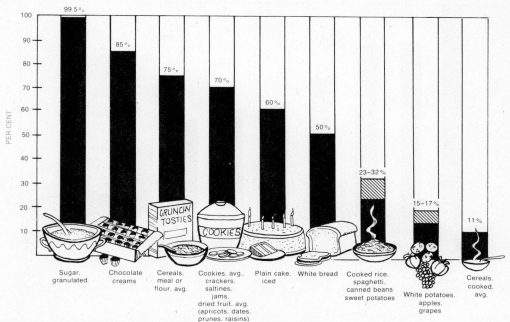

FIGURE 25-2 Typical carbohydrate-rich foods. (Bogert, Briggs, and Calloway: Nutrition and Physical Fitness, 9th. ed.)

food fats include margarine, butter, cream, shortening, salad and vegetable oils. The "invisible" sources (and the largest part of fat in the diet) come from meat, cereals, eggs, nuts, and dairy products.

Studies show that the amount of fat in the American diet has risen markedly—38 per cent in 1936 to more than 40 per cent at present. It is generally recommended that fat intake should be about 25 per cent to 30 per

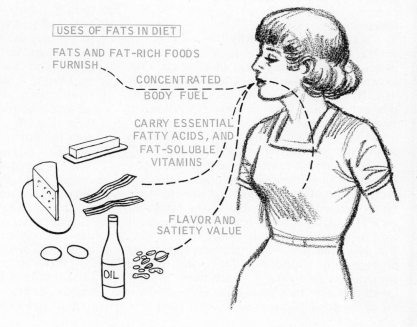

FIGURE 25-3 Uses of fats in diet. (Bogert, Briggs, and Calloway: Nutrition and Physical Fitness, 8th. ed.)

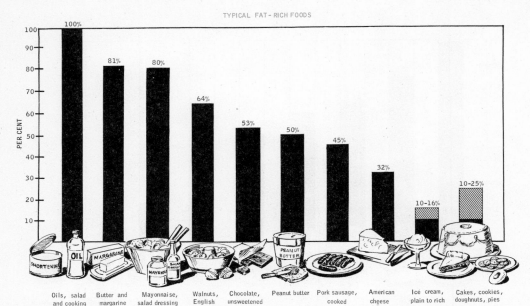

FIGURE 25-4 Typical fat-rich foods. (Bogert, Briggs, and Calloway: Nutrition and Physical Fitness, 9th. ed.)

cent of all food intake. The controversy about fats and their relation to arteriosclerosis (hardening of the arteries) has caused some changes in diet habits such as increased use of fish, poultry, milk, and cooking oils (replacing hard fats). For example, margarine (vegetable fat) has replaced butter (animal fat) in many households.

People are confused about the "fat controversy" perhaps because science has not yet found specific answers.

Saturated fat is usually the kind that is solid at room temperature, such as fats seen in meats, butter, lard and firm shortenings. One exception is coconut oil. *Unsaturated* fat is usually liquid at room temperature, such as oils (vegetable, fish, safflower, sunflower). Nuts are one exception.

Use Table 11–1 and follow fat digestion as you did carbohydrate digestion.

It should be remembered that the body can make fats from carbohydrates and proteins; it can also withdraw and deposit body fat as needed. When stored in the body, fat acts as padding around organs and glands; it aids in keeping the body temperature static. Fat assists in protein metabolism and in the absorption of vitamins A, D, E, and K. The presence of fat in the stomach tends to slow down digestion there, and this delays the feeling of hunger. Fats also add flavor to food.

Protein

The word protein means "first." All living tissue contains protein; because of this, it is considered *the most essential food nutrient.* Protein is found in every living cell and makes up almost one-fifth of body weight. (See Figs. 25–5 and 25–6.)

Proteins build and repair living tissues, furnish energy, and many carry needed vitamins and minerals. Before proteins can be absorbed and used, the digestive process breaks them down into *amino acids.* There are 23 known amino acids (commonly called "building blocks"); some 10 of them, known as *essential amino acids,* must come ready to use in the diet because the body cannot manufacture them through the digestion of proteins, as it does the others. This makes protein "intake" an especially important factor in health and illness. Besides having "building power," amino acids help regulate body processes through joint action with some vitamins, hormones, and enzymes.

Scientists are beginning to unlock some of the secrets of cell activities and the role amino acids play in living substance.

From 10 to 15 per cent of the daily calorie intake should be protein. When heavy demands for body protein occur (burns, fever, hyperthyroidism, pregnancy, growth, etc.), ad-

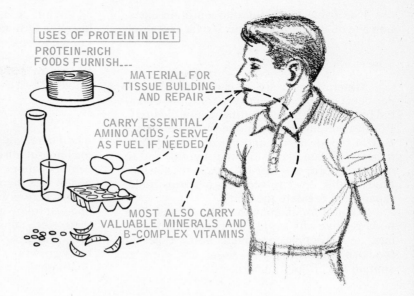

FIGURE 25-5 Uses of protein diet. (Bogert, Briggs, and Calloway: Nutrition and Physical Fitness.)

ditional protein must be added to promote healing and health, otherwise body tissue breaks down. This reminds one of the extreme importance of protein to the body and why the physician watches this factor so closely.

Proteins that contain all of the essential amino acids (in sufficient quantity) are called *complete* proteins. Examples are meats, fish,

eggs, milk (whole, dried, skim), and cheese. *Incomplete* proteins are those that do not contain all of the essential amino acids or are lacking in sufficient amounts for growth and repair purposes. Examples are beans, peas, nuts, peanuts, cereals, cereal products. (Soybeans are considered a complete protein but lack sufficient amounts of amino acids.)

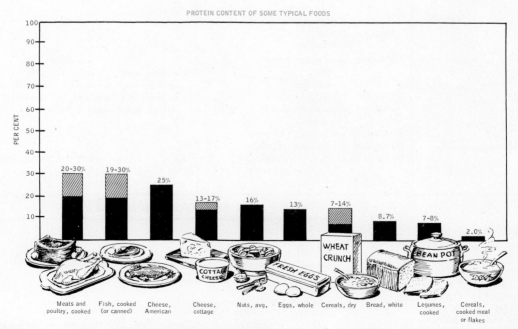

FIGURE 25-6 Protein content in some typical foods. (Bogert, Briggs, and Calloway: Nutrition and Physical Fitness, 9th. ed.)

Use Table 11–1 and follow protein digestion as you did carbohydrate and fat digestion.

Minerals

Minerals make up a small part (about 4
per cent) of body weight, yet form the essential framework (bones) for the rest of the body.
Besides building bones and teeth, minerals are
part of blood, nerve, and muscle tissue; they
help to regulate glands (iodine-thyroid) and to
maintain a proper water balance in the tissues.
Study Table 25–1 to see how minerals build,
repair, and regulate the body.

Natural foods contain mineral salts. The
body receives its supply from carbohydrates,
fats, and proteins consumed. Some types of
foods such as cornstarch, sugar, and pure fat
contain few, if any, minerals.

While some 19 or more minerals have
been found in the body, not all of them are yet
known to be essential to life. In time, research
may prove their necessity. Some minerals
known to be essential to life are listed in
Tables 25–1 and 25–2.

Vitamins

There are those who say that the most
meaningful discovery since the turn of the
century about food and its relationship to
health was the discovery of vitamins. Experiments were going on here and abroad prior to
and just following 1900 which pointed out that
there were substances besides carbohydrates,
fats, proteins, and minerals which regulated
body growth. These unknown factors (organic
compounds), tracked down by different scien-

(Text continued on page 252.)

TABLE 25–1. NEED FOR MINERAL ELEMENTS

	ELEMENTS ESPECIALLY NEEDED	*RESULTS OF LACK OF THESE ELEMENTS*
As Building Materials:		
Bones and teeth	Calcium and phosphorus	{ Stunted growth Weakened or soft bones Malformed or decaying teeth Rickets
Hair, nails, and skin	Sulfur	
Soft tissues — chiefly muscles	All salts, esp. { potassium phosphorus sulfur chlorine	
Nervous tissue	All salts, esp. phosphorus	
Blood	All salts, esp. { iron calcium sodium phosphorus copper	Lack of iron or copper results in less than normal amounts of hemoglobin in blood, a condition called nutritional anemia
Glandular secretions	Stomach secretions — chlorine Intestinal secretions — sodium Thyroid secretion — iodine	Lack of iodine results in enlargement of thyroid gland — simple goiter

	ELEMENTS ESPECIALLY NEEDED
As Body Regulators:	

To maintain *normal* Exchange of body fluids Contractility of muscles Irritability of nerves Clotting of blood Oxidation processes Neutrality of body	All salts
	All salts, especially balance of calcium with sodium and potassium
	Calcium
	Iron and iodine
	Balance between:
	    Basic elements — sodium, potassium, calcium, magnesium, and iron
	    Acidic elements — phosphorus, sulfur, and chlorine

TABLE 25–2. SOME COMMON MINERALS: THEIR SOURCES AND USES

Some Common Minerals and Their Use

Mineral	Sources and Uses
Sodium Potassium Chlorine	Work of one is related to work of another; found in all body tissues and fluid; help maintain normal fluid balance and proper movement of fluids in and out of cells. Maintain muscle tissue sensitivity. These 3 minerals are found in all natural foods; sodium chloride (table salt) is added to food in preparation.
Iron	A part of hemoglobin, the part of the blood carrying oxygen to all living cells; it aids in cell respiration, making it essential to the body as a whole. Amount in the body is very small and it is used over and over; the liver destroys old red blood cells and releases iron for future use. Some food sources are: organ meats (liver, kidney, heart, tongue), red meats, oysters, leafy green vegetables, dried beans, peas, whole grains, raisins, molasses, nuts.
Iodine	Essential to proper functioning of thyroid gland (metabolism). While this gland contains and uses about one-half of the iodine in the body, the rest is scattered through the cells and tissues. Water and vegetables supply iodine; so do seafoods. Iodized salt is another source and is needed especially in areas of the country where iodine is lacking in water and soil.
Calcium * (functions with phosphorus)	Almost all body calcium is found in bones and teeth. The remaining part (about 1%) is in tissue fluids. It aids in blood clotting; it influences muscle contractions (heart muscle) and responses of nerve centers and fibers. May be low in the diet. While it is necessary throughout life, it is needed in greater amounts during growth, pregnancy, and lactation. Lack of calcium is evidenced in deformed bones and in muscle spasms (leg cramps) due to an upset in response of nerve centers and fibers. Milk is the best source of calcium; lack of milk in the diet may cause a deficiency, because it is difficult to meet daily calcium requirements without milk. Adults should remember this and drink no less than 8 ounces of milk per day. The elderly adult, especially, is apt to have too little calcium in his diet. Other sources of calcium include: milk products, mustard greens, kale, broccoli, turnip greens, clams, and oysters.
Phosphorus * (functions with calcium)	When calcium is deposited in bones and teeth, phosphorus is deposited, too. It is found in body fluids and helps maintain acid-base balance of the blood. Like calcium, it aids in muscular contraction. While phosphorus comes from the same foods as calcium (milk, milk products, etc.), other sources include eggs, fish, cereals, meats, nuts, poultry, and legumes.

* These two minerals are present in larger amounts than are other body minerals.

TABLE 25–3. VITAMINS, THEIR FUNCTIONS AND SOURCES

VITAMIN	FUNCTION	FOOD SOURCES
Fat Soluble (not destroyed by usual methods of cooking)		
A	Essential for normal growth and development, normal night vision, health of eyes and mucous membranes. Guards against infections. Aids tooth formation.	Liver, sweet potatoes, carrots, squash, dark green leafy vegetables, cantaloupe, dried fruit.
D (sunlight helps body produce this vitamin)	Necessary for normal growth and development. Aids in the metabolism of phosphorus and calcium. Cures and prevents rickets. Aids tooth formation.	Vitamin D milk, milk fat, salmon, sardines, mackerel, tuna fish, egg yolk.
E	Use in man has not been clearly established. Thought to aid vitamin A in its work; also vitamin C. Aids tooth formation. Essential to animals for reproduction.	Available in many common foods: green leaves, cereal, germ oils, egg yolk, butter, milk, nuts, vegetable oils.
K	Essential for normal blood clotting (helps produce prothrombin). Promotes normal function of liver.	Available in many common foods: green leafy vegetables, liver, vegetable oils.
Water Soluble (readily destroyed in cooking water)		
Vitamin B Complex (not one, but a group of 12 or more known nutritive factors)	This group is essential to maintenance of health. Each factor identified with one or more functions has its own name, yet all factors work together. A deficiency of B complex usually means more than one factor is lacking. Some are included here.	
Thiamine (vitamin B₁)	Necessary for cell metabolism of carbohydrates to yield energy; helps maintain muscle tone of digestive system and thus promotes appetite and digestion; essential for healthy nerves.	Lean pork, liver, lamb, dry beans and peas, enriched cereals. Some in eggs, milk, other meats, vegetables, and fruit.
Riboflavin (vitamin B₂)	Essential for growth; aids in carbohydrate and protein metabolism. Prevents lesions at corners of mouth, on lips, nose, and around the eyes.	Liver, poultry, beef, veal, lamb, pork, oysters, milk, cheese, eggs, leafy green vegetables.

(Table continues on opposite page.)

Niacin (nicotinic acid)	Aids in metabolism of carbohydrates and proteins. Prevents pellagra, nervous depression.	Liver, fish, poultry, meat, whole grains, peanuts, peas, beans.
Folic Acid	Used in treating some types of anemia. While its function is not clearly understood, it is related to cell metabolism; thought to act on bone marrow to help produce normal red blood cells.	Widely available in foods: liver, meat, fish, green leafy vegetables, eggs, yeast.
Vitamin B$_{12}$ (cyanocobalamin)	Used in treating pernicious anemia. Thought to be important to the use of iron in the body.	Liver, kidney, milk, cheese, lean meat, eggs, fish.
Ascorbic Acid (vitamin C, works with folic acid and B$_{12}$, and possibly vitamin E.)	Essential to growth, healing of fractures and wounds. It is necessary in collagen production (has been likened to the cement that holds stones together in a wall), the holding substance in tissue such as: skin, bones, tendons, connective tissue. Prevents scurvy. Cannot be stored in the body so must be taken in daily. Apt to be deficient in the diet.	Citrus fruits, tomatoes, strawberries, cantaloupes, raw cabbage, dark green leafy vegetables, potatoes, green peppers. Easily destroyed by heat while cooking in a solution. Loses its value in cut or bruised fruit exposed to the air.
Pyridoxine Pyridoxal Pyridoxamine (vitamin B$_6$)	Aids in fatty acid metabolism. Used to treat dermatitis. Increased amounts needed during pregnancy.	Beef liver, fish, liver, whole grain cereals, Brewer's yeast, lean meats, peanuts, bananas, cabbage.
Panothenic Acid	Aids in metabolism of fats, anti-body formation. Lack of it contributes to some neurologic disorders, irritability, and skin disorders.	Lean meat, skim milk, egg yolk, Brewer's yeast, liver, kidney, wheat bran, oats, broccoli (manufactured in intestines by bacteria).
Biotin	Aids amino acid functions; needed in body to handle carbon dioxide "levels."	Beef liver, eggs, cauliflower, peanuts, and manufactured by bacteria in the intestines.
Choline	Aids Vitamin B$_{12}$ and folic acid in some aspects of proper liver function. Lack of it produces fatty infiltration of liver, hemorrhage, and death of liver tissues.	Liver, kidneys, beef brains, egg yolk, wheat germ, peas, skim milk, lean meats, peanuts, soybeans, asparagus, snap beans.

tists, were finally named vitamins in 1912. It had been determined that there were traces of certain accessory food substances which were vital to health and normal development. Today it is known that *vitamins are absolutely necessary to body metabolism*. For the most part, the body must rely on sources outside of the body to get these necessary substances. Knowing this about vitamins, it becomes clear that a person must have adequate types and amounts of these so-called body regulators if they are to enjoy good health and to have properly functioning bodies. One's daily diet must include foods which carry adequate vitamins if the body needs are to be met.

As a practical nurse, you should know everyday sources of the known essential vitamins and what happens to the human body if it is denied adequate amounts and varieties of these metabolism regulators. Likewise, you should know that there seems to be a limit to body vitamin needs, and "over-dosage" does no good and may even be harmful.

How Many Vitamins Are There? It is suspected that there are hundreds of such organic compounds awaiting discovery. Table 25–3 lists 14; some have long been known while others are newcomers to the list, which still continues to grow. Vitamins are classified into *water soluble* and *fat soluble* groups. The difference between the two groups is that water soluble vitamins are readily destroyed in cooking water and fat soluble vitamins are not. Table 25–3 shows these two groups, their functions, and natural sources. Man has learned how to duplicate these vitamins in the chemistry laboratory, and that is why they are available in stores. Easy access to vitamins can lead to misuse and overuse. People mistakenly use vitamins for almost any infirmity without the knowledge that indiscriminate "overuse" does no good and may prove harmful. Excess vitamins in the body that are water soluble are thrown off through the urine; in the case of fat soluble vitamins, they are stored with no value to the body and may cause toxicity. Any vitamin supplements to the diet should be taken only at the direction of a physician, because a healthy person who eats a well-balanced diet would have little need for them.

Functions of Vitamins in Health. Vitamins help to regulate the following:
1. Digestion
2. Cell metabolism
3. Growth and development
4. Reproduction
5. General good health
6. Appetite
7. Resistance to illness

Uses of Vitamins in Restoring Health and in Treatment of Some Diseases. Turn to Table 31–17 and locate the 14 vitamins covered in this chapter. Briefly notice in the "Use" column of that table the many deficiency conditions and therapeutic uses made of vitamins; this will help you understand the uses vitamins have in health and in illness.

Table 25–3 furnishes some detailed information about each of the 14 vitamins according to fat soluble and water soluble groups. Figure 25–7 lists them in a slightly different way but this illustration may help you use the table more effectively.

You will notice, as you study material in this chapter and Table 31–17, that much is known about some vitamins and very little about others.

Daily Requirements of Vitamins. Daily requirements vary from person to person and for the same person at different times. Requirements are influenced by individual metabolic condition and size; if a person is growing, or if he is exercising, he needs more vitamins. During illness, especially when fever is present, the requirement increases.

Cellulose

Often called "roughage," cellulose is the fiber found in plants. It is not digestible in the human body, but it is essential because *cellulose adds bulk to food and helps it move through the digestive tract*. Vegetables, fruits, leaves, stalks, hulls, and whole grain cereals furnish bulk in the diet.

Water

Water is essential to life—so much so that a person can live only a few days without it. You will recall (in Chapter 6) that water makes up the bulk of all living matter. In the body all fluids are chiefly water; it is found within and surrounding each cell. Review Tables 6–3 and 6–4 concerning factors which influence the body's need for water and what water does to assist the body.

Daily sources of water are liquids consumed, water in food, and water resulting from food metabolism. Figure 25–8 illustrates how the normal body maintains water balance.

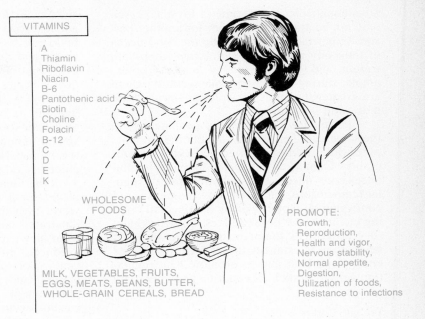

VITAMINS

A
Thiamin
Riboflavin
Niacin
B-6
Pantothenic acid
Biotin
Choline
Folacin
B-12
C
D
E
K

WHOLESOME FOODS

MILK, VEGETABLES, FRUITS,
EGGS, MEATS, BEANS, BUTTER,
WHOLE-GRAIN CEREALS, BREAD

PROMOTE:
Growth,
Reproduction,
Health and vigor,
Nervous stability,
Normal appetite,
Digestion,
Utilization of foods,
Resistance to infections

FIGURE 25-7 Different vitamins found in natural foods and their general functions in the body. (Bogert, Briggs, and Calloway: Nutrition and Physical Fitness, 9th. Ed.)

Factors Which Influence Nutritional Needs

Several factors influence the amounts of the seven basic substances required by the body.

Energy requirements vary within a 24-hour period, and they vary from person to person. The body requires less energy during sleep and rest; it steps up its demands during mild activity, and further increases these demands during strenuous exercise. Thus, what may be

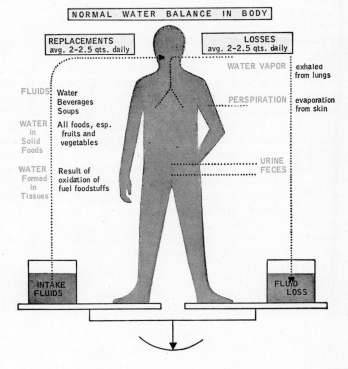

NORMAL WATER BALANCE IN BODY

REPLACEMENTS
avg. 2–2.5 qts. daily

LOSSES
avg. 2–2.5 qts. daily

WATER VAPOR : exhaled from lungs

PERSPIRATION : evaporation from skin

FLUIDS: Water
Beverages
Soups

WATER
in
Solid
Foods

All foods, esp.
fruits and
vegetables

WATER
Formed
in
Tissues

Result of
oxidation of
fuel foodstuffs

URINE
FECES

FIGURE 25-8 Normal water balance in body. (Bogert, Briggs, and Calloway: Nutrition and Physical Fitness, 9th. ed.)

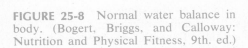

INTAKE
FLUIDS

FLUID
LOSS

an adequate diet at one time or for one person may not be at another time or for another person. Other factors influencing the food needs of the body are: *age, environment, optimum weight,* and *general state of health.* For example, during pregnancy and lactation there are greater demands for some minerals, vitamins, and proteins.

The elderly person needs a balanced diet, the same as the growing child, but the amounts of the different food nutrients can vary considerably. Climate (heat, cold, humidity) influences body needs. The body maintains a regular temperature, and, if the environment is not controlled by clothing or by heating and cooling facilities, the body utilizes its own regulatory powers to maintain its temperature. It needs food substances to produce the needed energy and heat and to promote heat regulation activities such as sweating and shivering.

Weight Control

Overweight makes a difference. It is an established fact that overweight people (especially men) run a greater risk of some serious illness than people of normal weight. "Dieting" or "weight control" is discussed almost as much as the weather in our society. "Crash" or "fad" diets can be dangerous to health. *Weight control, the need for it, and the means for accomplishing it are medical problems and require the direction of a physician.* Tremendous sums of money are spent every year by people seeking a "quick and easy way" to reduce the waist and hip measurements and eliminate the double chin. Body nourishment is a complicated process, as you can see from the roles played by vitamins, minerals, water, and the other food nutrients. Weight control "whys" cannot be answered without explanation; the problem is compounded by many factors such as not knowing how many calories are needed; lack of exercise; unwillingness to change eating habits; and not knowing how many calories, empty or otherwise, are in food and beverages consumed. The advice of a physician should guide all weight control efforts so that they are not harmful to the dieter.

AN ADEQUATE DIET

An adequate diet is also a balanced diet; it supplies the proper amounts of essential food substances for body growth and repair, heat and energy, and proper regulation of other body processes. These are the seven body needs just discussed. One is reminded, however, that no *one* diet serves all people. Adequacy varies from person to person. Food selection helps determine whether or not a diet will be balanced and adequate. Selection of proper food requires knowledge. The person untrained in food and its relative values to the human body needs ready information to guide his judgment in food selection. Government (national and local) agencies, private and professional organizations, and the business world provide almost unlimited printed and illustrated materials. The study of foods, of what they can and cannot do for the body, has produced many discoveries in the last 50 years. For example, knowledge of many vitamins and minerals and proper caloric requirements for children and for adults in various occupations has developed.

World War II pointed out the need to look at nutrition around the globe. Reports of studies started then (1941) and revised every few years since gave us what is called *Recommended Daily Dietary Allowances.* It lists, according to age, weight, and height, the number of calories needed by men, women, infants, boys, and girls (normally active in a temperate climate). This report is a detailed table, perhaps understood best by nutrition scientists, physicians, and nutritionists, but it serves as a reliable reference for others as well.

Following the World War II discovery that people needed guidance in planning balanced diets, the U. S. Government prepared a chart, "The Basic Seven Food Groups," for the housewife to use in meal planning. This guide was later changed in 1958 to the chart, "Basic Four Food Groups," to make it easier to use; it includes the same foods but it also includes the number of servings. Now it is known as the "Essential 4" food guide (see Figure 25–9).

1. Milk Group

Milk (or its equivalent in milk products):
3 – 4 glasses for each child through the growing (teen) period
4 – 6 glasses for the expectant or nursing mother
2 glasses (at least) for adults (including elderly)

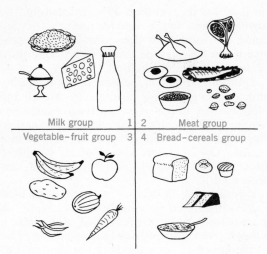

Milk group   1 | 2   Meat group

Vegetable–fruit group 3 | 4 Bread–cereals group

FIGURE 25-9 "Essential Four." (Schifferes: Essentials of Healthier Living, 3rd. ed., John Wiley and Sons, Inc.)

2. Meat Group

2 or more servings of meat, fish, poultry, eggs; dry beans, peas, nuts as alternatives

3. Vegetable and Fruit Group

4 or more servings of dark green or yellow vegetables, tomatoes; or citrus fruits (one raw vegetable and one good source of vitamin C fruit)

4. Bread and Cereal Group

4 or more servings of breads and cereals (enriched and whole grain)

The World Health Organization concerns itself with world-wide nutrition problems through its regional facilities. (See WHO, Chapter 24.) *The lack of food and the lack of proper food are serious world-wide problems.* The world food supply must double in the next 20 to 30 years just to meet the inadequacies we face today; therefore it means that the food supply must *more* than double if people are to have more adequate nourishment.

Meal Planning

Today, informed homemakers and meal planners are giving more thought to the quality of the food they purchase. The food industry pays attention to their buying habits and offers products accordingly. It is possible, despite weather, season, or distance, to find a wide variety of foods—fresh, frozen, dehydrated, dried, canned, etc.—in all parts of the country, at any time. These foods are distributed from all parts of the country.

One relative newcomer in the food family is the wide variety of "convenience foods." Agricultural scientists have discovered ways to prepare foods to save time for the busy homemaker (over one-third of whom now work outside the home). Examples of convenience foods include potato flakes (add hot water or milk and the result is mashed potatoes), sweet potato flakes, apple flakes, dry beans (30 minutes cooking time), frozen fruit juice concentrate, pre-cooked frozen whole meals, powdered milk, combination main dish foods (cooked in minutes), and full-flavored berry powders for sauces, pastries, and ice cream. The homemaker needs to know what her food dollar is buying when she uses convenience foods—cost per serving, quality, and basic nutrient worth.

Meal planning requires thought and knowledge. Balanced meals do not "just happen." The homemaker needs to know the critical foods, those essential to good nutritional status, and the proper amounts to be included in the daily diet; this takes time and planning. Likewise, it means keeping an eye on the food budget dollar. "Good food buys" are related to seasonal supplies; keep in mind that low cost foods can provide a balanced diet as well as (and sometimes better than) high cost foods.

Food needs to be attractive and appealing to the eater, whether he is a family member or a patient. Color, size of servings, arrangement of food, and surroundings can influence the appetite. It is one thing to plan a balanced meal, and it is another thing to have people eat and enjoy it.

Meal planning has a "togetherness" for the family today. Special foods are not thought essential for the varying age groups. Some variations may be used in preparing a given food for a meal, but that is all. For instance, applesauce may be served to elderly and younger members while the group between has apple pie. Or less seasoning may be added to one portion for some members. Size and number of servings vary according to individual needs.

FACTORS WHICH INFLUENCE DIETS AND FOOD HABITS

This list of factors includes *likes and dislikes, region and availability, income, pregnancy and lactation, religion, age, nationality and race.*

Likes and Dislikes.   Habit has a lot to do with our food likes and dislikes. What we "grew up on" tends to influence our attitudes toward food. While likes and dislikes are bound to occur, some things can be done to curb dislikes. How food is prepared often makes the difference. For example, a person may not care for vegetables but may find them easier to eat if they are used in good-tasting casserole dishes. A child is apt to mimic a parent's dislikes and continue this attitude as an adult. Schoolmates influence one another's eating habits. Social climate around the table should be pleasant. Punishment and argument related to food or at the time of eating should be avoided.

Region and Availability.   Region influences food habits. While there are national trends, such as an increased use of protein in this country today, there are regional variations to be considered.

In large cities, especially in the eastern section, it is common to find food specialties for groups with special tastes and needs (Italian, French, Poles, Jews, etc.). The Eastern Seaboard has long been known for seafood, fowl, "Boston baked beans," etc.

The South has its characteristic foods. Near the coast, seafood is common. Vegetable greens (collard, turnip, mustard) are cooked with salt pork (fat back). Greens, grits, and corn bread with sorghum or molasses may make up the diet when income is low. Vegetables and fruits are used. Milk consumption per person is not as high as in some other regions. Buttermilk is commonly used. One associates fried chicken, country ham with gravy, and hot breads with the South. Hospitality associated with food has long been a Southern tradition.

The Midwest is known for its bountiful meals. This area produces meat, dairy products, grains, vegetables, and some fruits. It is easy to see why this region is known for high consumption of these products.

Income.   Income has a direct influence on food habits and diet. Proportionately, the lower income family spends more of its income for food than does any other income group. On the average, one-fourth to one-third of income is spent for food.

Buying foods in season is an economy and a common-sense practice to stretch the food budget dollar. Luxury food specialties (caviar, paté, quail, etc.) are expensive delicacies often associated with social prestige and wealth. On occasion, the "not so wealthy" have prestige foods to satisfy the need that prompted it.

In a sense, this is a "prepackaged" food era. As discussed previously in this chapter an increasing variety of precooked, dehydrated, concentrated, frozen foods are available. The convenience of such foods is not denied, but they can be expensive substitutes without adequate nourishment unless meals are carefully planned.

Pregnancy and Lactation.   Both pregnancy and lactation make additional nutritional demands. During pregnancy the mother must eat to maintain her own health and provide for the growing fetus. Proteins (meat, poultry, fish, milk, cheese, eggs) are increased to provide necessary amino acids. Vitamins A and D and ascorbic acid often are added to the diet. Minerals such as calcium, phosphorus, iron, and iodine are needed for proper development of the fetus. Diet during pregnancy is planned with these needs in mind. Protein, well selected, usually helps the body of the pregnant woman meet the additional demands for minerals.

Religion.   Religious beliefs enter into diet restrictions and habits. Some foods may be forbidden entirely, others forbidden on certain days and for special occasions. A nurse needs to be aware of such dietary restrictions to appreciate and respect patients' needs.

Some *Jews* have specific requirements concerning meat. Pork may not be eaten. Four-legged animals (with cloven hoof) that chew a cud may be eaten. This group includes cattle, sheep, goats, and deer. Fowl are eaten (chicken, goose, duck, turkey, etc.) but both fowl and other animals must be inspected and prepared according to religious requirements before cooking. Blood is never eaten. Removing blood from meat or fowl before cooking makes it ritually clean (kosher). Other foods must be kosher, too, including those that are prepackaged.

Milk and meat are eaten at separate times in the orthodox Jewish home. Each may be eaten but not during the same meal. Fish with scales and fins are eaten, but shellfish are prohibited.

On the Sabbath (Saturday) no food is prepared. This is done the day before. During the year some religious holidays are observed either by fasting, or by feasting on specially prepared foods as may be required.

The *Roman Catholic* religious group is bound by dietary laws which include fasting and abstinence. Fasting means the allowance of one full meal and two light meatless meals per day.

When complete abstinence is called for this means no meat is eaten, nor foods such as soup or gravy made from meat. Partial abstinence means that meat (soup, gravy) may be eaten once a day.

Some other religious groups prohibit the use of any meat, or of a particular meat. Substances considered injurious to health are entirely excluded in some instances.

Age. Age varies the need for differing amounts of some food nutrients. See Growth and Development Factors Related to Nutrition in this chapter.

Nationality and Race. People of different nations and races have varying food habits which relate to tastes in food selection and preparation. Availability of food influences what is a "favorite" and is most commonly eaten. Here again, income also controls the diet. For example, in China where tea is the national beverage, income may prevent its use as often as the family would like.

People of a nation center their diets around the foods they can produce. For example, where the climate limits the production of vegetables, fruits, meats, dairy products, etc., this is reflected in the diets of the people who cannot avail themselves of these imported foods, if indeed such foods are brought in.

Food preparation varies from one nation to another. Perhaps more is done with meat than with most other foods. Some people prefer to stew it with vegetables (Bulgarians, Poles), some with noodles and dumplings (Germans). The Japanese put cereal products into the meat-vegetable stew. In various countries meat is dried, smoked, salted, braised, roasted, fried, broiled, and boiled. It is ground for sausage and it is pressed to make a wide variety of luncheon meats. Facilities for storage influence meat preparation in many countries.

With people moving about from one region, stage, or province to another, or from one country to another in this day of rapid travel, food habits tend to mix. One group more easily takes on the food habits of another. New ways to prepare foods are shared, yet there remains a pride in the specialty from one's own area.

GROWTH AND DEVELOPMENT FACTORS RELATED TO NUTRITION

If an adequate diet is essential for everyone, it stands to reason that people of all ages need the same nutritional substances. What is different among age groups is the amount and form of nutritional substances needed.

Following are some factors which relate to nutrition according to each of four age groups.

Infancy and Young Childhood

Food form goes from liquid to pureed foods to solids during this period of greatest growth. Energy requirements are proportionately higher than for other age groups and so are requirements for body building proteins, minerals, and vitamins.

Frequent daily feedings are required the first year; the need for water is established. By 12 months the child should be eating almost all foods (variety is desirable) and join the family at the table to start feeding himself with some help.

Within about 24 months, the child is eating three meals a day with the family, but his appetite is not as good as it was. Families vary in their food patterns due to habits, culture, money and so on, but this does not necessarily mean the small child will be poorly nourished. The range of food substances for the young child permits enough flexibility to fit most any family food pattern. The daily diet for the child should include:

1. Three or more cups of milk and milk products.

2. Two or more servings of meats, poultry, fish, and eggs.

3. Four or more servings of vegetables

and fruits, including a citrus fruit or other fruits or vegetables high in vitamin C, and a dark green or deep yellow vegetable for vitamin A at least every other day.

4. Four or more servings of bread and cereal of whole grain, enriched or restored variety.

5. Plus other foods as needed to provide additional energy and other food values. (Nutritionists sometime estimate an average serving for children as about one level tablespoon of meat or vegetables per year of age.)*

Middle Childhood Through Adolescence

Early in this period (6 years to 10 or 12 years) the growth pattern is slower and eating habits are usually established. It is now that food dislikes may become pronounced. If plumpness occurs, now is the time to adjust the diet so the child maintains a normal weight for his age.

Prepuberty and adolescence present quite another nutritional problem. Rapid growth and maturation mark this very active period. Boys especially are always hungry because their need for calories and other nutrients is high. Snacks as well as meals should include proteins (milk, meat), fruits, and vegetables.

Girls may have a tendency to put on weight faster than boys because they do not exercise as much, yet may continue to eat more than necessary. When underweight, eating habits may be to blame. Nibbling can reduce the appetite, resulting in inability to eat at regular meal times.

Girls should exercise as well as boys; it may not be as strenuous, but it should be included in daily living. Weight problems should be guided by the family physician and not tampered with by crash diet programs.

The upper limits of adolescence (early twenties) find eating habits established. To maintain proper nutrition, the young man continues his exercise and eats accordingly. More exercise calls for more calories. Less exercise than previously means less caloric intake. The diet should include lean meat, vegetables and fruit with a limited amount of starches and sugars.

---

*Breckenridge, Marian E., and Murphy, Margaret Nesbitt: *Growth and Development of the Young Child.* W. B. Saunders Company, 8th edition, 1969, pp 195–196.

The young woman is concerned about her figure. She wants to be attractive and to do this safely she must select proper foods (especially protective foods) and continue a regular program of exercise. Haphazard dieting can be dangerous.

Middle Life

The body is fully grown and continues to mature. Metabolism begins to slow down and proper food intake should be adjusted to supply only what the body needs to maintain itself if weight gain is to be avoided. Body organs seem less able to handle excess food and certain types of food (i.e., fatty foods).

Middle life calls for less food and a program of exercise. Food selection needs to include protective foods and less emphasis on empty calories of some carbohydrates and fats.

Later Life

Physical exertion usually decreases during this period, thus the body requires fewer calories. However, it is just as essential for this person to have an adequate diet as it is for any other age group. Adequate diet for this person means reduction in fats and moderation in carbohydrates with emphasis on high protein, vitamins, and minerals. Fluid intake is encouraged. Sensible eating can influence the state of health.

Metabolism is lower and appetites usually poorer. It is suggested that eating smaller amounts and eating more often helps the body use food to better advantage. Associated with consuming an adequate diet is the problem of loneliness or isolation during meal time. Community efforts are being made to locate elderly people living by themselves to determine if their nutritional needs are being met; this is a national problem involving the federal government.

PROTECTION OF OUR FOOD SUPPLY

Since 1883 the Federal Government has from time to time passed laws to help protect the public food supply. Early efforts (between 1883 and 1906) dealt with inspection of imported foods, false labeling, adding "foreign" substances to a product (adulteration), and inspection of animals for disease before they were slaughtered.

From 1906, when Congress passed the first Federal Food and Drug Act and the Meat Inspection Act, until 1938, the federal government established and carried out regulations that had to do with "misbranding" of foods that are transported across state lines. From time to time during this period, the original act was amended to broaden its scope and further insure safety and honesty in food processing and packaging. However, by 1938, it was felt necessary to write a new act which made it illegal to add any amount of an unsafe substance to food. When such a substance (additive) was needed to preserve or make food more attractive, the law set limits for the use of such additives. This new law, the Federal Food, Drug, and Cosmetic Act (FD&C Act, 1938) provided for standards to control additives, quality, identity, and proper filling of containers (to avoid deceiving the buyer).

The farmer's use of pesticides to grow more and better crops raised new problems. People began to ask questions about the effect these poisons would have on their health. Scientists were studying the problem. In 1954 Congress amended the FD&C Act to set limits on how much "left over" pesticide could remain on or in raw foods ready for market.

The federal government, in its "watchdog" role over food, drug, and cosmetic safety practices, has further amended the FD&C Act (1958 and 1960) concerning food additives (including colors) to be sure that no cancer-causing substance is used. The food manufacturer must now prove the safety of any additives he uses and the amount he uses is controlled. In 1967 Congress passed a stronger meat inspection law to insure cleaner, safer practices in meat processing and selling.

The Food and Drug Administration (FDA), part of the U. S. Department of Health, Education, and Welfare, has the chief responsibility for regulating food and drug safety, though it works closely with some other federal agencies.

To help you more fully appreciate the importance of food safety the following sets of questions and answers come from two federal government publications.

How Safe is Our Food?*

Why do we need laws to protect foods? Safe food is essential for life and health. Reliable food is essential to keep the consumer's trust.

What are the laws? Federal law states that food sold across state boundaries must be safe, sanitary, and honestly labeled, packaged, and prepared. Federal law also includes a number of standards that describe what certain foods must consist of, what the quality of certain foods must be, and how full the containers for certain foods must be.

When did the laws go into effect? Today's laws for food protection have a long history. The first broad act was passed in 1906. Other laws were added when new methods of farming, food processing, and marketing led to the need for regulation.

Who is responsible for carrying out the laws? The Food and Drug Administration (FDA), part of the U. S. Department of Health, Education, and Welfare, is responsible for enforcement of most of the Federal food protection laws.

How are the laws carried out? Many types of activities are needed to enable the FDA to carry out its responsibilities—investigational, scientific, administrative, legal, and educational.

What is the responsibility of the person who handles food? At home or on the job, any person who handles, stores, or prepares food should observe the same principles that underlie FDA's regulations.

Standards have been established for some foods; among them are: Wheat and corn flour products, chocolate and cocoa products, bakery products, milk and cream, cheese and cheese products, salad dressings, canned fruit and fruit juices, eggs and egg products, canned vegetables, canned tuna fish and shellfish.

Additives in Our Food†

What is a food additive? A food additive is any substance that becomes part of food, or

---

How Safe Is Our Food? FDA Life Protection Series, Publication No. 41. Food and Drug Administration, U.S. Department of Health, Education, and Welfare, 1967, p. 5.

†*Additives in Our Food.* FDA Life Protection Series, Publication No. 43. Food and Drug Administration, U. S. Department of Health, Education, and Welfare, 1967, p. 2.

affects the characteristics of food, through direct or indirect use and with useful intention.

Why do some foods contain additives? Substances may be added to food to preserve, emulsify, flavor, add nutritive value, color, or achieve other useful, desired purposes. Substances may also get into foods while they are grown, processed, or packaged; these are called incidental additives.

Who is responsible for the additives in foods? Before an additive can be used to improve a food product, it is subjected to toxicity studies by the food (or chemical) manufacturer, and it is evaluated and regulated by the FDA. Before a pesticide residue can be allowed to remain in or on food, the use of the pesticide on food crops must be approved by the U. S. Department of Agriculture. The pesticide is subjected to toxicity studies by the manufacturer, and is evaluated and regulated by the FDA.

How does the consumer know what is in a food product? Food products are labeled with required information to guide and protect the consumer.

What is the responsibility of the person who handles food? At home or on the job, any person who handles food should observe the same safety principles that underlie the Federal Food, Drug, and Cosmetic Act.

SUMMARY

Nutritional deficiency is a world-wide problem. In some areas of the world the problem is a lack of food or variety to provide a balanced diet. This is a serious problem now and it mounts with each passing month as world population increases. It is estimated that food production must double by the year 2000 if we are to even maintain our present already inadequate supply. Our country is blessed with great food resources, available in variety at all seasons of the year, but poor nutritional status is apparent none the less. Too often it is due to poor eating habits.

Food is one of the nine essential daily needs of people and continues to be an essential need when illness strikes. Food has a direct relationship to health and it plays a particularly important role during illness. Sometimes the most important need a patient has is getting proper nourishment and fluids.

Scientists have determined what substances the human body needs to maintain a state of good nourishment. They are seeking more information about how the body utilizes food and what goes on in cell metabolism. The seven basic food substances required in specific amounts by the human body are *carbohydrates, fats, proteins, minerals, vitamins, cellulose,* and *water.* Each one of these substances serves one or more purposes and works in cooperation with the others so that the body has heat and energy, grows, repairs itself, and regulates its activities.

Factors which influence diet needs are age, activity, environment, optimum weight, and general state of health.

Factors which influence what people eat are habits, customs, fads, religious laws, food supply, money, geographical location, season, weather, likes and dislikes.

Before the turn of the century the federal government was concerned with protecting the public from spoiled, contaminated, filthy food. In recent years its role has become more active and more restrictive.

GUIDES FOR STUDY AND DISCUSSION

1. In what way(s) does a good state of nourishment differ from a poor state of nourishment?

2. What does a state of good nutrition do for the body?

3. What basic food substances are needed by the body? What do they provide by themselves? Together?

4. As you study, make a list of things food scientists are trying to find out; have found out.

5. The word protein means "first" in a certain sense. According to this chapter and Chapter 6, protein is something special. What is special about it?

6. What are vitamins? How many are there? What do they do for the body? What is the source(s) for each common vitamin?

7. What is the difference between water soluble and fat soluble vitamins?

8. Where are minerals used in the body? What are some common sources of minerals?

9. Growth and development influence the body's need for nourishment. Under each age heading describe some of these influences.

> Early Childhood, Middle Childhood and Adolescence, Middle Adult Years, and Elderly Adult.

10. What factors influence what a person eats?

11. In what ways does the national government exert control over food?

SUGGESTED SITUATIONS AND ACTIVITIES

1. Certain facts about cells in Chapter 6 can be tied to one or more of the seven essential food substances. See if you understand the relationships well enough to explain them to your classmates. Prepare some visual aid to help you discuss this if you need to.

2. Take stock of your eating habits with the idea of seeing how you might improve them. To help you with your inventory, you might wish to consider such things as: *When* and how often? *What*—according to seven basic essentials? *Where*—under what circumstances? *How much*—amounts compared with normal intake for someone your age and height? *Why*—reasons for any of the above? What, if any, changes should you make in your eating habits? How are you going to proceed to change them?

3. Prepare a display which shows five or more good sources of each of the basic food substances needed by the body. See if you can include economical sources as well as more costly sources.

CHAPTER 26

NUTRITIONAL NEEDS DURING ILLNESS

TOPICAL HEADINGS

Introduction
The Patient's Diet
Diets for the Over-
    weight and Under-
    weight

Diets for Specif-
    ic Disorders
Responsibilities of
    the Nurse
Habituation to Bi-
    zarre Foods

Summary
Guides for Study and
    Discussion
Suggested Situations
    and Activities

OBJECTIVES FOR THE STUDENT: Be able to:

1. Explain why the physician prescribes the patient's diet.
2. Given a list of common house diets, describe the differences among them.
3. Compare the meaning of "house diet" with the meaning of "therapeutic diet."
4. Name five responsibilities of the LPN with respect to the patient and his diet.
5. Give two examples of dietary problems often associated with long-term illness.
6. Name four ways food is used to help the body during illness.
7. Explain how overweight can be injurious to health.

SUGGESTED STUDY VOCABULARY*

therapeutic
habituation
consume
enzyme
obese
malnutrition
malfunction
colostomy
hypoacidity
hyperacidity

peptic ulcer
duodenal ulcer
diagnosis
complication
bland foods
deficiency
anorexia
parenteral
feces
peristaltic movements

hypertension
hereditary
mucosa
cholesterol
cathartics
diarrhea
allergy
constipation
vascular lesions
arteriosclerosis

---

*Look for any terms you already know.

INTRODUCTION

Illness and abnormal conditions make special demands upon the nutritional status of the body. What is adequate in times of health may well be inadequate during illness, during pregnancy, or during the malfunction of some organ or gland. Thus, the basic ordinary living need of *food takes on additional importance when out-of-the-ordinary things occur in the body.* In fact, diet is of such importance that the physician always specifies (orders) what the patient should have to eat and drink.

Illness increases the body's need for the repairing of tissue and rebuilding of an energy supply. Food plays a vital role in meeting these increased demands. Food is also used to build body defenses to prevent complications from occurring and to correct faulty gland and organ functioning. Diets, like drugs, are ordered for special therapeutic purposes; in this sense diets are as important as drugs—a fact worth remembering.

The purpose of this chapter is to acquaint you with the importance of nourishment during illness and other conditions. It explains the two diet groups—house diets and therapeutic diets—to prepare you for accepting this aspect of patient care. The licensed practical nurse shares responsibilities for seeing that the patient's nutritional needs are met; therefore, you need to understand the importance of food to the patient and develop a high regard for your part in helping him meet this need. In addition, you need to know the responsibilities you carry in providing him this assistance.

Dietary information pertinent to the needs of the LPN accompanies specific patient needs in selected illnesses among all age groups; this chapter is a foundation for understanding dietary needs and relates this information to some common, yet special, conditions.

THE PATIENT'S DIET

From early Biblical times, man has seen a relationship between food and illness. Modern scientific methods are showing us that this relationship is very involved and complicated. As stated in the previous chapter, seven essential food substances have already been defined, but man is searching for more facts about cell metabolism. He wants to know more about the work of the cell: how it uses nutrients or refuses to use them. No period in medical history has placed as much emphasis on the role of nutrition as this one. Consequently, you will see and hear much discussion about nutrition with respect to patients' needs.

Based upon the information he has, the physician prescribes the diet, i.e., orders what, when, how much, and by what method, if necessary, the patient will eat.

In general, diets are divided into two groups: *the "house diet" group* and *the therapeutic diet group*. For purposes of economy of time, money, and planning, the hospital has a set of standard diets commonly known as "house diets." This group usually includes *general, light, soft,* and *liquid* diets. Each such diet features certain foods and it is designed for patients who need these foods at a particular time during their illness.

The therapeutic diet group is prescribed for patients with special nutrient needs. While these diets are based upon the house diets, they are modified to meet the specific therapeutic needs of the patients.

You will recall that regardless of age the body requires certain food substances in appropriate amounts. Whether well or ill the food intake must be adequate to meet body needs at a given time. The diet, regardless of its title, must furnish required nourishment. However, when certain illness conditions exist or there is faulty body function, it is essential for the physician to modify the diet to meet the nutritional needs of the patient. It is easy to forget that illness makes its own demands upon the body; to hold the diet at an adequate level of nourishment, it is often necessary to modify it.

The "House Diet" Group

This group has several variations— regular, light, soft, and liquid. The "regular" diet is sometimes called the "full" or "general" diet; the name varies from one institution to another. *This diet has no food restrictions.* It is a balanced, adequate amount (2000 to 2500 calories) of food containing proteins (70 to 80 Gm.), carbohydrates (200 Gm.), and fats (100 Gm.), and includes the protective foods, meat, eggs, milk, citrus fruits, vegetables, whole grain or enriched cereals, butter or margarine. Caution is used to avoid foods which could cause distress (cabbage, onions, fried pork).

The *light diet* is one step removed from the general diet. While it is an adequate diet in all respects, it does not contain the wide variety of foods found in the general diet. Foods in this diet are not highly seasoned; no fried or fatty foods or rich pastries are allowed; neither are roughage foods such as bran and celery. With these limits, this diet can become monotonous. However, a patient usually is not kept on a light diet long; it is used as a stepping stone to a general diet unless the patient has a limitation (few or no teeth, need for less roughage) which is helped by this diet.

The *soft diet* is used in place of the light diet in some hospitals and includes the same restrictions. This means there is no light diet as such, which may indicate that the differences between these two diets are so few that one can be used in place of the other. The soft diet, in that case, is one step removed from the general diet. Some hospitals have certain requirements for this diet, such as restriction of meat and the pureeing of vegetables. Others do not.

The *liquid diet* is easily digested. It takes little effort to consume it. The two main types of liquid diets are full liquid and clear liquid.

The *full liquid diet* includes carbohydrates, fats, and proteins (lower amounts than the general and soft diets) containing about 1500 calories. The number of calories can be increased and often is when a patient remains on this diet for a long period. Foods in this diet include: milk, cream, milk drinks, soups, cereal gruels, strained fruit and vegetable juices, beverages, plain gelatin, ice cream, sherbets, plain custards, sugar, oils, butter or margarine.

The *clear liquid diet* is most often used for patients following surgery. It is not an adequate diet but furnishes carbohydrates and water and does not form gas. The patient is not kept on this diet any longer than necessary because it is limited in its functions. The water in it helps the body restore its fluids; given at frequent intervals it relieves thirst. The foods allowed on the clear liquid diet are some strained fruit juices, tea, coffee, clear broth, gelatin, sugar, and carbonated beverages. No milk, milk beverages, or fats are included.

Increased knowledge about foods and digestion has led to fewer types of diets with less restrictions, keeping them as similar to adequate normal diets as possible. This is true of both house and therapeutic diets.

Therapeutic Diets

Food used for corrective purposes in the body is called a *therapeutic* diet. It can be an adjusted adequate diet (including foods allowed) or it can be calculated as to what amounts of nutrients are allowed, such as a diabetic diet. As stated earlier, the physician prescribes the diet; the LPN does not assume responsibility for making any modifications without specific instructions. *To serve its purpose the diet must be consumed; it is a nursing responsibility to help the patient accept his diet.* The LPN can help make the food service attractive, the environment acceptable, and assist the patient according to his state of dependency or independency. Observation of the patient accompanies all these acts.

Real progress has been made over the years in fighting such deficiency diseases as rickets, scurvy, beriberi, and pellagra. In this country they are so rare that for some years the U. S. Public Health Service has ceased to report them in their published statistics. Reasons for this progress include a better informed public, a public with more money to buy food, and active research programs finding new knowledge about how the body produces energy, performs its work, and repairs itself. New knowledge is pointing out the existence of more deficiency diseases and disorders. An example is the discovery of an unusual enzyme deficiency which is the cause of an hereditary condition affecting millions of people around the world. In general, research is looking at such things as overnutrition and its accompanying problems, the lack of nutrients in relation to disease, faulty metabolism present at birth, and the effect of chemicals (including "the miracle drugs") on normal digestion of food.

There is no question that nutrition plays a vital role in the prevention and treatment of illness. New knowledge about it makes diet as important as drugs in prevention and treatment. It has been found, for example, that there is a relationship between diet and how well burns and wounds heal, conditions of the heart and blood vessels, liver disorders, stress, and peptic ulcers, to name a few.

It is not essential to list the details of the many special therapeutic diets here because the practical nurse does not need this type of in depth knowledge to perform her assisting functions and tasks. However, it is essential that the practical nurse know where to gain the information she needs when involved in caring for a patient who has a special diet prescription. Sometimes this source is the hospital diet manual; sometimes it is the physician himself or the nurse in charge. There is safety in this approach because new knowledge about the body's use of food creates need for change in the therapeutic use of foods.

DIETS FOR THE OVERWEIGHT AND UNDERWEIGHT

The Reduction Diet

Overweight and obesity, growing health problems in this country, are commanding the attention of medical science because they can influence so many vital body functions and contribute to disorders of the heart, kidneys, pancreas, and lungs. In addition, obesity causes embarrassment, lethargy, inactivity, and difficulty in getting around.

A person is over his weight when he weighs more than he should for his height, age, and sex. The body has deposits of fat it does not need. When a person's weight is 10 per cent above what it should be, he is considered overweight. When he is 25 per cent above accepted weight, he is considered obese.

Excess fat accumulates in the body when the intake of calories exceeds the use of calories. Two main causes of obesity are eating too much and glandular disorder. Of the two, the first is by far the chief reason that people are obese. While many overweight people blame their condition on family traits or heredity or see it as a glandular disturbance upsetting body metabolism, records show that overweight due to glandular disorders is rare. There is disagreement about the part heredity plays in obesity. Many authorities say that it is simply a matter of eating too much and that heredity is not the cause of obesity.

Overweight presents health problems. During the growing years it is not frowned upon as much as it is in middle and later years but perhaps should be. Excess fat must be nourished the same as other body tissues. This requires more blood; the heart works harder and this encourages heart and circulatory disorders. Fat crowds organs and interferes with movements of the diaphragm; this, too, hampers the work of the heart and respiration.

It is a fact that obesity shortens the life span. Nine out of 10 slim persons reach the age of 60, but only six out of 10 obese persons do. Three times as many slim persons reach the age of 80 as do obese persons.

The physician usually requires an obese person to reduce to a certain weight before surgery, if possible, because excess body fat causes risks.

Persons with arthritis, heart disease, or circulatory diseases need to maintain normal weights or below. Other conditions such as nephritis and gout also make normal weight necessary.

If excess calories produce fat, the way to reduce weight is to decrease the calorie intake. In other words, eat less food. The problem is not a simple one, nor can it be solved with "crash" or "fad" diets alone. The obese person should have a physician prescribe and direct his plan for weight reduction. Curtailment of food intake can be harmful if the diet does not include basic essentials for adequate nourishment. Starvation as a means to lose weight is a hospital treatment requiring close medical management to avoid complications. Weight reduction followed by maintenance of proper weight is difficult to achieve because it means replacing old habits with new ones, and that is one reason that the obese public so readily "buys a new idea" about *easy* dieting. There are many causes of overeating. Studies show that two important ones are poor eating habits and emotional needs. Reducing diets usually range from 800 to 1500 calories. The physician determines the diet according to body requirements and the rate of weight loss desired.

The High Calorie Diet

A person is considered underweight when he is 10 per cent or more below the desired weight for his height, age, and sex. In a sense, he has a form of faulty nutrition (malnutrition). This condition may be due to insufficient intake of proper foods; poor or improper use of food by the body; poor or improper choice of food; a debilitating or wasting disease such as cancer or tuberculosis; nervous tension with anxiety.

The cause of underweight is determined before the diet is prescribed. If a disease condition is present or there is faulty function of some part of the body, the condition is treated and the diet is adjusted accordingly. If the cause is found to be the lack of proper quantities of necessary foods, the diet is so changed. Very often this requires helping the patient to understand what he needs and how these needs can be met within his means to do so.

In figuring how many calories an underweight person must consume to gain weight, the physician keeps in mind the number of calories required to meet body fuel needs and the number of extra calories needed to build fat tissue in the body. It could require as much as twice the number of calories the patient has been consuming to produce the desired weight gain. The average high calorie diet is about 3000 calories.

People differ in their eating habits and practices; king-size portions encourage some and discourage others. Between-meal eating is more popular with children than adults, as a rule. More meals than the usual three (with smaller amounts at each) suit some people better; for others the answer may be taking prescribed quantities of high calorie foods such as cream. In any event, every effort should be made to pattern the "underweight's" eating habits to his liking because, at best, he may find it difficult to make the weight gain he needs.

DIETS FOR SOME SPECIFIC DISORDERS

Disease and disorder can occur in a particular part of the body, a particular body system, more than one system at a time, or the body as a whole. In every instance the patient's nutritional needs are influenced and altered to meet additional demands. Diets used to help fight a disease, correct a deficiency, and relieve and prevent complications are rightfully called *therapeutic diets*. Their importance ranks with any other prescribed treatment.

There are two types of disorders which affect the body: organic and functional. In an *organic disorder* actual tissue changes occur. The following are some examples: skin lacerations, bone fractures, cancer, ulcers, fever, tumors, burns, and diabetes.

In a *functional disorder* everyday functioning is disrupted with no apparent tissue change. A functional disorder may be due to stress, fatigue, anxiety, fear, frustration, conflict, and the like. Some call a functional disorder a case of "nerves," which is a somewhat accurate label. Functional disorders may be due to a cluster of factors which together upset the normal nervous system control, thus creating the disturbance.

One cannot separate organic and functional disorders into two neat divisions because the body responds as a whole, with the nervous system and the mind being very much a part of this whole.

DIETS FOR DIGESTIVE DISORDERS

Gastric hypoacidity is a deficiency in the quality and quantity of gastric juice secretion. Treatment is instituted to bring the deficiency within the usual limits; this may be done either through the use of foods or drugs.

Gastric hyperacidity is a greater than usual amount of hydrochloric acid in gastric juice secretion. Here also something is done to bring the acidity within the usual limits with food or drugs.

Ulcers

A *peptic ulcer* is a lesion due to the loss of tissue on the surface of the mucous membrane lining of the stomach. A *duodenal ulcer* is a similar lesion in the duodenum. With surface tissue gone and the need for the stomach lining to heal, both types of ulcers require that food consumed contribute to the healing process and to the prevention of pain and complications. Diets today are more liberal and tend to allow the patient to eat more types of food, paying less attention to bland or nonirritating foods, but giving more serious attention to how often the patient eats.

Older therapy holds the idea that whatever is ingested should be smooth, nonirritating, and not excite the flow of gastric juice any more than possible. This diet plan usually has four progressive stages. First, a milk and cream diet is strictly adhered to, with specific directions as to mixture, amount, and time. Second, small feedings of bland foods are added to the milk and cream. Third, feedings of selected foods (in the mid-morning, mid-afternoon, and evening) are added to regular meal times. Fourth, there is a regular, three-meal, low cellulose diet of bland, non-irritating foods, or there may be six smaller meals.

The physician keeps close watch on the patient's need for essential amounts of nutrients to avoid complications. The licensed practical nurse has the responsibility to see that the patient receives—and consumes—the correct food at the prescribed times.

Gastritis

Gastritis (acute and chronic) is an inflammation of the stomach lining that is caused by irritating foods and drink, poisonous substances, gastric juice irritation, or bacterial inflammation. Contributing factors are anxiety, fatigue, and eating too quickly or too much. Symptoms include pain, burning sensation ("heart burn"), and belching accompanied by a burning sensation in the throat.

Sometimes no food is permitted for a period of hours to rest the stomach. Gradually there is a return to eating that generally starts with milk, cereals, and cream soups. A regular diet may be delayed for several days.

Cancer of the Stomach

Cancer of the stomach may go undetected in its early stages since the complaints of patients are sometimes vague, such as gastric distress and anorexia. However, a weight loss follows.

The stage of cancer development and its location influence the diet as well as the patient's personal preferences. Anorexia is common. Advanced, inoperable cancer poses a series of nourishment problems which become increasingly more acute as the patient's condition worsens. Liquid diets and parenteral fluids are often ordered.

Constipation

Constipation is present when the large bowel does not empty itself in a normal manner and retains the feces. Normal peristaltic movements are absent. Improper food and fluid intake, excessive use of body fluids (e.g., sweating, fever), and an organic (e.g., tumor) or functional (e.g., "nerves") disorder are some of the main causes.

Diet can influence peristalsis. Normally, diet should include fruits, vegetables, and whole grain cereal products to provide food bulk and roughage. The habit of regularity maintains good muscle tone. The use of cathartics does not.

Constipation due to overstimulation of the bowel lining (e.g., colitis) requires a diet prescription different from those mentioned above. Food must be non-irritating, smooth, and bland. Therefore, roughage (fruits, vegetables) is held to a minimum. Eggs, milk, white bread, fish, poultry, ground meat, butter, margarine, and oils are generally included. Patients need encouragement to eat, especially if pain is present.

Diarrhea

Diarrhea (acute or chronic) is the presence of abnormal, frequent, and liquid stools, It is a sign that something is seriously out of order in the intestinal tract. It is an especially grave disorder for newborn infants and calls for stringent emergency measures.

Dietary measures are aimed at getting the bowel back to normal as soon as possible. The cause must be removed; this often requires the use of drugs. The bowel is "put at rest" and food is withheld. The body fluid balance (electrolyte balance) is restored through parenteral means, and as early as possible the patient is returned to food by mouth. Small amounts of bland, easily digestible foods gradually lead to larger feedings and a normal diet.

DIETS FOR FEVER

It is now known that fever is a by-product of the metabolism of hormones. Fever is a sign that the body is reacting to something. This reaction increases the rate of heat production, the need for calories, and the need for fluids.

The body's need for more calories and fluids dictates their increase in the diet. Proteins repair and build tissue and therefore are important in the build-up of calories. Parenteral administration of food often supplements food taken by mouth.

Serious short- or long-term infectious diseases require careful diet prescription to help avoid complications by meeting the extra demands made upon the body. Anorexia is to be expected and therefore the nurse has responsibility to see that the patient consumes his diet.

DIETS FOR SKIN DISORDERS

Psoriasis is a usually chronic and recurring condition causing elevated, round, and scaly patches in the skin. Its cause is unknown. Alterations in diet are tried, sometimes with apparent success and other times not.

Acne is an inflammatory condition in and around the sebaceous (oil) glands, generally of the forehead, chin, and cheeks, which results in blackheads. It is most common in adolescents but it may occur at any age. The physician may or may not severely restrict the diet. There are differences of opinion on the role food plays in this condition. Foods most often mentioned for limited consumption include sweets and fats.

DIETS FOR ALLERGIES

An allergy is a total body response (change in body chemistry) to a "foreign substance" which may or may not be eventually outgrown. The circulatory system is affected, causing pressure to change, especially in the capillaries, which forces fluid into the tissues. Breathing is affected as the bronchioles become constricted (i.e., asthma). Skin rash, watering of the eyes, swelling of body parts, and sneezing are some common reactions.

While the "foreign substance" may or may not be a food, the physician tries to determine what, if any, foods are offenders and then eliminates them from the diet. The patient usually knows (if he is old enough) which foods bother him and such comments should be reported.

DIETS FOR BURNS

Extensive burns require serious nutritional attention because they rob the body of protein, fluid, and minerals. If infection sets in, additional calories are needed to fight the invaders, build resistance, and repair tissues. In addition, the act of eating may be difficult depending upon the location of the burns and the state of dependency of the patient.

To meet the immediate body need for proteins, fluids, and minerals, frequent feedings are ordered. Parenteral means are used to provide extra fluids, minerals, vitamins, and other nutrients to restore fluid balance and build resistance. Helping the patient may be time-consuming and require a high degree of skill to get him to consume the prescribed diet. Children pose a real challenge in this respect.

DIETS FOR METABOLIC DISORDERS

As the name implies, a metabolic disorder is an irregularity in body metabolism. Medical science is involved in research concerned with body chemistry and cell metabolism. *Gout, hypothyroidism,* and *hyperthyroidism* are all disorders that may require diet adjustments, often accompanied by drug therapy.

Diabetes Mellitus

Diabetes mellitus is a common type of metabolic disorder in which the body is unable to use carbohydrates in a normal way. Excessive amounts of sugar remain in the blood stream and are expelled in the urine. The offender is the pancreas, which fails to produce enough insulin to complete the metabolism of carbohydrates.

Treatment is directly related to diet. What, when, and how much food is to be consumed are all rigidly controlled. Insulin plus food control, or food control alone, helps the body to properly utilize carbohydrates and permits diabetic people to live normal lives.

All foods contain some sugar: starches become sugar(s) during digestion, proteins are partly changed to sugar, and about one tenth of fat consumed turns to sugar. Thus, all aspects of the diet must be considered by the physician. He takes into account the patient's age, size, activities, and results of laboratory tests (including urine and blood). Responsibilities of the practical nurse include helping the patient accept the fact that diet adjustments will help him keep well, seeking his cooperation in carrying out the diet plan, observing for any irregularities in eating which violate the diet, serving his food on time, and giving insulin as ordered. Since the diet is calculated by the physician, the LPN should have specific written instructions. Patients can and should learn about food selection according to their particular needs; here again the physician provides specific instructions.

DIETS FOR CARDIOVASCULAR DISORDERS

Diseases of the heart and circulatory disorders account for the highest percentage of deaths in the United States (more than in any other country). These disorders are known to be related to diet in some ways. For example, *obesity* creates a demand for extra blood because the extra weight needs nourishment via the blood the same as the rest of the body. Extra blood means extra work for the heart. Fat that is crowding the heart and diaphragm hampers heart action and breathing. Since the heart needs to exert itself as little as possible, a therapeutic diet should be such that additional strain is not put on the heart and the heart muscles. While a balanced diet is essential, proteins and fats are generally used at low minimum levels because they increase the work of the heart. Anything that overexpands the stomach (e.g., gas-forming food, too much bulk) can bring pressure on the heart, which is one reason why a patient with heart disease may eat numerous smaller meals per day rather than three regular meals.

Hypertension (high blood pressure) is more common in obese persons than those of normal weight. Fat deposits in the walls of the blood vessels are more common too; they may contribute to restricting the flow of blood through the vessels.

Authorities disagree about *cholesterol* (the "fat controversy") and the part it plays in fat deposits in blood vessels; it is found almost entirely in animal fats. Until more exact knowledge is available, various dietary treatments will continue. It *is* known that Americans consume more fat in their diets than is generally recommended.

The Low Sodium Diet

The body's use of sodium influences the amount of fluid in the tissues because sodium affects arterial pressure. Patients with heart disease need careful sodium regulation to relieve and prevent edema; excess fluid must be eliminated to relieve the work of the heart. The sodium diet is not a cure; it is a preventive and remedial measure. However, patients often show remarkable improvement (less edema) after sodium intake has been reduced.

Sodium diet restrictions range from *mild* and *moderate* to *strict* and *severe*. Diets for the first three ranges of restriction have standardized amounts of sodium permitted per day. The physician prescribes the diet in keeping with the individual patient's needs. *Severe* sodium restrictions are usually carried out in a hospital; the others can be carried out at home or may be ordered for the hospitalized patient.

Diets low in sodium are not too flavorful and patients often complain of this. Regular seasonings (spices) can be used to perk up the flavor unless otherwise indicated by the physician. The most important role of the LPN is to help this patient understand how his diet helps him so that he will accept the restrictions.

DIETS FOR RENAL (KIDNEY) DISORDERS

Kidneys and other related renal structures can dysfunction as well as any other part of the body. It is a serious matter when faulty waste removal occurs in the kidneys or when they are unable to regulate water balance (electrolyte concentration) in body tissues.

Normal kidney function is a complex process that goes on continuously to maintain the delicate mineral, nutrient, and water balance necessary for proper cell and tissue functions. Anything that upsets this delicate balance (i.e., infection, inflammation or obstruction such as a kidney stone) soon makes its presence known usually in a serious manner.

Diseases of the renal system include: nephrites (acute and chronic), scleroses, uremia and renal calculi (stones). While each condition calls for specific dietary treatment, the main reasons for dietary control are: (1) reduce the work of the diseased organ, (2) replace nutrients lost to the body, (3) exclude substances which cause the body to retain abnormal amounts of waste products and salt,

(4) maintain nutrition and weight at as nearly a normal level as possible, and (5) encourage appetite and improve morale.[1]

DIETS FOR NUTRITIONAL DEFICIENCIES

Nutritional deficiency is the result of "starved" body tissue that does not receive or properly use the essential food nutrients. The reasons are the following:

1. The diet lacks some nutrient(s).

2. The diet may contain all essential nutrients but in too small amounts to meet present demand.

3. There may be a malfunction of some part of the digestive system which prevents full use of the diet.

4. There may be a malfunction of some gland, organ, or part.

The following are various types of nutritional deficiencies: *Nutritional anemia* results from a lack of adequate amounts of protein, iron, or vitamins. A woman may find that she lacks adequate amounts of minerals, vitamins, or other essential nutrients *during pregnancy*. A lack of specific vitamins may cause *pellagra, scurvy,* or *beriberi*. A lack or faulty use of both vitamins and minerals causes *rickets* and *anemia*. A specific lack of minerals causes *hyperthyroidism* and *malformed teeth*. Specific *enzyme* (inborn) *deficiencies* result from a faulty metabolism that is present at birth.

Nutritional deficiency diseases are found in many parts of the world. In this country, malnutrition is present due to poor eating habits, lack of money to buy proper foods, and lack of knowledge of what to eat.

In each case of nutritional deficiency the physician prescribes the diet according to what the patient needs to replace the missing nutrients and to build, repair, and supply energy for the body. See Table 31–17 to note the relationship of diet and drug therapies in treating nutritional deficiencies.

Very often the patient from a low-income home has had limited opportunity to know about foods, much less have access to a wide variety of them. Sometimes the problem is one of poor judgment in eating, perhaps through lack of knowledge, but often it is through lack

---

[1]Adapted from: Krause, Marie V., and Hunscher, Martha A., *Food, Nutrition and Diet Therapy*. Philadelphia, W. B. Saunders Company, 1972, p. 472.

of concern for what is eaten and when. While the physician prescribes the diet, the nurse is called upon to help the patient understand and accept it.

As stated previously in this chapter, the matter of cell metabolism is of primary interest to scientists. When we know more about how a cell (all parts of it) does its work and what it takes to keep it in top working order, the therapeutic use of diets will take on even more importance than it does today.

RESPONSIBILITIES OF THE NURSE

The patient's diet is the concern of the physician, the dietitian, and the nurse. Prescribing the diet and preparing and serving it are important, but the story does not end there. The patient must eat it. The nurse has responsibilities for making eating as safe, effective, and pleasurable as possible, briefly outlined as follows:

Environment
1. Well ventilated, clean, and clear of unsightly objects.
2. Conveniently arranged for patient safety and satisfaction.

Patient's personal needs before eating
1. Toilet needs attended to well before tray arrives.
2. Hands washed (face, if necessary).
3. Comfortable, convenient position.
4. Any medicines required before or after meals, or both.

The tray
1. Proper diet to the right patient.
2. Hot foods hot and cold foods cold.
3. Attractive arrangement of moderate sized servings.
4. Correct arrangement of place setting.
5. Observation of restrictions (such as, no salt shaker on low-sodium diet tray.

Assisting Acts of Nurse:
1. For patient who feeds himself
1. Tray materials arranged for his specific needs.
2. Servings prepared, if necessary (bread buttered, meat cut, etc.).
3. Observation of appetite, and encouragement, if needed.
4. Sufficient time for eating.
5. Listening to comments about diet.
6. Removal of tray and arrangement of patient and environment soon after meal.

2. For patient to be fed
1. Provision of ample time; sit when possible.
2. Patient permitted to help any way he can.
3. Food and portions offered according to patient's preference.
4. Informing patient without sight what is on his tray, and letting him feel unhurried presence of nurse.
5. Helping family member who feeds patient.
6. Removal of tray and arrangement of patient and environment soon after meal.

Observations
1. Watch for state of appetite, comments made about food, whether all or part is consumed.
2. Report or record pertinent observations. Hospitals vary in means used for recording necessary information.

HABITUATION TO BIZARRE FOODS

Habituation is being possessed of a habit that results in dependency upon performing the action; it is something one cannot do without. Addiction means the same, but to some it is a not-too-acceptable term for ordinary, everyday habits of too much coffee, tobacco, candy, cola drinks, and the like because it has long been associated with narcotics, alcohol, and more recently with hallucinatory drugs (e.g., LSD).

No one knows how long people have been eating clay and dirt but studies show that people have cravings for and do eat such unnatural things as clay, coal, cornstarch, pure lard, baking soda, baking powder, newspapers, coffee beans, and dry oatmeal. They come to depend on these "foods" to the extent that, if not available, they have physical and mental symptoms something like narcotic withdrawal symptoms (cramps, nausea and vomiting, upset and disturbed, restless, sleepless).

The urge to consume bizarre substances is usually related to a deficiency of some dietary essential contained in it. Studies show that these habits create serious body imbalances that are hard to break.

SUMMARY

Young, middle-aged, or old—everyone requires adequate nourishment to maintain health. When illness strikes, the body needs extra nourishment or special diet modifications. Regardless of how the diet is altered, the patient must receive the essential nutrients. Long term and chronic illnesses pose their own unique problems due to the "everlastingness" of diet restrictions and adjustments.

New knowledge about food, its relation to health, and its use during illness make the patient's diet as important to him as the drugs he takes.

Diets are usually divided into two large groups: house diets and therapeutic diets. House diets are used for patients who do not have therapeutic nourishment needs; whether liquid, soft, or general diets, they are ordered to help the patient meet his regular nourishment needs in a form he is able to tolerate. Therapeutic diets are prescribed for patients who have particular nutrient needs. Such diets may increase the amount of one or more food substances or may reduce or eliminate a substance; in this way the diet is used for corrective purposes.

Faulty functioning of some organ or gland, trauma, allergies, disease, and symptoms accompanying disease can make it necessary to modify the kinds and amounts of food eaten.

The nurse has responsibilities to the patient concerning his diet. If he is to profit from his diet, he must eat it. Pleasant, clean surroundings, attractive trays and food arrangements, interest in his appetite, and help during the meal are needs calling for the attention of the nurse.

GUIDES FOR STUDY AND DISCUSSION

1. What is the difference in purpose between the house diet and the therapeutic diet?

2. Diet is an essential part of treatment for a person with diabetes mellitus. What can you do to help this person abide by his dietary restrictions?

3. What problems can long-term illness create for the patient?

4. If a person on a gastric ulcer diet asked why he ate so often and such small amounts, what would be your best answer?

5. What is your responsibility, if any, when a patient tells you he is allergic to a certain food on his tray?

6. Select one of your patients who is receiving a therapeutic diet. Why is he on this diet? List all nursing responsibilities you have to this patient because of this diet.

7. What is there in gastric juice that a bland diet tries to control?

8. Why is it that a newborn infant cannot withstand diarrhea as well as an older child or an adult?

9. At any age, patients often experience anorexia when ill. What can you do in such a situation? What difference does age make?

10. What type of assistance in meeting nourishment needs should the practical nurse be able to give a person who is severely burned? Consider the age of the patient, and the extent and location of burns as you prepare to discuss this question.

11. As you understand it, why is an overweight child less frowned upon than an overweight adult?

12. Regardless of the type of diet, what are your responsibilities to the patient?

13. The diet is ordered by the physician. Why is this so?

14. Illness makes special demands upon a patient's nutritional state. What are some of these demands?

15. What are the reasons for diet control when renal dysfunction is present?

16. In certain situations these patients must be fed. Think of two different states of dependency where this would be true.

17. Where are dietary observations recorded?

SUGGESTED SITUATIONS AND ACTIVITIES

1. Assume you are caring for a middle-aged female patient who has a diagnosis of inoperable cancer of the stomach. She is unaware of the cause of her gastric distress and talks about her lack of appetite a great deal. She all but refuses to eat. As a practical nurse what can you do to assist this person meet her need for nourishment?

2. List as many abnormal conditions as you can under each of the four reasons for nutritional deficiencies. Note how many seem to fit under more than one reason. Why is this so?

INTRODUCTION TO ILLNESS

In a sense, the two chapters in this unit could be called "forerunners" because they serve as a foundation for what will be more specific knowledge about illness and the needs of patients. You may need or wish to review this unit from time to time.

Many new vocabulary terms are introduced in these chapters; they will become quite familiar to you as you use and reuse them in future situations.

Chapter 27 provides a means for learning about the main factors which cause or contribute to illness and disorder. These factors are grouped under eight headings; each is discussed in a general way. This knowledge will deepen and broaden as you go along and put it to work.

Chapter 28 explains the purpose of the medical examination and how the physician "gathers" information about the patient. The nurse's role in this activity is pointed out to help you sense your responsibilities to the patient and to the physician. This chapter deals with the *what* and *why* of the medical examination. The *how to do* for the nurse is associated with patient care elsewhere in the text.

ILLNESS: CAUSES AND PREVENTION

TOPICAL HEADINGS

Introduction
Early Beliefs About
  Illness
Illness Today

Factors Which Contribute
  to Illness
Immunity
Inhibiting and Destroying
  Microorganisms

Summary
Guides for Study and
  Discussion
Suggested Situations and
  Activities

OBJECTIVES FOR THE STUDENT: Be able to:

1. Name three early contributions toward prevention of illness.
2. List two reasons why there has been rapid progress in medical science during the past twenty years.
3. Identify eight factors which contribute to illness.
4. Explain how microorganisms spread.
5. By giving examples, defend the statement: microorganisms are both harmful and helpful.
6. Describe the two chief causes of malnutrition.
7. Differentiate between a sterilized object and a disinfected object.
8. Tell how a sterile object may become contaminated.
9. Give five instances when a nurse should wash her hands.
10. Differentiate between immunity by natural means and by artificial means.
11. Explain why there must be several different means for sterilizing objects.
12. Name three ways a nurse can protect the patient from cross-infection.

SUGGESTED STUDY VOCABULARY*

microscope
microorganism
thermometer
stethoscope
asepsis
"germ theory of disease"
germ
anesthesia
protozoa
fungi
toxic agent
bacteria
electron microscope

Rickettsiae
pleuropneumonia-like organisms
viruses
malformation
congenital anomalies
statistics
gangrene
heredity
disinfection
sterilization
antisepsis
sanitation
immune

immunization
sterilized
contaminated
inhibit
destroy
trauma
antibodies
cross infection
direct contact
wound
shock
erythema
vaccination

*Look for any terms you already know.

INTRODUCTION

Scientific medicine had its start with the invention of the microscope about 300 years ago. Strange as it may seem, in the last 10 to 15 years more new medical knowledge has been uncovered than in all the previous years put together. Being able to miniaturize equipment makes it possible to explore the inside of the body as never before; using man-made materials to replace defective body parts and transplanting human tissues and organs from one body to another are not science fiction but a reality. Modern tools such as the electron microscope make it possible to explore living matter (the cell and its parts) in minute detail to learn how it performs its work harmoniously within itself and with its neighboring parts. The laser beam, capable of producing tremendous heat and power when focused at close range, is a new tool for performing surgery. As a result of new techniques, knowledge about body disorder and disease grows at a fast pace. The modern hospital provides new devices to perform its role and hospital personnel undergo on-the-job training to learn how to use them effectively; hence, "continuing to learn" is an urgent part of the life of people involved in health care.

Practically all nursing tasks, even the most simple, involve some general knowledge of the cause of disease or the spread of bacteria. The handling of bed linens, the cleaning and sterilizing of utensils and equipment, even the cleanliness of the floor in the patient's unit are important to the well-being of the patient, the nurse, and the patient in the next bed.

One does not have to know the extensive details of the cause of disease, its treatment, or its cure to help a patient feel that the physician and the nursing staff are working for his welfare. If the practical nurse can have an understanding of the causes of illness, its prevention and cure, it will enable her to give safe, effective care to her patients and make her work more meaningful and interesting. She will come to appreciate the importance of certain nursing care practices and techniques and the need to keep abreast of changes occurring around her.

EARLY BELIEFS ABOUT ILLNESS

The cause of illness has concerned mankind since time began. Early in history man had many fears and superstitions about the evil spirits he was sure caused illness. Some of the early beliefs are still around today. However, time has proven that the ancient (and not so ancient) ideas about the causes of illness were wrong. To the early physicians they seemed logical and correct, but as the centuries went by first one person and then another discovered new knowledge and presented new ideas and treatments. Sometimes the new knowledge and treatment spread over quite a large geographical area and then important events in history prevented their continued use and they were forgotten. The practice of medicine had its ups and downs through the many centuries; superstitions and theories about the body came and went.

It was not until 1676 that scientific medicine had its start, when a Dutch merchant by the name of Leeuwenhoek made one of the first microscopes. With his microscope Leeuwenhoek saw tiny objects moving about in drops of water, saliva, and urine. He did not know what they were or why they were there. Two hundred years later a French chemist named Louis Pasteur (1822-1895) determined that some of these tiny objects (microorganisms, bacteria) were causing certain diseases. This discovery by Pasteur was the real beginning of scientific medicine and its attempt to conquer disease.

Pasteur's name is perhaps most commonly used by the average person when he stops at the grocery store to buy a quart of pasteurized milk. This label on a carton means that the milk has been heated in a certain way to a certain temperature to prevent the growth of harmful bacteria in the milk. It is an indication of safe milk.

Robert Koch was the first man to clearly prove (1876) that certain organisms caused disease; thus the "germ theory of disease" was firmly established. Knowing that some microorganisms caused disease, many people became interested in finding out as much as possible about them. They also began to study body tissues and discovered that they are made up of very minute divisions called cells that grow and subdivide to make more cells.

The inventions of the thermometer and the stethoscope (during the 1800's) were two important tools for the physician to use in helping to make a diagnosis. Drugs at first were few and simple but years of research and study brought many new ones by 1900.

Surgery is an important part of medicine

today. This has not always been true. Living at the same time as Pasteur and Koch, Dr. Joseph Lister in England determined that wounds healed faster and with much less infection if special care was taken to avoid spreading contamination from one patient to another. This knowledge led to what is now called *asepsis,* or freedom from contamination. Dr. Lister is known as the father of modern antiseptic surgery. Along with improved techniques for surgery came the use of nitrous oxide, ether, and chloroform—the beginning of anesthesia.

The interest in *prevention* of illness also claimed the attention of early physicians. The first inoculations against smallpox (England 1798) by Edward Jenner and the successful work of Dr. Oliver Wendell Holmes, beginning in Boston in 1843, against the spread of infection during childbirth were outstanding contributions to safer living. Today all civilized countries try (with varying success) to guard against disease and illness; this is an age of prevention. Safe water, milk, and food, proper sewage disposal, and vast immunization programs prevent epidemics and keep people healthy. Though much progress has been made in some sections of the world, much remains to be done according to WHO and other international health movements.

ILLNESS TODAY

Today we know a great deal about causes of illnesses, the way to cure and to prevent many of them. This knowledge has come about through many years of experimenting with animals, and follow-up on humans, along with keeping accurate written accounts of progress made. But with all this there still remain many unexplained causes of illness. It may be recalled that nonofficial (voluntary) health agencies provide a great deal of money each year to help find causes and cures for illness conditions and to teach prevention as do local and national government agencies. In addition, government agencies have responsibilities for passing laws to provide measures to protect the health of the public.

Until the cause of an illness can be determined it may be difficult to treat the patient effectively. Careful observations, reporting, and charting by the nurse aid the physician as he seeks information about the patient. Before and after the cause is determined, the nursing care may include assistance with a variety of treatments and tests, including the use of therapeutic diets, special laboratory tests, different drugs, and complicated equipment.

The role of the practical nurse may be that of an "elbow to elbow" assistant to the registered nurse or the physician or it may be as simple a matter as observing a diabetic patient to make sure that he eats his whole meal on schedule. Whatever the tasks or functions, the licensed practical nurse with a general working knowledge of the causes of illness will be able to carry them out with skill and safety.

FACTORS WHICH CONTRIBUTE TO ILLNESS

Illness conditions may be due to many things. Following are some factors which cause or influence illness and body disorder. You will see relationships among many of these factors as you go along. For example, a wound is an open door for microorganisms. Or, a deformity in the alimentary tract can contribute to malnutrition.

1. Microorganisms.
2. Body deformities and abnormal functions.
3. Improper nourishment.
4. Trauma due to accidents.
5. Poisons and poisoning.
6. Housing as related to health and disease.
7. Heat and cold as related to illness.
8. Heredity.

MICROORGANISMS

Microorganisms are tiny living creatures of varying sizes and shapes which can be seen only with a microscope. Some are so small that it takes a special kind of microscope to observe them.

Some microorganisms are helpful and others are harmful. Each kind enters the body by many different means such as in air, on food, in water and milk; by *contaminated* objects placed in the mouth or to the lips; through breaks in the skin; and by way of the urinary tract, birth canal, and intestines. While

TABLE 27-1. FACTORS WHICH INFLUENCE THE SPREAD AND THE CONTROL OF DISEASE

SPREAD	CONTROL AND INHIBITION
1. Climate — warmer, humid climate is more favorable for growth of organisms.	1. Laws (local and national) — passed in relation to food purity, food handling and packaging, disposal of wastes, safe housing standards, inspection of public eating and sleeping places, and air and water pollution.
2. Season — some diseases are more common during the winter, others during the spring, etc.	2. Community facilities — sewage and garbage disposal, safe water and milk supplies, trash and litter clean-up requirements are a few such means.
3. Living conditions — slum areas (congested and with poor sanitation facilities) promote disease and often are starting places of epidemics.	3. Individual health habits — proper food, sleep, rest, elimination, exercise, and body cleanliness inhibit disease.
4. Large public gatherings — discouraged during epidemics.	4. An informed public — using every means of communication to inform people makes them aware of what to do or not to do.
5. Environment — polluted air, smog, lack of sunshine, poor ventilation all are contributing factors.	5. Immunization programs — these are made available and the public is urged to participate.

many types of microorganisms are present in the body and on its surface at all times, good health habits help the body to resist or eliminate them. Two groups of factors influence the *spread* and the *control* of microorganisms (Table 27–1).

Transportation of Microorganisms

One fact to remember about microorganisms is that they cannot travel about on their own; they need a means of transportation.

Air is one means. These tiny organisms cling to dust particles and settle on food, furniture, and floors. They are inhaled in air. Most of them are harmless. However, there is nothing to stop harmful bacteria from being spread by dust. The more dust there is in the air, the greater the number of bacteria. Thus proper ventilation of rooms with clean air and sunlight along with clean floors and furnishings, helps to control the spread of microorganisms. The air in crowded living quarters, buses, theatres, and the like is laden with all types of organisms. As people cough, sneeze, and breathe, the air is constantly being polluted.

Saliva and nasal discharges are known to contain harmful bacteria at all times.

Contact is another common means of spreading microorganisms; they are transported by clothing, books, and other articles. The human body, especially the hands and hair, carries microorganisms. Animals and insects are also ever-ready vehicles for these tiny passengers.

Hygienic practices are essential to the health of the individual and also of the community, regardless of size. To realize how disease can be spread or controlled will help you to maintain the best personal health habits and to appreciate why a clean, safe environment is essential for the patient. Such knowledge will make the techniques for handling soiled, clean, and sterile equipment more meaningful to you.

TYPES OF MICROORGANISMS.   There are many ways to group microorganisms. No one method satisfies all microbiologists as discovery of "new" organisms continues to add to the categories. The following list represents one means of grouping disease-causing microorganisms:

1. Protozoa.
2. Fungi—yeasts and molds.
3. Bacteria.
4. Rickettsiae.*
5. Pleuropneumonia-like organisms.*
6. Viruses.

The two most familiar groups are *bacteria* and *viruses*. These terms are used freely by the public along with the word *germ*. Germ is *any* one of the above microorganisms that cause disease.

1. *Protozoa* have harmful and harmless members in the group. They produce the well-known disease malaria. Protozoa live in the soil and digest material, thus making the soil more fertile.

2. *Fungi* is the name given to a class of vegetable organisms which produce toadstools, mushrooms, rusts, smut, yeasts, molds, and the like.

The two directly related to disease are *yeasts* and *molds*. Yeasts and molds are common in everyday life and some are very useful. Bread making is dependent upon a certain type of yeast. Harmful members of these two groups cause such illness conditions as skin infections (ringworm), lesions in the skin and lungs, and generalized body infections. Abscesses may occur in the lungs, kidneys, and other organs when a generalized body infection is caused by certain members of the yeast group. The illness conditions caused by yeasts and molds are called *fungus diseases*. They attack the skin or mucous membranes of the body. Healthy skin and mucous membranes usually resist the organisms. Fungus diseases are most frequently found in individuals with poor resistance. They sometimes appear as complications following some other disease. Improper diet, especially among children and older people, frequently causes them to develop fungus infections.

3. *Bacteria* are both harmful and helpful; some types cause disease and others are essential to healthful living.

Bacteria, the oldest known group of organisms, include a variety of sizes and shapes and each particular type of bacterium is recognized under the microscope by its size and shape. This identification helps to make the diagnosis.

A partial list of diseases caused by the many types of harmful bacteria includes *boils, carbuncles, impetigo,* several types of *pneumonia, scarlet fever, sore throats, inflammation of the heart valves (bacterial endocarditis), meningitis, gonorrhea, diphtheria, tuberculosis, typhoid fever, dysentery, plague, cholera, tetanus,* and *whooping cough.*

Many types of bacteria (and other microorganisms) are essential to human beings and to life itself. In fact, there are many more helpful types than harmful ones. If it were not for the work of helpful bacteria, refuse and dead plant and animal matter would accumulate and provide breeding places for the dangerous disease-causing bacteria. Bacteria help to purify sewage. Human excreta (urine and feces) carried to the sewage disposal plant through sewers is attacked by bacteria and other types of microorganisms. They use the sewage as food and thereby change it into harmless substances which collect as sludge. This sludge is a rich plant food and is used for garden fertilizer. Some types of bacteria in the soil help plant growth. In the preparation of certain foods like cocoa, spices, and pickles, in the making of some drugs, and in the preparation of leather from animal skins, helpful bacteria are necessary.

4. *Rickettsiae* compose a group of parasitic microorganisms named for their discoverer, Howard Taylor Ricketts. Rickettsiae resemble the viruses in some of their living habits. However, they can be seen with the ordinary microscope and the viruses cannot. They are much like bacteria in form, but smaller; this likeness causes some microbiologists to classify them as bacteria.

Rocky Mountain spotted fever and *typhus fever* are two of the most common diseases caused by the rickettsiae. These parasitic organisms are carried and spread chiefly by the bites of ticks, mites, fleas, and lice. Ticks and mites spread Rocky Mountain spotted fever by way of rabbits and rats. Fleas and lice spread typhus fever. This disease has produced some of the worst epidemics known to man. During famine and general disaster when hygienic practices are poor, typhus fever appears.

6. *Viruses* are the smallest of the microorganisms. A special microscope is needed to see them. Like the rickettsiae, they require living tissue for growth. For laboratory study, the chick embryo (growing in the shell) furnishes a suitable place for most viruses to grow.

---

*Resemble both bacteria and viruses in some respects.

Notice that viruses attack a wide variety of body locations and tissues. *Smallpox, measles,* and *chickenpox* are virus diseases affecting the skin. *Anterior poliomyelitis, rabies,* and *encephalitis* (sleeping sickness) are virus-caused diseases affecting the central nervous system. Viruses attack the respiratory system and produce the *common cold, influenza,* and *virus pneumonia*. These microorganisms frequently attack the liver, lymphatic glands, and gastrointestinal tract as well.

Virus-caused diseases spread very rapidly and produce epidemics. Successful immunization of human beings against virus diseases started with protection from smallpox and now includes rabies, yellow fever, and poliomyelitis among others.

BODY DEFORMITIES AND ABNORMAL FUNCTIONS

Congenital Anomalies

Deformities produced during the growth of the fetus (before birth) are due to the irregular division of the cells and are called congenital anomalies. The cells do not subdivide and follow a normal growth pattern, so that at birth the body is deformed. Some part(s) may be lacking, incomplete, or otherwise deformed. Most common among such deformities are harelip and cleft palate. Others include deformed spines, club feet, missing fingers and toes, shorter than usual extremities, etc.

Abnormal Functions and Malformations

Glands can be abnormal in their functions and cause unusual body growth and development. If, through a defect at birth or the growth of a tumor on or near the gland, the amount or strength (or both) of the secretion is changed, some part of the body is affected. An example of this is a faulty pancreas and the production of insulin. (See Chapters 12 and 14 for normal endocrine functions.)

Various types of malformation of the body, such as malformed bones, defective sense organs (eyes, ears, nose, etc.), defective heart, stomach, or intestines, cause people to seek medical care. Many people have minor deformities which do not seem to cause them difficulty or prevent them from carrying on normal living activities.

IMPROPER NOURISHMENT

Proper nourishment is directly related to health. (See Chapters 25 and 26.) A body which receives adequate amounts of essential nutrients and uses them in a normal way to build, restore, and maintain itself from day to day is in a much better position to ward off disease and stay healthy than a body receiving improper foods.

Two chief causes (there are many others) of malnourishment or undernourishment are:

1. The improper intake of essential nutrients.

2. The improper use of essential nutrients by the body.

Lack of Essential Food Nutrients

Undernourishment due to the improper intake of essential food nutrients is a condition found in every country of the world. It is more prevalent in some countries than others, especially where there is a large population and where drought and famine go hand-in-hand. This continent, while it is considered a land of plenty, has a great deal of undernourishment due to improper eating habits, lack of money, misinformation, and ignorance.

The lack of sufficient specific vitamins in the diet causes vitamin deficiency diseases, which have been known for centuries in some countries. Some of the more common of these diseases include rickets, scurvy, pellagra, and beriberi.

Mineral deficiency in the diet can cause such disease conditions as anemia and simple goiter.

Protein deficiencies due to loss of blood protein during hemorrhage, from severe burns, or during extensive operations must be treated to avoid complications the same as protein deficiencies due to the lack of sufficient protein in the diet.

Older people very often eat too many carbohydrates (starches and sugars) and too few proteins and minerals. Their appetites are poor and their inactivity does little to step up the desire to eat full meals with regularity. People of any age with poor eating habits (too much of one type of food to the exclusion of other types, etc.) can actually suffer from undernourishment without being aware of it.

Excessive and continued use of alcohol causes vitamin deficiencies and poor nutritional status. Likewise, the consumption of bizarre "foods" (See Chapter 26) creates serious body imbalances too.

The study of the relationship of diet to normal and abnormal cell metabolism is one of the liveliest research pursuits of our times. The electron microscope is a most helpful tool in this respect. Much has been learned about how the body utilizes the different food nutrients, but there are many unanswered questions in relation to certain diseases and conditions and how they might be influenced by body nourishment.

Improper Utilization of Essential Food Nutrients

Under certain conditions a person can consume proper amounts and kinds of nourishment and yet be undernourished. In such cases the body is unable to properly utilize the food nutrients due to some disease condition along the alimentary canal or the malfunction of glands producing digestive juices.

TRAUMA DUE TO ACCIDENTS

Trauma is a wound or an injury. Most trauma is due to accidents of one kind or another. Accidents account for about six out of every 100 deaths in this country, making them the nation's fourth-ranked killer, following heart diseases, cancer, and stroke. Home accidents, the nation's number one crippler and killer of children, take a high toll each year according to the National Safety Council. However, all age groups are victims but some have more accidents than others. For example, older people are more frequently involved in fatal accidents than any other group. Youth, between the ages of 15 and 24, experience accidents frequently, especially males.

Motor vehicle accidents, falls, burns, choking, poisoning, suffocation, explosions, and misuse of firearms all contribute to accidental deaths.

Through safety programs industry has cut its accident rate in half in less than two decades. Motor vehicle accidents have also been reduced despite the increased number of cars, but no statistic predicting the number of deaths, announced prior to a national holiday, is very inviting, nor is the final death and injured count when the holiday is over. The home accident rate remains about the same.

There is need for parents to be more keenly aware of home hazards and how to remove or control them. An aging population needs help to protect itself also.

Trauma to body tissues causes the body to react. If the injury is slight, the body reaction is usually of a local nature, such as a small cut or laceration which produces minor bleeding, soon clots, and heals under the protection of a crust or scab. Extensive body tissue trauma demands widespread reaction from the whole body. Several main factors influence the immediate reactions. The extent of damage to tissues, the loss of blood and body fluids, changes in body temperature due to exposure, emotional reaction, and the patient's general body condition influence not only the immediate but also the later needs of the patient. Shock, one of the frequent results of an accident, is a state of collapse of the circulatory system.

POISONS AND POISONING

Any substance which destroys or injures tissue when introduced into the body is called a poison. Poisons are grouped according to their origin and nature or according to the way the body reacts to them.

Certain gases, plants, metals, animals, and other substances can produce illness. The *amount of a dose* of any poisonous substance *greatly influences its effect on the body*. Some drugs considered to be poisons are very valuable as medicine when given in prescribed doses. A good example is digitalis, a medicine prescribed for certain types of cardiac patients.

One of the most common gaseous poisons is carbon monoxide. Faulty heating equipment causes many accidental deaths annually. It also serves as a means of suicide for people who intentionally inhale the exhaust fumes from an automobile.

Gases used for anesthesia during surgery are administered by highly skilled persons to avoid poisoning and explosions; the patient is watched very closely to avoid giving him more than is necessary or more than he can tolerate.

Certain types of acids and alkalis are sometimes taken for suicidal purposes, or they may accidentally or intentionally be placed in contact with the skin. When spilled on the skin, they produce severe burns which heal with heavy scar tissue. When swallowed, they cause severe damage to the membranes of the mouth, esophagus, and stomach. If the patient survives, the scar tissue resulting in the esophagus and stomach sometimes makes it impossible to swallow food.

Accidental poisonings occur in some industries. The white lead used in the manufacture of paint, the lead arsenate used in vegetable and fruit sprays, the lead materials used in automobile batteries, and gas poisoning due to leaky valves and containers are some of the common causes of accidental poisoning of workers.

Small children accidentally poison themselves by drinking such fluids as kerosene, liquid detergents, and cleaning solutions, and by consuming medicines left in easy-to-reach places. Adults need to be aware that the many modern cleaning materials, fertilizers, and pesticides are "killers" and should be stored in safe places. They can contaminate foods in some instances just by being stored beside them.

Foods can be contaminated by microorganisms due to improper handling and storage, "food additives" improperly used, and radioactivity ("fallout" from accidental or controlled testing sources). Approximately one million people in the U. S. experience definite food poisoning each year.

People with poor vision who cannot read labels accidentally swallow wrong substances. Such accidents account for many poisonings.

HOUSING AS RELATED TO HEALTH AND DISEASE

Standards have been established for food, drugs, pure water, and sewage disposal to protect the health and well-being of our people.

There is concern for adequate housing, too. In 1949 the National Housing Act was passed. It included this statement: "General welfare and security of the nation and the health and living standards of its people require a decent home and a suitable living environment for every American family."

Adequate shelter is a basic human need. Not only is poor housing related to the spread of communicable diseases, safety, and chronic illness, it is related to mental health as well. Poor ventilation, heating and lighting, dust, dirt, and microorganisms are responsible for physical ailments. Crowded quarters with no privacy, noise, and substandard living practices influence one's outlook on life in general. They influence attitudes toward acceptable living habits.

There are ways to control or improve housing conditions. For some years there have been building and housing codes. Health and fire departments work closely with building groups to see that certain safety and health standards are met in relation to space, heat, ventilation, light, and plumbing. Proper sewage disposal is vital. Special precautions are exercised where septic tanks are used. Health and safety hazards can be condemned and removal required by local health, police, and fire departments. Fast growing population areas — suburbs, new communities that seem to spring up in no time — often suffer from inadequate sewer-lines and water supply.

Local government in some fast-growing communities tries to control area growth by not permitting construction of new housing until adequate sewage-line, water supply, electricity, and gas are available. State governments are passing laws to bring local sewage treatment up to established standards before new housing can be built.

HEAT AND COLD AS RELATED TO ILLNESS

Extreme heat and cold can be dangerous. The normal body is equipped to maintain its normal temperature under average conditions. If exposed to extreme temperatures, the normal heat regulating mechanism of the body is affected and, in turn, the entire body reacts to the situation.

Heat

Excessive heat produced by steam, hot metal or oil, boiling water, or direct flames causes burns, usually of the skin and subcutaneous tissues. Under severe conditions other parts of the body are involved. *Burns are grouped into three classes.* The mild or *first degree burn* shows a redness of the skin (erythema). It is painful but heals without a scar. The *second degree burn* produces a blister filled with a clear yellow fluid. A reddened area usually surrounds the blister. Healing takes place rapidly and there is usually little or no scar. A *third degree burn* results when excessive heat is applied for a prolonged period of time destroying the outer layer of the skin (epidermis). From this denuded surface many hundreds of exposed capillaries release body fluid which can cause dehydration. The destroyed or burned skin can serve as a toxic agent (poisonous substance) as the body tries to absorb it. The denuded areas are open gateways for microorganisms to set up infection.

When more than half of the body surface has been exposed to second and third degree burns the patient's chances for survival are poor. Such burns heal slowly and during this process the body is subject to severe adjustments. The loss of fluids, the absorption of toxic substances, the possibility of infection, along with the patient's many anxious moments about himself.

Heat can affect the body as a whole. Conditions such as heat stroke, heat exhaustion, and sunstroke are results of exposing the body to high temperatures.

Heat stroke is the most serious and can cause death. Excessive temperature and humidity cause the heat regulating system of the body to work to full capacity in an attempt to cool the body. If this effort is not enough the blood slowly becomes overheated. At about 106° F. the heat regulation center begins to falter and the body temperature rises, sweating stops, and the final collapse of the heat regulating center produces convulsions and death.

Heat exhaustion is serious but should not be confused with heat stroke. In heat exhaustion the body has lost too much salt through excessive sweating. The patient faints and his blood pressure is low. Removal from the heat and replacement of the lost body salt usually cure the patient.

Sunstroke might be called a mild heat stroke. It occurs as a result of the direct effect of the sun. The heat regulating center is affected. Sweating ceases and there might be a feeling of lightheadedness. Unless the patient is removed to a cool place and the body cooled, *this can result in a generalized heat stroke with very serious results*. People who have recovered from heat and sunstroke usually have to be careful of re-exposure to heat.

Cold

Extremely cold temperatures cause frostbite. To protect itself, the body constricts blood vessels to conserve body heat. When the toes or fingers and other exposed parts of the body such as the nose, cheeks, or ears are subjected to low temperatures for a prolonged period of time, the blood supply can be shut off completely. The tissues then receive no food or oxygen, and there is danger of death of tissue and gangrene. A gradual warming of frostbitten areas is the treatment followed.

Death from freezing is due to an overall lowering of body temperature. Drowsiness and coma precede death as the body tissues and fluids gradually freeze.

HEREDITY

A disease or a disorder which is passed along generation after generation is called an hereditary condition. The inherited weakness may never be very pronounced or cause major trouble. On the other hand, as time goes by, it may develop into a full-blown trouble maker. Diseases with hereditary possibilities include, among others, numerous eye conditions (tumors on the retina, night blindness), pernicious anemia, progressive muscular weakness, migraine headaches, epilepsy, and mental deficiencies (e.g., feeble-mindedness).

As science further unravels the secrets of the cell, one can imagine that some inborn mistakes or weaknesses will be corrected either before birth or early in life.

IMMUNITY

Immunity is the power to resist disease; stated another way, it is the ability of the body to ward off infection. This ability may be the result of natural causes or a result of artificial means.

Natural Causes

Natural causes include several means: (1) a person may be born with a life-long resistance to some disease(s). (2) The body may naturally build up its own protection over a period of time by producing its own antibodies. This happens after exposure to a disease. The body with good natural resistive powers is able to build its own defenses (antibodies) against disease as time goes on. *Antibodies* are substances produced in the blood which tend to destroy organisms which attack the body. (3) If a person has had an infectious disease and recovered from it, he may have a natural resistance to that disease ever after. He has acquired this immunity by a natural means.

TABLE 27-2. PLAN FOR ROUTINE PROTECTIVE IMMUNIZATIONS*

APPROXIMATE AGE	IMMUNIZATIONS
6 to 8 weeks of age	First diphtheria, pertussis, and tetanus vaccine (DPT) and oral polio vaccine
1 month later	Second DPT
1 month later	Third DPT and polio vaccine
6 months of age	Last polio vaccine
12 months of age	Measles vaccine
15 months of age	Booster DPT and polio vaccine
4 years of age (preschool)	Booster DPT
8, 12, 16 years of age	Diphtheria and tetanus toxoid
Every 5 years thereafter	Tetanus toxoid
Approaching adolescence through adult group (not to young children)	Mumps vaccine**

*Adapted from Leifer: *Principles and Techniques in Pediatric Nursing,* 2nd ed., p. 197.
**Approval granted by U.S. Public Health Service, 1968. Further tests will determine how long beyond one year the single-injection vaccine will provide immunity.

This acquired immunity lasts a lifetime for certain diseases, such as diphtheria, measles, mumps, typhoid fever, scarlet fever, and smallpox. Some infectious diseases can be contracted many times. The common cold and influenza are two of these.

Infants are born with some antibodies in the blood stream. These have been passed along from the mother to the infant (fetus) before birth. She is able to share her supply of antibodies with her unborn child.

"Inborn" immunity is nature's way of protecting the baby the first several months of life. As this initial protection seems to disappear, the child is apt to have some of the many childhood diseases. Some are very serious and it is advisable to begin protecting a child early in life against certain diseases by using artificial means to establish immunity. Table 27–2 shows an immunization time schedule.

Artificial Means

When a person has a man-prepared substance introduced (by mouth or through the skin) into the body to help it produce protection (antibodies) against a specific disease, this process is called *vaccination*. This is considered an artificial means of providing immunity against disease and is more certain than natural means. Notice in Table 27–2 that some injections are given in a series; some require "booster shots" and some are needed every five years.

Vaccination substances have been produced for such diseases as smallpox, diphtheria, scarlet fever, whooping cough (pertussis), lockjaw (tetanus), typhoid fever, poliomyelitis, measles, mumps, and rabies. The list continues to grow. The newest vaccine in the preceding list is mumps, approved for use in 1968.

Vaccination helps to control the spread of disease because great numbers of the people can be protected.

In 1971 the World Health Organization (WHO) said it was now safe for *countries with extensive health services* to not require smallpox vaccinations because death from the vaccination is a greater risk than the possibility of the disease itself. There has been a 70 per cent worldwide decrease in smallpox since WHO started an extensive eradication program in 1967.

INHIBITING AND DESTROYING MICROORGANISMS

To destroy microorganisms *is to kill* them; *to inhibit* them *is to arrest or restrain* their activity.

The following terms, commonly used in reference to freeing an object from harmful organisms either by killing them or by inhibiting their growth, should be understood and properly used to give meaning to nursing practice.

Disinfection

This means the *destruction of disease-causing organisms*. Pasteurization of milk is an example of how a certain temperature for a specific period of time kills unwanted organisms. Chemicals (i.e., iodine, phenol) are sometimes used for disinfecting, and on occasion an article may be burned to be sure that it does not spread disease.

Sterilization

This process is more thorough because it *kills all (harmful and harmless) living organisms on or in an object*. However, some organisms (spore forming) have the ability to protect themselves with a tough outer covering and resist all killing methods except extremely high moist temperatures under pressure (autoclave) or prolonged periods of constant high temperatures of dry heat (oven).

Antisepsis

This is prevention of or fighting infection by destroying or inhibiting the action of harmful organisms. It is similar to disinfection, yet it does not *always* mean killing such organisms; it may only disable them.

The federal government has prohibited the use of the word antiseptic in advertising any product (i.e., mouthwashes, gargles, toothpaste) unless that product is *actually* capable of destroying harmful organisms.

Soaps and detergents, commonly classified as antiseptic agents, actually reduce microorganism activity, more through the rubbing or scrubbing process than through the antiseptic qualities of the products themselves.

Sanitation

An object is sanitary when it is free, or relatively free, from disease-causing organisms and is clean as well; this makes the object safe to use. Sanitation in public eating places provides clean, safe utensils and thereby safeguards the health of the public. Bedpans are sanitized and *not* sterilized in hospitals, except in cases of certain infectious diseases (i.e., amebic dysentery, typhoid fever) or whenever strict rules must be observed.

Certain factors influence the method (agent) used to sterilize an object: (1) the kind of organisms to be killed, and (2) the object to be sterilized. Because some organisms (spore forming) defy chemical methods and boiling and others (i.e., tubercle bacillus) resist chemical methods, too, if an object is to be entirely free from spores and other resistive organisms, sterilization under pressure in an autoclave (pressure cooker) is the safest method to use. However, some objects cannot withstand moist high temperatures, so dry heat (oven) over a long period of time is necessary. In other cases chemical agents are necessary.

METHODS OR AGENTS USED IN STERILIZATION

Heat (moist or dry) is a common sterilizing agent. Sterilization with dry heat takes longer than with moist heat, but it can be used for materials such as glassware, needles, syringes, powder, and oily substances. A closed oven at 170° C. for two to three hours will kill spores. A flame (dry heat) is used to sterilize small areas or objects. Incineration (complete burning) of burnable objects is sometimes used. A word of caution—half-burned, contaminated materials can be a dangerous source of disease (i.e., mouth wipes used by patients with tuberculosis).

Moist heating includes boiling, live steam, and steam under pressure. Spores are not killed by boiling, but other organisms are killed in 10 minutes or longer in actively boiling water. Live steam (free flowing, not under pressure) is as effective as boiling. Food processing plants (dairies, ice cream plants, etc.) use live steam to sterilize, disinfect, and sanitize equipment. See Figure 30–16 for home equipment used to sterilize a syringe by boiling.

The surest way to destroy any and all types of organisms is to use steam under pressure (autoclave). This tight-jacketed container allows steam to flow around each package or object carefully placed within it. The door is securely fastened and the air within the chamber replaced with steam under pressure. This vapor penetrates the packaged objects or materials (i.e., bandages, dressings, linens for the operating room, metal utensils and instruments, and some solutions).

Petroleum and oily substances need dry heat because they cannot withstand high moist temperatures, nor are they penetrated by moisture.

Operating an autoclave requires following very specific directions which are best learned when needed on the job.

If chemicals are used for sterilizing and disinfecting objects, care should be used in (1) having the proper strength of solution; (2) allowing sufficient time for solution to act; (3) selecting objects to be sterilized by this means; and (4) having objects free from organic matter (i.e., sputum, mucus, blood, feces, oil and grease).

Some chemicals used for cleansing, disinfecting, and sterilizing purposes are alcohols, iodine, Lysol, cresols, detergents, and bichloride of mercury (should be carefully labeled as being poisonous). Mercurochrome, Metaphen, and Merthiolate are mercury compounds used chiefly as skin disinfectants.

Electronic cleaning machines (ultrasonic cleaners) can wash, rinse, and dry objects (surgical instruments, glassware, etc.) better and faster than can be done by hand. These machines vibrate sound waves through a cleaning solution of water and detergent at a very high rate of speed (sonic vibrations), cleansing and even destroying some organisms on the objects in the process. It is presumed that the sound waves create tiny gas bubbles (in the solution) which pound or pepper the organism on all sides, upsetting its contents and rupturing its outside covering. However, due to the uncertainty about killing all and any type of living matter, the objects are then sterilized.

Table 27–3 divides the methods into two groups: *physical methods* and *chemical methods*. Some of these methods will become

TABLE 27-3

OUTLINE OF
STERILIZATION AND DISINFECTION

I. Physical Methods

    A. Radiation

        1. ultraviolet
        2. X-rays

    B. Ultrasonics
    C. Refrigeration
    D. Filtration
    E. Desiccation
    F. Heat
        1. dry heat
           (a) incineration
           (b) ovens (air)
        2. moist heat
           (a) boiling
           (b) free-flowing steam
           (c) pressure steam
        3. Pasteurization: heating to 60° or 65° for 30 minutes and then rapid cooling.

II. Chemical Methods

    A. Soap
    B. Detergents
    C. Alcohol
    D. Acids
    E. Phenol
    F. Alkalines
    G. Formaldehyde
    H. Metals
    I. Oxidizing Agents
    J. Dyes
    K. Oils
    L. Iodine
    M. Gas

quite familiar as you practice nursing; others are used in special situations (e.g., in a medical laboratory) which may never become part of *your* practice, as such.

APPLYING KNOWLEDGE TO PATIENT CARE

Knowing that microorganisms cannot move about of their own accord but that they have to be transported from one place to another, there are many precautions a careful nurse uses in protecting each patient from the others, and herself as well.

Keep in mind that the nurse (1) moves from patient to patient; (2) handles all types of equipment (handled by others); and (3) provides a ready means of transporting (hands, uniform, hair) organisms if she is not careful.

Cross-infection (from one patient to another) can occur because organisms can be spread by dust and moisture in the air or *direct contact* by physicians, nurses, aides, and visitors carrying organisms to the patient. This possibility in the nursery is especially frightening.

Handwashing

Handwashing—to curb cross-infection and self-infection—should be frequent and thorough. Plenty of soap and brisk washing action help to rid the hands of organisms. This is especially true if accompanied by thorough rinsing under running water. A safe nurse *always* takes time to wash her hands: before serving food or passing medications, before eating, after the care of each patient and before going to the next patient, after handling such equipment as urinals, bedpans, soiled dressings, linen and contaminated instruments, before changing dressings on a wound. Cleaning under and around the nails is a part of proper handwashing. Special handwashing or scrubbing techniques are used in some hospital areas, e.g., the operating room. (See Appendix III, Handwashing.)

Handling Equipment

Soiled equipment is handled so that it does not contaminate the uniform. For example, a bundle of soiled linen should be handled so that it does not come in contact with the uniform.

Shared Equipment and Safe Practice

Equipment used for first one patient and then another receives special attention. It is of the *utmost importance* that such things as thermometers (mouth and rectal), bedpans, urinals, syringes, needles, catheterization and enema equipment be properly handled, cleaned, disinfected, or sterilized. Using the proper cleaning methods, the proper agent for disinfecting or sterilizing, and allowing sufficient time for the agent to act on the organisms are exceedingly important nursing practices.

Today many items are made to be used once and discarded. These disposable articles when in use are handled with the same precautions and exact techniques to ensure patient safety against contamination.

The safe nurse recognizes that when a piece of sterile equipment comes in contact with a contaminated (nonsterile) object it needs to be resterilized (or discarded, if disposable) before it is used. The safe nurse also recognizes that improper storage of sterile equipment can contaminate it and make it unsafe for use.

Some objects are not sterilized but disinfected and sanitized. Here again the nurse is responsible for using proper methods to ensure the safety of her patients. Bedpans and urinals (if one is not provided for each patient) are stored in a common room on the hospital floor. They are used for any and all patients as necessary. Rigid cleaning and sanitizing methods should be strictly followed. You should be as conscientious about handling this equipment as you are about seeing that each patient receives drinking water in a clean glass or that he shares his towel with no one.

The widespread use of disposable equipment and prepackaged materials requires the nurse to know and use safe techniques for the same reasons as the reusable equipment. The nurse should remember that patients are often charged for each item used, hence wasteful, careless practices cost the patient money.

Clean Environment

A clean environment (floors, furniture, window sills) inhibits the growth and spread of organisms. Safe nursing care includes provision of a clean room whether in the hospital, clinic, or home. The conscientious nurse sees that the environment is clean and takes the responsibility for this if necessary.

SUMMARY

The practice of medicine became scientific during the 19th century when the "germ theory of disease" was established. Since then progress has been constant, if slow at times, except for the past 25 years. The present period is one of tremendous and rapid growth in new knowledge, tools, and techniques.

Safe nursing practice depends upon a working knowledge of the cause, spread, control, and prevention of illnesses and disorders. This knowledge includes the proper handling, cleaning, sterilizing, and disinfecting or disposing of equipment. Prevention (and rehabilitation) has become as necessary as cure, and such things as immunization, adequate housing, and proper nourishment number among the important problems facing people everywhere.

With respect to the "germ theory of disease," the conscientious nurse — the nurse who knows and uses acceptable practices — is a most valuable member of the health team. The safety of the patient in great measure depends upon the honest use of this knowledge by nursing personnel.

GUIDES FOR STUDY AND DISCUSSION

1. Inventions and discoveries during the 1800's made scientific medicine possible. What is *scientific* medicine? What inventions and discoveries of that period made medicine scientific? What had medical practice been before it became scientific?

2. When the public uses the word "germ," what do they mean?

3. When is an object sterile? How can it be contaminated?

4. The nurse provides a ready means for moving disease-causing organisms from one patient to another, or to herself. What practices should be followed to prevent this from happening?

5. Patients are often charged for disposable items used in their care. Consider the possibility of additional costs due to carelessness. What does this mean to the nurse using disposable sterile equipment?

6. What must you do to help prevent cross infection as you assist patients?

7. Why should a nurse wash her hands so often? Compose one overall rule about the frequency of handwashing that would provide for safety.

8. How may a person become immune against a certain disease?

9. What means are included in moist heat sterilization? Dry heat sterilization? Chemical sterilization?

10. Complete this chart by providing information as indicated.

FACTORS CONTRIBUTING TO ILLNESS

1. Microorganisms	Five diseases:
2. Deformities and abnormal functions	Two examples:
3. Improper nourishment	Four causes:
4. Trauma due to accident	Body reaction to:
5. Poisons/Poisoning	Ten examples:
6. Housing	How responsible for illness?
7. Heat and Cold	Types of Burns: Body reaction to extreme cold:
8. Heredity	Four conditions:

SUGGESTED SITUATIONS AND ACTIVITIES

1. Visit the service area(s) of the hospital where equipment is sterilized to find out what methods are used for what types of objects and for what purposes. Find out how objects can be ruined through careless handling. If possible, borrow some ruined equipment to set up a classroom display. Label each object telling what errors had been made.

2. Evaluate your handwashing practices. Consider *how* you do it, *how thoroughly* you do it, *when* you do it, and *why*. (See Appendix III, Handwashing.)

3. Prepare some type of visual aid showing how two or more of the eight illness-causing factors are related to each other.

CHAPTER 28

ILLNESS: DETECTION AND THE MEDICAL EXAMINATION

TOPICAL HEADINGS

Introduction
The Medical Examination
Techniques to Obtain
　Information

The Patient's History
Examination of the Body
Summary

Guides for Study and
　Discussion
Suggested Situations
　and Activities

OBJECTIVES FOR THE STUDENT: Be able to:

1. Explain how a medical examination is related to a diagnosis.
2. State two reasons why a regular examination is valuable.
3. Name five techniques used by the physician to obtain information.
4. Name six instruments a physician might use to obtain information.
5. Describe the responsibilities the nurse has to the patient during a physical examination.
6. Describe the responsibilities the nurse has to the physician conducting a physical examination.
7. Name five diagnostic tests.

SUGGESTED STUDY VOCABULARY*

diagnosis	sphygmomanometer	urine
detection	ophthalmoscope	sputum
inspection	otoscope	feces
auscultation	audiometer	nausea
palpation	cystoscope	holography
percussion	proctoscope	laser beams
manipulation	x-ray	scanning
thermometer	percussion hammer	cerumen
stethoscope	microscope	speculum

*Look for any terms you already know.

INTRODUCTION

Detection means uncovering or revealing something that is hidden or not readily seen. In the practice of medicine, early detection of a disorder or illness may be the factor that prolongs normal life.

When the patient seeks medical advice, the physician begins a series of actions to help him make a diagnosis (determining the nature of illness). He bases his conclusions on what he sees, hears, feels, and concludes from laboratory reports and from conversations with the patient or family member; the starting place in determining a diagnosis is a medical examination. The practical nurse often assists the physician in this exploration.

This chapter is designed to help you understand *what a medical examination is* and *what its purpose is*. The various means the physician uses to get specific information about the patient are discussed. Pointed out is the role of the nurse who assists, but the *"how to do"* to carry out these various measures is discussed in Chapter 34 where it relates to *any* patient, not just to one receiving a medical examination.

THE MEDICAL EXAMINATION

The medical examination is used to determine one's state of health. The physician has more means at hand today for detecting illness and disorder than ever before. A complete medical examination consequently generally involves many different types of tests and even more than one doctor, if the need arises. This is true particularly if some out-of-the-ordinary sign or symptom is detected.

Regular Examinations

Today prevention is an essential part of health care. People are urged to have regular medical check-ups not only to help maintain their health but to detect any early signs of body disorders. When such signs are found by the physician early treatment is far more helpful to the person than treatment that comes too late. This has particular meaning in the case of long-term illness conditions. If some of these conditions can be detected before they get too far along, chances for halting their progress are much improved.

People are more health conscious and follow preventive measures to a greater extent than in times past, but the need for constant reminding still exists. Mass communications media (television, radio, newspapers) help with this. Some heed the advice; others do not.

In some types of occupation, regular medical examinations are required because the nature of the work itself demands healthy workers. A good example of this is air transportation. Members of a flight crew need to be in top physical and mental condition to safely perform their duties. Food handling is another such occupation. Nursery school personnel—those caring for pre-school children—also need regular examinations.

Diagnostic Examinations

To determine the cause(s) of a patient's complaints, the physician uses whatever means he needs or has at hand. One means is the *diagnostic test*. This is any one of many special tests used to examine or investigate a particular structure or function of the body. There are many tests for blood, urine, feces, and body tissues to say nothing of a host of common other ones such as x-rays of parts of the body, analysis of stomach contents, timing the action of the digestive tract, recording brain and heart performance patterns, and studying body metabolism rates.

The results of any single test may not mean too much by themselves, but when all results are compared and used with the information gathered from examining the body and talking with the patient or family member, the physician is in a much better position to make a possible diagnosis. This may be a simple, rapid process or it may take a long time. The physician may find that he is still unable to make a clear-cut, firm diagnosis and lists a tentative one instead. Further information may confirm or change it.

TECHNIQUES TO OBTAIN INFORMATION

Very often the practical nurse is present and assists the physician during the medical examination by seeing that the patient is properly draped (his privacy protected) and that necessary equipment is assembled. Providing privacy is reassuring to the patient and dispels some of his anxiety. The patient has a right to expect privacy.

The physician uses his special senses to gather information with the aid of some small tools and techniques, and his specially trained senses listen, look, and feel for any abnormalities. The following terms describe these techniques.

INSPECTION. This is examination by observation. The physician sees swellings, discoloration of the skin, scars, rashes, general state of nourishment, and body alignment and contour. Some patients "look" sick; others do not.

AUSCULTATION. This is examination by

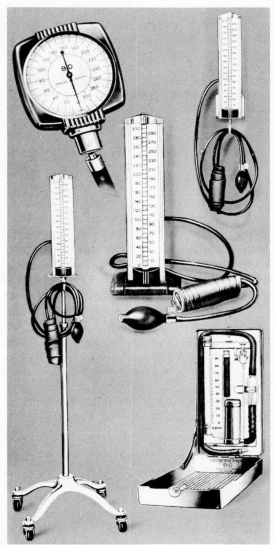

FIGURE 28-1 Different types of sphygmomanometers. (Riehl: Family Nursing and Child Care, Charles A. Bennett.)

PERCUSSION. This is examination by tapping. Short, gentle, and sharp tapping blows are applied to parts of the body (i.e., chest, abdomen). The sounds produced by this tapping are meaningful. For example, under normal healthy conditions the chest has a certain characteristic sound when tapped; with the presence of fluid and swelling the tapping sounds are different. The doctor may use one hand or two, or he may use an instrument (percussion hammer) for this purpose.

MANIPULATION.   This is the act of moving a part of the body. Very often the physician will move a hand at the wrist, a foot at the ankle; or he may bend the knees and move the thigh to help determine normal or abnormal movements or stiffness. He will note any patient remarks about pain or soreness as he does this. Manipulation is sometimes used as a treatment to restore body movement.

Instruments Commonly Used for Examination

Thermometer—for taking temperature.

Stethoscope—for listening to internal sounds of the body.

Sphygmomanometer—for taking blood pressure (Fig. 28-1).

Ophthalmoscope—for examining the eye.

Otoscope—for examining the ear (Fig. 28-2).

listening for sounds within the body and is usually done with the aid of a stethoscope. Sometimes the ear is placed in direct contact with the body. The lungs, abdomen, and heart are examined by auscultation.

PALPATION. This is examination by feeling with the hands. Taking the pulse is an example. The rate and quality of the pulse are felt through the finger tips. By applying finger tip pressure on the abdomen the physician can determine shape, size, and location of many of the organs. He will know if they are swollen or their location has changed.

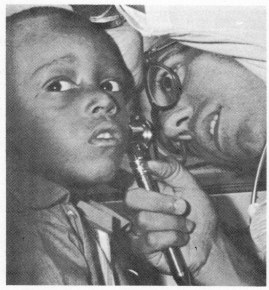

FIGURE 28-2 Examination by looking with an otoscope. (U.S. Department of Health, Education and Welfare: Promoting the Health of Mothers and Children, 1971.)

Audiometer—for testing hearing ability.

Cystoscope—for examining the urinary bladder.

Proctoscope—for examining the rectum and lower bowel.

X-ray—for taking internal pictures of bones, teeth, organs.

Percussion hammer—for tapping body surfaces.

Microscope—for examining fluids, tissues, sputum, feces, etc., under magnification.

Not all of these instruments are located in the ward in the hospital. Various departments (x-ray, laboratory) are set up within the hospital to provide needed services.

Common Diagnostic Tests

The physician needs accurate, reliable test results if he is to arrive at a correct diagnosis and order the correct treatment. As stated previously, medical science has many complicated techniques for studying body tissues, discharges, and functions. Thus, the physician has available and may use a wide variety of diagnostic tests as he studies the patient. Many different trained personnel (including nurses) are involved in seeing that the test results are accurate and reliable.

The patient is charged for all tests and their cost often represents a major part of his bill. He puts his trust in all involved; he has every reason to expect that any tests ordered by the physician will be carried out as directed.

As a practical nurse, you may be involved in assisting with collecting specimens, making observations, reporting, and recording certain results. Your accuracy and dependability are just as important as those of other personnel.

Following are some of the more usual types of tests ordered by the physician.

URINE. The urine specimen (amount, etc.) varies according to how it will be used. Sometimes only one specimen is necessary, or a series of specimens may be ordered. Collecting the specimen is usually a nursing responsibility.

The most common examination of urine (routine) includes measurements of volume, specific gravity, odor, turbidity (clearness), color, and reaction (acid or alkaline). The presence of either sugar or albumin indicates abnormal body function (see Chapter 13, normal urine).

Urine specimens need to be sent to the laboratory as soon as possible because bacteria can change the elements in urine within a few hours. Delay can also make the reaction alkaline and cause the specimen to become cloudy.

When a quantity of urine is to be analyzed, a 24-hour specimen is ordered. This means that all urine voided during this period is saved in a large container. The nurse measures the total amount and records it on the chart.

When you are responsible for collecting urine specimens, determine any specific directions ahead of time. For example, if the physician wants a urine culture to determine presence (or absence) of microorganisms in the urinary tract, it is most important to provide a specimen which has not been contaminated by any outside means (genitalia, placement in a nonsterile container, careless technique, and so forth). Procedures are set up for carrying out such measures, and you should always check your course of action prior to starting it.

SPUTUM. This is matter expectorated from the nose, throat, and lungs. Normally there is little or no sputum. During illness it may need to be examined to determine the presence of any microorganisms. Specimens are collected in paper cartons or cups which should be incinerated afterwards. Recording includes the appearance as to color, consistency (may be frothy fluid to heavy and tenacious), and odor. Amount is sometimes important; if so, this is measured on a 24-hour basis.

Variations are indications of certain diseases; therefore, accurate observation and recording are essential to diagnosis.

VOMITUS. This is matter which is forcibly expelled from the stomach through the mouth due to physical or emotional causes or both. Often it is preceded by nausea. Recording the time of vomiting (whether immediately after meals, etc.), the frequency and type (forceful, projectile, etc.) is as important as the description of the color, amount, and consistency. Patients' complaints in relation to nausea, pain, etc., should be included.

FECES. Frequently in diagnosing gastrointestinal disorders, stools are examined. The microscope is used to determine presence of microorganisms. The frequency, amount, color, form, and consistency of feces are noted and recorded.

Diet influences the amount, color, and consistency of stools; tension can influence frequency and form; some medications influence the appearance and consistency of feces (i.e., iron makes stools very dark).

Collection of stool specimens must carefully follow written directions. If a warm stool specimen is ordered, it is the responsibility of the nurse to see that the laboratory receives a warm specimen. If the stool is to be collected in a sterile container for a bacteriological examination, precautions should be taken and directions followed to see that requirements are met.

GASTRIC ANALYSIS. Gastric contents and secretions are sometimes examined for pus, blood, microorganisms, fecal odor, and acidity. The stomach contents are removed by passing a rubber tube (Levin tube) through the mouth or nose into the stomach. A large glass syringe is used to aspirate a sample of the stomach contents. Patients usually experience no difficulty as the tube is passed, although some may gag as the tip is being swallowed, but they may be tense or frightened; it may help the patient if the process is first explained to him.

Special test meals, sometimes ordered to study the action of the digestive tract, are certain amounts and kinds of food given at specified times. Nurses are responsible for seeing that the test meal procedures are carried out accurately and recorded. Here again, if the patient is capable of understanding, an explanation should be given.

BLOOD TESTS. Blood tests of many kinds are used in making diagnoses. The most common is *a complete blood count.* The red and white cells are counted, the amount of hemoglobin (oxygen-carrying red pigment in red cells) and a count of the various forms of white cells (lymphocytes, neutrophiles, etc., given in per cents) are included. This routine blood test is usually done upon admission and the laboratory findings are recorded on the patient's chart. Blood counts may be repeated frequently. The blood for this test is obtained by a trained medical laboratory worker who pricks the ear lobe or finger tip of the adult or the heel or toe of the infant.

When a larger amount of blood is needed, a sterile syringe and needle are used to enter a vein (venipuncture). The large vein in the bend of the elbow is usually used. The blood is withdrawn and placed in a glass test tube with a substance to prevent coagulation. The trained medical laboratory worker or the doctor is responsible for obtaining such blood samples.

Blood tests are done to determine *clotting time, blood type, presence of microorganisms, presence of antibodies, the "complete count,"* and for other reasons.

SPINAL TAPS. Spinal fluid is removed from the spinal column for examination. The physician may also use this procedure to relieve pressure on the brain. Often the nurse assists the physician. A knowledge of instruments, equipment, and aseptic technique is required to skillfully assist with this test.

The appearance of the extracted fluid and the manner in which it comes through the needle are carefully noted by the physician. He is aware of any unusual color, odor, or consistency. The laboratory examines it for white cell count, bacteria, and amounts of certain substances (sugar, salts, protein) normally found in spinal fluid.

Special Laboratory Tests

Smear and culture specimens are obtained from the eyes, ears, nose, throat, mouth, vaginal orifice, wounds, abscesses, and sinuses. Many types of microorganisms are present in or on the body at all times. Close cooperation among personnel is generally needed in getting accurate results. Sometimes the identification of the organism is what actually determines the diagnosis and the treatment.

THYROID FUNCTION TESTS

Tests used to determine thyroid function are varied. Following are three of the common ones:

NAME	NORMAL RANGE
1. Basal Metabolic Rate (BMR)	From −10 percent to +10 percent. (below −10 percent: hypothyroidism; above +10 to +15 percent: hyperthyroidism.)
2. Serum Protein-Bound Iodine (PBI)	3.5 to 8.0 mcg./100 ml.
3. Butanol-Extractable Iodine (BEI)	3.2-6.4 mcg./100 ml. (Above this level indicates that the thyroid is discharging abnormal products into the blood stream.)

Examination by "Pictures"

Until now, and including the present practice, the method commonly used to "see and study" the shape of a broken bone, the presence of fluid in the chest, or abnormal growths in the intestinal tract or within the skull was to *x-ray* the part. A new method of taking pictures is being developed; it is called *holography*. Each method is discussed briefly.

X-ray pictures are taken for many different reasons. A bone may be fractured and the extent of the fracture needs to be determined before treatment is started. The physician may order an x-ray picture of the chest to determine the presence of fluid or the position of the heart. To obtain a picture of soft tissues (stomach, intestines, bladder) certain substances must be taken by mouth or injected into the veins so that the form of the organ can be readily seen. Bone shows up in x-ray pictures because it is dense and thick; soft tissues need additional substances to make them denser so they will show form.

HOLOGRAPHY. Holography is the new science of taking three-dimensional pictures with sound waves instead of light as in x-ray photography. In this new process sound-wave energy is converted into light. Laser beams are used to produce three-dimensional images (holograms); the ordinary photograph has two dimensions. Holograms can be made in color. One of the real advantages of using sound waves instead of light waves is that they can penetrate and photograph all types of tissue, hard or soft, and provide an immediate, detailed, three-dimensional picture of any part of the body. For example, being able to locate a small tumor growing in the brain immediately will make a speedy diagnosis possible and treatment can be arranged accordingly.

Radioisotope Scanning

A relatively new means for diagnosing disease is the use of radioiostopes in a method called "scanning." Usually the patient receives an oral or intravenous type of radio nuclide, a substance that disintegrates, throwing off electromagnetic "rays." These rays are detected by a Geiger counter, or more recently by a more sensitive instrument (i.e., rectilinear scanner). The scanner moves a "counter" across the body area being studied and exposes film showing where the radioactive material is concentrated. This shows the physician an image of the intensity of radioactivity within the body. The information gained by scanning is used in conjunction with other diagnostic findings; it is not considered a short cut to faster diagnosis.

THE PATIENT'S HISTORY

Knowledge of the patient's personal and medical history helps the physician establish a diagnosis. Every means possible is used to get accurate information from the patient or from a family member.

A record (history sheet) of such information becomes part of the patient's chart in the hospital or the clinic. The history sheet usually includes the following:

1. *Present complaints.*
2. *Personal data*—date and place of birth, where living and how long.
   a. Parents—ages, living or deceased; if deceased, cause of death.
   b. Brothers and sisters—ages, living or deceased; if deceased, cause of death.
   c. Habits—eating, sleeping, exercise, use of tea, coffee, alcohol, drugs, and tobacco.
   d. Occupation.
   e. Education.
3. *Past illnesses*—what and when; diseases, operations, accidents.
4. *Present illness*—specific information about when it started and what the patient experienced; what, if any, treatment for it.
5. *Any family history* related to hereditary conditions, long-term or chronic illnesses (diabetes, epilepsy, heart disease, cancer, tuberculosis, etc.).

EXAMINATION OF THE BODY

The following information is usually included in a complete physical examination:

TEMPERATURE, PULSE, RESPIRATION. The nurse usually takes care of obtaining this information.

HEIGHT, WEIGHT. This, too, is usually the responsibility of the nurse.

EYES. With a head mirror, ophthalmoscope, and light (natural or artificial) the physician observes eye movements, the change in the size of the pupil as it reacts to light, and the condition of the interior of the eye.

EARS. A head mirror may or may not be worn by the physician as he examines the ear by inspection with an otoscope. Cotton-tipped applicators may be used. The ear canal and ear drum are examined for discoloration, growths, discharges, ear wax (cerumen), and swollen or bulging ear drums (tympanic membranes). Hearing is tested in a variety of ways. The audiometer is a machine for that purpose. Listening to a ticking watch held at different distances from the ear is not a very exact method, but it has some use.

MOUTH, NOSE, THROAT. Inspection is the chief method for examination. The condition and number of teeth, the condition of the tongue, throat, and gums, and the odor of the breath are all noted. The air passages in the nose are checked for adequate breathing spaces, discharges, and growths.

NECK. Scars, growths, enlarged thyroid glands, and lymph nodes are determined by inspection and palpation.

CHEST. This includes breasts, lungs, and heart. Breast tissue is examined by palpation for growths. The condition of the lungs is determined by listening (auscultation) and tapping (percussion). The stethoscope is placed in various locations on the chest and the patient is asked to breathe through his mouth to determine normal or abnormal air sounds within the chest cavity. The location and size of the heart are determined by percussion, and heart sounds are noted with the aid of a stethoscope. A chest x-ray may be ordered.

ABDOMEN. Examination is by means of inspection, percussion, and palpation. The physician looks for scars, growths, or abnormalities. The presence of gas or fluid is determined, as well as that of any tumors, and tender or sore areas.

GENITALIA AND RECTUM. For the female patient the cervix, vaginal canal, uterus, and ovaries are examined. The most common procedure for this is called a bimanual examination. The physician places one hand on the abdomen and one or two fingers of the other hand in the vaginal canal. By using pressure he determines the location and size of the ovaries and uterus and the presence of any growths.

A vaginal speculum may be used to examine the vagina. A proctoscope permits inspection of the lower bowel while a rectal speculum is used to examine the rectum.

EXTREMITIES. (Arms, hands, legs, feet.) Inspection includes the condition of the skin, nails, fingers, presence of deformities, varicose veins, scars, growths, and enlarged joints.

SPINE. Observation of the spine when the patient is standing helps to determine presence of deformity, curvature, and hip alignment.

During the entire examination close observation is made of the general body posture and stature, the skin (color, blemishes), general state of nourishment, and total body development.

To pinpoint or narrow down a possible disorder, complicated tests and inspections are used by the physician. The modern medical laboratory and new types of tools (e.g., miniaturized instruments, scanning) plus the long-used x-ray techniques are often useful (and vital) in diagnosing a patient's ills. These means frequently reveal what "outside" inspection—palpation, percussion, and listening—fail to reveal. Information comes from many sources when a diagnosis is made.

SUMMARY

The medical examination is used to determine a person's state of health. People are urged to develop the habit of having regular medical check-ups as a preventive measure. If some disorder is detected early, treatment can follow sooner and one's chances of recovery or cure are that much better.

Diagnosis is the determination of the nature of a patient's illness; this determination is made after tests and all manner of inspections have been done and the findings fitted together in relationship to one another. Many different "specialists" are involved in working on tests and specimens and making observations, recording and reporting findings. The physician needs accurate results if he is to do his work well. This means that *all* personnel involved in any and all phases of information gathering must work with skill, accuracy, and honesty.

In particular, the nurse who assists the physician during a medical examination should keep two main things in mind: (1) *Obligation and responsibility to the patient:* providing for and protecting his privacy, remaining with the patient, readying and explaining to him what to expect, providing for his safety and physical comfort, showing acceptance of him regardless of the situation at hand, and taking care of his needs following the examination. (2) *Obligation and responsibility to the physician:* knowing what he will want to have at hand, having these materials available and convenient for use, assisting with positioning the patient, handling the equipment, and recording any information before, during, or following the examination.

GUIDES FOR STUDY AND DISCUSSION

1. As you understand it, what is your role with the patient during a physical examination? With the physician?

2. Think of reasons why a patient might be nervous during a physical examination. Be ready to discuss how a nurse could be helpful to such a patient.

3. What is the purpose of a physical examination during apparent good health? During a disorder?

4. Certain types of occupations require regular medical examinations. In addition to the three listed in this chapter, list as many more as you can.

5. In addition to various instruments, how does a physician gather information about a patient?

6. The physician uses certain instruments or equipment when doing a medical examination. Complete the following:

Name of Instrument   Purpose of
   1.
   2.
   3.
   4.
   5.
   6.
   7.
   8.

7. What is a diagnostic test? How many can you name? Where, in the patient's chart, are diagnostic test results located?

SUGGESTED SITUATIONS AND ACTIVITIES

1. A patient has just seen his hospital bill; he complains to you that he is unhappy with the charges made for "a lot of tests" he feels he did not need because the physician had told him the test findings were all negative. How will you handle your responsibilities in this situation? You may wish to role-play this scene with a classmate so other class members can assess your response.

2. The word-form *scope* combines with other word-forms to build words which indicate instruments to view things or hear things. The same is true of the word-form *meter* which measures things too. Make a list of "scope" words. Tell what each is. Do the same for "meter" words.

3. Assemble a display of instruments used by the physician to obtain information about a patient. Print the name of each instrument on a separate card. Shuffle the cards and test your ability to match cards with instruments. Have a classmate check your results.

DRUGS: THEIR ADMINISTRATION AND ACTION

Unit VIII is an introduction to the world of drug therapy. The contents of the three chapters form a foundation of general knowledge and source material useful to the practical nurse within the defined limits of Role I and Role II. This general knowledge is not sufficient (nor intended) to make a "medicine nurse" out of the practical nurse, but rather to arm her with information that points up the importance of *what not to do* as well as *what to do* in the matter of assuming responsibility for drug administration.

The story of drugs is as old as man himself. Early man used many of the things around him for relief from illness, and some are used in medical treatment today. No period in history has given us more knowledge of drugs than the present one, in which each day produces new efforts and results to help man live a longer life freer from disease and suffering. The list of drugs will continue to grow.

This unit discusses the use of drugs, how the public and the patient are protected, safety factors the nurse uses in giving drugs, specific points in administering them, and the action and use of some common drugs.

The practical nurse today is involved in the administration of drugs in patient care. This is an earnest and serious responsibility for the practical nurse considering the limitations of her preparation which do not equip her to administer all types of drugs. To handle safely the drugs that are entrusted to her requires a working knowledge and skills equal to the responsibilities. As responsibilities change, so must knowledge and skill. No practical nurse can predict what her future practice will be, so it behooves her to learn that which is basic to Roles I and II. Uppermost in each of these roles is the need to seek assistance from the physician or the charge nurse when responsibilities exceed her understanding and judgment.

CHAPTER 29

DRUGS: GENERAL USE, CONTROL, AND TYPES

OBJECTIVES FOR THE STUDENT: Be able to:

1. Name four ways drugs serve the patient.
2. Explain how drugs get their names.
3. Identify one source of drug information.
4. Give two reasons why narcotics are under strict government control.
5. Criticize the statement—a nurse is respected for what she knows when giving advice about medicines to take.
6. Explain the difference between a pill and a tablet.
7. Give three examples each of solid, semisolid, and liquid drugs.
8. Identify the four sources of drugs.
9. Tell why suppositories come in different shapes.

SUGGESTED STUDY VOCABULARY*

drug	lozenges	emulsions
drug dependency	capsules	infusions
diagnose	powders	spirits
vaccine	extracts	milks
pharmacy	ointments	mixtures
pharmacology	plasters	solutions
prescription	pastes	syrups
channel of administration	poultices	tinctures
dosage	suppositories	narcotic
pills	elixirs	synthetics
tablets		

*Look for any terms you already know.

INTRODUCTION

There are many ways to treat a patient's disorder—rest, diet, exercise, surgery, even a vacation or a change of work, and drugs, to name a few. One of the most popular means is by drugs. Today, the physician has a very wide range of drugs to choose from and the number is increasing rapidly. On first thought, one might think of this as real progress and it

298

is, to a large extent. But rapid drug production raises problems, too. The physician must *know* and *know about* the drugs he prescribes for patients; he has to depend on drug producers to furnish evidence of the therapeutic worth of the drug he prescribes.

Scientists must experiment (mainly with animals) to determine the effectiveness of a drug before it is given to humans. Every now and then a laboratory tested drug does not live up to predictions or expectations; it produces unplanned for or undesirable side effects. In the case of a drug with undesirable, dangerous side effects, steps are taken to control or abolish the use of the drug. This was not true in ancient times. Decisions then on the use of drugs were reached through trial and error. Little was known about the cause of disease and less was known about treatment. People kept track of what was a remedy and what was not. In this way knowledge slowly grew. Some of those early remedies (drugs) are still in use today because they "proved themselves" over many years.

Scientists can reproduce some drugs in the laboratory. This means that, after experimentation, they can create chemical substitutes which are called *synthetics*. The drug tables in Chapter 31 include examples of synthetic drugs which have been widely developed. However, we still know too little about how the cells of the body use drugs; this part of drug knowledge is in its infancy compared with drug production.

This chapter contains general information about how drugs serve the patient, where they come from and how they get their names, who sets drug standards, and how drugs are controlled. You will come to know that the practical nurse is not expected to have the depth of knowledge about drugs that the registered nurse has. However, you will need to know how to use current sources of information if you are to keep up-to-date with the drug responsibilities you will have.

HOW DRUGS SERVE

Drugs serve in several ways. They are used to:
1. Diagnose or investigate.
2. Treat symptoms.
3. Cure disease.
4. Prevent illness.

DIAGNOSTIC AID. The cure and recovery of many patients have been speeded up by use of drugs to help diagnose or investigate. For example, substances such as barium, iodine, and bismuth do not give out light. When taken internally, an x-ray picture shows the outline of the internal organs containing the substance. The doctor can determine if the size, shape, and location of these organs are within normal limits.

TREAT SYMPTOMS. Some drugs relieve symptoms, give supportive care, and regulate needed substances which are lacking or over-abundant in the body. Examples are pain, sleep, cough medicines, hormones, insulin, and blood plasma.

CURE DISEASE. Many diseases are cured by drugs. They may alter the chemistry of the body in some way, depress or stimulate the functioning of a system, or act directly on the cause of illness. For example, antibiotic drugs have markedly reduced the death rate in respiratory infections.

PREVENT ILLNESS. Vaccines and serums are used for disease prevention. Whooping cough, smallpox, poliomyelitis, and diphtheria are some of the diseases prevented by inoculation. Small doses of certain drugs taken regularly prevent some diseases (e.g., malaria).

DEFINITIONS, NAMES, STANDARDS

Definitions

A *drug* is a substance or mixture of substances used to aid in diagnosis, treat or prevent illness, control symptoms, or replace or add needed substances.

Pharmacy is concerned with preparing drugs.

Pharmacology is the study of drugs, their preparation, and their action.

Names of Drugs

A drug may have more than one name.

Chemical name—given by the chemist(s). It may combine names of chemicals in the drug.

Trade name—given by the manufacturer to catch the public eye and ear.

Common name—used by the physician.

Very often it is the same as the trade name.

Generic name — refers to the animal or plant classification of the drug. This may be similar to the chemical name.

Standards

As stated in the Introduction, drugs are produced in laboratories. Any company producing drugs must do so according to government standards for purity and strength. They must follow certain regulations which are based upon laws (local, national, or both).

Lists of effective drugs are published periodically to provide source material for physicians, dentists, pharmacists, nurses, and veterinarians. Following are some of the most commonly used sources of information about drugs. Some are called "official," others "non-official."

United States Pharmacopeia (U.S.P.) — revised by the government about every five years. Drugs which have been proven effective are listed. This is known as the official list of drugs.

A.M.A. Drug Evaluations — The Council on Drugs of the American Medical Association publishes this book at regular intervals for physicians. It replaces *New Drugs* and *New and Nonofficial Drugs* (N.N.D.).

The National Formulary (N.F. — published about every five years by the American Pharmaceutical Association. This book describes commonly used drugs not listed in the U.S.P. It is considered an official listing because each drug has met standards set by the association.

Physicians' Desk Reference (PDR) — published yearly by a private company. Drug manufacturers cooperate in the preparation of this book. Major products of the companies are listed in several ways.

American Hospital Formulary — issued by the American Society of Hospital Pharmacists at various times throughout the year. An individual drug is discussed (loose leaf sheet) as to action, use, and dosage.

British Pharmacopoeia (B.P.) — a British listing of standard drugs used in Canada.

Pharmacopoeia Internationalis (VI-I) — published by the World Health Organization (WHO), is an attempt to standardize and control important drugs in this world wide health effort.

Laws, both federal and local, control the strength and purity of most drugs to protect the public. In the case of certain drugs (e.g.,

narcotics) special laws are passed to provide specific controls on distribution and use. Local laws can be more strict than federal laws. This does not mean that state regulations are contrary to federal regulations, but rather that more safeguards are required within state, county, or city boundaries.

Federal Food, Drug, and Cosmetic Act

Passed in 1938, this law strengthened the original law of 1906. Federal legislation in 1962 measurably strengthened the controls again. Tragedy or near tragedy often occurs before such changes are made. In 1937 about 100 people died in this country because of the use of one drug, and in 1962 a drug not officially approved for general use in this country was found to be responsible for infant deformity at birth. These tragedies prompted tightening of regulations. Some important requirements of the Act are:

1. Drug labels must clearly state the contents in understandable words.

2. "Warning — may be habit-forming" must appear clearly on the label of a medicine containing habit-forming drugs. The name and the strength of the drug must be included.

3. Labels must include clear directions for use of drug. Dosage for children must be specified. Any limitations in use of drug must be included. No label may contain false information.

4. The Department of Health, Education, and Welfare must give permission before new drugs can be released to the general public. The *effectiveness* and *safety* of any drug must be proved before such approval is given.

5. Certain drugs are available only with a prescription. The label must state: "Caution: Federal law prohibits dispensing without a prescription."

The 1970 Comprehensive Drug Abuse Prevention and Control Act

This act became effective May 1, 1972; it is sometimes called the *Controlled Substance Act.*

The purpose of this law is to provide more rigid control over dispensing and administering addictive drugs and narcotics. It repeals previous narcotic laws and drug abuse amendments to the *Federal Food, Drug, and Cosmetic Act.* Substances controlled by the 1970 Act are divided into five schedules

(I,II,III,IV,V); drugs listed in Schedule I are those not used for medical purposes yet have the potential for abuse and drug dependency (heroin, LSD, marijuana, etc). The remaining schedules take care of barbiturates, amphetamines, narcotics, and so on.

The Canadian General Food and Drug Act

Under the supervision of the Department of National Health and Welfare, Canada controls all drugs through the dominion law known as the *General Food and Drug Act*. As in the United States (Federal Food, Drug, and Cosmetic Act), Canada's law covers the production, sale, and importation of foods, drugs, and cosmetics. Additional laws cover special drugs as in the case of narcotics (*Narcotic Control Act*), patent medicines (*Proprietary and Patent Medicine Act*), and drugs shown to be dangerous such as barbiturates (*Controlled Drug Act*). Unlike the United States, Canada requires that patent medicines must be examined, approved, and the seller licensed before they can be sold.

THE PRESCRIPTION AND SELF-MEDICATION

Writing a prescription for any drug the patient needs is the responsibility of the physician and the dentist. Such a prescription has several parts:

1. Patient's name (in full).
2. Date and hour the prescription was written; it indicates the time the use of the drug may be started.
3. Name of drug or combination of drugs.
4. Strength of the dose.
5. Amount of drug to be given.
6. Frequency with which drug is to be given.
7. Channel of administration.
8. Physician's signature.

Taking drugs yourself or advising others about them is an unsafe practice. A nurse simply does not have enough knowledge to prescribe medicines for herself or for anyone else. And, legally, she has no authority to do so. Diagnosing, prescribing, and treating are part of medical practice. Preparing and giving drugs according to the physician's orders is one thing; doing this without such an order is quite another thing. A nurse becomes quite familiar with drugs, dosage, and the like as she gives medicines to patients, but such knowledge is only a small part of what must be known about a patient (or herself) before a drug is prescribed. Each person is different. These differences are taken into account by the physician when he prescribes medicine.

A nurse is respected for what she knows, and "advice seekers" may ask her for help. Family members, neighbors, and friends are apt to seek help from the nurse because they feel she should know. This responsibility is one which must be met honestly each time it occurs. People should be helped to understand that the physician (not the nurse) is the person able to piece the information (complaints, signs, symptoms, age, size) together in a safe, meaningful way. Respect for you as a nurse will grow and endure in your community as you help others go to the proper source for their medical answers.

DRUG ABUSE

Drug abuse goes back to the beginning of drugs. No part of the world has been without its problems caused by the misuse of drugs.

The abuse of drugs occurs when a person uses a drug he does not need; taking the drug becomes a habit and all too soon he has to depend upon the drug (Drug Dependency). Drug dependency includes physical and emotional dependence the same as Addiction and Habituation.

A person may become drug dependent as the result of taking a medicine due to illness. After the illness is over, the craving for the drug remains. Another way to develop a drug dependency is to use the drug to see what happens. This is especially true of marijuana, hallucinogenic drugs (LSD), and narcotics such as heroin.

The drug abuse problem today is present among teenagers and even preteens, as well as young adults; one involves the other. Not all become drug dependent, but too many do.

The person who gives way to drugs may have one or more tendencies including: rebelling against authority, not wanting to face life as it is, seeking a thrill, wanting to live in a fantasy world, and emotional problems.

Drug abuse has no regard for age or for any particular economic group. Users range from very young to old; an astounding number are members of the health team.

WHERE DO DRUGS COME FROM?

Today most drugs are manufactured and prepared for use by pharmaceutical laboratories even though some of the substances used come from outside sources. Substances used in drugs come from four sources:

1. Plants—roots, bark, stems, leaves, seeds, flowers, sap, buds.
Examples: digitalis made from powdered leaf of the foxglove plant, quinine made from cinchona bark.

2. Animals—chiefly glands, organs, body fluids, although other parts may be used.
Examples: insulin from the pancreas, cortisone from adrenal glands.

3. Minerals—all types are used.
Examples: table salt (sodium chloride), epsom salt (magnesium sulfate), baking soda (sodium bicarbonate).

4. Synthetic drugs—made in the laboratory. Chemists knowing the various substances in drugs can sometimes make them artificially. They may use any or all of the above sources in combination to get the substance they seek. Sometimes important drugs are found by the scientist stumbling onto them while seeking something else. Penicillin was discovered in this way in 1928. The use of Antabuse for chronic alcoholism also was an accidental discovery.

COMMON TYPES OF DRUG PREPARATIONS

Drugs are given in *solid, semisolid,* or *liquid* form, depending upon the method of administration and the drug itself (Figs. 29–1, 29–2, 29–3, and 30–10). Table 29–1 describes and gives examples of some common solid, semisolid, and liquid drugs.

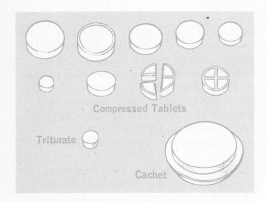

FIGURE 29-1   Types of tablets.

FIGURE 29-2   Sizes of capsules.

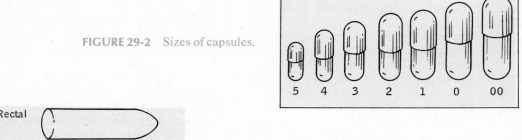

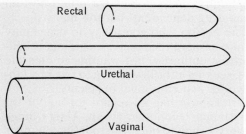

FIGURE 29-3   Types of suppositories.

TABLE 29–1.   COMMON TYPES OF DRUG PREPARATIONS

TYPES	BRIEF DESCRIPTION	EXAMPLE	INTERNAL/ EXTERNAL USE
Solid-semisolid			
Pills	Small pellets, usually coated.	Strychnine	Internal
Tablets	Powdered drugs compressed into disks; vary in size, not usually coated; may be scored to break easier.	Aspirin	Internal
Lozenges	Round or oblong disks, drug usually mixed with sugar; dissolve in mouth.	Cough drops	Internal
Capsules	Hard gelatin casings used for holding unpleasant tasting drugs; sizes vary.	Sleeping powders	Internal
Powders (simple and effervescent)	Finely ground substance; mixed with liquid or taken in capsule.	Chalk powder compound	Internal
Extracts	Solid or semisolid concentrated preparation from plant or animal drug.	Extract of liver	Internal
Ointments	Semisolid substance (lard, lanolin, petrolatum) holding a drug.	Boric acid ointment	External
Plasters	Mixture spread over a fabric and applied to the surface of the skin.	Mustard plaster	External
Pastes, Poultices	Soft mixture of a drug in starch or dextrin.	Zinc oxide paste	External
Suppositories	Drugs mixed with lanolin, gelatin, glycerin, or cocoa butter to form a solid at room temperature; body temperature melts it when inserted into vagina, rectum, or urethra.	Glycerin suppository	Considered external though inserted into body opening
Liquids			
Elixirs	Clear, sweetened solutions; usually water and alcohol mixed with a drug.	Elixir of phenobarbital	Internal
Emulsions	Small droplets of fat or oil suspended in a substance such as water.	Cod liver oil emulsion	Internal and external
Infusions	Products made by steeping drugs in water (hot or cold).	As in making tea	Internal
Milks	Suspension of fine particles in small amount of water; thick milky substance.	Milk of magnesia	Internal and external
Mixtures	Tiny particles of a solid suspended in a watery solution or one fluid mixed with another fluid; usually marked "Shake well before using."	Magnesia mixture	Internal and external
Solutions	Liquid, watery preparations consisting of a substance dissolved in another substance.	Boric acid solution, saline solution	Internal and external
Spirits	Alcoholic solutions which evaporate quickly.	Aromatic spirits of ammonia	Internal and external
Syrups	Sweet, watery solutions often used to disguise the disagreeable flavor of a drug.	Cherry syrups	Internal
Tinctures	Mixture of a drug and alcohol (about 10% solution of drug).	Tincture of belladonna; tincture of iodine	Internal and external

SUMMARY

Today most drugs are manufactured. Research and experimentation in drug laboratories produce a continuing supply of new drugs. As helpful as the new and better drugs may be, they pose challenges to the physician to inform himself of their effectiveness, limitations, and dangers. Likewise, the nurse is challenged to know what observations to make and what precautions to take in administering them. Up-to-date source material should be available and used.

To ensure drug purity and strength and to ensure that proper claims are made for effectiveness, governments set standards and controls backed up by laws. The nurse needs to be aware of any local or federal regulations which might involve her practice.

Drugs serve to diagnose or investigate illness, treat symptoms, cure diseases, and prevent illness. They come in solid, semisolid, and liquid forms which are used externally, internally or, in some instances, both ways.

GUIDES FOR STUDY AND DISCUSSION

1. Drugs serve useful purposes. What are they?

2. Imagine that you have been practicing as a private duty LPN for five years. What means have you used to keep up-to-date in drug therapy?

3. Narcotics are controlled by the government. Why is this necessary? What might you be expected to do (about narcotics) when you are practicing?

4. Prescriptions are made out by a physician, a dentist or a veterinarian. The pharmacist must prepare the medicine by following the doctor's directions. What information is essential on the prescription?

5. As a nurse, be ready to discuss how you can best help people who might come to you for "free advice."

6. Drugs come in solid, semisolid, and liquid forms. Study Table 29–1 so you can name some examples of each form.

7. Why are there pharmaceutical laboratories? What do they do? Where do they get their materials?

8. What are suppositories? Why do they come in several sizes and shapes?

9. How may a person become drug dependent? What are some common tendencies among young drug abusers today?

10. What is a scored pill? Find an illustration of one in this chapter. What is a tablet?

SUGGESTED SITUATIONS AND ACTIVITIES

1. You have been taking care of an elderly patient in his home for two months prior to his death. The physician had ordered a narcotic to relieve his pain. When the patient expired, you had a supply of this narcotic on hand. What do you need to know

about your responsibilities concerning the narcotic? How are you going to proceed to carry out your responsibilities?

2. Laws control narcotics. Visit the hospital pharmacy and find out how that department abides by the laws. Visit a nursing service unit and see what happens to narcotics when they are under the control of the nursing staff. Be ready to discuss with your classmates what you have learned that will make you a more careful nurse.

3. Explore at least two clinical areas to see how many sources of drug information are available. Make note of the name(s) of every source.

4. Prepare an exhibit of materials being used to fight drug abuse.

DRUGS: PREPARATION AND ADMINISTRATION

OBJECTIVES FOR THE STUDENT: Be able to:

1. Identify one problem the LPN may have with respect to drug administration.
2. State three reasons why medication errors occur.
3. List the four channels for administering drugs.
4. Describe the main factors which determine drug effectiveness.
5. Describe six practices for the care and storage of drugs.
6. Use the conversion tables for metric and apothecary measurements.
7. Given a list of official abreviations for drug administration, state the meaning for each.
8. Name the six rights to observe in drug administration.
9. List the essential requirements for charting a drug administered.
10. Give two examples of adjustments made in giving a medicine to a baby.
11. Using an assortment of syringes and needles, identify the size of each.

SUGGESTED STUDY VOCABULARY*

local action
systemic action
allergic
anaphylaxis
idiosynerasy
tolerance
abrasion
immersion
inunction

inhalation
instillation
intradermal injection
subcutaneous injection
hypodermic injection
hypodermoclysis
intramuscular injection
intravenous infusion
parenteral
addiction

infusion
sublingual
suppositories
lumen
ampule
vial
dosage
untoward results
contraindications
toxic

*Look for any terms you already know.

INTRODUCTION

As stated in the beginning of Unit VIII, the licensed practical nurse carries certain responsibilities related to giving patients their medicines. Her basic preparation does not equip her to administer all types of medicines using all channels of administration. Drug therapy is so involved and complex that in addition to the licensed practical nurse, the registered nurse assumes responsibility for some administrations and the physician for other administrations. In this respect, one could think of drug administration as a shared action. Sometimes it is difficult for the student practical nurse to "see" where her responsibilities begin and end because many situations are not very clear-cut. Judgments on the part of the charge nurse or physician must precede the assignment of drug administration to the licensed practical nurse. This means that the LPN should not be asked or expected to carry responsibility she is not equipped to carry safely. In turn, the LPN should not assume responsibility she is unable to carry safely. Such statements would seem to have little meaning when one views what is apt to happen in hospitals and nursing homes during the night hours when the staff is fewer in number than during the day. Nonetheless, there are legal and moral responsibilities which the licensed practical nurse must face in situations which demand judgment that she is not equipped to render.

Perhaps no aspect of patient care causes more concern than the mounting errors made in drug administration. This serious problem has many "faces." You will see many reasons why errors can occur when you observe a busy nursing service in action, view the contents of the medicine cabinet, notice the location and size of the area where nurses prepare medications, observe how many different drugs a single patient might be getting, or notice the system for "taking" the physician's order and carrying it out. You will become a part of this situation and be expected to carry varying responsibilities in it. The purpose of this chapter is to introduce you to some techniques of preparing and administering drugs. It spells out guidelines to follow so that you can perform your responsibilities safely.

FACTORS WHICH DETERMINE EFFECTS OF DRUGS

Scientists do not yet understand how many drugs accomplish their work in the human body, but this kind of precise knowledge is growing.

Three factors chiefly influence the effects of drugs:

1. Route of administration.
2. Reacting power of the drug.
3. The patient.

ROUTE OF ADMINISTRATION. The effect of any drug depends upon how concentrated it is when it arrives at the place it is to go to work. This means that the "route of administration" should be one that allows as much of the drug as possible to get to its intended site of action.

REACTING POWER OF THE DRUG. Drugs react upon the body in two ways:

1. *Local reaction*—the drug influences only the area where it is applied (e.g., ointment applied to the skin).

2. *General (systemic) reaction*—the body reacts as a whole. The drug is absorbed into the circulatory system and carried to cells throughout the body.

THE PATIENT. Patients may react quite differently to the same drug even though the physician has made allowances for size, age, condition, and weight in the dosage ordered. The cells in one individual's body can reject or turn against a drug while the cells in another person are able to use and profit normally from the same drug. One has heard of a person being allergic to certain foods. If a person is allergic, the body sets up a reaction; there may be sneezing, watering of the eyes, hives, etc. The same can be true of drugs; sometimes the reactions are much more severe. An exaggerated reaction is called *anaphylaxis*. Another term which means abnormal susceptibility to a drug is known as *idiosyncrasy*. In rare instances, people have died within minutes after receiving an injection of a drug such as penicillin. Physicians often ask a patient if he is sensitive to a certain drug (e.g., penicillin) before he administers or orders it.

The power of the body to excrete (throw off) a drug, to build up a reserve supply, or to

TABLE 30-1. DRUG REACTIONS

TYPE OF REACTION	EFFECT ON THE BODY
Depressive	Slows down a physical activity, such as to produce sleep.
Stimulating	Speeds up a physical activity, such as to step up the function of the kidneys to produce more urine.
Irritating	Local stimulation of cells or organs to function more actively, such as healing a decubitus ulcer by promoting cell growth at the site.
Salt action	A term given to certain solutions which change the internal pressure in body cells.
Cumulative	Not completely eliminated from the body; there is a "storing up" effect which could produce a toxic condition harmful to the patient.
Demulcent	Protects the surface of the skin or mucous membrane from irritation, such as a lotion applied to the feet and legs.
Additive	One drug used in combination with another to increase effectiveness
Selective	The power to act on a certain part of the body, such as a drug that stimulates the "breathing center" in the brain.
Tolerance	Loss of effectiveness when doses are repeated over a long period of time.
Addictive	A need or craving for certain drugs which have been taken to relieve some condition, such as narcotics.
Side effects	A "by-product" reaction or one other than the main result sought.
Untoward	An unwanted side effect, such as a skin rash resulting from taking a drug.

develop a tolerance (loss of effective response) to it over a period of time can also make a difference in the effectiveness of a drug in the body (see Table 30–1).

CHANNELS OF DRUG ADMINISTRATION

If a drug is to be effective, it must reach its destination with enough strength (concentration) to do its work. To make this possible, it is necessary to use several different body channels of "ports of entry." They are:
1. The skin
2. Mucous membranes
3. Parenteral means
4. The alimentary canal

Any body channel that prevents a drug from reaching the site of action in sufficient concentration would be considered an ineffective channel. For example, while many drugs are taken by mouth (orally), not all can be administered that way because the alimentary canal prevents them from reaching their site of action (cells where needed) in "full strength." This can be caused by the digestive juices destroying part or all of the drug strength, the lining of the intestines acting as a barrier to

absorption, or the drug irritating the stomach and intestines causing vomiting and diarrhea.

Another factor the physician considers in choosing the drug channel is: how fast is action needed? If a patient needs "results" at once and the drug is compatible with the blood, it is injected directly into a vein (intravenous). Or, it may be injected into the layers of the muscles (intramuscular) for rapid pickup by the circulatory system. The patient with small veins (difficult to locate and use) or who lacks muscle tone or muscle size creates problems for intravenous (I.V.) or intramuscular administration.

If local action is needed, the drug is applied to the affected areas as in the case of painting a skin abrasion with iodine.

The four channels of drug administration are listed in Table 30–2, including examples of the different methods.

GENERAL PRACTICES FOR CARE AND STORAGE OF DRUGS

Every agency has its policies and regulations concerning drug storage; however, some

TABLE 30–2. CHANNELS OF DRUG ADMINISTRATION

CHANNEL	MEANS USED
Skin	1. *Applying* plasters, poultices, or moist dressings to the skin. 2. *Immersing* a part into a solution, sometimes called a local bath. 3. *Painting* or *spraying* the skin. 4. *Rubbing* a drug into the skin (inunction).
Mucous Membranes	1. *Applying* drug directly to the membrane by swabbing or painting the area. 2. *Breathing* in air, steam, and smoke containing suspended particles. (inhalation) 3. *Dropping* the drug upon the affected area. (instillation) 4. *Spraying* a drug into the nose, the mouth and throat, or either. 5. *Washing* or *irrigating* a body cavity with a continuous flow of water containing drugs; gargling is a form of irrigating.
Parenteral (a broad term including all methods of general or systemic administration outside the alimentary canal)	*INTRADERMAL INJECTION:* Small amount of drug is injected between the upper layers of the skin. It is often used for diagnostic purposes. The most common site is the inner surface of the forearm. Study Figure 30-7 for equipment used and needle position in the tissue. *SUBCUTANEOUS INJECTION:* Drug is injected into the layer of fatty tissue beneath the upper layers of skin. Two common names for types of subcutaneous injections are: hypodermic (Fig. 30-8) and hypodermoclysis (Fig. 30-11). Hypodermic injection is a much-used means for depositing a small amount of drug in the body. Condition of patient, action of digestive juices, and need for rapid action are reasons for using this means rather than oral means. The upper, outer arm is a common injection side. Study Figure 30-12 for equipment used and needle position in the tissue. *Hypodermoclysis* is used to introduce a large quantity of fluid into subcutaneous tissue. It may be a means of getting fluid with or without a drug into the body. Common sites are the upper surfaces of the thighs, under the breasts, and in back tissues. Study Figure 30-11 for equipment and needle position in the tissue. It is a slow method and is used when veins cannot be used.

TABLE 30–2.   CHANNELS OF DRUG ADMINISTRATION (Continued)

INTRAMUSCULAR INJECTION: (Study Figures 30-12, 30-13, and 30-14.) The drug is injected down into the layers of the muscle. This route is used: when rapid action is needed, when a larger amount of a drug needs to be deposited and absorbed over a longer period of time, when a drug cannot be taken by mouth, when a drug would irritate upper layers of tissue. While there are numerous sites for this injection, the buttocks are the most common except for babies. Caution is used in selecting a site to avoid large nerves and large blood vessels and to prevent discomfort.

INTRAVENOUS INJECTION: (Fig. 30-15.) The drug is injected directly into the vein. This is a direct route for getting a drug into the blood stream. Common sites are the veins at the bend of the elbow and on the surface of the ankle. In infants the "soft spot" in the skull is used. Note the size of needles and syringes commonly used and the position of the needle in the vein.

OTHER less commonly used parenteral means include: intraperitoneal, intracardial, intrapleural, intraspinal.

Alimentary Canal

1. *Oral* administration means that the drug is swallowed. It enters the stomach (may be acted on and absorbed there) or it moves on to the intestines and is absorbed there. Of all channels, this is most frequently used. Physician may or may not specify oral channel; other channels are always specified. One should be aware of this difference.

2. *Sublingual* administration means that the tablet is placed under the tongue. It is dissolved and absorbed here.

3. *Other body cavities* (vagina, rectum, urethra). *Suppositories* are inserted into these cavities. See Figure 29-3 for proper shapes used to conform to different cavities.

TABLE 30–3. GENERAL PRACTICES FOR THE CARE AND STORAGE OF DRUGS

GENERAL PRACTICE	REASON
1. Drugs are kept in a special area; within the area they are usually arranged in a definite way.	To insure safekeeping and to make it easier for the nurse to prepare medicines accurately.
2. Some drugs, such as addictive drugs, are stored in a special locked compartment; the key is the responsibility of a designated person.	To meet legal requirements. Federal control of narcotics makes this a requirement. This supply of drugs is counted regularly and accurate records are kept.
3. A special area is set aside for poisonous drugs.	To avoid confusion with less dangerous drugs.
4. Drugs are placed in containers and labeled by the pharmacist.	To insure accuracy and safety.
5. Certain drugs are stored in refrigerator (antibiotics, vaccines, etc.)	To prevent them from becoming useless or less effective.
6. Old, rancid, and discolored drugs are discarded.	To maintain a fresh drug supply. Many types of drugs deteriorate with age.

common practices are followed wherever drugs are used. These practices are discussed in Table 30–3.

COMMON ABBREVIATIONS, WEIGHTS, AND MEASURES

A type of "medical shorthand" has been used many years to save time and space in recording drug and other administrations on the patient's chart. Appendix I lists acceptable abbreviations in common use. Sometimes terms are abbreviated when they should not be. Haste and "local practice" are the excuses often given for fractured terminology when a question arises in the courtroom or in the hospital.

Drugs must be measured accurately. Two different systems are used: *metric* and *apothecary*. Hospitals use one system or the other. Household measurements are not considered as accurate as the other two systems, but household measurements are sometimes used in home situations, especially in relation to drugs given externally.

Table 30–4 lists some basic comparisons; the inside back cover gives the entire table of metric and apothecaries systems. You will need to *learn how to use the comparison table for reference* to ensure accuracy in your work.

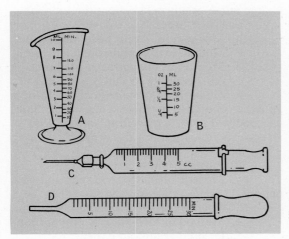

FIGURE 30-1 Equipment for drug measurement.

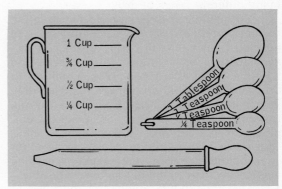

FIGURE 30-2 Household measuring equipment.

TABLE 30–4. COMPARISON OF MEASURING SYSTEMS

METRIC	APOTHECARY	HOUSEHOLD
Volume — Liquid		
	1 minim (m.)	1 drop
1 cubic centimeter (cc.)	15 m.	15 drops
4 cc.	60 m. or 1 fluid dram (fl. dm.)	60 drops or 1 teaspoonful (tsp.)
30 cc.	1 fluid ounce (fl. oz.)	2 tablespoonfuls (tbsp.) or 8 tsps.
250 cc.	8 fl. oz.	1 measuring cupful
500 cc.	1 pint (16 fl. oz.)	1 pint (2 measuring cupfuls)
1000 cc.	1 quart (32 fl. oz.)	1 quart (4 measuring cupfuls)
Weight — Dry		
60.0 milligrams	1 grain (gr.)	
1 Gram (Gm.)	15 gr.	¼ tsp.
4 Gm.	1 dram (dr.)	1 tsp.
30 Gm.	1 ounce (oz.)	2 tbsps.

SAFETY IN DRUG ADMINISTRATION

No nursing activity requires more attention to details and safety precautions than preparing and administering medicines. The possibility of error in drug administration is constantly present and becomes more acute as drugs continue to change, when personnel changes occur, and when patients receive so many different types of drugs.

You will need to pay particular attention to some safety factors from the start so as to develop right habits in carrying out your responsibilities as a student and later as an LPN. A word about your responsibilities in drug administration: no one can tell what they will be in the future. The LPN carries varying responsibilities at present; the place of employment and the time of day seem to influence these responsibilities. However, legal responsibilities remain the same regarding negligence. "If you did it, you're responsible." Knowing this should emphasize the need to develop right habits. Following are some guidelines that will serve in any situation:

1. *Agency policy is developed for a reason.* Follow the policies and directives of the hospital or agency.

2. *The order should be written.* Give *only* those medications for which the physician has written and signed the order.

3. *Avoid chance-taking.* Check with the charge nurse or physician about the following:
   a. Exact order.
   b. Medication, its purpose and action.
   c. Method of preparing the medication.
   d. Method of giving the medication.
   e. Observations to make.

4. *Know about the medication.* Inform yourself and ask questions ahead of time, especially if it is a new drug or one that is strange to you. Find out the drug's:
   a. Type.
   b. Purpose and action.
   c. Dosage (usual for the type and size patient?).
   d. Channel or route of administration.
   e. Method or technique of preparation.
   f. Desired results to expect.

g. Unwanted effects which could result.

h. Precautions to take.

i. Contraindications (when you should not proceed).

j. Calculations (have them checked).

5. *Lock the medicine cabinet* (or drawer) before leaving for any reason. Remove the key and return it to the authorized person.

6. *Observe these six "rights".* Make sure you have the:

a. Right patient.

b. Right medication.

c. Right dosage.

d. Right channel or route of administration.

e. Right technique or method.

f. Right time.

7. *Prepare and give the medicine.* Give *only* those medications you have prepared; prepare *only* those medications you are to give.

8. *Work alone.* Do not converse unless seeking help. Attention to detail requires complete concentration.

9. *Start with clean hands.* Wash thoroughly. (See Fig. 30–3).

10. *Use the medicine card.* Be sure it is accurate. Assemble all cards and materials *before* you start to "pour" medicines.

11. *Read the drug label three times* and compare it with medicine card:

a. *Before taking* container from location.

b. *Before pouring* (or removing) drug from container.

c. *Before returning* container to proper location (see Fig. 30–3).

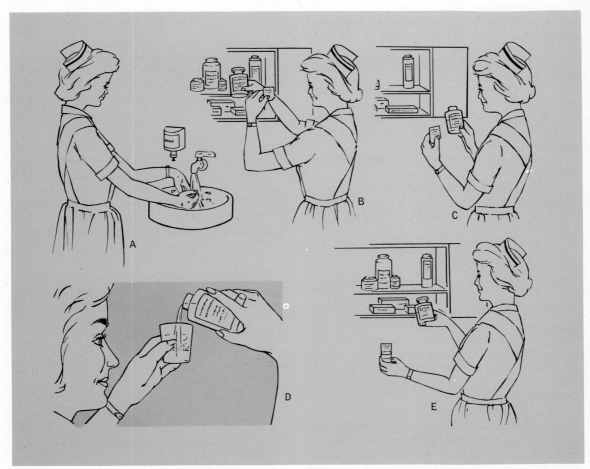

FIGURE 30-3　Safety precautions in preparing medicines.

12. *Be accurate in drug measurement.* Use proper equipment (e.g., calibrated measure) and proper technique (e.g., eye level).

13. *Some special "do nots."* **Do not:**

a. Use medications from containers with labels that are not readable.

b. Change label or relabel any container.

c. Change a drug from one container to another.

d. Mix two or more drugs, except when ordered.

e. Return a drug, or portion of a drug, to container, or save a drug taken from container by mistake (e.g., too much poured or a medication refused by the patient).

14. *Some special "do's."* **Do:**

a. Carry measured and prepared medication with the medicine card *together* on the medicine tray.

b. *Stay with* the patient until the medication is administered (e.g., swallowed, injected, applied).

c. *Remove* medication from bedside if it is not administered (e.g., patient refuses it, is absent from bedside, is sleeping).

d. Make any exceptions *only* when ordered by the physician.

e. Carry and keep the medicine tray with you.

15. *Make positive patient identification first.* Use the medicine card to read and compare with:

a. Name and number of room, ward, or unit.

b. Identification band on the wrist or ankle of patient (Fig. 30–4).

c. Bedcard on the patient's bed.

PARENTERAL ADMINISTRATION

Four channels or passageways for drugs to become useful to the body are through the *skin,* through the *mucous membranes,* by *parenteral means,* and by way of the *alimentary canal.* These channels and the methods used to make drugs useful to the body are described in Table 30–2.

Parenteral means is a broad term; it includes all methods of general or systemic administration outside the alimentary canal. To make drugs available to the body by this route calls for special skills in the use of equipment that penetrates the skin, thus making available

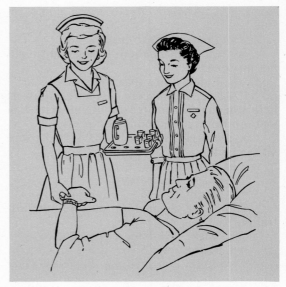

FIGURE 30-4 Identifying patient with medicine card.

underlying layers of tissues, a blood vessel, or a closed body cavity.

The LPN gives some medicines by this route (Role I) and may be called upon to assist the physician and registered nurse with others (Role II).

The Syringe and the Needle

The equipment that is of primary concern to the practical nurse (in parenteral administration) is the "syringe and the needle."

Syringes (to measure cubic centimeters) come in many sizes, ranging from 1 cc. to 100 cc. and are marked accordingly along the barrel. Study Figure 30–5 and notice the dual

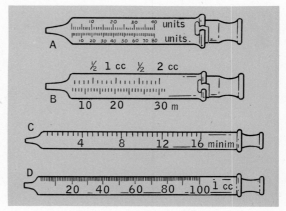

FIGURE 30-5 Some types of syringes.

markings on syringes A and B. Also, notice that syringes A and C are not marked off in cc. but one (A) is in units and one (C) is in minims. This tells you that certain syringes are made to handle some drugs that are measured in other than cc.

A syringe is made up of a barrel and a plunger made to fit perfectly. Each piece bears the same number, so they can be readily matched. Some syringes are manufactured so that the parts of one fit the parts of others like it. Sterile, disposable syringe and needle units are available now and are in common use.

The life of a glass syringe is lengthened when promptly and properly rinsed to remove foreign material after use. While procedures for cleaning and sterilizing these items vary according to sterilizing equipment and delegation of responsibility, immediate rinsing after use is essential.

Needles are hollow (the lumen) to permit the drug to pass from the syringe into the tissues; this passageway in the needle must be clean and free from foreign matter; hence, the need to rinse it right after use.

Needles are made in *regular* and *special* sizes:

1. *Regular needles* come in various sizes and lengths. The smallest gauge is 27 G. and the largest 13 G. Lengths run from three-eighths of an inch to three and one-half inches.

2. *Special needles* are made to serve special purposes; its purpose determines how long it is, how large its gauge is, and what type of point it has. (Fig. 30–6).

Disposable needles and syringes should be discarded immediately after use to avoid mistaken reuse; bend the needle as a safety precaution to prevent reuse.

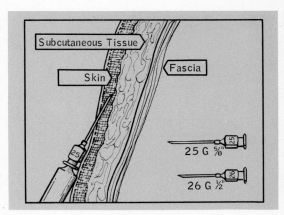

FIGURE 30-7   Intradermal injection.

THE INTRADERMAL INJECTION

When a very small amount of drug—usually for diagnostic purposes—is introduced just under the outer layer of skin (above the subcutaneous tissue) it is called an *intradermal injection*. It actually means that the small amount of drug is deposited "sandwich style" between the upper and lower layers of the skin where it is slowly absorbed. Notice the location of the point of the needle and the angle of the needle in Figure 30–7.

THE SUBCUTANEOUS INJECTION

Subcutaneous injection gets its name from the fatty (subcutaneous) tissue where the drug is deposited through the needle. Notice the location of the point of the needle and the angle of the needle in Figure 30–8. Absorption is rapid and this makes it a good, common means for getting a drug to the cells in a hurry (Fig. 30–9).

The most common of all subcutaneous injections is the *hypodermic*. Drugs used for hypodermic injections are in tablet form or in sterile solution in vials or ampules (Fig. 30–10). A procedure for preparing and administering this type of injection is found at the end of this chapter.

The *insulin injection* is similar to the hypodermic injection in that the insulin is injected into the same layer of tissue. The syringe is special; it is marked off in units (Fig. 30–5, Syrine A). The technique for preparing and administering is the same as for withdrawing a drug from a vial.

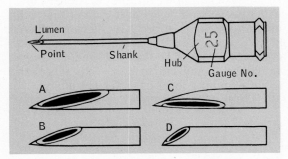

FIGURE 30-6   Parts of a needle and some types of points. Each has a gauge number (e.g., 25). A dull or damaged needle can injure tissues and be painful to the patient.

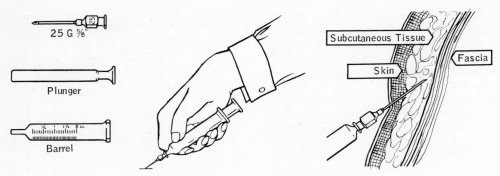

FIGURE 30-8   Hypodermic injection.

The *hypodermoclysis* is the introduction of large amounts of fluids (with or without drugs) into the subcutaneous tissues. Notice in Figure 30–11 the manner in which the equipment is anchored to the upper aspect of the thighs. Other sites include under the breasts and under the arms.

The role of the LPN in this procedure is to assist (Role II).

THE INTRAMUSCULAR INJECTION

The intramuscular injection deposits the drug in the layers of muscle (fascia) where it is absorbed; some types (aqueous) absorb more quickly than others. The larger the amount of drug the longer it takes to absorb. Intramuscular equipment is larger than subcutaneous equipment. Study Figure 30–12 for equipment size and the position of the needle in the tissues.

A variety of sites (see Figs. 30–13, 30–14) are available for use in children and adults. Buttocks muscles of small children are not yet well developed, so the gluteal site is not generally used. *The chief concern is to avoid large nerves and large blood vessels in any type of patient.* Selecting a proper site may require assistance in some instances and it should be sought without hesitation if the need arises. See the end of the chapter for procedure with common variations and adaptations.

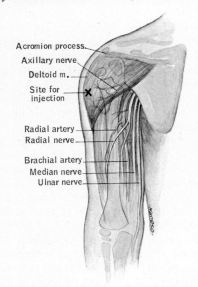

FIGURE 30-9   The site for injection when the deltoid muscle is used. (Hughes: Pediatric Procedures, W. B. Saunders Company.)

THE INTRAVENOUS INJECTION

Some medicinal substances are introduced directly into the blood stream by penetrating a large blood vessel with a needle. Figure 30–15 shows the angle of the needle in the blood vessel. This procedure is generally done by a physician; however, the registered nurse with special training is performing this technique, too. Some states have declared this a legal practice for the registered nurse, and others have not. The licensed practical nurse would be ill-advised to carry out this technique without a legal basis for her action.

DRUG ADMINISTRATION IN THE HOME

Drugs are prescribed for the patient in the home the same as in the hospital. The physi-

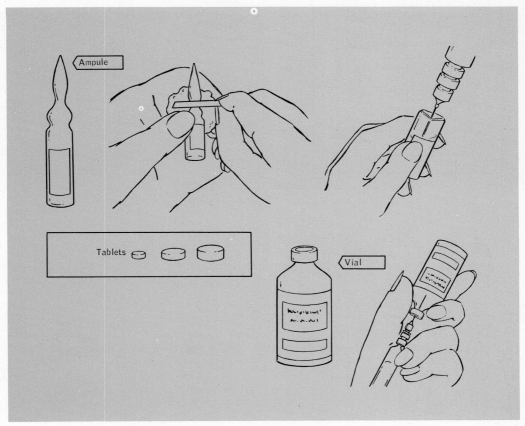

FIGURE 30-10   Forms of drugs for hypodermic injections.

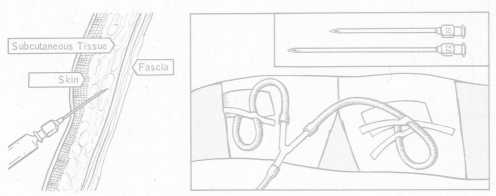

FIGURE 30-11   Hypodermoclysis.

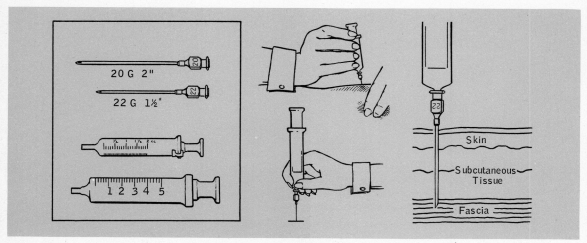

FIGURE 30-12   Intramuscular injection equipment and needle position.

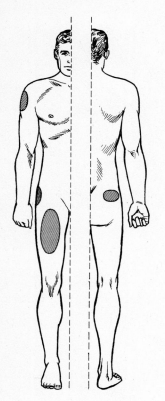

FIGURE 30–13   Intramuscular injection—four sites. (Kozier and DuGas: Introduction to Patient Care, W. B. Saunders Company.)

FIGURE 30-14 Intramuscular injection sites appropriate for a baby. (Leifer: Principles and Techniques in Pediatric Nursing, 2nd Ed., W. B. Saunders Company.)

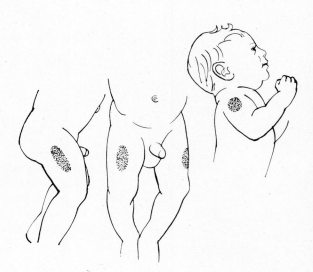

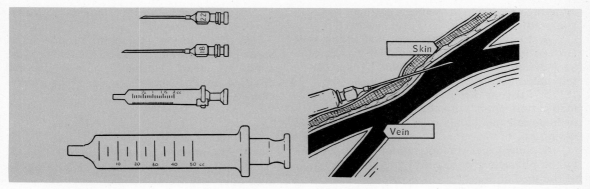

FIGURE 30-15 Intravenous injection.

cian prescribes the drug and the pharmacist prepares it. Giving a drug in the home means following the same rules in preparing, administering, and observing as in the hospital or other agency. Special problems in the home are providing a safe storage place, writing specific directions for giving, instructing family members who help, recording the administration, and disposing of unused narcotics. Confer with the physician regarding proper disposal of any unused narcotics. The nurse has responsibility for the safety of drugs in her charge. When they are disposed of, there should be a written record of this action.

Sterilization of syringes and needles in the home most often means using improvised equipment. Figure 30–16 explains how this can be done. Keep in mind that you handle

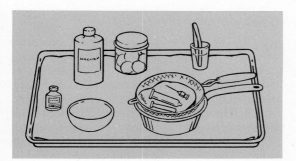

FIGURE 30-16 Tray, equipment, and supplies for injection at home. Sterilize syringe and needle by boiling for 10 minutes. Place barrel and plunger with needle on gauze strainer; place in pan and cover with water. Heat water and boil rapidly for 10 minutes. Lift strainer from water and pour water from pan; replace strainer in pan for contents to cool.

and use the sterilized syringe and needle with the same respect for surgical asepsis as in the hospital.

SPECIAL NURSING PROCEDURES

APPLICATION OF TOPICAL MEDICATIONS

Purposes: Provide for either a local or systemic action (e.g., antiseptic, astringent, emollient, counterirritant, etc.) depending on the drug used.

Equipment:
Medicine card
Tray, as indicated
Medication
Suitable container
As appropriate or needed:
 applicators
 tongue blades
 brush
 old muslin or linen
 rubber glove
 dressing

Course of action:

1. Know and follow directions and safety precautions for giving any medication as given at the beginning of this chapter.

2. Use medical asepsis or surgical asepsis, as directed or indicated.

3. Make certain by which method medication is to be applied: painting, spreading,

spraying, rubbing, swabbing, patting, or by some other method.

4. Leave stock supply of medication in storage location; use an individual packet or an individual container designated for a certain patient.

5. Prevent using bare hands to apply medication; apply with appropriate equipment or material; use hands only when ordered or permitted.

6. Select site for application as ordered by the physician, or according to the purpose of the medication.

7. Cleanse sufficient area of skin before making application, if necessary, unless contraindicated.

8. Cleanse area of skin between frequent applications by appropriate means, unless contraindicated; then remove applications at prescribed intervals with the solvent ordered.

9. Make certain skin is *dry* as well as *clean*.

10. Apply medication at specified site(s) or area indicated or appropriate; rotate sites, as indicated.

11. Apply measured and exact amount of medication ordered, or know how much should be used for therapeutic effect; avoid excess that can cause stickiness, caking, crusting, discomfort, or waste.

12. Cover medicated area with a suitable dressing *only* as ordered, or if permissible and necessary.

13. Instruct patient and use appropriate means to protect bedding and clothing of patient.

Application of Lotion

1. Shake container to mix thoroughly before removing cap or cover to pour or spray; always read directions on pushbutton, spray, or aerosol cans *before* shaking or using.

2. Use firm, gentle pressure to apply lotion.

3. Use old muslin or linen to apply lotion on area, *not* cotton or gauze.

4. Use small, flat brush to *brush* lotion on area.

5. Hold aerosol container upright at a distance of three to six inches from skin to *stream spray* lotion on area; use quick, short pressure (two to three seconds) on nozzle to apply smoothly and evenly; shield to protect any area not to be covered with medication.

6. Hold container inverted next to skin to apply a *foam* aerosol.

7. Pour lotion into palm of one hand, spread to other palm to *rub* on area; make sure hands are clean; use hands *only* if safe and directed to do so, otherwise, wear rubber gloves.

Application of Oil

1. Warm oil in a water bath.

2. Pour measured amount or portions as necessary into a small container.

3. Use cotton balls to spread and rub oil on area.

4. Pour oil into palm of one hand, spread to other plam to spread and apply oil on area; make sure hands are clean; use hands *only* if safe and directed to do so.

Application of Ointment

1. Remove ointment from jar with a tongue blade; use a fresh tongue blade each time ointment is removed; squeeze ointment from a tube onto a tongue blade and apply on skin area.

2. Use a tongue blade to spread ointment directly on area, or to spread ointment on a dressing to be placed directly over area.

3. Use gloved fingers to rub the ointment into the skin area according to drug or as directed (e.g., certain length of time, amount).

4. Apply ointments carefully and in small amounts at a time.

Application of Powder

1. Tap or shake powder from container or packet carefully onto appropriate material to be applied on skin area; shake powder into palm of one hand, then spread to other palm if hands may be used safetly to apply powder.

2. Hold container inverted over surface site to spray powder packaged in aerosol.

3. Avoid excessive use; make certain skin is dry before applying powder to skin; spread smoothly and evenly.

After application: Make observations important to the purpose of the application and the drug(s) for the desired or any undesired effects; observe especially the area of application for any change in color or the appearance of any irritation(s), lesion(s), swelling; *report* and *record* following each application.

Some common variations and adaptations:

1. Use appropriate restraints to protect patient adequately, especially a child.

2. Apply a medication by spray to an infant or young child *only* if the physician has so direcred in his written order; if ordered and used, take every precaution to avoid injury and to achieve the desired results.

ORAL MEDICATIONS

Purpose: Give medication by an easy, economical, effective, acceptable way.

Equipment:
Medicine card
Medicine tray
Medications
Medicine glass (minim glass)
Medicine dropper
Paper cups
Pitcher of water
Drinking tubes or straws
Paper towels or wipes

Course of action: Know and follow directions and safety precautions for giving any medication, as given in beginning of this chapter.

Preparation of Tablets and Capsules

1. Shake or pour required number of tablets or capsules into container cap; empty medication into medicine glass or cup; replace cap on container at once.

2. Select the single packaged, commercially prepared, completely labeled tablet, if available; place tablet intact with the medicine card on the medicine tray; open wrapper at bedside to remove tablet when ready to give to patient.

Preparation of Liquids

1. Grasp bottle in palm of hand and shake carefully, as needed.

2. Remove cap and hold with little finger (or between two fingers) without touching the inside of the cap.

3. Face the light to hold medicine glass at eye level; place thumbnail on line of desired measurement.

4. Hold bottle to protect label; pour medication until base of meniscus reaches the line marked with the thumbnail; use clean wipe to wipe rim of bottle and replace cap at once.

5. Place poured medication with medicine card on the medicine tray.

6. Use minim dropper or glass to measure dosage if required.

After medication is prepared:

1. Take medicine tray to bedside.

2. Make identification of patient.

3. Give medication(s); offer fresh water, unless contraindicated.

4. Instruct patient to hold a *troche* in mouth and suck until dissolved; instruct patient to place and hold medication under the tongue to be dissolved slowly and absorbed if medication is ordered, or is to be given, by *sublingual administration* (e.g., nitroglycerin).

5. Record administration; observe for action and effects of medication, and report or chart if needed.

Some common variations and adaptations:

1. Avoid use of any restraint; use only when directed or necessary.

2. Give one tablet or capsule at a time if there are several, if they are large in size, or if the patient has difficulty in swallowing.

3. Instruct patient how to properly swallow a tablet or capsule.

4. Use firm kindness, encouragement, and patience with a patient of any age who resists taking medication; use of force, threats, scorn, bribery, or coaxing is not condoned.

5. Crush tablet or empty capsule and mix in small amount of water or approved liquid to disguise taste and odor, if necessary, for an infant or small child.

6. Raise head and shoulders of patient; bring child to a sitting position; hold infant on lap, if permissible and possible.

7. Use a medicine glass, cup, or tip of a spoon to give appropriate medication to a child; allow child to hold glass or cup; provide straw for child.

8. Pour liquid or diluted medication into a small disposable bottle for infant to suck; use a plastic- or rubber-tipped dropper to place medication on middle of infant's tongue and give very small amounts *slowly,* with time to swallow before giving more.

9. Check mouth of infant or child to make certain medication has been swallowed.

10. Report any loss of medication or vomitus after medication has been taken; measure, if possible, or estimate amount; chart hap-

pening; repeat medication, or any part of it, *only when ordered.*

SUPPOSITORIES

Purpose(s): Give a drug, or a mixture of drugs, for local effect on the lining of the rectum or the vagina, or for systemic effect after being absorbed.
  Equipment:
  Medicine card
  Medicine tray
  Suppository
  Small paper cup
  Rubber glove or finger cot
  Lubricant
  Course of action:
  1. Know and follow directions and safety precautions for giving any medication, as given in beginning of chapter.
  2. Lubricate suppository with warm water before insertion; use a lubricant *only* when directed.
  3. Wear rubber glove or place finger cots on the thumb and forefinger of the hand used to hold and to insert suppository.
  4. Lubricate inserting finger with warm water; prevent any dry surface coming in contact with sphincter or orifice.

Rectal Suppository

  1. Have patient use the bedpan or the commode, if ambulatory.
  2. Place patient in left Sims' position, if possible.
  3. Turn or fold top bedding to expose anal region.
  4. Remove wrapper from suppository and lubricate.
  5. Insert suppository gently, point first, into rectum past the internal anal sphincter muscle approximately two and one-half to three inches into the rectum or one finger length; ask patient to breathe through mouth as suppository is inserted; remove finger.
  6. Apply pressure over anus; hold buttocks together for a short time.
  7. Instruct patient about retaining suppository; hold for at least 20 minutes and 30 minutes, if possible, for purpose of defecation; hold until absorption is completed, according to purpose of drug and effect desired.
  8. Record immediately, as for any medication; report and observe, as necessary.

Vaginal Suppository

  1. Have patient use the bedpan, or the commode if ambulatory.
  2. Place patient in the dorsal recumbent or the Sims' position; provide proper drape.
  3. Remove wrapper from suppository and lubricate.
  4. Insert suppository gently, point first, into vagina; make certain suppository is inserted full length.
  5. Instruct patient about retaining suppository until absorption is completed; ask ambulatory patient to remain quietly in bed.
  6. Record immediately, as for any medication; report and observe, as needed.
  Some common variations and adaptations:
  1. Hold small child or infant on lap or raise buttocks as for taking a rectal temperature.
  2. Hold and coddle infant or small child until suppository is dissolved.

SUBCUTANEOUS INJECTION

Purpose(s): Give a medication when it cannot be taken orally and when a more rapid and complete absorption is desired than if taken orally.
  Equipment:
  Medicine card
  Hypodermic tray
  Medication
  File for ampule
  Sterile lifting forceps
  Sterile syringe—two cc. usually
  Sterile needle—one half inch to one inch; No. 24 to 26 gauge
  Sterile cotton balls or gauze sponges
  Antiseptic solution
  Course of action:
  1. Know and follow directions and safety precautions for giving any medication, as given in the beginning of this chapter.
  2. Use surgical asepsis.
  3. Assemble syringe and fit needle; touch only barrel of syringe, knob of plunger, and hub of needle. Or, carefully open wrapper of a disposable unit with sterile syringe and needle already assembled.
  4. Protect sterile needle with *dry* sterile cotton ball or sponge.
  5. Draw medication into syringe pre-

pared in solution from the tablet, vial, or ampule.

Preparation from Tablet

1. Using vial of sterile distilled water place "H" tablet on sterile field; use tablet of exact dosage, if possible; if tablet for exact dosage is not available, check your calculation with the charge nurse.

2. Use cotton ball or gauze sponge moistened with approved antiseptic solution to cleanse rubber cap of vial; discard the cotton ball or sponge.

3. Pull plunger of syringe to mark for desired measured amount (usually 1 cc); remove protector from needle; insert shaft of needle through center of rubber cap of vial; push plunger to force the air into the air space in the vial.

4. Invert vial; withdraw desired amount of the distilled water; expel any air bubbles; withdraw needle from vial; provide bubble of air, and protect sterile needle with dry sterile cotton ball.

5. Dissolve tablet in the distilled water:

   a. One method—carefully remove plunger from barrel of syringe; place tablet in barrel of syringe; carefully replace plunger and gently rotate or shake barrel until tablet is completely dissolved; expel any necessary amount for correct dosage, avoiding air bubbles.

   b. Another method—place tablet in a small sterile container provided for this purpose; expel measured amount of sterile distilled water from syringe over the tablet; make certain tablet is completely dissolved; draw required measured amount for the desired dosage of medication into the syringe, avoiding air bubbles.

6. Provide bubble of air and protect sterile needle.

Preparation from Vial

1. Obtain help from nurse-in-charge when vial contains a form of medication (e.g., powdered) which must be prepared with a sterile solution into a liquid form before using.

2. Follow this method for using a vial with a single or multiple dose of medication already in liquid form.

3. Use sterile cotton ball or gauze sponge moistened with the approved antiseptic solution to cleanse rubber cap of vial; discard the cotton ball or sponge.

4. Pull plunger of syringe back to point for the desired, measured amount of dosage for medication to be withdrawn; remove protector from sterile needle; insert shaft of needle through center of rubber cap of vial; push plunger to force air into air space in the vial.

5. Invert vial and syringe and hold syringe at eye level; withdraw desired measured amount of medication into syringe; expel any air bubbles; withdraw needle from vial; provide bubble of air; protect sterile needle with dry sterile cotton ball.

6. Check label on vial with medicine card before vial is replaced or empty vial is discarded.

Preparation from Ampule

1. Hold ampule upright and tap the stem (neck) to get solution into bottom of the ampule; make certain none is trapped in the stem.

2. Use dry sterile cotton ball or gauze sponge behind stem of ampule and hold firmly; open ampule by breaking off top at stem into the cotton ball or sponge and discard.

   a. Use pressure at the so-called "blue-line" of the stem of some ampules to break off top into the cotton ball or sponge.

   b. Use ampule file to score around stem of some ampules well above level of solution; break off top into the cotton ball or sponge.

3. Place ampule on firm, flat surface.

4. Insert needle into ampule; avoid touching needle to edge of glass; withdraw desired measured amount of medication into syringe, avoiding air bubbles; withdraw needle from ampule; provide bubble of air; protect sterile needle with dry sterile cotton ball.

5. Discard ampule after checking with medicine card.

After injection is prepared:

1. Place syringe with medication on the hypodermic tray with the medicine card; keep the needle sterile with a *dry* sterile cotton ball (a sterile needle holder may be available); carry tray to bedside.

2. Select site for injection; assist patient into position; expose area and prepare site for injection.

3. Cleanse the skin at injection site with fresh sterile cotton ball or gauze; use well-moistened sponge with the antiseptic solution. Use an individually packaged ball or sponge already moistened with an antiseptic, if such is provided and available; open package when ready to use.

    a. Start at center of area, the injection site; cleanse with a firm, circular, outward motion for about two inches.

    b. Allow skin to dry.

4. Remove protector from needle; hold syringe upright and carefully expel air bubble.

5. Hold syringe at 45 degree angle with one hand, with the bevel of the needle upward.

6. Grasp tissue firmly with the free hand so that skin is taut at site of injection.

7. Insert needle quickly and firmly; release grasp on tissue; draw back gently with plunger; continue with injection if no blood appears with aspiration; follow policy of agency for course of action to take if blood appears.

8. Inject solution slowly; use smooth, steady pressure with plunger.

9. Remove needle rapidly at the same angle of insertion.

10. Apply dry sterile cotton ball at site and massage with gentle pressure for several seconds.

11. Record immediately; indicate route according to policy, or with the word "subcutaneous" or the letter "H."

Some common variations and adaptations:

1. Read the discussion and study the illustrations in this chapter regarding subcutaneous injection of medications.

2. Apply proper and adequate restraint of an infant or young child, as necessary, to assure a safe and correct administration of injection; obtain assistance of a second nurse to hold and help restrain young child; hold and coddle infant or child after giving injection.

3. Check with nurse-in-charge to make certain of site for the safety of such patients as a child, one thin or emaciated, one with different or unusual needs.

4. Use a three-quarter inch, 25-gauge needle for an obese patient, if needed, in order to inject solution into the subcutaneous tissue.

5. Pinch skin firmly into a fold between the thumb and index finger to inject solution into the subcutaneous tissue of a *thin* patient or child.

INSULIN INJECTION

1. Know and follow directions and safety precautions for giving any medications as listed in this chapter.

2. Use an *insulin syringe,* graduated in insulin units equal to or totalling one cc.

3. Make certain the insulin syringe corresponds to the strength or dosage of insulin ordered; match the correct scale on the syringe to the bottle of insulin and the ordered dosage on the medicine card.

4. Follow method for subcutaneous (hypodermic) injection to prepare from vial and administer the insulin.

5. Make certain of site, especially in relation to the rotation of sites for frequent injections of insulin.

6. Record administration of insulin on the forms and places designated; indicate type of insulin, number of units, time, and observations.

INTRAMUSCULAR INJECTION

Purposes: Give a medication when it cannot or should not be taken or given by mouth or subcutaneous injection; it is irritating or more irritating to other tissues; a more rapid and continuous absorption may be desired or a larger quantity must be given by injection.

Equipment:
Medicine card
Hypodermic tray
Medication
File for ampule
Sterile lifting forceps
Sterile syringe—two cc. to five cc., usually
Sterile needle—one and one-half inch to two inches;
No. 19 to 22 gauge
Sterile cotton balls or sponges
Antiseptic solution
Course of action:

1. Know and follow directions and safety precautions for giving any medication, as given in Chapter 30.

2. Use surgical asepsis.

3. *See* Subcutaneous Injection, p. 315; *follow* course of action steps, numbers 3, 4, 5. (See also use of tablet, vial, or ampule.)

4. Provide for small air bubble (0.2 to 0.3

cc.) as syringe is held in upright position: steady or anchor plunger.

5. Use free hand to press tissue at site area and hold skin taut.

6. Hold syringe with the needle at a right (90 degree) angle; insert needle quickly and firmly; insert needle to reach the muscle tissue.

7. Release grasp on tissue; draw back gently with plunger; continue with injection if no blood appears with aspiration; follow policy of agency for course of action to take if blood appears.

8. Inject solution slowly; use very slight but smooth pressure with plunger; allow time to make certain needle is empty of medication before withdrawal.

9. Remove needle quickly; apply dry sterile cotton ball at site and massage with gentle pressure for several seconds.

10. Record immediately; indicate route according to policy or by using "I.M."

Some common variations and adaptations:

1. Read the discussion and study the illustrations in this chapter regarding intramuscular injection of medication.

2. Use proper syringe and needle, suitable in size to type of medication and patient.

a. Select length of needle appropriate to site, age, and condition of patient.

b. Select needle with a gauge according to type or thickness of solution.

3. Check with the nurse-in-charge to make certain of site and the method to determine exact site for the safety of such patients as an infant, a child, one thin or emaciated, and one with different or unusual needs.

4. Seek instructions and directions from the nurse-in-charge or physician when an irritating drug is ordered, or any drug is ordered to be given by intramuscular injection using the "Z-Track Method."

5. Obtain assistance of second nurse to hold or help restrain, if necessary, an infant or young child; hold and coddle infant or child after the injection.

6. Apply a small, dry, sterile dressing over site if there is oozing or the patient is a child.

SUMMARY

The role of the LPN in drug administration is not clear-cut when it comes to listing what she does and does not do. What is clear is that she carries legal and moral responsibilities and can be held accountable for any alleged acts of negligence on her part. The practical nurse (just as anyone who officially administers drugs) must have knowledge of the drug, know why it is being given, know the dosage to be given, and what to observe for in relation to the patient receiving the drug. She is expected to know and use the safety precautions in preparing and giving drugs. All of these facts place the practical nurse in the unique position of having constantly to decide when to seek advice, when to refuse to administer a medicine that is beyond her capabilities to do so, and how to maintain good relationships in the process.

It is possible for you to gain certain selected background knowledge and beginning skills related to drug administration which can serve as a sound foundation for continued growth as a licensed practitioner, but this foundation in no way represents the depth of knowledge needed to administer all drugs under all circumstances. It is as essential for you to know your limitations in drug therapy as it is to know your capabilities.

GUIDES FOR STUDY AND DISCUSSION

1. What are the four main channels for administering drugs. What factors help to determine which channel is used? Who decides the channel to be used?

2. List the official abbreviations for oral, hypodermic, intramuscular, and intravenous methods of administration.

3. Write the meaning for each of the following:

a.c.	h.s.	Gm.	c̄
p.c.	p.r.n.	gr.	s̄
q. 3 hr.	stat.	gtt.	sol.
q.i.d.	C.	m.	tbsp.
t.i.d.	F.	os.	tsp.
b.i.d.	cc.	oz.	elix.

4. If you mistakenly give a medicine to a patient, what should you do?

5. List the "six rights" to observe in drug administration. Be ready to discuss how each is carried out in safe practice.

6. The essential facts for charting include medication, dosage, route, method, and time plus pertinent observations made at time of administration. Use the following orders to practice charting (omit observations) with appropriate abbreviations:

 a. Aspirin grains 10 every three hours.

 b. Phenobarbital grains one-half four times a day.

 c. Demerol fifty milligrams every four hours.

 d. Seconal grains one and one-half at hour of sleep.

7. Use chapter illustrations to study the position of the needle in body tissue for the following injections: (1) intradermal (2) intramuscular (3) subcutaneous (4) hypodermoclysis (5) intravenous. How do they differ?

8. Why are there different sizes and types of syringes and needles?

9. Study the sites of intramuscular injections for a baby and for an older person in figures 30–13 and 30–14. What is alike about them? What is different?

10. What three factors influence the effect of a drug? Be ready to discuss each factor.

11. What precautions must you take when asked to administer a drug strange to you?

12. Why should you administer only the drugs prepared by you?

13. How can you be sure you are giving the drug to the right patient?

14. What precautions are taken in the care and storage of drugs?

SUGGESTED SITUATIONS AND ACTIVITIES

1. You have just come on duty at 11:00 P.M. and have been asked to prepare and administer a medication that is new to you. The patient had been admitted at 2:00 P.M. How would you proceed to meet this assignment?

2. Arrange for a classmate to work with you; carry out one of the following observational assignments in a clinical situation:

 a. Observe a nurse giving either a hypodermic or an intramuscular injection: observe the preparation and the administration of the drug. Compare the procedure with the one in this chapter for similarities and differences. Be ready to share this learning experience in class.

 b. Visit the place in the hospital where syringes and needles are cleaned and sterilized. While you are in that area find out if disposable syringes are used and for what purposes. Determine the cost to the patient. Be ready to share this learning experience in class.

c. Examine the Order Sheet in a medical patient's chart. Count the number of drugs the patient is receiving. How many are to be given orally? At what time(s) are they given? Does he get more than one at a time? What is the maximum number he can receive at one time? What other channels of administration are used for his drugs? Be ready to tell about this patient's drug orders in class.

d. Observe the "medicine nurse" at work preparing a tray of medicines. Pay particular attention to the environment where she does this: Is it quiet? Does she have ample room to work? What, if anything, happened to distract her from her work? Was it well lighted? Did she seem to have the things she needed or was it necessary to go someplace to get something? In your opinion, could anything have been done to improve conditions to promote safety practices?

3. Prepare a display of assorted types of syringes and needles (reuseable and disposable). Label each item as to its size, possible use(s), and cost.

4. Make medicine cards for the drugs listed in study guide item number 6.

CHAPTER 31

SOME COMMON DRUGS: ACTION AND USE

OBJECTIVES FOR THE STUDENT: Be able to:

1. Give two ways drugs may be grouped for study.
2. Explain the difference between results that are therapeutic and results that are untoward.
3. Differentiate between a local drug reaction and a systemic drug reaction by using
   an example.
4. Name two sources to locate drug information.
5. Give one reason why drug information from a source may be out of date.
6. Given a selected list of drug actions, state the general use for each.
7. Tell why drug administration by the L.P.N. is becoming more prevalent.
8. Compose three rules to promote safety by the L.P.N. in drug administration.

SUGGESTED STUDY VOCABULARY*

diagnostic
reaction
analgesic
narcotic
addictive power
parenteral

nebulizer
palpitation
euphoria
anoxemia
agitation
cathartic

hemorrhage
antacids
emetics
antiemetics
expectorant
diuretics

suppository	antiseptic action	hematuria
sedative	disinfectant action	oliguria
hypnotic	caustic	ophthalmic
tranquilize	astringent	mydriatic
toxic	anti-infective	miotic
stupor	vasodilators	hyperactivity
antipyretic	vasoconstrictors	hypoactivity
diaphoretic	hematinics	hormones
hyperirritability ·	hemostatics	fluid retention
apprehension	anticoagulants	vitamins

*Look for any terms you already know.

INTRODUCTION

If you examine a number of books containing drug information, you discover several different ways drugs can be grouped for study because there is no *one* best way to group them for this purpose. Sometimes they are grouped according to the body part(s) they treat (e.g., Drugs Which Affect the Kidneys), sometimes according to the diseases or disorders of the patient (e.g., Drugs Which Fight Cancer), sometimes according to the symptoms relieved (e.g., Drugs Used to Relieve Pain), and sometimes according to the results they produce (e.g., Drugs Used to Stimulate).

Many drugs serve the body in more than one way; that is to say, a drug may have more than one favorable (therapeutic) influence upon the body. Likewise, a drug can produce several unfavorable results as well. Along with the wanted results may come some unwanted results (sometimes called "untoward" results). The fact that there is always possibility of unwanted results makes it vital that close observation occur before, during, and following any drug administration. At best, the practical nurse can master only the gross or general body reactions, the obvious favorable body reactions and the obvious unfavorable body reactions. The subtle (diagnostic or specific) reactions are observations made by the physician and the registered nurse.

As you become familiar with the general ways a patient reacts to various drugs, you will be reminded time and again that the human body functions as a unified, whole organism. For example, if the physician orders a drug to improve the ability of the blood to carry more oxygen and the results are favorable, the patient feels better "all over." Or, if something is prescribed to relieve pain and the results are favorable, the patient turns his thoughts to something other than his previous discomfort. Knowing that the body is apt to respond as a "whole," you learn to observe accordingly, watching for both local *and* overall reactions occurring in the patient.

Accurate reporting and recording of reactions are a vital part of drug administration. The skill to do this comes in doing; in other words, skill in observing, recording, and reporting continues to develop through nursing practice. The practical nurse learns certain terms which describe such things as pain, skin, pulse, feces, vomitus, urine, apetite, frame of mind, etc. She learns how to use this descriptive vocabulary economically to appropriately describe patient complaints and her own observations prior to, during, and following drug administration. The skill to do this improves with time and practice, but you should recognize now that never is there a time when one knows "all about drugs." New drugs are constantly appearing and sometimes their effectiveness or ineffectiveness is not actually known for months or even years after they appear. Under these circumstances, the practical nurse should be doubly sure that she works with the greatest care and uses the strongest possible precautions to protect the patient and herself as a licensed practitioner. Time in the basic program allows for only an introduction to some of the more common drugs used today; daily practice acquaints one with others. Knowing the importance of *not* administering "strange" drugs or "experimental" drugs and of getting needed help from the charge nurse or the physician are lessons that should be learned early and practiced every day. No single responsibility carried or shared by the practical nurse is more discussed than that of administering medicines.

This chapter is arranged in tables for easy

use and reference. The *Drug* column includes some commonly used drugs; it is not possible or practical to make the lists exhaustive, as references are always needed. The *Use* column lists some of the chief ways the drug is used and indicates what some results might be. The heading *Reactions* is used to include specific information about the drug, especially the unwanted results. This column guides the observations of the nurse. The fourth column, *Dosage—Administration*, may or may not specify dosages. In instances where dosage is given it is the usual dosage cited but does not include a range. This is understandable when one considers the age, size, and needs of patients, varying opinions among physicians,

and the newness of some drugs. The last column, *Remarks*, lists some general and some specific information which can be helpful in observing the patient, in using appropriate nursing measures, and in providing some background for judgment.

There is no intent to say here that the following tables include all you will need or want to learn about drugs. They represent only an introduction to this vast subject. New drugs appear with great rapidity; sections of the country may show preferences for using some drugs above others; and research points out new uses for older drugs. All of these factors make a drug list incomplete, with supplementary information necessary to its use.

Tables 31–1 to 31–18 are shown on the following pages.

TABLE 31-1. DRUGS USED TO RELIEVE PAIN

Drugs which relieve pain are known as analgesics. Some of these drugs – narcotics – act by depressing certain brain cells which control pain perception. Narcotics are habit forming and controlled by law. Other analgesics are coal-tar products such as aspirin; they work well alone and in combination with some narcotics.

DRUG	USE	REACTION	DOSAGE – ADMINISTRATION	REMARKS
Acetylsalicylic acid, U.S.P. (aspirin)	Relieves headache, ache and pain in muscles, reduces fever.	Dizziness, ringing in ears, nausea, vomiting, skin rash.	0.3-0.6 Gm. (5-10 gr.) Oral. Suppository. Experimenting with I.V.	The most commonly used pain reliever. Common cause of accidental poisoning in children.
Codeine sulfate, N.F. Active principle of opium yet milder than morphine.	Relieves mild pain; encourages sleep; acts on cough center of the brain.	Slightly constipating; high dosage causes restlessness.	1/4 gr. (15 mg.) - 1.0 gr. (60 mg.) Oral; parenteral.	A narcotic controlled by Harrison Narcotic Act. Small amounts in some cough syrups available without prescription. Often used in combination with other pain and fever reducing drugs. May be addictive.
Dihydromorphinone hydrochloride, U.S.P. (Dilaudid) – a preparation of morphine.	Relieves severe pain; sedative; hypnotic.	Slows respirations; somewhat constipating; nausea.	1/30 gr. (2 mg.) Oral or parenteral; rectal suppository.	A narcotic controlled the same as above. Its addictive power is about the same as that of morphine.
Levorphanol tartrate, N. F. (Levo-Dromoran, Levorphan)	Relieves pain; produces sleep quickly.	Similar to morphine but less severe.	2-3 mg., 3-4 h. p.r.n. Oral or parenteral.	Used instead of morphine. Unlike morphine can be given orally. Under control of narcotic control laws.
Meperidine hydrochloride injection, N. F. (Demerol, Dolosal) – a synthetic substitute for morphine.	Relieves severe pain; sedative; hypnotic.	Some nausea and vomiting; moderate degree of dryness of the mouth, perspiration, dizziness.	20-100 mg. (1/3 gr. - 1½ gr.) Oral; parenteral.	Addictive. Pain relieving effects do not last as long as those of morphine. A narcotic controlled the same as above.

(Table 31-1 continues on the following page.)

TABLE 31–1. DRUGS USED TO RELIEVE PAIN (Continued)

DRUG	USE	REACTION	DOSAGE – ADMINISTRATION	REMARKS
Morphine sulfate, U.S.P. Derived from opium. (Opium is obtained from juice of poppy.)	Relieves severe pain; produces sleep quickly.	Slows respirations; constipation; nausea; vomiting; pin-point pupils; moderate slowing of heart rate; reduces kidney output.	Average adult dosage 1/8 - 1/4 gr. (8 - 15 mg.) Hypodermic; I.V.	Addictive. If patient remains quiet, nausea is less likely. A narcotic controlled the same as above.
Pantopium hydrochloride (Pantopon) – a concentrated form of opium.	Relieves severe pain.	Slows respirations.	1/12 - 1/3 gr. (5 - 20 mg.) Oral or parenteral.	Addictive. More expensive than morphine. A narcotic controlled the same as above.
Papaverine hydrochloride, U.S.P. (Active principle of opium poppy.)	Relieves smooth muscle spasms, painful contractions in the stomach, bile duct, and the ureters. Depresses cough.	Slows respirations.	1/2 - 1 gr. (30 - 60 mg.) Oral or parenteral.	Not a narcotic but controlled as a narcotic; it is reportable.
Acetophenetidin, U.S.P. (phenacetin)	Relieves minor aches and pain. Used in combination with other drugs. Helps reduce fever.	Not very toxic but can produce skin rash, weakness, perspiration, weak pulse and respiration, nausea under some conditions.	5 gr. (0.3 Gm.) Oral.	Used in combination with other drugs. May be harmful (kidneys) if used over long period of time. Required warning: not to take longer than 10 days without direction from physician.
Dipyrone (Dimethone, Diprone, Methapyrone, Pyralgin)	For pain and fever, antirheumatic agent.	Can produce dizziness, skin rashes, and chills.	0.3 - 0.6 Gm. q3 - 4 h. Oral 0.5 - 1 Gm. q 3 h. p.r.n. Parenteral	When given over long periods frequent blood counts essential.
Phenazocine (Prinadol)	For a wide variety of pain, including cancer.	Observe for depressed respirations.	2 mg. every 4 - 6 h. p.r.n. I.M.	Is not used when certain condition(s) present: coma, convulsions, liver disease, alcoholism, hypothyroidism.

TABLE 31-2. DRUGS USED TO INFLUENCE FRAME OF MIND OR MOOD

Ataractics come from the Greek word "ataraxia" which means peace of mind. The drugs in this group do more than tranquilize, in some instances. They are used in combination to relieve pain and to treat some disorders.

DRUG	USE	REACTION	DOSAGE – ADMINISTRATION	REMARKS
Ataractics "Tranquilizers," a commonly used term to cover an expanding group of drugs.	Muscle relaxers; produce "peace of mind." Calm overactive patient without causing great drowsiness or confusion; lessen irritability and body tension; make sleep possible.		Dosage varies depending upon effect desired and physician plans for using these drugs.	Addictive powers. A new drug group which needs study and research to furnish additional information about it.
Diazepam N.F. (Valium)	See Librium	Drowsiness, fatigue, withdrawal symptoms noted.	2-5-10 mg. Daily. 25-50 mg. I.M.	Dosage adjusted to individual.
Chlordiazepoxide hydrochloride (Librium)	Calms the anxious mind but due to reactions may affect ability to work.	Feeble action in moderate dosage. Some toxicity in large doses. drowsiness, dizziness, ataxia.	15-40 mg. (1/4 to 3/5 gm.) Oral, I.V., I.M.	Not generally used with debilitated or elderly.
Chlorpromazine hydrochloride, U.S.P. (Thorazine)	Used to calm overactive mentally ill patients.	Acts rapidly, followed by decreased depression and drowsiness.	Wide range of dosage used. Tablets, capsules, syrup, suppositories, ampules.	More rapid action accounts, in part, for widespread usage.
Prochlorperazine, N.N.D. (Compazine)			Tablets, capsules, suppositories, ampules. 15-150 mg. (¼ to 2¼ gm.)	
Rauwolfia (a plant from India; the root is used). Reserpine, U.S.P. (Serpasil)	Same as above but now commonly used to treat hypertension.	May cause serious depression; nasal congestion; dryness of mouth; drowsiness; sense of weakness.	Wide range of dosage used. Tablets, ampules. Oral, parenteral.	The first available group of tranquilizers, but not now used as much as some others.

(Table 31-2 continues on the following page.)

TABLE 31–2.   DRUGS USED TO INFLUENCE FRAME OF MIND OR MOOD (Continued)

DRUG	USE	REACTION	DOSAGE — ADMINISTRATION	REMARKS
Meprobamate, U.S.P. (Miltown) (Equanil) (Meprospan) (Metrotabs)	Muscle relaxers; lessen body tension; unworried frame of mind promotes sleep.	Some reported reactions include: skin rash, edema, chills, fever, gastrointestinal symptoms. People using this drug should avoid hazardous occupations.	Adult dosage: 6 gr. (400 mg.) Single dose for sleep: 6 – 12 gr. (400 - 800 mg.) Tablets, capsules, suspension.	Considered a limited sort of tranquilizer. Continued use can cause dependence. Not very toxic but overdose can cause stupor. Sold without prescription in Japan. Widely used around the world.
Azacyclonol hydrochloride, N.F. (Frenquel)	For anxiety and tension.		Wide range of dosage used. Oral, I.V.	More effective in acute psychotic states. Not useful at all in some types of disorders.

TABLE 31–3. DRUGS USED TO AFFECT BODY TEMPERATURE

Drugs listed here serve as pain relievers, too. Reference is made to Table 31-1 for further information. The roots *Anti* (meaning against) and *pyretic* (pertaining to fever) join to make the word antipyretic – "against fever." *Diaphoretic* is an agent that promotes profuse perspiration (diaphoresis).

DRUG	USE	REACTION	DOSAGE – ADMINISTRATION	REMARKS
Antipyretics	Lower abnormal body temperature by causing increased perspiration. (heat elimination).			
Acetophenetidin, U.S.P. (phenacetin)	See Table 31-1.			
Acetylsalicylic acid, U.S.P. (aspirin)	See Table 31-1.			
A combination of caffeine with the 2 drugs above is called APC.	Same as above.		Tablets, capsules.	
Diaphoretics	Increase perspiration. Dilate cutaneous blood vessels, thereby promoting perspiration.			This action sometimes accompanies other drug actions. For example, phenocitin reduces pain as well as fever.
Neostigmine bromide, U.S.P. (Prostigmine bromide)	Increases perpiration, reduces fever; increases urinary and intestinal peristalsis. To treat myasthenia gravis.	May cause slow heart action, lowered blood pressure, nausea, vomiting, muscular twitching.	15 mg. Oral	Severe reaction may require artificial respiration.

TABLE 31–4. DRUGS USED TO RELAX (SEDATIVE) AND TO PRODUCE SLEEP (HYPNOTIC)

Drugs in this group can produce either relaxation or sleep; the size of the patient and the amount of dosage make the difference. A wide variety of so-called "sleep-producing" drugs are available without prescription; an overdose can cause death.

DRUG	USE	REACTION	DOSAGE – ADMINISTRATION	REMARKS
Barbiturates (four common ones discussed)	Used to depress central nervous system to relax and produce sleep. They long have been the most widely used drugs for this purpose. Tranquilizing drugs are also being used to relax the patient and put him in a frame of mind to sleep (Table 31-2)	In general this group of drugs produces some listlessness following sleep. A hangover effect is often experienced, and restlessness and skin rash may occur. Slow respirations. Two long-acting drugs in this group (mebaral and gemonil) are used to treat patients with epilepsy. Continued use may result in gastrointestinal difficulty, loss of appetite, anemia.		Some act faster and some act longer than others (see below). Some have addictive power.
Secobarbital sodium, U.S.P. (Seconal)			100 - 200 mg. (1½ - 3 gr.) Oral; I.M.; rectal.	Acts rapidly; duration of action about 3 hours.
Amobarbital, U.S.P. (Amytal)			20 - 40 mg. (1/3 - 2/3 gr.) Oral.	Duration of action 3 - 6 hours.
Pentobarbital sodium, N.F. (Nembutal)			100 - 200 mg. (1½ - 3 gr.) Oral; rectal.	Usually patient is asleep within 30 minutes; duration of action 3 - 6 hours.
Phenobarbital, U.S.P. (Barbipil, Barbita, Eskaborb, Lixophen, Luminal)			30 mg. (1/2 gr.) Oral.	Slow to act, but duration of action is longer (6 hours or more).

(Table 31–4 continues on the opposite page.)

TABLE 31-4. DRUGS USED TO RELAX (SEDATIVE) AND TO PRODUCE SLEEP (HYPNOTIC) (Continued)

DRUG	USE	REACTION	DOSAGE – ADMINISTRATION	REMARKS
Bromides	Depress central nervous system, resulting in mental slowness, indifference, and sleepiness; slow respirations and pulse.	Slow to act; sedation comes through prolonged use in small doses. Large doses or "bromide intoxication" produce unwanted reactions including skin rashes, headache, dizziness, irritability, impaired memory, slurred speech. Bromides leave the body slowly through the urine; it may take days for a single dose to leave.		The public can buy bromides without prescription; there continues to be danger of bromide intoxication due to the wide and "free" use of this drug.
Sodium bromide, U.S.P.			Sedative dosage 300 - 600 mg. (5 - 10 gr.) t.i.d. Oral.	
Chloral hydrate, U.S.P.	Depresses central nervous system; produces refreshing sleep.	Irritates gastrointestinal tract. May aggravate the stomach for a short time. Dilution of the drug in plenty of flavored solution helps prevent stomach distress. Lowers blood pressure; causes perspiration.	0.6 Gm. (10 gr.) in flavored solution to disguise the disagreeable taste. Retention enema containing drug sometimes used with children.	Addictive power. Commonly used hypnotic before barbiturates were available. A liquid is not as handy to take as a pill, hence barbiturates and tranquilizers are used more commonly. Patient should have sufficient covering to prevent chilling.
Paraldehyde, U.S.P.	A powerful hypnotic drug. Acts within 10-15 minutes; produces sleep even in excited, agitated patients.	Coughing, nausea, dizziness, headache.	Oral dosage ranges from 5 - 20 ml. (1 - 4 tsp.) given in shaved ice or iced drinks. I.M. dosage smaller; irritates the tissues. Liquid taken by mouth; also available in soft gelatin capsule for rectal use; ampules for parenteral use.	Addictive power. A colorless, odorous liquid. Leaves patient with a bad breath.
Alcohol, ethyl, U.S.P.	Has limited hypnotic effect; sometimes prescribed as a bedtime medicine.	May be particularly helpful to elderly patients who resist stronger hypnotics.	Brandy, wines, whiskey.	Addictive power. Other types (denatured, methyl alcohol) are not used internally.

TABLE 31–5. DRUGS USED TO STIMULATE

To stimulate means to spur on or arouse. Drugs included here stimulate the underactive nervous system; reduce fatigue; increase heart rate, blood pressure, and blood circulation; and strengthen respiration.

DRUG	USE	REACTION	DOSAGE – ADMINISTRATION	REMARKS
Amphetamine sulfate, U.S.P. (Benzedrine)	Stimulates central nervous system; produces feeling of exhilaration, reduces fatigue; increases desire to work; reduces appetite; nasal decongestant.	Headache, insomnia, dryness of mouth, constipation; hyperirritability; profuse perspiration; increased blood pressure.	5 - 10 mg. (1/12 - 1/6 gr.) Tablets, ampules, capsules. Oral.	Generally considered to be habit forming. Sometimes called "pep pills." Commonly misused.
Dextroamphetamine sulfate, U.S.P. (Dexedrine)	Same as above.	Same as above.	Same as above.	Used to control appetite.
Methylphenidate hydrochloride, N.F. (Ritalin)	Alerts "underactive" nervous systems without causing euphoria, loss of appetite, or insomnia.	Dizziness; dryness of mouth; palpitation.	5 - 20 mg. Two or three times daily. Oral; parenteral.	Used with elderly patients who have lost interest in everything. Causes wakefulness if taken too late in the afternoon.
Pipradrol hydrochloride, N.F. (Meratran)	Much the same as above In both instances dosage and frequency are observed to keep stimulation in bounds		1 - 2.5 mg. Two or three times daily.	Care is used not to "overdose" and cause anxiety or agitation.
Epinephrine hydrochloride, U.S.P. (Adrenalin)	Increases heart rate and blood pressure; shrinks nasal passages and promotes free breathing; relaxes smooth muscle; saliva and tear flow increased.	Fast acting; patient may cease to get desired results with continued use. Excessive dosage may produce apprehension and tremor as pulse and blood pressure increase.	Dosages vary according to form of drug used. Ampules; vials for inhalation; suspension in oil for I.M.'s. Not given orally due to action of digestive juices.	Commonly used to treat asthma. While this drug has many uses, care is taken not to give to patients with certain types of circulatory conditions and overactive thyroid glands. Observe pulse and blood pressure.

(Table 31–5 continues on the opposite page.)

TABLE 31-5. _ DRUGS USED TO STIMULATE (Continued)

DRUG	USE	REACTION	DOSAGE — ADMINISTRATION	REMARKS
		As a nasal decongestant may cause tearing and sneezing.		
Nikethamide, N.F. (Coramine)	Chiefly used in cases of circulatory and respiratory failure.	Can produce convulsions.	Most often used parenterally. I.M. and I.V.	Commonly used stimulant.
Caffeine and sodium benzoate, U.S.P.	Commonly used together as a general body stimulant; used for shock, barbiturate poisoning, heat exhaustion. Strengthens respirations; quickly excreted through the kidneys.	Restlessness; wakefulness; nervousness; nausea; vomiting; palpitation.	0.5 Gm. (7½ gr.) Oral; I.M.	Toxic symptoms are rare. Most people use coffee and can tolerate caffeine.
Oxygen, U.S.P. (gas, compressed form in steel cylinders)	Stimulates the respiratory system to relieve "oxygen want" in patients with pneumonia, pulmonary edema, cardiac disorders, shock, and other conditions which promote anoxemia.	Nose and throat irritations, ear discomfort, leg muscle pains, light-headedness.	Amount and method of administration vary. Catheter, mask, tent.	Supports combustion. Safety precautions observed in patient area when in use.
Carbon dioxide with oxygen, U.S.P. (gas, compressed form in steel cylinders)	Expands lungs by increasing rate and depth of breathing when such is needed. Used to treat hiccup.	Prolonged use causes severe circulatory and respiratory changes.	Small amounts given for short periods of time.	The home remedy of breathing and rebreathing into a paper bag often relieves hiccup.

TABLE 31-6. DRUGS USED AS EXPECTORANTS AND TO RELIEVE COUGH (ANTITUSSIVE)

Expectorant drugs liquefy respiratory secretions so that they are more easily expelled. Antitussive drugs affect the cough center in the brain and the nerve impulses which go to that center in such a way as to reduce cough.

DRUG	USE	REACTION	DOSAGE – ADMINISTRATION	REMARKS
Expectorants	Aid in the expelling (spitting) of secretions from the trachea and lungs. Aid in increasing the amount of such secretions.			
Ammonium chloride, U.S.P.		A diuretic for some patients.	0.3 - 1.0 Gm. (5-15 gr.) every 4 hours with plenty of water. Oral.	Disagreeable tasting, yet commonly used.
Ipecac, U.S.P.		Causes nausea in larger doses.	½-1 tsp. syrup for young children; 2 tsps. for older children and adults. Syrup, extract, tincture, powder. Oral.	Commonly used for children. Follow dosage with tepid water.
Iodides Potassium iodide, U.S.P. Sodium iodide	Make secretions more liquid.		A few drops in water or juice every 2 or 3 hours; varies with size of patient. Physician specifies.	Considered an effective drug.
Cough Medicines	Affect the cough center in brain and act on the respiratory tract to slow down impulse to cough.			
Codeine sulfate, N.F.	See Table 31-1		Small doses every 3-4 hours are ordered.	A narcotic often used in a mixture with other drugs (terpin hydrate, fruit flavored syrups).
Dextromethorphan hydrobromide, N.F. (Romilar)	Used almost exclusively for cough.	No apparent side effects.	Adult dosage 20-30 mg. 3 or 4 times a day. Tablets and syrup.	Seems to have no addictive power. A synthetic type of morphine.
Benzonatate, N.N.D. (Tessalon)	Relieves cough and eases respirations.	Nausea, some drowsiness, dizziness, skin rashes.	50-100 mg, (3/4 - 1½ gr.) 3-6 times daily. Oral. Capsules to be swallowed intact.	Acts in about 15 minutes, effect lasts 2-8 hours.

(Table 31-6 continues on the opposite page.)

TABLE 31–6. DRUGS USED AS EXPECTORANTS AND TO RELIEVE COUGH (ANTITUSSIVE) (Continued)

DRUG	USE	REACTION	DOSAGE – ADMINISTRATION	REMARKS
Opium compound and glycyrrhiza mixture, N.F. (Brown mixture)	Has a sedative effect upon respirations and thus reduces cough.		4.0 ml. Oral.	
Alevaire Trade name for a mixture of superinone (detergent) and water	Increases production of respiratory tract fluid in bronchial and pulmonary diseases.	Seldom any. Observe for signs of pulmonary edema.	Inhalation. Special equipment, nebulizer.	Commonly used. Other brands are available.
Terpin hydrate elixir, N.F.	Soothing to mucous membrane; decreases secretions; relieves cough.		4 ml. every 4 hours p.r.n. Oral.	Often used in a mixture with codeine.
Cough Syrups (Flavored syrups raspberry, chocolate, cinnamon, etc., mixed with expectorants).				There are many "cough medicines" available without prescription.

TABLE 31-7.   DRUGS TO AFFECT BOWEL ACTIVITY

Perhaps no group of drugs is used so widely and misused so frequently as cathartics. There is danger in using cathartics, and their wide use suggests that people need to be aware of this. Undiagnosed abdominal pain should not be treated with a cathartic unless this is ordered by the physician. Proper diet, exercise, and regularity promote normal bowel activity. Those people who make cathartics a habit need to know this.

DRUG	USE	REACTION	DOSAGE – ADMINISTRATION	REMARKS
Cathartics	Stimulate intestinal peristalsis and thus remove wastes from lower intestine.			Actions range from mild to very severe.
Bulk Agar, U.S.P.	Adds bulk and moisture to feces. Not digestible.	Colic-like pain may result if powder is too fine.	Tablespoon dosage is usual. Coarse powder or shreds dissolved in hot water.	May be added to food at the table.
Psyllium hydrophilic mucilloid, N.N.D. (Metamucil)	Furnishes bulk.		Stirred into a glass of water, fruit juice, or milk followed by glass of water.	
Bran	Furnishes bulk.	Overeating dry in large amounts can be constipating.	Ordinary bran foods (cereals, bread, etc.) are common and adequate source for many people.	
Irritating Cascara sagrada, U.S.P.	Increases peristalsis by irritating the lining of the bowel.	Usually causes no griping discomfort when taken at bedtime.	Dosage varies with age. Fluid extract, tablets. Oral.	Mild and reliable. May be habit forming.
Castor oil, U.S.P.	Same as above.	May cause nausea and griping.	1/2 – 1 fluid ounce.	Liquid stools produced in a few hours.
Saline Magnesium magma, U.S.P. (milk of magnesia)	Attracts water into bowel and retains it to make stool watery.	Rapid action of drug suggests taking in the morning. Griping and loss of fluid.	Suspension. Taken directly or stirred in cold water. Tablets. Oral.	
Magnesium sulfate, U.S.P. (Epsom salt)			White crystalline powder dissolved. Oral.	Effective; distasteful unless dissolved in fruit juice.

(Table 31–7 continues on the opposite page.)

TABLE 31–7. DRUGS USED TO AFFECT BOWEL ACTIVITY (Continued)

DRUG	USE	REACTION	DOSAGE – ADMINISTRATION	REMARKS
Mercury preparation Mercurous chloride mild, (calomel) N.F.	Delays the ordinary absorption of water in the bowel, thus producing semifluid stool.	Griping pain; severe diarrhea. Systemic mercury poisoning can occur through absorption.	0.12 gm. (2 gr.) in the evening followed the next morning by a saline cathartic to rid the bowel of mercury. Oral.	Stool may have a greenish color. Seldom used.
Other Bisacodyl (Dulcolax)	Irritates the lining of the colon, thus stimulates peristalsis.	May cause some gastrointestinal distress to elderly patients. Suppositories used for elderly patients.	1 or 2, 5 mg. enteric coated tablets. 10 mg. suppository. Enteric coated tablet; suppository. Oral, rectal.	Found effective (and time saving) as a preoperative and postoperative laxative and in preparing a patient for x-ray procedures.
Dioctyl sodium sulfosuccinate (Doxinate, Colace)	Softens fecal material by assisting water and fats to mix with stool.		10–20 mg. daily for children; 60–100 mg. daily for adults.	
Lubricants Liquid petrolatum, U.S.P. mineral oil (Nujol) (Albolene)	Bland, odorless oil used to coat the lining of the bowel so feces move along more easily.	May be leakage from the anus. Oily coating of feces covers rectal lining. Interferes with absorption of some vitamins.	Amount and frequency vary. Oral, rectal (to soften fecal impaction).	Many flavored preparations available.
Olive oil	Coats the lining of the bowel causing soft stools.		30 ml., divided doses. Oral.	
Carminatives Some are used alone and in combination. Peppermint spirits Spearmint spirits Ginger Wintergreen Anise Bile salts Turpentine	To rid the bowel of gas.	Are irritating to the gastrointestinal tract.	The mixture is designated. Oral. Tablets. Oral. Ordered as enema or abdominal stupe.	Seldom used. Seldom used.

(Table 31-7 continues on the following page.)

TABLE 31-7. DRUGS TO AFFECT BOWEL ACTIVITY (Continued)

DRUG	USE	REACTION	DOSAGE — ADMINISTRATION	REMARKS
Antidiarrheics	To control diarrhea and protect the lining of the bowel.			
Bismuth subcarbonate, U.S.P.	Coats the intestinal tract.	Seldom causes unwanted reactions.	1.0 Gm. (15 gr.) Suspension. Oral.	
Opium tincture, U.S.P. (laudanum)	Retards peristalsis and relieves pain. Used for the discomfort of acute diarrhea.		0.6 ml. (10 minims) Oral.	
Opium camphorated tincture, U.S.P. (paregoric)			4.0 ml. (1 fluid dram) Oral.	Distasteful. Children resist taking it.
Anthelmintics	Treatment for worms in intestinal tract.			
Quinacrine hydrochloride, U.S.P. (Atabrine)	Effective treatment for tapeworm infestation, also for malaria.	Headache, dizziness, and gastrointestinal distress.	0.1 Gm. (1½ gr.) Dosage and frequency vary. Oral, I.M.	Temporarily discolors skin (yellow) and urine.
Piperazine citrate, U.S.P. (Antepar) (Parazine)	Effective treatment for pinworm and roundworm infestation.	Rarely toxic; slight gastrointestinal disturbance, skin rash.	Body weight determines dosage. White crystals soluble in water; syrup; tablets. Daily for a week, omit for a week, resume for a week. Oral.	Rarely given to people with impaired kidney function.

TABLE 31–8. DRUGS USED TO AFFECT SKIN AND MUCOUS MEMBRANES

Drugs in this group are used for a number of purposes: as an antiseptic or disinfectant, to promote healing, harden skin, reduce inflammation, increase or decrease local blood supply, reduce irritation, protect, and lubricate. The type and strength of preparation used depends upon the tissue treated and the purpose of the treatment. Some of these same drugs are used to disinfect and store equipment.

DRUG	USE	REACTION	DOSAGE – ADMINISTRATION	REMARKS
Phenol – Carbolic Acid	Antiseptic action and mild local anesthetic action in weak solutions.	Tissue can be damaged if solution is too strong.	Weak solutions (0.5 – 1.0%), ointments.	
Resorcinol, U.S.P.	For some skin disorders.		1 – 10% solution, topical. 5 – 20% ointment, topical.	
Hexachlorophene, U.S.P. (pHisoHex)	Skin disinfectant. To combat some skin conditions.		0.5 – 3% used in detergent soaps and creams.	Its use is being questioned.
Detergents (synthetic)	To cleanse and disinfect with some power to destroy bacteria.			Not used with soap.
Benzalkonium chloride, U.S.P. (Zephiran chloride)	Skin disinfectant; to irrigate wounds, mucous membranes, eye, urinary bladder.		1 : 1000 – 1 : 40,000 solutions, depending upon use.	
Chlorine Solutions	Antiseptic and disinfectant; to irrigate wounds.	Very toxic; irritates skin. Odor can be disagreeable to patients.		Skin should be rinsed after use.
Diluted sodium hypochlorite solution, N.F. (Dakin's solution)			0.5% solution, topical.	Great care is used to protect skin around wound.
Iodine	For infected wounds, and skin disinfectant.	Strong solutions irritate skin. Tincture is not used in severe wounds.	Tincture, solution, powders, ointments.	
Mercury Compounds	Local application: skin, nasal cavities, eyes, vagina.		Solutions, tinctures, jellies, ointments, suppositories.	
Merbromin, N.F. (Mercurochrome)			1 – 2% solutions, topical.	
Nitromersol, N.F. (Metaphen)			1: 2000 – 1: 5000 solution, topical.	
Thimerosal, N.F. (Merthiolate)			1: 1000 tincture.	
Yellow oxide of mercury ointment.	Eye infections.		1% ointment, topical.	

(Table 31–8 continues on the following page.)

TABLE 31–8. DRUGS USED TO AFFECT SKIN AND MUCOUS MEMBRANES (Continued)

DRUG	USE	REACTION	DOSAGE – ADMINISTRATION	REMARKS
Astringents	Constrict blood vessels, thus reduce swelling and inflammation.			
Ethyl alcohol, U.S.P.	Disinfectant and astringent. Lowers body temperature, toughens skin.		70% solution.	Some antiseptic and disinfectant power.
Boric acid, N.F.	Reduces swelling of inflamed tissues. Gargle, douche, eye irrigations.	Rarely produces toxic conditions when used as directed.	2 – 5% solution and ointment. Powder.	
Sodium borate, N.F. (Borax)	Reduces swelling of inflamed tissues. For gargles, wounds, burns.		1 – 5% solution, topical. Powder, ointment.	
Nitrofurazone, N.F. (Furacin)	Stimulant and antiseptic. Has healing qualities.	Toxic reactions rare. Caustic if solution is strong.	0.02 – 1.0% solutions and ointments, topical.	
Potassium permanganate, U.S.P.	Antiseptic action.		Strength of solution ranges from 1: 1000 – 1: 10,000 depending upon use.	Stains everything it touches; deodorizing power.
Silver nitrate, U.S.P.	Antiseptic and disinfectant actions.	Caustic in strong solution.	Strength of solution ranges from 0.5 – 2.0% to 1: 2000 – 1: 10,000 depending upon use. 1% solution dropped into eyes of newborn to prevent blindness.	Stains black.

TABLE 31–9. DRUGS USED AS ANTI-INFECTIVES

These drugs act against infections in the body. Some act against certain specific organisms and others act in general against a wide range of different organisms. Anti-infective drugs are widely used. While their discovery has brought about changes in the treatment of many disorders, they do not cure everything. On the contrary, their use raises some new questions and problems.

DRUG	USE	REACTION	DOSAGE – ADMINISTRATION	REMARKS
Antibiotics *Penicillin*	Kills bacteria and inhibits growth of bacteria. Especially useful in treating diseases caused by streptococcus, staphylococcus, pneumococcus, gonococcus.	If reactions occur they range from local burning sensations and skin rashes to chills, fever, shock symptoms.	Penicillin comes in forms for parenteral and oral use.	Observation of patient is particularly important, especially in relation to reactions.
Some of the types are: Benzathine penicillin G, U.S.P. (Bicillin)			Aqueous suspension, tablets.	
Hydrabamine phenoxymethyl penicillin, N.N.D. (Compocillin – V)			Tablets, suspension.	
Phenoxymethyl penicillin, U.S.P. (Pen – Vee)			Capsules, drops, tablets, suspension. Oral only.	
Potassium penicillin, U.S.P. crystalline buffered (Dramcillin) (Dropcillin) (Penalev) (Pentids)			Capsules, ointments, powders, suppositories, tablets (buffered and soluble type added to infants' formula).	
Procaine penicillin G, U.S.P. aqueous suspension (Crysticillin) (Duracillin)	Long lasting.		Parenteral. Sterile oily suspension does not need refrigeration. Dry form when mixed with water requires refrigeration.	Widely used.
Synthetic penicillin Ampicillin (Polycillin)	To treat a variety of infections.	Pain at the injection site. Allergic reactions.	250 – 500 mg. q.i.d. Oral I.M.	A "broad spectrum" drug.
Cephalothin (Keflin)	Same as above.		0.5 – 1 Gm. I.M. 2 – 6 Gm. I.V.	

(Table 31–9 continues on the following page.)

TABLE 31–9.   DRUGS USED AS ANTI-INFECTIVES (Continued)

DRUG	USE	REACTION	DOSAGE – ADMINISTRATION	REMARKS
Bacitracin Bacitracin ointment, U.S.P. Bacitracin solution, U.S.P.	Inhibits growth of bacteria. Most commonly used locally.	Severe pain is common at site of injection. Toxic.	Oral, I.M., topical. Powder, solution, tablets, troches, ointments.	Most often given by I.M. injection.
Streptomycin	Effective in many conditions where penicillin is not. Highly effective killer of bacteria.	Dizziness, temporary hearing loss, skin rashes, fever. Can be dangerous to persons sensitized to this drug.	Powder, solution, inhalation form.	
Dihydrostreptomycin sulfate, U.S.P. (Doramicin)			0.5 – 1 Gm. I.M.	
Chlortetracycline hydrochloride capsules, N.F. (Aureomycin)	Convenient for patient at home. Infections of mouth, throat and skin disorders.	Seldom see undesirable side effects of gastrointestinal upset and diarrhea.	Capsule (50 – 250 mg.) usually given 3 or 4 times a day.	Oral route is most common one. Schedule is set to avoid awakening patient for night doses. Also in troche, ointment, and I.V. forms.
Chloramphenicol U.S.P. (Chloromycetin) (Chlorphenol, Mycinol, Enicol) (Chloromycetin succinate)	Used for diseases of the intestinal tract and urinary infections.	Inflammation of tongue and mouth. May attack bone marrow, causing blood abnormalities.	Capsules, ampules, cream, powder, ointment. Oral, I.V., I.M.	Strong caution (by federal government) about use of this drug.
Oxytetracycline hydrochloride, N.F. (Terramycin)	Effective for many types of infections.	Might cause gastrointestinal disorders with diarrhea.	Oral. Parenteral, rectal.	
Other Chemotherapeutic Action Drugs	These drugs act more specifically on selected diseases than do the antibiotics; they inhibit bacterial growth.	They yield some toxic results which tend to limit their usefulness.		

(Table 31–9 continues on the opposite page.)

TABLE 31-9. DRUGS USED AS ANTI-INFECTIVES (Continued)

DRUG	USE	REACTION	DOSAGE – ADMINISTRATION	REMARKS
Sulfonamides. This is the name of a large group of synthetic compounds.	To treat bacterial infectious diseases (except syphilis).	Toxic reactions include: dizziness, skin rash, fever, nausea, vomiting, diminished urine output. Jaundice is a serious though rare reaction. If a patient reacts the second time this reaction is likely to be more severe and rapid.	Dosage and frequency of administration vary with drug, patient, and condition being treated. Oral, parenteral, rectal routes, and local application are used. Doses are prescribed to maintain a certain level of drug in the body.	Antibiotics are used in place of many sulfonamides; however, they remain the drugs of choice for certain disease conditions and in others are used in combination with the antibiotics. Organisms may develop resistance to the drug, thus making it necessary to discontinue it. The nurse should maintain exact time schedule in giving drug. Patient will be awakened unless ordered otherwise. Fluid intake and output are measured and recorded. Ambulatory patients should be cautious of working machines and driving a car while taking these drugs.
Some of these drugs are: Sulfadiazine, U.S.P. Sulfamerazine sodium injection, N.F. Sulfamethazine, U.S.P. Sulfacetamide, N.F. (Sulamyd) Succinylsulfathiazole, N.F. (Sulfasuxidine) Sulfamethizole, N.F. (Thiosulfil)	Systemic infections. Systemic infections. Systemic infections. Systemic infections. Local action in gastro-intestinal tract (orally). Urinary tract infections (orally).			
Isoniazid U.S.P. (Hyzyd, Lanizid, Rimifon).	Used with other drugs (streptomycin, PAS) to treat some types of tuberculosis.	Constipation, dizziness, difficulty voiding.	50-200 mg. t.i.d. or b.i.d. Oral.	Sometimes used as a preventive measure for persons with recently converted positive tuberculin test.
Erythromycin (Erythrocin, E-Myain, Ilotycin).	To treat certain organisms, especially penicillin-resistant staphylococci.		100-250 mg. every 6 h. Oral.	Also given I. M. and I. V. Also for topical use.

TABLE 31-10. DRUGS WHICH AFFECT THE HEART AND BLOOD VESSELS

Drugs which affect the heart may be grouped as stimulants and depressants; those which affect the blood vessels are called vasodilators and vaso- constrictors. Notice the types of reactions which can occur and the necessary measures cited in the Remarks column.

DRUG	USE	REACTION	DOSAGE – ADMINISTRATION	REMARKS
Heart				
Stimulants				
	Increase the force with which the heart muscle contracts.	Blood circulation generally improved.		
Digitalis preparations	Stimulates heart muscle. The beat is stronger; the rate is slower. Used as an emergency drug and for maintaining long term cardiac conditions.	Slow pulse (if below 60 report it), headache, nausea, general body discomfort, loss of appetite, arrhythmia, vomiting, blurred vision, diarrhea.		Urinary output is increased. Most often given by mouth, as these drugs irritate tissues. Observe patient for reactions. Physicans may order that dosage be skipped at certain intervals. Patient is kept quiet.
Some of these preparations are: Digitoxin, U.S.P.			Oral, 0.1 - 0.2 mg. (1/600 - 1/300 gr.)	Also injection form for I.V.
Digilanid			Liquid, tablets, suppository. Oral, I.V., rectal.	
Digoxin, U.S.P.			Oral, 0.25 - 0.5 mg. (1/250 - 1/120 gr.)	Also injection form for I.V.
Digitalis powdered, U.S.P.			Oral, 0.1 Gm. (1½ gr.)	
Depressants	Slow the heart rate and change the irregular rapid beat to a more normal one.			A rapid change in rate of heart beat can be frightening to a patient.

(Table 31-10 continues on the opposite page.)

TABLE 31–10. DRUGS WHICH AFFECT THE HEART AND BLOOD VESSELS (Continued)

DRUG	USE	REACTION	DOSAGE – ADMINISTRATION	REMARKS
Quinidine gluconate, U.S.P. (Quinaglute) Others: (Cardioquin) (Quinidate) (Quinidex)		Headache, dizziness, ringing in the ears, visual disturbances, nausea, vomiting.	0.2 - 0.4 Gm. (3 - 6 gr.) Oral, I.M., I.V.	
Procainamide hydrochloride, U.S.P. (Pronestyl)		Low blood pressure may occur.	Oral, I.V.	Blood pressure should be checked frequently.
Blood Vessels *Vasodilators* There are many such preparations available. A few of them are:	Cause blood vessels to enlarge and thus allow the blood to flow more freely.			
Nitrites	Reduce cardiac pain by enlarging coronary vessels.	Flushed face, blurred vision, irregular pulse, headache, dizziness, vomiting, diarrhea, cyanosis, mental confusion.		
Amyl nitrite, U.S.P.			A clear, yellow, inflammable, pungent liquid (fragile ampule) by inhalation.	Physician is careful to individualize dosage to prevent over-dosage during self-medication, if possible. Ampule is crushed and fumes inhaled.
Octyl nitrate (Octrite inhaler)			Available in inhalers.	
Glyceryl trinitrate, U.S.P. (nitroglycerin)			0.4 mg. (1/150 gr.) Sublingual, oral.	

(Table 31–10 continues on the following page.)

TABLE 31–10. DRUGS WHICH AFFECT THE HEART AND BLOOD VESSELS (Continued)

DRUG	USE	REACTION	DOSAGE – ADMINISTRATION	REMARKS
Pentaerythritol tetranitrate (Angicap, Circulin, Metranil, Pentafin, Vasodiatol)	Used to relieve anginal attacks, asthma, and chronic hypertension by lowering blood pressure.	Same as above.	5 - 20 mg. Oral.	Dosage may be changed from time to time.
Papaverine hydrochloride, U.S.P. See Table 31-1	To dilate blood vessels and relieve spasms in gastrointestinal and urinary tract.	Oral administration seldom causes side effects, but there may be mouth and throat dryness; constipation.	Dosage varies according to need. Oral, parenteral.	
Aminophylline	Has direct relaxing action on blood vessel walls. Increases flow of urine.	Sometimes causes nausea, vomiting, dizziness, headache. I.V. injection may cause a peculiar sensation around mouth and in the face.		
Aminophylline, U.S.P.			Oral, 0.1 - 0.2 Gm. (1½ - 3 gr.)	
Aminophylline injection, U.S.P.			I.M. or I.V., 0.2 - 0.5 Gm. (3 - 7½ gr.)	
Aminophylline supposi- tories, U.S.P.			Rectal, 0.25 - 0.5 Gm. (4 - 7½ gr.)	
Beta-pyridylcar binol (Roniacol)	Dilates peripheral blood vessels.	Rare.	25 - 50 mg. Oral.	
Dioxyline phosphate (Paverone)	Relaxes muscles.	Rare.	0.2 - 0.5 Gm. Oral.	

(Table 31–10 continues on the opposite page.)

TABLE 31–10. DRUGS WHICH AFFECT THE HEART AND BLOOD VESSELS (Continued)

DRUG	USE	REACTION	DOSAGE – ADMINISTRATION	REMARKS
Vasoconstrictors	Cause blood vessels to constrict and thus decrease flow of blood to a part of the body.			
Epinephrine Epinephrine hydrochloride, U.S.P. (Adrenalin supranol)	Treatment for asthma, shock, cardiac failure, and congestion of breathing passageway.	Tremors, palpitation, apprehension.	I.V., I.M., Spray.	Note: this drug is never given orally.
Levarterenol bitartrate, U.S.P. (Levophed)	Constricts peripheral vessels and is used to combat some types of circulatory shock.	Irritates subcutaneous tissues, apprehension, tremors, palpitation. Raises blood pressure.	I.V. (given slowly), 10 - 15 drops per minute at start. Regulated according to blood pressure.	Patient must be watched carefully; frequent blood pressure readings necessary.

TABLE 31–11. DRUGS WHICH AFFECT THE BLOOD

Drugs affecting the blood may be grouped as hematinics — increase red cells, anticoagulants — prevent clotting, and hemostatics — control bleeding. Notice the essential precautions related to these drugs.

DRUG	USE	REACTION	DOSAGE — ADMINISTRATION	REMARKS
Hematinics	Help to increase the number of red blood cells, thereby increasing the hemoglobin.			
Iron salts	To help correct iron deficiency, thus stimulating red blood cell production.	Black stools, constipation, skin rash.	Liquids, tablets, syrup, capsules.	Liquid form should be taken through a tube to reduce staining of teeth. Syrup preparations are used for children.
Ferrous sulfate, U.S.P.			0.3 Gm. (5 gr.) enteric coated tablets.	Most widely used.
Ferrous gluconate, U.S.P. (Fergon)			0.3 Gm. (5 gr.) Oral.	
Vitamin B12 Cyanocobalamin, U.SP.	To treat some types of anemia. Stimulates proper production of red cells in bone marrow.		Oral, parenteral.	Appetite improves.
Folic acid, U.S.P.	To treat some types of anemia.		Oral, parenteral.	Usually given in combination with other drugs. Seldom used now.
Liver extract	Increases production of red blood cells.	Local irritation to tissues at site of injection.	Oral, parenteral.	Watch for any signs of internal or external bleeding.
Anticoagulants	Prevent clotting of blood.			
Sodium citrate	Especially useful in blood collected for transfusion; it must not coagulate. Used for patients having open heart surgery, to treat thrombophlebitis. Used in blood collected for transfusion.			
Heparin sodium, U.S.P. (Liquaemin, Metarin, Panheprin)	Prolongs clotting time. Acts rapidly. Effect stops shortly after drug discontinued.	Observe for any signs of internal hemorrhage.	I.V.	Follow physician's orders closely for patient activity while drug is being given and discontinued.

(Table 31–11 continues on the opposite page.)

TABLE 31-11.   DRUGS WHICH AFFECT THE BLOOD (Continued)

DRUG	USE	REACTION	DOSAGE – ADMINISTRATION	REMARKS
Bishydroxycoumarin, U.S.P. (Dicumarol) (Cumopyran)	Prolongs clotting time.	A dangerous drug. Reliable laboratory findings (prothrombin determination) are essential. Bleeding can easily occur.	Dosage is carefully individualized for each patient. Single daily dosage given at the same time each day. Oral.	Cheaper than heparin but acts more slowly. Careful observation for any signs of internal or external bleeding is essential.
Fibrinolysin (Actase, Thrombolysin)	To dissolve thrombi. Breaks down blood clots.		50,000 - 100,000 units I.V.	
Warfarin sodium (Coumadin sodium, Panwarfin, Prothromadin)	Prompt action. Prolongs clotting longer than heparin.	Watch for signs of hemorrhage.	2 - 25 mg. Oral, I.V.	
Hemostatics	To control bleeding and stop hemorrhages (especially in oozing capillaries and veins).			
Thrombin	Promotes clotting.		Dry sterile powder; solution in vials.	
Absorbable gelatin sponge, U.S.P. (Gelfoam)	Used locally to stop bleeding.		A porous, dry packing which is soaked with thrombin solution and applied directly to the bleeding area. Oral, parenteral.	Is absorbed in 3 or more weeks and leaves little evidence.
Vitamin K	Elevates low prothrombin factor of the blood to control bleeding. Used with the newborn and to prevent postpartum hemorrhage.			

TABLE 31–12.   DRUGS WHICH AFFECT THE STOMACH

Drugs in this group are divided into the following categories: antacids (relieve stomach distress due to acidity), emetics (cause vomiting), antiemetics (prevent vomiting and nausea), and drugs with the ability to reduce gastric mobility and stomach spasms.

DRUG	USE	REACTION	DOSAGE – ADMINISTRATION	REMARKS
Antacids	Neutralize the acid contents of the stomach and give general systemic relief.			Antacids are widely used. There are many such drug combinations available without prescription.
Sodium bicarbonate, U.S.P. (baking soda)	To reduce stomach acidity	Can produce alkalosis. The symptoms include: dry mouth, thirst, headache, nausea, vomiting, loss of appetite.	1–2 Gm. (15–30 gr.). Oral.	
Magnesium oxide, U.S.P.	More effective than sodium bicarbonate.	Can be a cathartic.	0.25 Gm. (4 gr.). Oral.	
Magnesium magma, U.S.P. (milk of magnesia) (magnesium hydroxide)		Can be a cathartic See Table 31-7.	4.0 ml. (1 fluid dram). Oral. Also in tablet form.	
Aluminum hydroxide gel, U.S.P. (Amphogel) (Creamalin)	Both aluminum compounds are used in the treatment of peptic ulcers; they inhibit the action of the pepsin and coat the ulcer surface.		4.0–8.0 ml. (1-2 fluid drams). Oral.	Flavoring is usually added to improve the taste. To be given with plenty of water.
Aluminum phosphate gel, N.F. (Phosphaljel)			15.0 ml. (4 fluid drams). Oral.	
Precipitated calcium carbonate, N.F. (Calcibarb)	Protective to irritated stomach	May cause constipation.	1–2 Gm. Oral.	Long-lasting neutralizing action.
Emetics	Used to intentionally cause vomiting.			Little occasion to make patient vomit; may be needed in case of swallowing some poisonous substance.

(Table 31–12 continues on the opposite page.)

TABLE 31–12. DRUGS WHICH AFFECT THE STOMACH (Continued)

DRUG	USE	REACTION	DOSAGE – ADMINISTRATION	REMARKS
Ipecac, U.S.P.	To cause vomiting. Larger doses given than when used as an expectorant. See Table 31-6.		0.5 Gm. (7½ gr.) Oral.	
Ipecac syrup, U.S.P.			8.0 ml. (2 fluid drams). Oral.	
Antiemetics A good number of drugs have some antiemetic power. (Tranquilizers and antihistamines.)	Used to prevent and overcome nausea and vomiting.			
Pipamazine (Mornidine)	Used for nausea and vomiting associated with pregnancy and for postoperative nausea.		5.0 mg. (1/12 gr.). Oral, I.V.	
Meclizene hydrochloride, U.S.P. (Bonamine)	Used for nausea, motion sickness, and for dizziness associated with improper balance.		25 mg. (3/8 gr.). Oral.	
Dimenhydrinate, U.S.P. (Dramamine)	Same as above.		50 - 100 mg. (3/4 - 1½ gr.). Oral.	
Reduce Gastric Mobility and Pain Belladonna Atropine Sulfate, U.S.P. (Synthetic)	Decreases secretions, relaxes smooth muscles.	Dryness of mouth and skin, blurred vision, urinary retention, constipation.	0.25 - 0.5 mg. Oral. Parenteral.	Dilates eye pupil. Patient may express "uneasiness."
Propantheline bromide, U.S.P. (Pro-Banthine)	Relaxs stomach spasms.	See atropine.	15 mg. Oral. 30 mg. I.M., I.V.	Results are similar to atropine.

TABLE 31–13.   DRUGS WHICH AFFECT THE KIDNEYS

Drugs affecting the kidneys may be grouped as: diuretics (increase excretion of urine); urinary antiseptics (control infections); urinary anti-infectives (drugs specific for treating urinary infections).

DRUG	USE	REACTION	DOSAGE – ADMINISTRATION	REMARKS
Diuretics	**Increase excretion of urine from kidneys. Used to relieve edema and ascites due to cardiac, kidney, and liver disorders.**			
Ammonium chloride, U.S.P. (Amchlor) (Dalitol, synthetic)		May cause acidosis; elderly patients are more susceptible. The symptoms are weakness, nausea, vomiting, changes in respirations.	1 - 2 Gm. (15 - 30 gr.) Oral. Enteric coated tablets and capsules. Solutions for oral and I.V.	See Table 31-6. I.V. is given with caution due to toxicity of drug carried directly to circulating blood.
Aminophylline, U.S.P. (Aminocardol, Diophyllin, Metaphyllin)	In common use to reduce edema by increasing urine flow; lowers blood pressure, relieves asthma.	Seems to stimulate the heart muscle; relaxes smooth muscles. May cause headache and stomach distress.	0.1 - 0.2 Gm. Oral.	Irritates tissues, hence given by mouth in most instances. If given I.V. observe pulse rate and signs of distress (nausea, rapid breathing, fall in blood pressure).
Meralluride, U.S.P. (Mercuhydrin)	Produces diuretic action in the kidney.	Sometimes causes nausea, vomiting, mouth soreness, diarrhea, albumin and blood in urine. Patient can develop resistance to this drug.	1.0 ml. (15 minims). I.M., I.V. 0.6 Gm. Suppository	Physician may alternate type of drug to preserve effectiveness.
Mersalyl (Salyrgan)	Same as above.	Same as above.	80 mg. (1⅓ gr.). Oral.	Not given to patients having acute nephritis.
Mercurophylline (Mercupurin)	Same as above.	Same as above.	0.2 Gm. (3 gr.) I.M.	

Table 31–13 continues on the opposite page.)

TABLE 31–13. DRUGS WHICH AFFECT THE KIDNEYS (Continued)

DRUG	USE	REACTION	DOSAGE – ADMINISTRATION	REMARKS
Chlorothiazide, U.S.P. (Diuril)	Effective oral diuretic; edema responds well to this drug.	Little or no toxicity.	0.5 Gm. (7½ gr.) Oral.	
Urinary Antiseptics	Used to control urinary tract infections.			
Methenamine mandelate, U.S.P. (Mandelamine), a combination of two drugs.	Is an acidifying agent used for controlling many common urinary tract infections.	Seldom toxic; on occasion there may be urinary burning and frequency and slight gastric disorder.	250 mg. (3¾ gr.) Tablets. Oral.	
Methenamine, N.F. (Urotropin)	Given in combination with an acidifying drug. Same as above.	Seldom toxic.	0.5 Gm. (7½ gr.) Oral.	
Urinary Anti-infectives				
Sulfonamides Two common ones are:	Used for severe bladder infections.	Toxic symptoms include: nausea, vomiting, hematuria, oliguria, cyanosis, skin rash, dizziness.		Observe accurate time schedule for giving.
Sulfadiazine	See Table 31-9.	Not as toxic as some sulfonamides.		
Sulfisoxazole, U.S.P.		Effective but tends to be toxic.	Oral. First dose is usually larger than following ones; ointment.	Observe for sufficient urinary output.
Chloramphenicol (Chloromycetin)	See Table 31-9.			This drug is under investigation.

TABLE 31–14: DRUGS WHICH AFFECT THE UTERUS

Some drugs *stimulate* the uterine muscle so that its contractions and the chance of abortion during pregnancy. The drugs included here are more powerful; others *depress* the contractions to reduce pain act upon the uterus during labor and in other ways.

DRUG	USE	REACTION	DOSAGE – ADMINISTRATION	REMARKS
Stimulants				
Oxytocin injection, U.S.P. (Pitocin)	Shortens labor when it is prolonged and when it is slow in starting; helps prevent severe post-partum bleeding.	Can cause uterus to rupture.	I.V., I.M., and by nasal pack.	Oxytocin comes from Greek and means "swift birth." I.V. administration most frequently used.
Ergonovine maleate, U.S.P. (Ergotrate) (Ergosterine)	Acts on the uterine muscle to cause strong contractions, helps prevent severe postpartum bleeding.	Acts rapidly; observation is made for "overaction"; changes in blood pressure may occur.	I.V., I.M., Oral	I.V. method commonly used.
Ergot Methylergonovine maleate, U.S.P. (Methergine)	Used for postpartum bleeding; causes strong uterine muscle contractions.	The physician observes for over-active, excessive, stimulation of uterus.	0.2 mg. Oral. I.M., I.V.	Physicians vary in how they use this type of drug.
Depressants	Depresses the uterus during dysmenorrhea and threatened abortion.			
Isoxsuprine hydrochloride, N.N.D. (Vasodilan)	Relaxes smooth muscle. Effective in treating dysmenorrhea.	Seldom any toxic results. Occasional dizziness and palpitation.	10 – 20 mg. (1/6 – 1/3 gr.) Oral, I.M.	A wide range of preparations available.

TABLE 31-15. DRUGS WHICH AFFECT THE EYE

For some types of treatment the pupil of the eye needs to be enlarged (dilated); drugs for this purpose are *mydriatics*. In other treatment, the pupil of the eye needs to be smaller (contracted); drugs for this purpose are *miotics*. Drugs prepared specifically for eye treatment are labeled "ophthalmic."

DRUG	USE	REACTION	DOSAGE – ADMINISTRATION	REMARKS
Mydriatics	Dilate or enlarge pupil.	Vision disturbance occurs while pupil is dilated, but gradually disappears.	Solutions are applied in drops (1 or 2) at certain intervals depending upon the need.	
Atropine sulfate solution	An effective, long lasting action drug to dilate the pupil; this rests this part of the eye structure.	Vision disturbance lasts longer in younger children (7 – 10 days).	0.5 – 1.0% solution, topical.	
Cyclopentolate hydrochloride, U.S.P. (Cyclogyl)	Rapid action mydriatic with moderate lasting action.	Not as irritating as some mydriatics.	0.5 – 2.0% solution, topical.	
Miotics (myotics)	Contract or make the pupil smaller. This causes increased drainage through canals and reduces inner eyeball pressure as in glaucoma.	Vision blurred. When ointment is used in treatment, it adds to this blurring. With severe contraction there may be pain and nausea.	Solutions are applied in drops (1 or 2) at certain intervals depending upon the need.	
Pilocarpine nitrate solution, U.S.P.			0.25 – 2.0% solution, topical.	Constriction appears in 10 to 15 minutes. Stronger solutions effective for nearly a day. Ointment available.
Physostigmine salicylate, U.S.P. (eserine salicylate)			0.25, 0.5, 1.0, and 2.0% solution. 0.11 and 0.65 mg. (1/600 – 1/100 gr.) disks or tabloids. 0.25, 0.5, and 1.0% ointment.	Constriction starts shortly and lasts for a day or more (12 – 36 hours).
Others				
Yellow oxide of mercury ointment	To treat and prevent eye infections.		1.0% ointment, topical.	See Table 31-8.
Boric acid (boracic acid), N.F.	For eye irrigations.	Nonirritating to membranes when properly used. Can produce poisoning effect when taken internally.	2 – 5% solution, ointment, topical.	See Table 31-8.
Silver nitrate, U.S.P.	To prevent blindness in newborn.			See Table 31-8.

TABLE 31–16. DRUGS USED FOR ENDOCRINE DISORDERS

Hormones are chemical substances (animal substances or synthectic sources) which influence the work of the body cells. They work in harmony in the healthy body. Treatment for hypoactivity or hyperactivity of one gland can influence the work of hormones from other glands. This table deals with drugs used for a few common conditions of hyperactivity and hypoactivity of some of the endocrine glands. It points out drugs used in replacement therapy, as prophylactic measures, and for therapeutic effects.

DRUG	USE	REACTION	DOSAGE – ADMINISTRATION	REMARKS
Drugs Used to Affect the Thyroid Gland				
Depress the Activity of the Thyroid Gland	To treat hyperthyroidism or hypersecretion of the gland.			
Thioamides				
Propylthiouracil, U.S.P.	To prepare thyrotoxic patient for surgery; to treat hyperthyroidism.	Skin rash, sore throat, malaise, fever.	0.1 Gm. (1½ gr.) Oral.	Drug should be stopped at once if reactions appear; less toxic.
Methimazole, U.S.P. (Tapazole)	Same as above.	Same as above.	5 - 10 mg. Oral.	More potent than propylthiouracil. Acts more rapidly.
Iodides				
Strong iodine solution, U.S.P. (Lugol's solution)	To prepare thyrotoxic patients for surgery.	Toxic reactions seldom occur but may cause symptoms similar to those of common cold, also skin rash.	0.3 - 1.0 ml. (5 - 15 minims) Oral. Give with drink (milk, cream, juice) to disguise disagreeable taste.	Patient shows improvement while on drug.
Iodized salt	Used as a prophylactic measure to prevent goiter.			A food supplement when iodine is lacking in food and water.
Assist in the Absence or Shortage of Thyroxin	To treat hypothyroidism or hyposecretion of the gland.			

(Table 31–16 continues on the opposite page.)

TABLE 31–16. DRUGS USED FOR ENDOCRINE DISORDERS (Continued)

DRUG	USE	REACTION	DOSAGE – ADMINISTRATION	REMARKS
Thyroid, U.S.P.	A substitute for thyroxin in the body.	Observe for signs of overdose: nervousness, palpitation, rapid pulse, sleeplessness, dizziness, excessive warmth.	Dosage varies according to individual needs. 15-300 mg. (¼-4½ gr.)	
Thyroxin	Same as above.	Same as above.	0.5 mg. (1/120 gr.)	
Sodium levothyroxine, U.S.P. (Synthroid)	Same as above.	Same as above.	Dosage begins about 0.1 mg. (1/600 gr.) and is increased at intervals depending upon patient's need. Oral.	Physician seeks correct metabolic balance.
Sodium liothyronine, U.S.P. (Cytomel)	Same as above.	Same as above.	Initial dosage 5 to 25 micrograms depending upon patient's need. Oral.	Acts rapidly but not as long as Synthroid.
Drugs Used to Treat Diabetes Mellitus				
Insulin as a drug is a replacement of that substance in the body	Affects body metabolism of carbohydrates; holds blood sugar within normal levels; working ability is measured in units.	See Chapter 45 for diabetes mellitus, its treatment and nursing care, including symptoms of diabetic coma and hypoglycemic shock.	Dosage is individualized as determined by tests. Hypodermic administration is most commonly used.	Dietary control accompanies use of insulin. I.V. administration sometimes used.
Some types are: Insulin injection, U.S.P. (regular insulin)	Used most commonly when fast action is needed as in emergencies.	Fast action; shorter duration requires more frequent injections.	10 ml. vials of 40 and 80 units per ml.	Acts within an hour; peak action 2-3 hours, lasts 6-8 hours.

(Table 31–16 continues on the following page.)

TABLE 31–16. DRUGS USED FOR ENDOCRINE DISORDERS (Continued)

DRUG	USE	REACTION	DOSAGE – ADMINISTRATION	REMARKS
Globin insulin with zinc, U.S.P.	Medium rate action. Absorption is retarded at site of injection.	Effects diminish quite rapidly; can lead to glycosuria before and after breakfast.	10 ml. vials of 40 and 80 units per ml.	Acts within 1-2 hours; peak action 8-16 hours, lasts 18-24 hours.
Insulin protamine zinc suspension, U.S.P.	Slower action. Absorption is retarded at site of injection.	Glycosuria may appear after meals; hypoglycemia may occur during the night.	10 ml. vials of 40 and 80 units per ml. A single daily injection may be used in moderate cases.	Acts within 4-6 hours; peak action 16-24 hours, lasts 24-36 hours. Shake preparation thoroughly before giving.
Insulin isopane suspension, U.S.P. (NPH Iletin)	Medium rate action. Absorption is retarded at site of injection.	Young patients usually need a faster action insulin.	10 ml. vials of 40 and 80 units per ml.	Acts within 1-2 hours; peak action 10-20 hours, lasts 28-30 hours.
Insulin zinc suspension, U.S.P.	Medium rate action. Absorption is retarded at site of injection.	Controls effectively; is less likely to cause allergic reaction than other delayed action types.	10 ml. vials of 40 and 80 units per ml.	Acts within 1-2 hours; peak action 10-20 hours, lasts 28-30 hours.
(Lente insulin)	Used the same as other insulins. Various forms may be combined into one injection.			Length of action varies depending upon the size of particles in the drug. Comes in three forms: short, medium, long acting. Lasting action may be 36 hours or more.
Synthetic noninsulin drugs now available to treat diabetes mellitus are given orally.	For mild types of disorder. Convenient for older people or those with failing eyesight and tremor.		The following dosages are listed to show commonly used amounts. The range is from less to more than shown here. Dosage must be individualized.	A fairly new treatment with obvious advantages in taking a pill instead of injection. The chief disadvantage is the tendency of patient to be lax about taking the pill as directed.

(Table 31–16 continues on the opposite page.)

TABLE 31–16. DRUGS USED FOR ENDOCRINE DISORDERS (Continued)

DRUG	USE	REACTION	DOSAGE – ADMINISTRATION	REMARKS
Tolbutamide, N.N.D. (Orinase)		Few severe reactions to date. Mild reactions include: headache, skin rashes, ringing in the ears, weakness, gastric disturbances.	2 Gm. (30 gr.) per day, usually in divided doses.	Acts within an hour; peak action in 5-8 hours.
Chlorpropamide (Diabinese)		More toxic than Orinase. Serious toxic actions related to the liver and the blood have occurred.	250 mg. given once per day.	Acts within an hour; peak action reached more quickly than with Orinase and lasts longer.
Other Hormones and Hormone Substitutes	Drugs included here are used as replacement therapy for patients with: adrenal insufficiency, metabolic disorders, and for an increasing variety of other conditions not related to endocrine disorders.	Edema, restlessness, insomnia, moon face, feeling of well-being, body fluid imbalance.	Orders to be followed with extreme care to avoid serious results.	Salt is apt to be restricted. Intake and output are measured. Blood pressure is taken frequently (low blood pressure is a sign of adrenal insufficiency). Observe for early reaction signs.
Adrenal cortex injection, N.F.	To treat adrenal insufficiency as in Addison's disease.		2-10 ml. (50 units per ml.) Parenteral.	
Cortisone acetate, U.S.P. (Cortogen) (Cortone)	Affects metabolism of carbohydrates, fats, and proteins; stimulates the adrenal cortex.		5-300 mg. Oral or I.M. Oral dosage divided into 3 or 4 doses. 0.25-2.5% ointment.	
Corticotropin injection, U.S.P. (ACTH) (Cortrophin)			10-100 units. Single or divided doses. I.M., I.V.	

(Table 31-16 continues on the following page.)

TABLE 31–16. DRUGS USED FOR ENDOCRINE DISORDERS (Continued)

DRUG	USE	REACTION	DOSAGE — ADMINISTRATION	REMARKS
Ovarian hormones (Animal or synthetic) Estrogens Benzestrol, N.F. Estrogenic substances (Estrifol, Premarin)	This group is large and has a wide variety of uses: relieve symptoms of menopause and prostatic cancer; reduce uterine bleeding, pruritus, senile vaginitis.	Nausea, vomiting, dizziness, headache	1 - 25 mg. Oral. 2.5 - 2.75 mg. Oral.	May cause fluid retention.
Tissue Building Hormones				
Methandrostenolone, N. F. (Dianabol)	Repairs tissues and promotes new tissue growth; used in aging, convalescence.	Low toxicity; edema may result under some circumstances.	5 mg. q̄.d. Oral	Used with caution in some disease conditions: kidney disorders, pregnancy, prostatic cancer.
Methandriol (Stenediol)		Menstrual disturbance may result.	5-10 mg. Oral	

TABLE 31–17.   DRUGS WHICH AFFECT NUTRITION AND GROWTH

Vitamins ordinarily are thought of as food nutrients; however, they are used as drugs when the body requires more than the diet supplies and when they can perform a specific function for the body. Frequently, they are ordered along with other drugs. Minerals are inorganic nutrients essential to normal body function, and are used to treat patients with certain disorders; they, too, are used in a variety of combinations with other drugs.

DRUG	USE	REACTION	DOSAGE — ADMINISTRATION	REMARKS
Vitamins				
Vitamin A Fat soluble. Synthetic preparations, also derived from fish liver oils. (Fish liver oils also contain vitamin D)	Necessary to growth and development of children. Signs of deficiency are: skin changes, night blindness and other eye signs, vaginitis, upper respiratory disorders.	Excessive intake may produce irritability, dry skin, loss of hair, loss of appetite, contraction of pupils, tender extremities.	Dosage varies according to age and need.	The use of this substance should be directed by a physician.
Vitamin B complex Water soluble. Has 12 known nutritive factors. Some commonly used for therapeutic purposes are:	To treat patients with beri-beri and nerve disorders; to improve appetite and aid body building in in general.			There are many available preparations.
Thiamine (B₁) hydrochloride, U.S.P. (Betalin) (Betaxin)	For some types of neuritis as with pregnancy, pellagra, alcoholism.		20–30 mg. 3 times a day. Oral. 50 mg. twice a day I.M. in more severe cases.	Oral preparations usually given with meals.
Riboflavin, U.S.P. (B₂) (Flavoxin) (Vitamin G)	To treat a deficiency marked by lesions on the lips, around the nose, eyes, and at corners of the mouth.		5–10 mg. daily. Oral, parenteral.	Usually accompanied by a high vitamin B content diet.
Nicotinamide, U.S.P. (Nicotinic acid amide) (Niacinamide)	Used with other vitamin B drugs to treat pellagra.	Does not cause flushing of the skin as does nicotinic acid.	50 mg. Oral, parenteral.	
Nicotinic acid injection, U.S.P. (Naotin) (Niacin)	Same as above.	Large doses cause flushing of the skin. Dilates peripheral blood vessels. May cause nausea, vomiting, urticaria.	50 mg. Oral, parenteral.	
Pyridoxine hydrochloride, U.S.P. (B₆) (Beadox)	To treat convulsions in children, hyperemesis with pregnancy, gastrointestinal disorders, nausea, vomiting.		5.0 mg. Oral, parenteral.	

(Table 31–17 continues on the following page.)

TABLE 31–17.   DRUGS WHICH AFFECT NUTRITION AND GROWTH (Continued)

DRUG	USE	REACTION	DOSAGE – ADMINISTRATION	REMARKS
Cyanocobalamin, U.S.P. (B₁₂) (Bevidox) (Crystamin) (Rametin)	To treat pernicious anemia.	Mouth soreness disappears within a few days; skin color improves, appetite returns for patient taking this drug.	1 microgram to 1 mg. Oral, parenteral.	There are many preparations available.
Folic acid, U.S.P. (Folvite)	Aids in the treatment of some anemic conditions; generally used in combination with other drugs.		10-20 mg. Oral, parenteral.	
Vitamin C Water soluble. Ascorbic acid, U.S.P. (cevitamic acid)	To prevent and treat scurvy; hastens wound healing; increases resistance to infections (virus).	Does not seem to be toxic.	0.1 - 1.0 Gm. (1½ - 15 gr.) Oral.	Injection form for parenteral use.
Vitamin D Fat soluble. Obtained from fish liver oils. (See also vitamin A)	To treat rickets, infantile tetany, fractures, calcium deficiencies. Ointments used for burns of face, neck, head, genitalia.	Excessive dosage and use can produce nausea, vomiting, diarrhea, dehydration, polyuria, mental confusion.	Dosage varies according to age, purpose, and preparation.	Often used with parathyroid extract and calcium salts in treating rickets and infantile tetany. The use of this substance should be directed by a physician.
Cod liver oil, U.S.P.				Disagreeable taste and lower vitamin D content.
Halibut liver oil, U.S.P. Percomorph liver oil Oleovitamin D, synthetic, U.S.P.				Bland tasting, light yellow, oily liquid.
Vitamin E (eggs, milk, whole grains, wheat germ, leafy vegetables)	To treat abortion, thrombosis, muscular dystrophy, symptoms of menopause.	Seldom any side effects or contraindications.		The deficiency in animals has been established but not the specific results in man.
Tocopherols, mixed concentrate (Esprolin, Gelseals, Toxafin, Vitamin E Concentrate			10-200 mg. Oral or I. M.	

(Table 31–17 continues on the opposite page.)

TABLE 31–17. DRUGS WHICH AFFECT NUTRITION AND GROWTH (Continued)

DRUG	USE	REACTION	DOSAGE – ADMINISTRATION	REMARKS
Vitamin K Fat soluble. Two forms: Vitamin K1 Vitamin K2	Aids in blood clotting to prevent hemorrhage and control tendency to bleed.	Seldom shows toxic reactions.	Dosage varies.	
Vitamin K-5 (Synkamin) Menadiol sodium diphosphate, U.S.P. (Kappadione) (Synkayvite)			Oral or parenteral.	
Menadione, U.S.P. (Kappaxin) (Kayklot)			Oral or parenteral.	
Menadione sodium bisulfite, U.S.P. (Hykinone)			Oral or parenteral.	
Vitamin P Water soluble. A substance from paprika and lemon peel.	To treat the condition of blood escaping from the vessels into the tissues (increased capillary permeability).			
Rutin, N.F.		No evidence of toxicity.	20–50 mg. Oral	Usually accompanied by ascorbic acid.
Panothenic Acid Calcium pantothenate, U.S.P. (Pantholine) (Panthoject)	For types of neurologic disorders, irritability, and skin disorders.	Seldom causes side effects.	250–500 mg. P.R.N. I.M.	Also comes in oral preparation. (Pantholin).
Biotin (Vitamin H)	Thought to be necessary for cell metabolism. Knowledge of deficiencies in man is lacking.		Dosages have not been established.	Thought to be "manufactured" by bacteria in the intestines.
Choline	Thought to be necessary for cell metabolism. Aids B12 and folic acid in proper liver function to prevent "fatty liver," hemorrhage, and death of liver tissue.		Dosages have not been established.	
Inositol	Thought to help the removal of fats from the liver.		Dosages have not been established.	

(Table 31–17 continues on the following page.)

TABLE 31–17. DRUGS WHICH AFFECT NUTRITION AND GROWTH (Continued)

DRUG	USE	REACTION	DOSAGE – ADMINISTRATION	REMARKS
Minerals *Calcium and phosphorus*	To treat disorders of bones and teeth, during pregnancy, tetany, and some disorders of mucous membranes and nerves.			
Calcium gluconate, U.S.P.			Oral and I.V.	
Calcium glycerophosphate, N.F.			Oral.	
Calcium lactate, U.S.P.			Oral.	
Dibasic calcium phosphate, U.S.P.			Oral.	
Calcium chloride, N.F.			I.V. 5% aqueous solution.	Very irritating to tissues.
Iodine See Table 31-16.				
Iron See Table 31-11.				

Table 31–18 SOME DRUGS FOR SPECIFIC CONDITIONS

Some drugs are known as specific treatment for certain disorders and diseases. As noted in the *Reaction* column, they influence the body and body systems in many ways.

DRUG	USE	REACTION	DOSAGE–ADMINISTRATION	REMARKS
Protamide U.S.P.	For herpes zoster, neuritis, chicken pox, tabes dorsalis	Sensitivity may occur.	Usually twice a week, I.M.	
Ephedrine Sulfate U.S.P.	To treat asthma, allergies, myesthenia gravis, increases hypotension, to dilate eye pupil.	Increases rate and strength of heart beats, increases blood pressure, sweating, palpitation, anxiety.	25–50 mg. q̄ 3–4 h. p. r. n. Oral, 3% solution. Topical.	Also paranteral preparations.
Ambenomium Chloride, N. F. (Mytelase, Mysuran)	For myesthenia gravis (exhaustion of voluntary muscles).	Signs of overdose vary: epigastric distress, abdominal cramps, urinary urgency, diarrhea, vomiting, pallor, excessive salivation.	Oral dosage individualized; every 3 or 4 hrs.	Oral absorption good. Long duration of action. Amount of activity influences dosage requirements.
Desipramine hydrochloride, N. F. (Norpramin Petrofrane).	For depression due to psychogenic origin.	Works rather quickly; mouth dryness, sweating, dizziness, constipation.	25–50 mg. t.i.d. Oral	Prolonged use usually means that liver and blood should be tested for toxicity.
Levodopa (Dopar, Larodopa)	Parkinson's disease to relieve rigidity and slowness of movement. Sometimes helps tremors and swallowing difficulty.	High incidence of untoward reactions.	Dosage individualized.	Great care is taken by the physician to determine whether or not to use. Patient usually hospitalized to start treatment.
Chlorphenoxamine (Phenoxine)	For allergies and Parkinson's disease.	Drowsiness, dryness of mouth and the throat, gastrointestinal distress, insomnia, nausea, vomiting.	20–40 mg. q.i.d. Oral. May be a delayed action tablet and taken once or twice a day.	Patient cautioned about driving a car.
Carbamazepine (Tegretol)	For pain due to trigeminal neuralgia called tic douloureux.	Used cautiously with patients with cardiac difficulties. Dizziness, drowsiness.	200–1200 mg. every 24 hours.	A powerful drug used with caution. Complete blood and platelet counts should be done early and frequently.
Glacagon, U. S. P.	Given for hypoglycemic coma (any cause).	Increases the concentration of blood glucose. Excessive dosage may cause hyperglycemia.	0.5–2 mg. Parenteral	Dosage individualized. Overdosage may require insulin treatment.

SUMMARY

There is no one best way to group drugs to study them. They are grouped according to the disease being treated, the part of the body involved, the symptoms to be relieved, the results they produce, and so forth. A drug given for one purpose may have additional therapeutic side effects, as well as unwanted side effects or untoward reactions. The two main factors in drug administration are *accuracy* and *meaningful observations before, during, and following the giving of the drug*. Because it is impossible to "know all about drugs," current source materials should be used and help should be sought when indicated. Nothing should be left to chance. Knowledge of and skill in drug administration expands and develops through careful practice.

GUIDES FOR STUDY AND DISCUSSION

1. What is meant by the following: the therapeutic reaction of a drug, an untoward reaction, a local reaction, and a systemic reaction?

2. Make a list of as many sources of drug information as you can find.

3. Make a list of drugs to suit your learning needs. Check it with your teacher for adequacy. Learn how to spell each name and know (in general terms) the use of each.

4. What observations do you make prior to giving a drug? During the giving? Following it?

5. Why is it difficult to keep up-to-date with drug information? What can be done (by a nurse) to try and keep up-to-date?

6. What is each? Give an example.

    a. sedative
    b. analgesic
    c. tranquilizer
    d. antipyretic
    e. nebulizer
    f. cathartic
    g. disinfectant
    h. astringent
    i. vasodilator
    j. vasoconstrictor
    k. antacids

    l. anticoagulant
    m. emetic
    n. antiemetic
    o. expectorant
    p. diuretic
    q. mydriatic
    r. miotic
    s. hormone
    t. vitamin
    u. diaphoretic
    v. anti-infective

7. What must an L.P.N. do to protect the patient and herself when responsible for drug administration?

8. There is a difference in depth of observations made by the L.P.N. and the R.N. or physician. How might they differ?

SUGGESTED SITUATIONS AND ACTIVITIES

1. Select one patient you are caring for and list the drugs ordered for him; describe (in general terms) the purpose of each drug. Are there any in your list a practical nurse would not administer? If so, what are they? Why would you not administer them?

2. Select one of the tables in this chapter and compare the drugs listed with those used for the same purpose in your hospital.

3. Prepare a classroom exhibit of source materials for drug information. Find out what source materials are available in the clinical situation.

4. Prepare a visual aid to point up an important factor in observation as it relates to drug administration.

NURSING CARE IN GENERAL

This unit introduces you to the patient and *uses him as the reason for the care given.* The focus is on the patient and his ten daily living needs. These ten needs provide a way for you to learn how to plan for and provide patient-centered nursing care for any patient at any age. Diseases are not in the forefront in order to give you time to learn what is meant by "daily living needs" and how you use them to give assistance to the patient *according to his need for assistance* (i.e., dependent or more independent).

To help you move into the development of nursing skills in an orderly manner, the ten basic needs approach is used first with the most independent patient—the ambulatory patient. Next it is used with a bed patient who is "mildly" ill—more dependent upon the nurse for some types of assistance. Following that, the ten basic needs approach is used with the seriously ill patient (very dependent upon the nurse for assistance) where you will see Role II activities appear for the LPN. This same approach is then used with the long-term patient followed by its use with the elderly patient. Each step of the way the ten basic needs are used to size-up the individual patient, his need for assistance and a plan for his care. It is a gradual approach moving from the more simple nursing situations toward the more complex ones.

The last chapter discusses responsibilities in caring for the patient prior to and following death.

CHAPTER 32

MEETING DAILY NEEDS OF PATIENTS

OBJECTIVES FOR THE STUDENT: Be able to:

1. Compare the basic needs of a well person and a sick person by showing what is different.
2. Describe one patient circumstance for each basic need which could influence how nursing care would be provided.
3. Explain this statement: "All patients have common basic needs regardless of age."
4. Tell why the patient needs to feel confident about his care.
5. Give two examples of nursing actions which indicate "personalized care."
6. Name at least four workers involved in providing total patient care.

SUGGESTED STUDY VOCABULARY*

confidence
fatigue
nutrition
privacy
nursing need

physiological functioning
habit
disoriented
contractures

atmospheric conditions
muscle tone
unconscious
diversion
rehabilitation

---

*Look for any terms you already know.

INTRODUCTION

This chapter could be called the "nursing foundation" chapter because the ten basic needs approach to nursing care presented here is useful in every patient situation regardless of age or degree of infirmity. It furnishes you a tool to learn how to plan and provide nursing care. To say it another way—the ten basic needs approach is a structure for learning how to personalize patient care.

The basic needs approach is somewhat

familiar to you. Return to Figure 22–1 and review the list of nine essential needs for health. Compare that list with the ten essential needs for any patient (Fig. 32–1). A quick glance points up the noticeable fact that the basic needs remain about the same. The key difference comes in *how* the person meets these needs when he is sick. He needs assistance to take care of his basic needs because he is unable to meet them the same way he does when he is well or independent. *When you "nurse" a patient you assist him.* You help him do what he is unable to do for himself.

The purpose of this chapter is to furnish you with a structure for assisting patients; it is based on *10 daily needs* common to all patients regardless of age. Each basic need is described with some simple examples of things which can influence the assistance needed.

The ten daily needs approach is useful knowledge you can apply later when you study the nursing needs of mothers and newborn infants, sick children, the disabled elderly patient, the sick adolescent, the young or middle-aged adult, the mentally ill person, or the large category of patients commonly called "the medical-surgical patients."

Some factors about the patient cause you to alter how you assist him; these can be called "modifying factors."

Most important in assisting patients is your ability to establish confidence. A patient needs to feel confident that he is getting what he needs and, besides that, he needs to feel that the person(s) giving him assistance cares about him and his well-being.

THE MEANING OF TOTAL PATIENT CARE

It is difficult to say exactly when and how all of a patient's needs are met. In nursing, we do know that there is *far more* to a patient's well-being than his daily personal hygiene, the food tray, elimination, and a chart that reads "Slept well" and recites the long list of drugs received. More and more is being said about other factors which personalize his care, rehabilitate him, and return him to society at his best. An individualized approach to him, his

need for assistance and his seemingly "hidden needs" is beginning to appear. This may be due in part to the patient's plea for attention. He wants somebody in authority to care about him and his plight; he wants to sense or feel *that caring*, even when he realizes every one is very busy and there are many other patients to care for. This is not as unreasonable as it may seem when you first think about it. Recall your last illness. If it kept you in bed, you appreciated the attention given to your necessities, and more than that you especially liked the feeling of someone who showed he was concerned about you as well as cared for you. This calls to mind the influence of relationships, those invisible elements which flow back and forth between patient and nurse.

Bringing totalness to patient care involves more than the nurse. Others must be involved, but the nurse is just about the most important person at hand to see that good care happens. She is in the situation more than other workers and consequently can make a great deal of difference in the overall patient care. Providing totalness takes the person-patient into account—his individual differences, age, likes, dislikes, disability, dependence, independence, habits, beliefs, anxieties, complaints, and peculiarities. Knowledge of these things, seasoned with appropriate good judgment, is used in planning and giving assistance.

To date, progress in this direction has been slow because nursing the whole person—the patient—requires new thinking and a shift in emphasis from the procedure-disease thinking habit in nursing to a broader view of all needs the patient presents. This view recognizes that a nurse cannot be all things to a patient; she can do only so much in meeting his needs, and then gets help for those needs which are better met by others. By recognizing the patient's needs, she brings "totality" to his care, though she herself may provide only a part of that care.

TEN GENERAL DAILY NEEDS

The following general daily needs are essential to all patients:
1. Personal Care and Hygiene
2. Sleep and Rest
3. Nutrition and Fluids

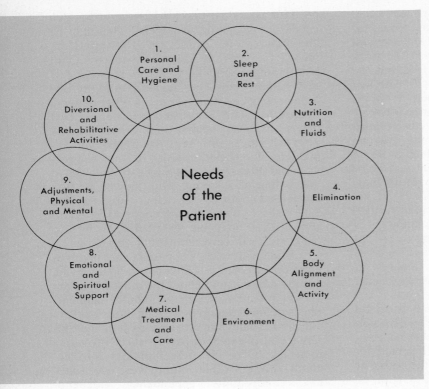

FIGURE 32–1 Essential daily nursing needs of any patient.

4. Elimination
5. Body Alignment and Activity
6. Environment
7. Medical Treatment and Care
8. Emotional and Spiritual Support
9. Adjustments, Physical and Mental
10. Diversional and Rehabilitative Activities

A nursing *need* may be thought of as any requirement or want of the patient; it may be physical, emotional, or spiritual in nature. The safety, comfort, and well-being of the patient depend upon how effectively these needs are met. *All nursing* is concerned with these needs (see Fig. 32–1). Each one is discussed briefly to point out what it is and how it influences the patient's well-being.

Personal Care and Hygiene

All patients require daily nursing care for personal hygiene. This includes bathing and care of the skin, mouth, hair, and nails. For some patients, it may be necessary for the nurse to give most of this care; for other pa-

tients, the nurse may give only a part, or very little, if the patient can care for himself. Others will require no direct help at all from the nurse with their bathing and grooming; self-care will help them to become or remain more independent.

Most patients have regular habits for bathing and care of the mouth and hair. Being able to follow these habits, they enjoy their normal feeling of cleanliness. Careful personal care also protects the patient against infection by keeping the skin clean and in good condition. Safety measures are used to protect the patient, whether he is caring for himself or is cared for by others. If a patient brings his own toilet articles, clothing, and accessories with him, they should be used, if possible, and handled properly.

Sleep and Rest

Adequate rest and sleep are even more necessary in illness than in health. A certain amount of rest and sleep must be provided to prevent undue fatigue, to repair worn tissues, and to rest body organs. The patient's need for sleep will depend upon his age, habits, and physical condition. Additional rest and sleep may be very important to the recovery of the patient.

Certain factors help to promote rest and sleep. Usually the patient will be able to get sufficient sleep if he is *relaxed* and *comfortable*, both *physically* and *emotionally*. The condition of the bed, the position of the patient, the control of unnecessary noise and light, proper ventilation, and relief from pain help the patient to relax. Acquainting the new patient with his surroundings and answering his general questions may often be all that is necessary for him to feel secure enough to sleep.

Nutrition and Fluids

The role of nutrition in relation to health and disease is considered in Unit Six. All patients have specific requirements for food and fluid, and their recovery may depend upon proper food and fluid intake as much as or more than upon anything else.

Being able to wash the hands before eating, the attractiveness of the tray, and the choice and preparation of the food are some of the factors which help patients enjoy their meals.

Certain foods or diets are prepared according to the physician's orders and are related to the physical condition of the patient. Fluids and nutrients may be limited or increased in quantity or kind. Observance of any religious beliefs and practices is important to the patient's peace of mind.

Although the practical nurse may not cook the food or even serve the tray, she may feed the patient. Observing appetite and appropriateness of food in relation to the patient's ability to chew or his acceptance or rejection of food, and deciding how to be most helpful during mealtime are other practical nurse responsibilities.

Certain physical and esthetic elements play an important part in helping to improve food habits, increase the appetite, and bolster the mental and emotional well-being of the patient. They include an attractive tray served in surroundings free from unpleasant sights, sounds, and odors and one that is convenient for him to use if feeding himself.

Elimination

Body function, diet, fluids, temperature, exercise, habits, privacy, pain, discomfort, and surroundings all may affect the patient's elimination.

The safety and comfort of the patient depend upon the observations of the nurse and how she uses care to prevent injury and complications. For instance, the bedpan that is clean, in good condition, and used with proper care will help to protect the skin against injury and possible infection or irritation. Careful attention to promptness and the provision for privacy necessarily help any patient feel more comfortable about using the bedpan or urinal.

Needs for elimination vary with age and physical condition. The very young are unconcerned; the disoriented may be unaware, while the oriented but very sick person may be helpless to control these body processes. Patients' attitudes toward this basic need will also vary. Some people worry about bowel elimination; others have never concerned themselves with regularity or irregularity. Illness may help the patient understand better the meaning of normal elimination and the importance of good bowel habits.

Body Alignment and Activity

Good body alignment (standing) is present when body segments squarely rest upon one another. Body alignment for the bed patient keeps the body segments in line and supported to maintain that alignment; it further means that there should be nothing to interfere with proper alignment such as bed covers that are so tight over the toes that they cause foot drop. Proper alignment helps the body (sick or well) perform its functions better (e.g., breathing, balance, elimination, sleep, etc.).

Safe nursing care includes attention to the body alignment of the patient whether he is ambulatory or in bed. Unless the circumstances are unusual, there is likely to be no physician's order for this nursing action; therefore you will be expected to help the patient maintain proper body alignment to the best of his ability to do so. A change in position, raising the back rest, or placing a pillow roll under the knees are examples of nursing measures which may be needed to provide for proper body alignment and to afford comfort to the patient. Turning and changing the position of the helpless patient not only help to make him more comfortable but also help to prevent fatigue and protect him against complications. Change of position furnishes some exercise and joint motion to prevent loss of muscle tone and the development of contractures, such as foot drop.

Environment

A patient's surroundings are related to his health and well being. At home or in the hospital his immediate surroundings need to be clean, quiet, attractive, comfortable, and convenient for his needs.

One could broaden the meaning of this basic need to include oxygen because it certainly is essential to life; however, it becomes a treatment when ordered by the physician and as such it is discussed as oxygen therapy in Chapter 42.

A clean environment, the room and its furnishings, helps to protect the patient from disease infection and to promote recovery.

The control of temperature and ventilation in the patient's room affects his safety and comfort. The room temperature that is too high or too low can be uncomfortable and even detrimental. Fresh air, or a change of air, in the room is refreshing and helps the patient rest or sleep better. Properly regulated light, natural or artificial, is needed. Some patients have definite preferences concerning the amount of light they want or like. In a ward with several beds, solving this problem takes good judgment.

A quiet, attractive environment helps the patient relax and rest. Unnecessary sounds or noise are disturbing to most people and during illness they are more so. Most noise is caused by carelessness and can be prevented. Patients often complain of noise in the hospital.

The arrangement and order of a room can make for attractiveness as well as contribute to the convenience and safety of the patient. Chairs, tables, lights, wastebaskets, and personal belongings of the patient should be placed for his convenience and comfort. A chair that is too far away or a signal light that is out of reach may be the cause of a fall, an injury, or both. Color, odors, flowers, and the general order to the room affect some patients. They can be quite unhappy and uncomfortable until adjustments are made. A room that is adequately furnished, is clean and in good order, has correct atmospheric conditions, and that provides for use of some of the patient's personal belongings will usually be sufficient.

Environment takes on much importance during illness. Because the practical nurse has many responsibilities for various aspects of the patient's environment, Chapter 33 discusses this need in detail.

Medical Treatment and Care

The physician prescribes or orders the things he wishes the patient to receive. For example, he wants the patient to receive a certain diet, specific medications or treatments, and he writes the order(s) on the "order sheet" in the patient's chart. The nursing staff carries out these orders in a manner helpful to promoting the results sought by the physician.

All patients have some medical orders; they are under the care of physicians in the hospital who prescribe specific things to aid recovery, to determine diagnosis, to prevent complications, or to keep the patient comfortable if recovery is not possible.

Emotional and Spiritual Support

Personalized nursing care includes consideration for the patient's feelings of worry, loneliness, and uncertainty about himself and what might happen to him. The manner in which these needs are recognized and handled has much to do with the patient's frame of mind and his peace of mind. If these needs are overlooked or disregarded, the patient may well become quietly upset within himself or openly disagreeable.

The patient's emotional and spiritual needs are often closely related. Sickness has a way of sometimes bringing a patient's feelings out in the open and if uncertainties occupy his mind, he may express the need to talk with someone about them. Careful observation may reveal the names of people the patient wishes to see. These observations should be called to the attention of the charge nurse.

His religious habits and practices should be respected and opportunity provided for carrying them out, if possible. It is often much easier to recognize and meet the physical needs of the patient than to recognize and meet his emotional and spiritual needs.

Adjustments, Physical and Mental

Any patient with a disability or illness condition has certain physical and mental adjustments to make, whether he is at home or in the hospital. Some of these are closely related, and one adjustment may involve another.

Illness limits a person's "world." The patient must rely upon others and, in many respects, fit into their schedule. He realizes he is living in a scheduled existence (unless he is too young, disoriented, or unconscious) and that a schedule is essential, but the patient is apt to accept these facts in a better frame of mind if he knows what to expect. For example, most patients ask some of the following questions about daily activities: When are the meals served? Do I have any choice in selecting my menu? When are visiting hours? When does my doctor usually make rounds? When is mail delivered? Do I have to use a bedpan? Can't I get up and go to the bathroom? Do I have to wear this hospital gown?

The patient who "fusses" about too much regimentation (things too well organized for him) *needs* to have someone listen to him. People usually adjust to regimented living in one manner or another. They try to find out what to expect and ask questions of almost any personnel who come their way. The answers they receive may or may not be accurate.

By listening to the patient, you can often obtain clues to his needs; frequently some simple, thoughtful act on your part satisfies his need. This goes back to the nurse's ability to establish confidence.

Diversional and Rehabilitative Activities

Complete care of the patient gives attention to the need for certain activities which will divert his attention, help in his recovery, or help him make an adjustment to his limitations.

Many activities of the average person's day are recreational in nature, that is, they serve "to refresh strength and spirit after toil." Patients need recreation too. This need is supported by diverting attention and energies into purposeful activities (conversation, listening to the radio or television, reading, handicrafts, writing, or developing a bedside or room interest such as plants or an aquarium) which pass the time and hold their interest.

Age, individual differences and interests, and physical and mental capacities or incapacities all enter into the selection of suitable diversional activities. Keep in mind that for some patients, doing even a simple act may be very rewarding.

Rehabilitative activity is a selected act aimed at restoring a specific function to its former capacity, if possible. The physician prescribes activities (planned therapy) which aid in the patient's recovery. Sometimes there is full recovery; sometimes partial recovery is all that can be gained.

Persons specially trained in rehabilitative therapies include the physical therapist, occupational therapist, and recreational therapist. Large hospitals usually have some or all such therapists on their staffs as well as special "departments" or facilities.

In the home or the hospital where there is no provision for the trained recreational, occupational, or physical therapy worker, the nurse may be responsible for carrying out a program of activities planned by the physician.

Encouragement from the nurse very often aids the patient's recovery by helping him to be as independent as possible during his illness. This may be especially true in the nursing care of the child, the aged, or the patient with a long-term illness or a severe physical handicap.

MAIN FACTORS WHICH DETERMINE PATIENT CARE

Although all patients have essentially the same basic needs, the nursing care required to meet one individual's specific needs may be quite different from the nursing care given to the patient in the next bed. Many conditions or factors modify the way the patient's needs are met. Some of them are discussed briefly to help you understand why it is necessary to *plan* each patient's care. Methods of giving safe care are based on certain facts which guide the nurse's actions. As long as the nurse observes these guidelines, she can safely modify or adjust her actions to suit the patient's needs. The practical nurse will need to discuss modifications with the charge nurse prior to making changes if there are any questions in her mind.

Nursing care (planning for it and carrying it out) is always influenced by:
Medical Management
Disease and Illness Conditions
Situation Conditions
Personal Facts
The Patient's State of Dependency

Medical Management

The physician's orders for the treatment and care of the patient are factors in determining the nursing needs of any patient. It is easy to understand that nursing care would be influenced if the physician ordered restricted fluids for one patient on complete bed rest and forced fluids with the temperature taken every hour for another patient who also was on complete bed rest. The bath, diet, position, activity, and even the environmental conditions may be affected by the orders of the physician treating the patient.

Disease and Illness Conditions

The patient's disorder influences the type of nursing care required. For example, a patient with a communicable disease is nursed under conditions quite different from a patient with a non-communicable disease. A blind patient needs types of assistance a seeing patient does not. A disorder affecting breathing may necessitate having certain equipment available at the bedside, or require that the patient be kept in a particular position.

The duration of the illness alters nursing care needs; therefore, meticulous attention to skin care and turning the patient may be the most important assistance the nurse can give the patient.

Situation Conditions

Certain life situations may influence both immediate and long-range patient needs. The patient who has been injured in an accident has nursing needs different from one whose illness has not been so abrupt or unexpected. Lifesaving measures command first attention. Prevention of shock, control of hemorrhage, and avoidance of further injury are of first importance. The type and extent of the injury influence the patient's physical and emotional reactions. The possible loss of sight or a limb could be a severe emotional, as well as physical, shock. Accidents require extreme adjustments on the part of the victim. Total nursing care takes this into account. Sometimes there are legal complications; patients worry about suing or being sued.

The season of the year or the region of the country, with differences in seasonal conditions, may also alter the nursing needs of the patient. Such conditions may influence the temperature of the room or the visits of relatives.

While daily basic needs are the same, regardless of where the patient finds himself, the nursing care to fulfill those needs may differ. The patient who is at home, for instance, may have no difficulty sleeping and resting. Being at home in quiet, familiar surroundings with members of his family may be enough to promote sleep without medication. The greatest need for the aging patient in a nursing home may be diversional and recreational activity and purposeful living rather than daily "front porch complaining."

Personal Facts

There are certain individual circumstances about every patient, over and above his illness condition, which may have a bearing on how his total nursing needs are met. They include age, sex, marital status, race, nationality, religious practices, beliefs, and economic and social status. To individualize the care a patient receives, the practical nurse will need to have some general information. She should seek help from the nurse in charge to determine some information about the patient if it is not available through observation or on the chart. Great care should be used to avoid the impression of prying into personal facts or misusing information.

The *only* reason for gathering any personal facts about a patient is to enable you to personalize his care; knowing about him will guide your actions and will improve your judgment in listening, observing, and planning his care. Here again, patient confidence is involved. Respect for the individual (his habits, expressed wishes, right to privacy, etc.) is displayed through your manner of planning and carrying out his care.

The Patient's State of Dependency

The patient's state of dependency or independency affects the total plan for meeting his needs. Consider these two contrasting situations: A bath is usually considered a daily need under ordinary circumstances. If the patient is ambulatory, he may well be able to take his own bath and require little direct attention from the nurse. If the patient is in bed with a "complete bed rest" order on his chart, the nursing care plan will provide sufficient time (and skill) to give the patient his bath and prevent undue patient fatigue as well. In the first instance, the patient is reasonably independent of the need for "on the spot" nurse assistance; in the second situation, the patient is entirely dependent upon skilled assistance. In both instances the need is the same—a bath.

Keep in mind, too, that a patient's state of dependency may not remain the same hour after hour or day after day. Consider how dependency changes in these situations and how nursing plans are affected as well as who gets involved: An ambulatory patient has been convalescing well, when suddenly his condition worsens critically and he is moved to the intensive care unit. A patient has just been moved from the operating room to the recovery room still under the influence of a general anesthetic; one day later he has bathroom privileges. A 25-year-old male patient is making a good recovery from an accident which requires that his right arm be put in a cast below the elbow to the wrist and his left leg in traction. He is feeling better every day and wants to do all he can for himself even though use of his right arm is limited and his left leg is in traction.

In each of these three examples, "change" in patient dependency is evident. The first patient became immediately dependent upon highly skilled personnel and lifesaving equipment. The second moved from complete dependence (in fact, unconsciousness) to bathroom privileges within 24 hours. The third gradually moved toward independence, hampered only by a cast and by traction which kept him in bed.

Think about the newborn and his state of dependency to give you further evidence of need for assistance and how dependency or independency of the patient influences what you do to assist him.

PLANNING DAILY NURSING CARE

So far in this chapter, a 10-part structure for approaching nursing care has been discussed. This structure is built upon 10 daily needs of patients; we know, too, that these basic daily needs during illness are not too different from daily needs during health. The difference comes in how they are met and what adjustments are made due to age, physician's orders, and the state of dependence or independence of the patient. You are now aware that patients have common needs, but one might say that at this point "commonness" ceases; now the nurse has to consider "the person-patient" and his individuality and uniqueness. This requires planning based upon knowledge of "Who is *this* patient?" "What are his age, state of dependence or independence, disorder, physician's orders for medical management, likes and dislikes, family attachments, and beliefs and feelings?

Personalized care requires planning. It is not enough to know *about* a patient. You need to know *what to do* with the facts you have gathered. This requires planning or scheduling your assistance to the patient.

In the work situation as a licensed practical nurse, you will be called upon to provide assistance to several patients during a tour of duty. In fact, the several become many at particular times during the 24-hour schedule. For instance, during the night hours there are not as many personnel on duty; therefore, responsibilities for patient care are generally arranged in a manner different from the daytime hours. During the night, presumably patients are asleep or resting and activities are at a minimum. Yet observation and needed care never cease.

Following are some guidelines which will be helpful in planning and carrying out patient care.

1. Get acquainted with the facts about each patient for whom you are responsible. Ask yourself, "Who is this patient? What are his special needs?"

2. In particular, *know* the physician's orders for his medical management. Be certain you understand which orders are your responsibility. Pay close attention to orders which have a "time" element involved. Clarify any

questions you have; in other words, *be sure you understand your responsibilities*.

3. Take time to look over your total assignment once you have acquainted yourself with the needs of each patient. Arrange what you are going to do into a logical schedule or order. First, write down all those things which include a time element so they will be placed appropriately in your plan. Next, continue planning by listing activities (some may have a written order, some may not) which must be carried out for and with each patient *in light of his needs*. Be guided by such things as:

a. Painful or disagreeable treatments should *follow* mealtime whenever possible.

b. Patients able to do some or all things for themselves need your early attention so they can proceed while you are working with others.

c. Patients who are slow, tire easily, or are hesitant (even resistant) need more time either alone to work at their own ease or with your assistance.

d. All patients need to feel that the nurse is available. Your presence is important, even if it is only for a few minutes to get them started or to let them know when you plan to return. This helps them know what to expect.

e. Acquaint yourself with a procedure before you start it. You will save time and effort in assembling materials, carrying it out, observing the essential things, and cleaning up afterwards. It may be something that should be completed *before* the bath and *before* the bed is changed, e.g., a cleansing enema. It could be something which is more appropriately done during the bath or after the bath.

f. Keep in mind your responsibilities for providing patient safety and privacy as you carry out your plan.

g. Organize materials and patient environment so that he can help himself (if he can and should) or for you to help the patient in a manner to his liking and comfort.

h. Learn to relate to your patient in a manner so that you will "be well-received"; do this by using your knowledge of what makes good relationships. Assess what you do in this respect so that you will improve with practice.

i. By all means try to stick to your schedule, if possible; however, when adjustments need to be made, make them and proceed from there. Ability to make adjustments improves with practice as you become more secure in what you do and how to judge your time.

j. Report unusual observations at once. Report or record other pertinent observations and information as soon as possible after completion of activities so that other personnel using the patient's chart will have this information to use if needed.

k. Compare your plan with the manner in which you carried it out. How could you have improved upon it? What were its strengths? Its weaknesses? What factors interfered? What could you have done to prevent this interference? What have you learned from this experience that will make your plan more effective next time?

Guide for any Nursing Procedure

Some nursing measures require a physician's written order before they are carried out; many other nursing measures require no "order" as such, but are part of every patient's care. Regardless of whether the procedure is one requiring a physician's order or not, the nurse can use the following guides or "standards" to assess effectiveness of either type of nursing measure.

1. Provide safety for the patient, the nurse, and any others involved. Accuracy and correctness of action protect against injury, infection, error, and poor results.

2. Achieve effective and desired results. Know what the measure is supposed to do (what are the desired results). Observe during and following to see if desired results were achieved. If not successful, decide why not.

3. Provide the greatest possible comfort to the patient without the prevention of desired results, as described above. Often the effectiveness of results depends upon the physical and mental comfort of the patient.

a. Prepare patient—inform him about the procedure, provide for his privacy.

b. Allow sufficient time.

c. Carry out at appropriate time.

d. Carry out measure accurately (i.e., position, time, temperature, solution or materials, proper equipment, etc.).

4. Provide for economy of time, effort, and materials, yet do not deny any safety, comfort, or effectiveness factors in the process.

SUMMARY

All patients have the same basic needs of personal care and hygiene, sleep and rest, food and fluids, elimination, physical comfort in desirable surroundings, and the need to feel secure and be respected as people. Medications and treatments are usually required also.

Patients need to make adjustments to illness, hospitalization, staying in bed, or being incapacitated. The nurse can do many simple yet thoughtful things to help the patient accept his infirmity and cooperate fully in the nursing care plan for his recovery.

Basic needs of patients are met in many ways. The nurse adapts her care to the patient according to his age, sex, and illness condition and gives consideration to him as a person who is ill rather than as a disease to be treated or a surgical condition to mend.

Personalized nursing care requires planning. The licensed practical nurse needs the ability to plan because she carried responsibility for many types of patient-oriented functions and tasks during a "tour of duty." To make full use of time, to consider the patient's unique needs, and to carry out nursing measures with safety, comfort and effectiveness, a well-planned schedule is necessary. The ability to do this improves with practice.

Each patient is unique, yet somewhat like every other patient. Skillful nursing takes the individual patient into consideration first and adapts nursing measures to meet his needs next. Patients like to feel they are receiving special attention, and they will be if their nursing care is planned with them in mind.

GUIDES FOR STUDY AND DISCUSSION

1. Copy the following chart in your notebook. Leave enough space so you can add information as you go along.

Needs of the Patient	Facts Worth Remembering
Personal Care and Hygiene	
Sleep and Rest	
Nutrition and Fluids	
Elimination	
Body Alignment and Activity	
Environment	
Medical Treatment and Care	
Emotional and Spiritual Support	
Adjustments, Physical and Mental	
Diversional and Rehabilitative Activities	

2. Factors which modify nursing care: In addition to the examples given, see how many more you can think of under each heading.

Medical Management　　　　　　　*Situation Conditions*
Disease and Illness Conditions　　　*Personal Facts*
Patient's State of Dependency

3. The nurse is with the patient more than most other health workers. Who are some of the other workers? Why is the patient apt to depend upon the nurse more than the others?

4. Imagine you are helping a 40 year old female patient with her bed bath. This is the first time you have helped this patient. What could you do to help her have confidence in you?

5. If patients have common daily needs, what is it that makes their care different?

6. If a patient is worried about his sickness and asks you questions you cannot or should not attempt to answer, what should you do to help him?

7. Why do you need to know some things about your patient? Where do you get this information? Once you have this information, how do you use it?

SUGGESTED SITUATIONS AND ACTIVITIES

1. You have a means (10 basic needs) for learning how to "personalize" patient care. Visit two patients for the purpose of looking for factors which could influence how their basic needs are met in the hospital (i.e., a patient in traction—how would that factor influence his basic needs and assistance from the nurse?) After you have visited the patients, use a list of the ten basic needs to make notes about what would (might) need to be considered in planning the nursing care for each patient.

2. Choose any patient illustration in the text for this activity. Plan some diversional activity for this patient, Be ready to explain why you selected what you did and how you would proceed to get the patient involved in it.

CHAPTER 33

NURSING RESPONSIBILITIES FOR THE PATIENT'S ENVIRONMENT

TOPICAL HEADINGS

Introduction
Factors Related to
  the Environment
The Patient's Room
  and Unit

Preparation and Care
  of the Patient's
  Environment
Bedmaking
Summary

Guides for Study and
  Discussion
Suggested Situations
  and Activities

OBJECTIVES FOR THE STUDENT: Be able to:

1. Name nine environmental factors which influence the patient's well-being.
2. Give three examples of environmental situations which could be upsetting to the patient.
3. Explain why precautions must be taken in caring for the environment.
4. List the equipment usually found in the patient's unit; the supplies.
5. Describe a situation which shows how nurse action concerning environment can strengthen patient confidence.
6. Write four safety rules useful in protecting patient environment.
7. Distinguish between daily cleaning of a patient unit and terminal cleaning.
8. Tell what the well-made bed provides for the patient.
9. Support this statement: regardless of the size of a bed or its use, certain guidelines apply to all bedmaking; name five such guidelines.

SUGGESTED STUDY VOCABULARY*

environment
manipulate
esthetic
disposable

humidity
privacy
hazardous
multiple bed units

emesis basin
dentures
organic matter
diversional materials

*Look for any terms you already know.

INTRODUCTION

The word "environ" means to form a ring around or surround. The word *environment*, as used here, includes the things (not people) that surround or encircle patients. We recognize that people influence environment in a broader sense through relationships and interaction, but this chapter concerns itself with things rather than people insofar as this is possible.

The word "esthetic" is often used to describe desirable surroundings for patients. Here, esthetic means in good taste, appealing and appropriate for sick people. It is a known fact that a patient can be favorably influenced by pleasant, comfortable surroundings; they can make him feel less anxious about the situation as he thinks of his safety and comfort. The patient can imagine, "If personnel are this careful about my unit and room, they are careful in the other things they do for me too."

This chapter discusses, in some detail, various things you can do about environment. In fact, you will have considerable responsibility for maintaining safe, comfortable, and clean patient surroundings. Environmental "things" include furnishings that are clean, convenient, and comfortable; proper light and ventilation; control of the noise factor; and all aspects of safety. You need to know what the factors in a patient's "world" are so that you can carry your responsibilities in helping to maintain it in a suitable manner.

FACTORS RELATED TO THE ENVIRONMENT

In today's hospital, maintaining the physical environment is a shared responsibility. Housekeeping departments and maintenance departments take care of regular cleaning, and general repair. Heating, cooling, and ventilating buildings belong to the engineering department. The nursing staff will, in some circumstances, call attention to specific things needing repair, cleaning or inspection (e.g., broken equipment, faulty plumbing, dirty floors). Likewise, the nursing department may be required to supervise housekeeping activities at certain times or places. Perhaps most important to remember is the fact that there are instances when the nurse herself must participate in cleaning and in orderliness because safety factors are involved. In other words, a situation may be hazardous if ignored or left to be remedied by other personnel who are not immediately available.

Nine environmental factors which relate to the patient's well-being are *temperature, humidity, air circulation, lighting, odor, noise, orderliness, privacy* and *safety*.

Indoor climate control is a reality in the most modern hospital building. It provides for the first three environmental needs: air is freshened, heated, cooled, and its moisture content is controlled. Individual rooms have their own controls to permit adjustments. In older buildings or in some regions climate control is not as specific. Heating systems are provided and individual cooling units may be used. Open window ventilation is still popular, either by necessity or choice.

Temperature

Patient response to temperature varies. Room temperatures ranging between 68 and 72° F. are comfortable for most people. Certainly the patient should not feel chilly, nor should he perspire. Unless a room is temperature controlled, it may be difficult to keep the patient as comfortable as he would like. During the summer temperatures soar, and unless the room is air-conditioned patients may be quite uncomfortable. When temperatures are in the 80s and above, patients perspire and, consequently, they have less energy and may chill more easily.

Humidity

Humidity has a great deal to do with patient comfort. When there is excessive moisture in the air, some complain of breathing difficulties, evaporation of skin moisture (perspiration) is slowed down, and patients may experience a chilly sensation. When both temperature and humidity are high, the patient can be extremely restless and complain of discomfort. High temperatures with little moisture in the air are more easily tolerated than high temperatures with excessive humidity.

Air Circulation

Circulation or ventilation is necessary in both health and sickness. Drafts should be avoided to prevent chilling. Open windows permitting air movement directly across a patient's bed, or the direct flow of air from an electric fan or cooling unit, may be sufficient to cause chilling. Stale, foul air, on the other hand, can contribute to restlessness and be a source of infection when laden with air- and dust-borne microorganisms.

Indirect ventilation through open doors is

one means of providing air movement. Windows open at the top and bottom may also help if the patient is not in a draft. (See Oxygen Therapy).

Lighting

Improper lighting causes eyestrain and fatigue whether a person is sick or well. A patient's surroundings should be cheerful. Proper lighting helps. Patients are apt to feel lifted in spirit, and say so, when their rooms are brightened with sunshine. Shades and blinds help to control the amount and direction of the light in relation to the patient. Certain illness conditions (i.e., eye surgery, measles) may require limited light in the patient's room. Reduced light during periods of rest (sleep) is helpful.

Artificial light is a necessity for carrying out some nursing measures and providing the patient with adequate, well-directed light to carry on activities he may pursue (writing, reading, handwork). It should be placed for convenience and proper use.

Odor

Proper ventilation helps to control odors. Patients react to odors but do not always feel free to talk about them to the nurse. This is especially true if disagreeable odors are brought to the bedside by the nurse (strong perfume, bad breath, perspiration, soiled uniform, etc.). Not only is the odor disturbing, but it may upset the patient that the nurse has used such poor judgment or is so careless. He may wonder if she is equally careless in ways that may affect his well-being and care.

Offensive odor due to the patient himself may embarrass him whether or not he mentions it. A ventilated room helps keep this patient relaxed. The manner of the nurse during his care can help him too; he observes the way the nurse handles his situation.

Some people are more sensitive to odors than others, especially when ill. Every effort should be made to keep the surroundings free from all food and waste materials which may cause odor.

Noise

Noise irritates patients. It is difficult for most of them to accept it because they feel they have come to the hospital to rest and get well. Studies show that patients complain of noise and inappropriate timing of activities as much as or more than anything else.

Nursing personnel have a responsibility to the patient to keep his environment as quiet and restful as possible; they should conduct their activities with the least amount of disturbance and be watchful that other workers and visitors do likewise. People and equipment account for most hospital distrubance. If the people responsible for the noise are members of the hospital family of workers, one could say they should know better. They should be aware that noise causes fatigue, disturbs rest and sleep, and aggravates patients. If the people are other patients or their visitors, steps need to be taken to curb the noise by every reasonable means.

Timing has a great deal to do with the effect noise has on patients. Clattering activity during regular rest and sleep periods is especially difficult for patients to accept. The sounds from radio and television sets, loud talking and laughing, slamming doors, noisy elevators, dripping faucets, and utensils dropped on the floor are just some of the noise-makers that get on patients' nerves. What is considered ordinary hustle and bustle of human activity during the day can become unbearable during the night.

Orderliness

Things well arranged and in good order are pleasing to look at. In addition, good order can make the patient's environment convenient for him and the nurse; orderliness can promote safety. Tasteful arrangement of the patient's personal items contributes to his sense of well-being.

Privacy

Privacy is necessary to everyone under certain circumstances. It is especially important to the patient because he is apt to be among strangers. He may not ask for it because he is shy or has come to expect that in a hospital he has no say over such matters. The patient unit in a ward has curtains which should be drawn when nursing care indicates that the patient needs or wants no "onlookers." Closed doors and screens provide privacy, too. The practical nurse who is careful to provide privacy for her patients will be respected, but more than that she will be protecting the feelings of her patients.

Safety

Safety is the basis of all care. The importance of cleaning, disinfecting, sanitizing, and sterilizing equipment and supplies is discussed in Chapter 27.

Other safety factors which need mentioning are the following:

1. *Use equipment that is in good condition* (e.g., avoid cracked or chipped utensils, damaged electric cords, etc.).

2. *Keep the floor cleared of hazardous materials* (e.g., broken glass, spilled liquids, flower petals).

3. *Observe all safety regulations concerned with oxygen equipment, steam producing devices, heating pads, siderails, and other appliances.*

4. *Provide assistance to ambulatory patients who have poor vision or are unsteady on their feet.*

5. *Arrange beside table so that things are within easy reach of patient.*

6. *Keep hazardous objects out of reach of children* (e.g., safety pins, medicines, instruments, etc.). Use the same precautions with adults who might misuse such items.

7. *Observe directions for proper temperature* of water, enema solutions, wet dressings, infant feedings, and other liquids.

Carelessness and ignorance are not acceptable excuses to the patient and his family when accidents occur, or to the court in case of lawsuit.

THE PATIENT'S ROOM AND UNIT

The patient's room or unit may be in a private home, nursing or convalescent home, or in the hospital. He may or may not share the room with others.

In the hospital, private, semiprivate (two beds or units), and multiple (more than two beds or units) accommodations are generally found. Daily rates to patients depend upon the type of accommodations selected. Very often the patient's condition influences his location (e.g., intensive care unit, close to the nurse's station for close observation). The quiet and privacy of a single room may be essential to patient recovery.

Some patients need and want someone to talk with; they may feel that a semiprivate room not only saves them money but also provides company for them.

Multiple bed units (wards) are the least costly, yet the same quality of nursing care and consideration should and does prevail as in the more costly accommodations. Indigent or charity patients are assigned to ward beds unless their illness condition requires other accommodations. Patients who need to keep hospital costs to a minimum and who do not require private rooms select semiprivate or ward accommodations with the assurance that the care could not be better even if they spent more.

A patient's unit includes his bed, bedside table, other furnishings, and equipment set aside for his use. This may be in a private room which he has to himself or it may be in a room accommodating other patients' units.

The most important piece of equipment in the unit is the bed. Hospital beds are higher than beds used in the home for the convenience of physician and nurse as they treat and care for patients. When patients are being cared for in the home, the bed should be raised on blocks to a convenient height for the nurse so as to avoid fatigue and body strain. Back rests and knee rests are a part of the modern hospital bed. They are operated by hand or by electricity. Some electric models permit the height of the bed to be raised or lowered according to the needs of the patient or the nurse. Back and knee rests can be improvised for the home bed patients. A box of sufficient size may be arranged behind pillows to give support to the patient's back, shoulders, and head. Pillows, blanket rolls, or both may be used under the knees to relieve strain and add to the patient's comfort.

A firm, comfortable mattress contributes to good body alignment, rest, and sleep. It may be innerspring, foam rubber, or horsehair construction. Pillows (large and small) should be suited to the patient's needs.

The bedside table serves as a working space for the nurse and a storage place for the patient's personal equipment.

Mouth care materials (toothbrush, toothpaste, container for dentures), cosmetics, deodorant, soap, and such are kept in the drawer.

The bath basin, emesis basin, urinal, and bedpan are kept below. The top is used while giving nursing care and otherwise serves to keep things convenient for the patient.

An over-bed table is a common and useful piece of unit equipment. Sometimes called a tray table, it extends over the bed, is on casters, and moves about to serve the patient. Its chief use is to hold the tray while the patient eats. With the back rest raised, the over-bed table is pulled up to a convenient position for the patient. Some tables have a compartment in the top surface, the cover of which can be raised to expose a mirror, located on the underside of the cover. Patients able to comb and care for their own hair, shave, use cosmetics, or engage in diversional activities find this very useful.

A foot stool and a chair are other common pieces of unit equipment. A place to hang clothing may or may not be close at hand. Patients like to know that their personal belongings are safe and nearby, if possible.

Each unit has its own light or lamp. Improved artificial lighting provides for indirect, nonglare light. Lamps attached to the wall are safer than floor lamps, and save floor space around the bed. Night lights (subdued source of light) are important to the nurse as she observes her patients and assists them during the night. They may also help the patient to adjust to his strange surroundings.

Modern hospital room equipment may include individual units which provide oxygen, suction, light control, bed position control, call signals as well as television control.

Supplies in Each Unit

Linens for the bed include spread, sheets, pillowcases, and a drawsheet. A moisture proof cover protects the mattress. A bath blanket (soft, lightweight cotton blanket) protects the patient during the bed bath. It replaces the upper sheet and covers the patient, keeps him warmer, and affords privacy as well as protection. The upper sheet is used when a bath blanket is not available. A hand towel, washcloth, and bath towel are also part of the patient's daily linen supply.

Utensils (some may be disposable) for the patient include wash basin, emesis basin, cup for mouth care, soap dish, bedpan, and urinal.

Skin care supplies include soap, powder, and alcohol or lotion. Mouth care supplies include toothbrush, paste or powder, and denture cup when needed.

Mouth wipes and a waste container (wastepaper basket or paper bag fastened to the bed) are essential items.

Many personal care items and other individual supplies (e.g., thermometer) are prepackaged and provided for each patient. He is charged for all supplies and treatment equipment issued to him.

The patient's unit, its order, cleanliness, and adequacy, is a nursing responsibility. While the nurse may not do the housekeeping, it is her responsibility to see that the unit is clean and equipped, whether in the hospital or in the home.

PREPARATION AND CARE OF THE PATIENT'S ENVIRONMENT

Keeping a hospital clean and safe for one patient after another requires rigid standards for cleaning and preparation of utensils, equipment, and the rooms themselves.

Each unit should be clean, orderly, and equipped. Before a patient is admitted to the room and put to bed, the bedside table should be checked for needed utensils and equipment.

Daily Care and Cleaning

A patient's unit needs daily attention. It should be kept clean and in good order (floors, furniture, utensils, bathroom) to help prevent the spread of infection and for esthetic purposes.

The bedside table serves many useful purposes during the course of a day, being a place to set the food tray, bath basin, emesis basin, mail, water glass, pictures, cosmetics, treatment tray, medicine cup, linen, and so forth. The lower portion stores the utensils for bathing and elimination. Used for so many purposes (and being close to the patient), it should receive close attention so that it remains sightly and harbors no offensive odors or pests.

The bath or washbasin, soap dish, and emesis basin require cleaning after each use. Organic matter (feces, vomitus, sputum, blood) should be washed off equipment with cold water and the utensil then washed thoroughly with soap and warm water. Soap and detergents dissolve fatty substances such as petroleum jelly and mineral oil; clean water will not. Sterilization may then be necessary. Most stains can be scoured from metal equipment, but harsh abrasives should not be used.

Care of Flowers and Plants

When arranging flowers, put them into the vase one at a time. Plan to have them at irregular heights. Mixed flowers arranged so they look as if they came directly from the garden are more attractive. Very often patients have too many flowers in the hospital during illness and too few when convalescent at home where they are more able to enjoy them. With care, plants can be kept fresh and attractive to be sent home with the patient.

Proper care of fresh cut flowers preserves their beauty. Plunge the stems into a large amount of water and cut them diagonally under the water so that water can flow into the stem instead of air; this preserves freshness.

Some patients, with help, can take care of their flowers. They may enjoy rearranging the bouquets and trimming dead leaves and stems from plants. Protect the area where the patient will work. For a bed patient, newspapers or a waterproof pad can be arranged on the bed or over-bed table. The container should be conveniently placed to avoid over-reaching and the danger of falling.

Flowers and plants represent the thoughtfulness of friends. Patients appreciate the thoughtfulness of hospital personnel who help them enjoy these gifts.

After Discharge of the Patient

Terminal cleaning is the complete cleaning of a unit after a patient leaves it. He may leave because of discharge, transfer, or death. Regardless of the reason, every part of the unit needs attention to ensure the cleanest possible room and equipment for the next patient.

All soiled linens are carefully gathered to avoid any further spread of dust or lint and consequent spread of microorganisms. All utensils in the bedside table are removed to the utility room for proper washing, sterilization or disposal.

The bed, mattress, bedside table, and chair(s) should be cleaned. Lint and dust on the mattress, in the crevices and around the tufts, may be a source of infection if not removed. Vacuum cleaners quickly remove the loose surface dust and dirt. A small brush and damp cloth will help if a vacuum cleaner is not available. Waterproof mattress and pillow protectors should be thoroughly washed with warm soapy water, rinsed, dried, and then aired. Avoid folding these protectors to prevent cracking. Floors, window sills, and baseboards harbor dust and dirt. Daily attention should keep them reasonably clean, but terminal cleaning needs to be thorough and complete. Metal furniture should be washed. Furniture made of wood cannot tolerate much water but should be wiped well with a damp cloth, and all organic matter removed.

BEDMAKING

The Patient's Bed

The word "bed" has many meanings, but for our purposes it refers to the piece of furniture used by the patient for rest and sleep. Even so, the patient's bed comes in a great variety of sizes and shapes with many different adjustments, safety features, and accessories. Mention should be made of special beds such as the CircOlectric which allows patients with limited motion (e.g., paralyzed in lower extremities) to change to a wide range of positions at intervals, or the oscillating (vibrating) bed which can be controlled as to time of vibration and the "tilt" it takes to improve blood circulation.

Beds are manufactured according to the purpose they are to serve. For example, the bassinet for the newborn is small, easily cleaned, and built to keep the baby out of drafts. The premature infant has a special, covered bed that controls the immediate environment to protect and assist him. The "crib" in the pediatric department is smaller than a regular bed and has high siderails as part of standard equipment.

Hospitals have their own names for beds according to the way they are made or the purpose they serve. Some of these common names include:

Closed bed is an unoccupied bed; it is unassigned to a patient.

Open bed refers to one ready to receive a patient; the top bedding has been turned down.

Occupied bed is taken to mean the patient is in the bed.

Postoperative bed is made to receive a patient immediately following surgery; it has been called an "ether bed."

Fracture bed generally refers to something special about the bed. It may have to do with overhead frames, pulleys, grab bars, a special type of mattress, or bed frame. Examples of special types of frames are the Stryker frame and Foster bed.

Making the Bed

Regardless of the name of the bed or the kind of bed, certain facts should be kept in mind when making it if the patient is to be comfortable, if the making itself is to last reasonably well until the next making, and if the nurse is to be economical with time and energy. There is nothing difficult about learning how to make a bed. It seems slow at first but after practice one soon develops the necessary skills. The nurse considers the well-made bed a vital part of the patient's need for a comfortable environment and not just a procedure to be done.

From *the patient's point of view*, a bed should provide:

1. *Comfort*—it should be clean, dry, smooth, litter-clear, and wrinkle-free; the patient should have room to move around in it and not feel mummified. Lightweight bedding should be used, but enough so that he will be warm. A backrest is supplied as desired or as allowed.

2. *Convenience*—it should be located within reach of things needed or wanted (the call light, intercom system, reading light, bedside table, diversional materials, etc.).

3. *Safety*—it should be clean, with things within reach, with properly working bedside devices and accessories.

From *the nurse's point of view*, the bed-making should include:

1. Economy of energy, time and materials.

2. Protection of herself (and subsequent patients she cares for).

3. Protection of the bed from bodily discharges.

4. Esthetic appearance of the unit when finished.

It does not matter whether the bed is small, large, special or ordinary; *certain guidelines apply to all bedmaking.* You will find them useful from the beginning of your practice and in all types of situations.

1. Assemble all necessary linen before starting and arrange it in the order to be used.

2. Place it in the most convenient place to save steps and time.

3. Unfold clean linen on the bed, working from the top of the bed to the bottom, and from the far side to the near side.

4. Handle clean linen as little as possible without shaking or fanning it.

5. Handle soiled lined to protect self and environment.

6. Adjust the bed, if possible, to a convenient height and position for working.

7. Practice good body mechanics.

8. Develop a system for removing and sorting bedding:

   a. Straighten top bedding and loosen the top and bottom bedding from under the mattress.

   b. Fold each piece separately (work from head to foot of bed) while it is on the bed.

   c. Sort the bedding as it is removed; stack the discarded linen by itself or drop directly into a container for laundry.

   d. Arrange reusable bedding in order for remaking the bed. See Bedmaking Procedure.

SUMMARY

The patient's environment influences his recovery. If it is clean it helps to protect him from infective factors; if it is convenient and free from hazards it is safer for him. And if it is attractive and pleasing to him it influences his frame of mind. All of these have a bearing on his recovery.

While the nurse may not do the housekeeping, she is responsible for the cleanliness, good order, convenience, and completeness of the patient's unit. She has further responsibility for the general environment, that is, to see that it is safe from hazards which cause accidents and contamination.

The patient's bed is the most important part of his environment. Bedmaking skill comes with practice and regardless of the size or type of bed, one can learn how to make a comfortable, durable bed. The guidelines remain the same; adaptations are made to suit the siutation and circumstances.

GUIDES FOR STUDY AND DISCUSSION

1. There is such a thing as "patient's environment." What nine factors must be considered? Give an example of things you will be responsible for in the patient's room.

2. The nurse's own personal health habits can influence the patient. What does this mean?

3. Imagine a patient's unit where a piece of ordinary equipment is hazardous.

4. Why is the nurse responsible for the patient's environment? Why not some other hospital department?

5. Why can it be said that "safety is the basis of all care"? How can patient safety be protected?

6. How does providing privacy for the patient show that the nurse is protecting his feelings? Why should a nurse ever need to be told to "draw the curtains around the bed"?

7. What are the nurse's responsibilities for daily cleaning? Why is terminal cleaning of a patient unit more extensive than daily cleaning?

8. Ordinarily, what equipment and supplies are in a patient's unit? In your hospital what, if anything, is considered disposable?

9. Imagine you are a patient in an unsightly room. What things might cross your mind about the care you are receiving?

10. The patient has the right to expect certain things with respect to his bed. What are they? What must the nurse keep in mind?

SUGGESTED SITUATIONS AND ACTIVITIES

1. Practice bedmaking at home and in the laboratory, using adult beds, cribs, and bassinets. Evaluate your own work; see if it measures up to your expectations. What can you do to improve your skill? See Appendix III — Bedmaking.

2. Visit the hospital for the special purpose of noticing as many different types of beds as possible. Find out the names of any you do not know. Take enough time to "study" a bed situation that is different. Try to imagine what new problem(s) it might present if you were asked to make it while it is unoccupied.

3. Visit the clinical area to observe: sources of noise, evidence of respect or lack of respect for patient privacy, safety factors.

CHAPTER 34

OBSERVATIONS: SKILLS FOR EFFECTIVE PATIENT CARE

TOPICAL HEADINGS

Introduction
Definition of Observation
Developing Observation Skills
Defining Signs and Symptoms
Vital Signs and Blood Pressure
The Patient's Chart

Admission of the Patient to the Hospital
The Medical Examination
Collecting Specimens
Diagnostic Tests
The Transfer of the Patient in the Hospital

Discharge of the Patient from the Hospital
Summary
Guides for Study and Discussion
Suggested Situations and Activities

OBJECTIVES FOR THE STUDENT: Be able to:

1. Tell why observations are an essential part of patient care.
2. Name the personal capacities used in observing the patient.
3. Explain the statement: "Observations are related to relationships and communication."
4. Distinguish between objective and subjective symptoms.
5. Describe a patient situation which provides for his privacy.
6. Define temperature, pulse and respiration.
7. Name six body positions used for examination, treatment and comfort.
8. Describe the role of the practical nurse assisting with a medical examination.
9. State three reasons why the patient has a chart.

SUGGESTED STUDY VOCABULARY*

observation
coherence
disorientation
cyanosis
fatigue
edema
fissures
anomalies
nares
Cheyne-Stokes breathing
rales

contractures
untoward signs
lacerations
decubitus ulcers
cerumen
flatus
ankylosis
sputum
mucus
pus
vomitus

frame of mind
vital signs
rate
rhythm
graphic sheet
stethoscope
sphygmomanometer
specimen
privacy
projectile vomiting
recurrent vomiting
cyclic vomiting

*Look for any terms you already know.

INTRODUCTION

The term *observation* is a sort of family name for a whole group of skills and actions on the part of the nurse (and others) which have a great deal to do with whether or not the patient receives effective care. One thing about this cluster of skills is that they cut across *all* manner of nursing actions and measures. They are not skills you learn in a vacuum, apart from doing something for or with a patient; observations invade all interchanges between patient and nurse. They occur in the presence of the patient and even when he is not present as, for example, when you examine the appearance of urine as you prepare a specimen for the laboratory.

A nurse is trained to use personal resources to gather information which, in turn, is passed on and becomes useful evidence for the physician as he plots the medical plan for the patient. These personal resources include seeing, listening, feeling, and sensing—all with a purpose. All are personal resources you, in fact, have been using for observation purposes all your life. In nursing, it becomes necessary to use these personal possessions in a special way. You learn to "look" with a purpose to see if something is "normal" or if it has the earmarks of something abnormal. The same holds true for use of other resources.

This chapter is designed to help you think about your resources so you can begin to develop some skill in purposeful observations of patients.

DEFINITION OF OBSERVATION

By general definition, *observation* means gathering data, noting facts and happenings. It means taking notice. When a person takes notice, gathers facts, and pays attention to happenings, he is said to be *observant*. He is careful, mindful, attentive to detail, and heedful. All of these terms apply to a nurse who is trained to gather facts and notice happenings related to the patient.

Observation Has A Purpose in Patient Care. In fact, it has several major purposes:

1. It is essential in making a diagnosis, or in keeping track of a patient's progress—diagnosis or no diagnosis.

2. It gives purpose and direction to patient care.

3. It aids others (therapists, social workers, clergy) in their work with the patient and the family.

Observation actually is the key to patient care because it dictates what should or should not be done. The physician observes, orders, and treats the patient according to the evidence he has at hand. The nurse observes, reports, and records noteworthy facts which the physician needs. In addition, the nurse observes things which call for some nursing measures which do not require a written order by the physician. An example of such an observation would be seeing a bed patient in an uncomfortable position and making the necessary adjustments to the bed and pillow, and assisting the patient to a "new" position or posture. Or another example would be giving the type of skin care that prevents pressure sores.

The facts gathered by all involved form a cluster of evidences which become a compass which points the direction for medical management and the accompanying patient care.

You can tell from the preceding discussion that some observations are *vital, required,* and very *essential* to the physician's judgment while other observations might not be considered vital, but in their small, on-the-spot way, can make a big difference to the patient's comfort and well-being. There is too much of a tendency to think that observation relates only to what the doctor specifies. This is not so; effective nursing care includes many nursing measures which never have a physician's order written for them, yet they are very much a part of assisting the patient to meet his needs. Observation is ongoing with every patient contact. It can even make the difference between happiness or unhappiness of the patient regardless of how effective the physician's management is.

The practical nurse plays a valuable role in the vital fact-gathering *and* in the small, on-the-spot observations and actions. This is true because she is apt to be with the patient as much as or more than other nursing personnel, especially when patients are not critically ill or are attached to some complicated electronic machine which is recording its own observations. Therefore, the practical nurse needs to develop keen observational skills, keeping in mind that some acts of observation involve the ability to be accurate and precise in making and reporting the findings. Other skills and sensitivities may not have the same need for being mindful and attentive to detail. Actually, the good display of mindful attention to "small" observations may do as much as anything else to help the patient's need for emotional support. He is pleased to be in the hands of people who care enough to pay attention on their own.

To be this "looker," "listener," "senser," "reporter," and "recorder" calls for various uses of one's personal resources, but the practical nurse should recognize that her role in this does not require that she know the underlying factors responsible for what was seen, heard, or sensed. She is the supplier of facts which in turn are used by the physician and the professional nurse. In other words, do not underestimate the importance of what you do, but keep in mind that it does not require that you know the detailed ins and outs of the pathology (science of the nature and cause of disease) involved because you do not use that depth of information in fulfilling your responsibilities.

DEVELOPING OBSERVATION SKILLS

One might start by saying that patient observation cuts across and relates to relationships and communications. Relationships and interaction (positive or negative) flow between patient and nurse. They go together; the one can hardly exist without the other. You cannot very well be conversing with someone and not be making mental note of some things about that person. You have feelings about him, too. If it appears that the other person is not listening to what you have to say, how does this influence the contact? Now turn this situation around. The other person is making observations, too, and develops feelings as the interaction and observation proceed. This interchange, then, is a mixture of observation, communication, and relationships. These same factors are present when you are with patients. It is understandable that the newborn or the person so ill that he seems not to register your presence is not involved in this interchange to the same degree nor in the same way that another type of patient may be. But who is to say what is the sensation experienced by the newborn or the critically ill

comatose patient as the nurse makes observations?

Personal Resources Involved

As pointed out, the practical nurse learns to use personal capacities (ability to talk, listen, see, feel, and hear) in a unique way in her observing role. Skill and judgment in observing develop with practice, patience, and the will to improve, the same as with any other skill. It takes time and exposure to one situation after another to know what to look for as well as how to gather and report the data. To help you understand and accept the fact that observation skills are something that grow and improve as you experience actual situations, imagine how much more quickly a person can recognize a patient in shock when that person has already seen, felt, and sensed the cold, clammy skin, rapid, thready pulse and colorless face expressing fear. This experience sets up a picture in the mind's eye that becomes useful from then on.

One learns what is normal first and then what is abnormal. As knowledge accumulates, one also sharpens one's skill to observe because she knows what to look for.

Ways the Practical Nurse Will Observe

Following is a discussion of five personal resources which take on new meaning when used as "tools" for observing the patient.

1. LOOKING. The sense of sight is in constant use and is the gateway for observing the patient, his surroundings, and factors related to his condition.

In looking at the *patient*, take particular note to detect the usualness or the unusualness of the following: (1) *Facial expression*—note alertness or lack of it, expression of pain or discomfort, agreeableness, worry, satisfaction, and the like. (2) *Skin*—note whether it looks hot, dry, cold, clammy, rashy, red, discolored (particularly the lips, fingers, feet, toes, arms, and legs), and also check for the evidence of pressure on some part of the body, breaks in the skin, and general color tone. One of the best opportunities for making total skin observations is while bathing the patient; however, there are almost endless ways to observe the patient's skin and color tone when doing things for and with him. The skin can be a "general index" to the patient's well-being. Touching as well as looking is involved. (3) *Body posture and use*—note whether the patient is ambulatory or in bed, and the position, stiffness, moveability, use or disuse of his hands, arms, legs, and feet.

One looks to see if the *patient's immediate surroundings* are arranged to his convenience, safety, and liking. The patient's state of dependence upon others for meeting his daily living needs helps to dictate what is safe and convenient. Eye-appealing (esthetic), pleasant surroundings can influence a person's well-being. That is why the practical nurse provides surroundings that are as appealing as possible, with utensils for personal hygiene, elimination, nourishment, treatments, and such kept out of sight except when in use. Light, ventilation, temperature, and noise all come under the topic "surroundings." Notice, too, that in addition to looking other resources (feeling, smelling, hearing) are at work at the same time.

In checking the *patient's condition,* one must look at such things as the amount, character, and color of drainage; appearance of dressings; and amount and character or urine, feces, vomitus, and sputum. Looking includes seeing if the diet was consumed and if "off limits" foods, tobacco, beverages, and articles which might be dangerous or attract pests are in the patient's unit.

2. LISTENING. Some people know how to do this better than others; it is the most important half of conversation. Listening is something worth practicing when conversing with patients. Purposeful listening during conversation is a means for gaining such information as coherence, disorientation, satisfactions, worries, fears, uncertainties, needs, and interests of the patient. Patients appreciate being listened to. If you can train yourself to give "full-stop" attention even during a short patient contact, the patient has the feeling you do listen. This bit of confidence helps to strengthen the relationship between you.

Listening plays other important roles. At night when "making rounds," one listens for rate, depth, and character of respirations, and signs of restlessness, wakefulness, and disorientation in patients. If equipment is in use and it makes sounds while running, one listens for the characteristic sound or absence of it.

Use of the stethoscope and the sphygmomanometer requires special listening skills developed with repeated practice over a period of time.

3. SMELLING. Unusual odors are an index to circumstances and they capture the attention of the alert nurse. For example, the observation of a sweet odor on a patient's breath might be a valuable aid to the physician. Dressings and drainage have characteristically foul odors, yet a change in this odor may be significant. This is also true of human excreta—urine, feces, and perspiration.

4. TALKING. Chapter 3 pointed out the importance of showing acceptance and "being well-received." This fact is particularly essential when talking with a patient for the purpose of gaining essential information. Keep in mind that *how* something is said or asked (tone of voice, language used, facial expressions, attention "full-stop," etc.) makes a difference in the way the patient responds.

Talking will include asking the patient questions about how he slept and about his appetite and elimination. The nurse may discuss his complaint of pain or discomfort with him and find out if he is warm enough or would like to change position. The skill in *talking* for observation purposes comes when the nurse develops judgment in how she asks questions and seeks information as to what is important to report and record and what is not. You may need to confer with the professional nurse because of the variety of means used today to record and report information.

5. TOUCHING OR FEELING. Taking the pulse is a good example of observing through touch. Here one learns to locate the pulse and sense its quality, rate, rhythm, and the pressure used to count it. Placing the hand on the brow detects fever or perspiration. During the bath the sense of touch may locate abnormalities of the skin or scalp, detect skin dryness, or abnormal temperature.

Skill in the Observer's Role

The practical nurse has many opportunities to use personal resources in observing; the challenge comes in continued motivation to develop these abilities within her knowledge and her responsibilities. The role is one of supplying accurate, specific information to the physician and to the professional nurse. It is a vital role, but should not be confused with the responsibilities and judgments of the physician and the professional nurse who must render judgments based upon such observations.

DEFINING SIGNS AND SYMPTOMS

The two words *sign* and *symptom* are used one for the other most of the time. Beyond a simple definition of each supplied here, they will not be considered separate and apart from each other.

A *sign* is an indicator or a fact that points out evidence of something. These indicators are things that can be seen, heard, felt, smelled, etc. For example, you could take your temperature, read the thermometer, and see whether or not there was a sign of fever present.

A *symptom* is evidence that the patient shares or tells, such as nausea, headache, dizziness, fatigue, thirst, fear, and chilliness.

Types of Signs and Symptoms

Keeping these definitions in mind, it can be said that signs and symptoms are generally grouped under one of two headings: *objective,* those readily sensed by the nurse or physician; or *subjective,* those the patient tells about. They are equally important.

OBJECTIVE SYMPTOMS. (Skills chiefly used: looking, listening, touching, smelling, talking.)
 1. Cyanosis.
 2. Fatigue.
 3. Edema (general or local).
 4. Sleep habits.
 5. Appetite.
 6. General appearance of patient: facial expression, deformities, state of nourishment.
 7. Condition of the skin (general and local).
 8. Fever, chills.
 9. Respiration, coughing, sneezing.
 10. Color and amount of urine, feces, sputum, vomitus.
 11. Mental state (depressed, disoriented, etc.).
 12. Character and amount of drainage on dressings.

SUBJECTIVE SYMPTOMS. (Skills chiefly used: listening, looking.)
 1. Dizziness (vertigo).
 2. Ringing in the ears (tinnitus).
 3. Fatigue, malaise.
 4. Nausea.
 5. Pain, aches, discomfort.
 6. Feelings or sensations (chilliness, thirst, anxiety, loneliness, fear).

What should be reported? In general, *change* should be reported: any observable change in the patient's condition, for either better or worse, any new sign or symptom, or one that is different in intensity. Evidence, subjective or objective, may be misleading or not run true to form, but the judgment of that is the responsibility of the physician, not the nurse.

Guidelines in Recording Observations

The following guidelines are not necessarily numbered in order of importance, nor would all nine items apply to each recording. However, the time something was observed must accompany the remarks. Good reason for this is pointed out later on in this chapter when the patient's chart is discussed. *The nature of what is recorded is determined by what is important for the physician to know.*
 1. Time (when observed).
 2. Location of abnormal sensation (exactness insofar as possible).
 3. Duration (how long it lasted, i.e., a chill).
 4. Frequency and intensity (i.e., whether pain was constant or intermittent, severe, mild, throbbing, etc.).
 5. Relief obtained from nursing measures (whether or not they seemed to help).
 6. General appearance of patient (if this has changed).
 7. Amount, color, character of discharge (urine, feces, vomitus, sputum, drainage).
 8. Exact words of patient (when indicated).
 9. Complaints (as to eating, sleeping, pain, etc.).

Observation of the patient's general condition and behavior goes on without the patient's knowledge of it. All recordings should be made away from the patient's bedside if possible. This helps to prevent anxiety and worry which might arise if the patient watched the nurse making notations about himself.

(*Text continued on page 402.*)

TABLE 34–1. OBSERVATIONS: BASIC NEEDS—GENERAL COMMENTS

Basic Need	What to Notice	What to Report	Comments
Personal Care and Hygiene			
Skin	Moistness, dryness, heat, coldness, discoloration (pale, red, cyanotic, flushed, bruises), abrasions, lacerations, swellings, rashes, growth, pressure areas, bed sore (decubitus ulcers).	"Normal" appearances are not usually recorded unless they indicate a change that is useful information for the physician or charge nurse. This would be the case when "a word picture of progress" is indicated.	Opportunity for thorough observation comes while assisting the patient with personal care and hygiene. Every patient contact is "observation time."
Ears	Crusts, swellings, scabs, wax (cerumen), discoloration.	New developments are reportable and will be recorded if the charge nurse or team leader so decides.	Circumstances in the situation dictate what is recorded; specific process can be set forth for what to or what not to chart. Your ability will continue to develop as you practice and observe local charting policies (rules, forms to be used, etc.).
Eyes	Size of pupils, discharges, swelling of the lids, edema, discoloration, sensitivity to light.	Same as above.	Same as above.
Nose	Skin around nares, discharges, fissures.	Same as above.	Same as above.
Lips and mouth	Dry, parched, blisters, fissures, color, sores; appearance of tongue — coated, color, sores, swelling.	Same as above.	Same as above.
Teeth	Natural, dentures, removable bridges, braces, absence of, discoloration.	Same as above.	Same as above.
Hair	State of cleanliness: oily, matted, presence of pediculi (lice), nits, blood, other foreign matter.		
Scalp	Scabs, scales, growths, bruises, lacerations, rashes, swelling.	Same as above.	Same as above.
Hands and nails	Condition of skin: dry, moist, breaks, sores, discolorations, fissures, deformities, state of cleanliness and length of nails.	Same as above.	Same as above.
Sleep and Rest	Habits: daytime napping or drowsiness; duration — uninterrupted or short periods; position — need for additional pillow(s), elevated back rest.	If this is a problem for which a relief measure(s) is ordered, you would record the measure and results.	Routine charting of "a good night" or "slept well" is considered nonessential *unless* it indicates progress the physician is seeking.
Nutrition and Fluids	Diet as ordered; appetite; type and amount of food consumed; likes, dislikes; texture of food relative to ability	Diet is *always* ordered. Follow practices of local agency for routine, nonspecial diets. Record any essential	Routine charting of "ate well" tells the physician little unless "poor appetite," or something else has been

(Table 34–1 continues on the opposite page.)

TABLE 34-1. OBSERVATIONS: BASIC NEEDS—GENERAL COMMENTS (Continued)

Basic Need	What to Notice	What to Report	Comments
	to chew, swallow; if special orders, note specific things related to orders.	information related to special orders; agency forms and policies dictate the manner for recording diet information.	a problem or if diet is serving therapeutic purpose. As you learn more about such disorders as diabetes you will begin to develop ability to record pertinent, essential information.
Elimination *Normal Discharges:* Urine	Color, amount, odor, frequency.	Normal appearances are not (usually) recorded unless they indicate a change that provides useful information; record abnormalities.	To be able to observe abnormalities, use your knowledge of "what is normal."
Feces	Amount, form, character of, frequency, presence of flatus.	Same as above.	Same as above.
Abnormal Discharges: Sputum, mucus, pus, vomitus, blood	Source, color, amount, character of, frequency.	Reportable and are recorded.	Abnormal discharges are signs of body disorder the physician needs to know about.
Body Alignment and Activity Posture, Contractures, Position in bed and walking, exercise, moving and turning	Presence of any abnormalities. Ease of doing, willingness to do, frequency of, ability to use hands and arms in assisting with personal hygiene, feeding self, etc.	Normal alignment and activity are not recorded; new developments indicating a change (i.e., seems to use left hand more or less than before) are reportable, as are beginning signs of poor alignment, body support, or lack of exercise such as "foot drop," inability to straighten legs, bend knees, move fingers.	Many actions by the nurse not reportable including making a comfortable bed which allows freedom of movement, turning or repositioning a patient, getting him involved in helping with his daily hygiene, and eating unless indicated otherwise by medical orders. This area of nurse observation and action needs more attention called to it. What excuse is there for a long-term bed patient developing abnormal immobility and "solid" joints (ankylosis)?
Environment Noise, light, ventilation, convenience, safety factors, eye appeal, cleanliness	Factors surrounding the patient which keep him as comfortable as possible, which do not work to his disadvantage or cause irritability, and which provide for safety (his, yours, others).	Most environmental factors noted and adjusted by the nurse without "orders," or recording; report hazards which require the attention of another worker (e.g., a poor electrical connection, a malfunctioning air conditioner).	Seldom are environmental "orders" written. It is the responsibility of the nurse to notice and take steps to provide surroundings conducive to patient safety and satisfaction. In some instances, common sense will dictate that the nurse do at once what *(Table 34-1 continues on the following page.)*

TABLE 34-1. OBSERVATIONS: BASIC NEEDS—GENERAL COMMENTS (Continued)

Basic Need	What to Notice	What to Report	Comments
			needs to be done rather than report it to Housekeeping, Food Service, or some other hospital department.
Medical Treatment and Care	Physician orders diet, drugs, treatments, and specific measures to be received or not received.	Most orders recorded as having been carried out including when (time), what, how (medicine, in particular), and results (if pertinent). Some may not be recorded but are observed (e.g., No visitors, No salt shaker on tray).	What to record is related to specific orders. For example, for preparing and passing or giving medicines by mouth, you will learn how to record what you have done. The same is true for preparing and giving a cleansing or a retention enema.
Emotional and Spiritual Support Well-being, worries, frame of mind, wishes	Facial expressions and posture communicate as well as words. Listening and looking provide clues. If the patient cannot speak, looking is essential. Your questions should reflect good judgment lest they be mistaken for prying curiosity.	Report any undue, repeated expressions of concern. The charge nurse would be the guide for what to include in the record. Normal reactions, under ordinary circumstances, would not be reported or recorded except if they represent a change from past reactions.	These items seldom call for a physician's orders, but they are very real and do influence the total person; thus they are related to his progress. It is especially interesting to note the posture and facial expressions of the newborn who is clean, dry, and being held (or rocked) while eating. While you have responsibility for observing patient well-being, you would not go from patient to patient looking for unhappiness; know the indications when you encounter them.
Physical and Mental Adjustments	Recognize the need for patients to know what to expect while in the hospital. Notice how you can help them get acquainted with the hospital "routines," related to food service, mail, visitors, special restrictions such as "nothing by mouth after midnight," how to get to a department to receive a certain treatment, etc.	Many observations and nurse actions are neither reported nor recorded because they represent your helping patients. If one observes unusual curiosity and repeated requests for a particular thing, it should be discussed with the charge nurse.	This factor has close relationship to the emotional factor mentioned above and is a good example of how difficult it is to "divide up" a person and discuss his parts.

(Table 34–1 continues on the opposite page.)

TABLE 34–1. OBSERVATIONS: BASIC NEEDS—GENERAL COMMENTS (Continued)

Basic Need	What to Notice	What to Report	Comments
Diversional and Rehabilitative Activities	How a patient spends his time; compare this with his general well-being. Notice what may or may not interest him. Know about the therapeutic measures he receives. Find out what you should watch for or help promote prior to and following such measures.	Reporting and recording ordinary activities not done; they are part of total care. If activities are planned seeking certain outcomes, then observations would be reported and recorded.	Consider what you can appropriately suggest or provide. Patients (certain ages, at least) may enjoy helping to plan activities.

The preceding information is arranged to provide you with a means for beginning to see that observation relates to all manner of patient needs. Some things are reportable and are recorded; some are not, but this in no way makes them unimportant. Keep in mind that any of the factors are subject to what the patient does and says, too. He has complaints, comments, requests, his own judgments and expressed satisfactions.

This is good practice to follow: *make your recording (or report) as soon as possible following the observation.* Two main reasons for this are: (1) it may be information that should be shared at once, and (2) time has a way of causing one to forget or overlook some essential facts.

VITAL SIGNS AND BLOOD PRESSURE

The body has a "ready reference" system made up of three related signs which indicate the immediate condition of the patient. They are *temperature, pulse,* and *respiration.*

Normal body regulation includes maintaining the body at a fairly even temperature; the heart continues to beat at much the same rate unless influenced by age, rest, exercise, or eating, and the same is true with the rate of breathing. When illness strikes, the body begins to make self-adjustments to cope with its needs and these three related vital actions (abbreviated TPR) are quick to reflect these body adjustments. For example, for every degree (F.) the temperature increases, the heart beat steps up about 10 beats per minute. Thus, they serve as one of the first (and most ready) means for observing the patient's condition.

Review normal physiology related to heat production, pulse, respiration, and blood pressure. *Normal adult ranges* of vital signs are:

Mouth temperature—97 to 99° F. (average, 98.6° F. or 37° C.).

Pulse—60 to 80 per minute (average, about 72).

Respirations—14 to 18 per minute.

The vital signs are such an important index to a patient's condition that they are usually taken and recorded at least twice a day, and more frequently, if indicated. It is a hospital requirement that vital signs be recorded frequently in certain situations (after surgery, during critical illness, and with the use of some drugs or some treatments).

Taking the Temperature

This is the measurement of body heat by use of a clinical thermometer. Presently there are two main types of thermometers: (1) mercury-in-glass (Fig. 34–1) showing two scales), and (2) electronic (Fig. 34–2).

While the electronic thermometer provides an accurate reading much faster (five to seven seconds in contrast to three to five minutes) than the mercury-in-glass type, the latter is still the more commonly used instrument. It is a short, triangular, hollow glass shaft with mercury in one end. The end holding the mercury is a variously-shaped bulb (slender, round, pear-shaped) which is inserted or secured at the selected site. Body heat expands the mercury (and glass) and it pushes into the hollow glass shaft. The glass shaft is marked with a Fahrenheit or centigrade scale. The Fahrenheit scale is in common use in Canada and the United States. However, the centigrade scale is becoming more widely used. Figure 34–1 explains how to change one scale to another.

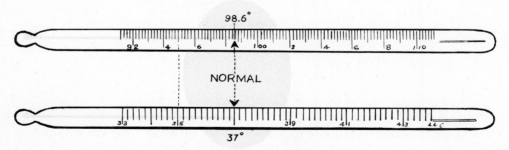

FIGURE 34–1   Fahrenheit (F.) and centigrade (C.) scales are used to measure body temperature. To convert Fahrenheit to centigrade, subtract 32 from F. reading and multiply by the fraction 5/9. To convert centigrade to Fahrenheit, multiply the C. reading by 9/5 and add 32; (adapted from Kozier and DuGas: Fundamentals of Patient Care.)

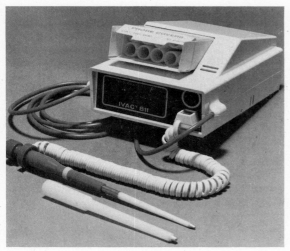

FIGURE 34–2 Electronic thermometer. (Courtesy of IVAC Corporation, La Jolla, California.)

It is of historical interest that a hundred years ago, the thermometer was a foot long and placed in the axilla. At the turn of the century the thermometer was in the personal possession of the physician or locked in the hospital safe between his visits.

Sites for taking temperature include mouth (oral), rectum, axilla, and groin. Oral and rectal temperature readings are more nearly accurate because they indicate a "within-the-body" temperature which is less influenced by the environment than if taken in the axilla or groin. However, circumstance may be such that it is impossible to get an oral or rectal reading; in such cases the other sites are used.

Factors which can influence readings are:

1. Time of day — highest in mid-afternoon and lowest during the night.

2. Site — rectal reading about 1° F. above oral reading; oral reading about 1° F. above axillary reading.

3. Hot or cold foods or fluids consumed just prior to an oral reading.

4. Crying — when a baby cries hard the temperature increases.

5. Mouth breathing — during the taking of an oral temperature.

See Fig. 34–3 for a "close-up" reading view of the Fahrenheit thermometer.

Taking the Pulse

The pulse is observed by "feeling through the finger tips." It is a throbbing (pulsating) sensation you feel when you press your finger tips against an artery.

You will recall that with each beat of the heart, blood is forced through the circulatory system. After the blood has been resupplied with oxygen in the lungs, it returns to the left side of the heart (entering the upper chamber and then going on to the lower chamber) which contracts and relaxes to pump the blood into the systemic circulation system. For the person taking the pulse, it is a "finger tip picture" of this pumping action which is felt. The vehicle carrying the impulses is the moving blood in the arteries.

FIGURE 34–3 Clinical thermometer measures body temperature to nearest tenth of a degree. The arrow shows normal temperature when taken by mouth. (Notice below normal range, fever and high fever or heatstroke.) (John Henderson: Emergency Medical Guide. New York, McGraw-Hill Book Co., 1963.)

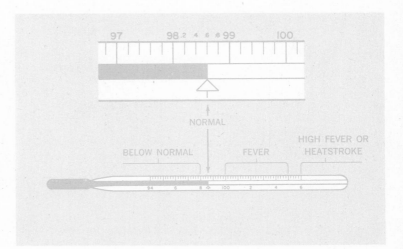

Three characteristics of the pulse:

1. *rate*—the beat by beat count over a one-minute period of time. The normal rate for a child is higher than for an adult. When the child's rate is below 70 beats per minute and the adult's rate below 60 beats per minute they are considered slow (bradycardia). When the infant's rate goes over 200 beats per minute and the adult rate over 100 beats per minute they are considered rapid (tachycardia).

2. *rhythm*—the evenness or unevenness of the beat. Ordinarily the spaces between beats are even. When they are uneven the rhythm is called arrhythmia.

3. *quality*—the thrust or bounce of the blood against the vessel wall as the beat comes through: it may be strong and bounding or only moderately so; or, the thrust may be weak, feeble or even thready and seem to trail off into nothingness.

Learning to count the pulse is the easiest of the three things to learn about it. Rhythm and quality come next; here practice is needed to gain the ability to "estimate" them. (See Appendix III, Taking Pulse.)

There are several sites where the pulse can be felt. The one most commonly used is the radial site; pulse count here is called *radial pulse*. Study Figure 34–4 and locate the radial site and the seven other places where a pulse can be felt.

Sometimes it is necessary to compare the heart beat from two sites at the same time to see if there is a difference between the two counts (such a difference is called *pulse deficit*). One site is the apex of the heart; the other is the radial site. It requires two people, using the same watch, counting at the exact same time. This process is called *taking the apical-radial pulse*.

Observing Respirations

Respiration is the act of breathing including the inspiration and the expiration of air. Counting respirations takes place while the fingers are still in position to take the pulse; this avoids calling attention to the process. A patient could alter his rate of breathing if aware it was being counted.

As with the pulse, respirations have rate, rhythm, and quality. Breathing in and out (normally) is a regular, even, and quiet process. There are many patterns of irregular breathing. Sometimes one observes this when listening to a person in sound, deep, natural sleep, when (perhaps due to body position) there are full, deep inspirations followed by long intervals before expiration.

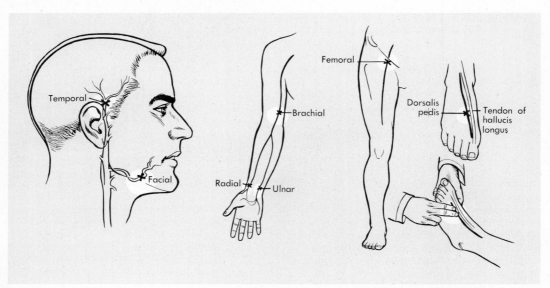

FIGURE 34–4   The pulse may be located at a variety of body sites. Age and patient condition sometimes make it necessary to use other than the radial site. (Kozier and DuGas: Introduction to Patient Care, 2nd ed.)

There are many medical terms to describe various rhythms and qualities of respirations. Some common ones include:

1. *Apnea*—temporary cessation of breathing followed by forced breathing.

2. *Dyspnea*—labored or difficult breathing.

3. *Bradypnea*—slowness of breathing.

4. *Cheyne-Stokes breathing*—(named for two physicians, John Cheyne and William Stokes) uneven breathing from strong to weak with intervals of apnea.

5. *Stertor*—abnormal snoring sounds during breathing.

6. *Artificial breathing*—breathing maintained by means outside the body.

7. *Diminished breathing*—partially suppressed breathing sounds.

8. *Interrupted breathing*—jerky inspirations distinctly separated from irregular expirations.

(See Appendix III, Taking Respirations.)

Taking Blood Pressure

Blood pressure means the force blood exerts against a vessel wall as the heart beats. The practical nurse needs *to know how to take and record an accurate reading*. The ability to do this represents real skill that comes after *much* practice (see Appendix III, Taking Blood Pressure).

The commonly used instrument for measuring blood pressure is called a *sphygmomanometer*. Figure 34–5 shows two types: (1) the mercury manometer, and (2) the aneroid or spring manometer. These instruments have been in use since the turn of the century and provide accurate readings when blood pressure is steady. However, new electronic devices are used to keep track of rapidly changing blood pressure; in this respect they are more useful than the slower mercury manometer.

Arterial blood pressure is always measured at the same body site unless age or some other condition prevents it. That site is the brachial artery (inner aspect of the arm). Notice in Figure 34–5 where the stethoscope is placed in each illustration; notice also where the cuff (wrapping) is located above the elbow.

Blood pressure is recorded by using two numbers (such as 120/80) which represent the two points where the mercury stands (or the needle points) when two distinctly different sounds are first heard with the stethoscope.

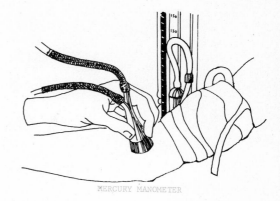

MERCURY MANOMETER

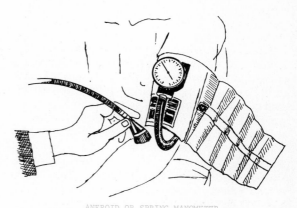

ANEROID OR SPRING MANOMETER

FIGURE 34–5 Two common types of blood pressure measuring instruments. (Seedor: Aids to Diagnosis: A Programmed Unit in Fundamentals of Nursing.)

The first number (in this example, 120) represents the *systolic* reading—the first clear, sharp, thumping sound heard through the stethoscope as you gradually open the valve. The second number (in this example, 80) represents the *diastolic* reading—the point where the clear, sharp sound suddenly changes to a dull thump or muffle. In this example the reading is said to be "120 over 80." It is easier to get accurate readings on persons other than infants and toddlers (under two years of age) because the two different sounds are more distinct. In infants, the first sound (systolic) is audible but the second sound (diastolic) is not easily picked up; it is not as well defined. For this reason infant blood pressure readings are usually taken by the physician.

Immediate factors which influence blood pressure readings include the site used (see Fig. 34–6), exercise, emotions, crying, painful

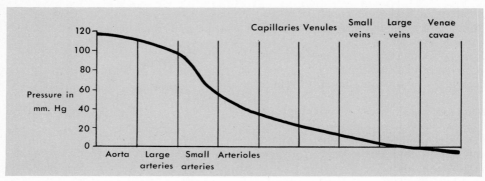

FIGURE 34–6   Notice the differences in pressure in various types of blood vessels. (Dienhart: Basic Human Anatomy and Physiology.)

experiences, sleep, and rest. Explain the process to the patient if he is not familiar with it and can in any way understand what you are going to do. He needs to know what to expect and how long it takes. If some immediate happening has upset or altered the blood pressure, this fact should be taken into account.

Other things which account for differences in blood pressure include age and disease or disorder. One of the common signs of the aging process is increased blood pressure. The physician observes this closely and provides treatment and advice to help guard against it. Certain illnesses or disorders (e.g., accidents involving head injuries) readily show blood pressure changes which the physician needs to know about.

Charting the Vital Signs and Blood Pressure

A special form located in the front of the patient's chart, usually known as the "graphic sheet," is used to record temperature, pulse, and respiration. There is a place for recording blood pressure readings and other pertinent information as well.

Accurate recording of temperature, pulse, and respiration on graphic sheets requires practice.

Unusual temperature, pulse, and respiration observations are recorded in the section of the chart usually called "nurses' notes." For example, if, as the nurse was taking the temperature, pulse, and respiration, the patient showed evidence of labored breathing or complained of pain while breathing, these observations would be recorded there.

THE PATIENT'S CHART

Purposes of the Chart

The patient's chart is a continuous, record of his illness because it:

1. Provides a detailed account of treatment, medications, and nursing care received by the patient and includes the results of such care.

2. Shows the physician what, if any, progress is being made by the patient and guides his judgment in planning future medical care.

3. Serves as a guide for planning nursing care.

4. Furnishes valuable statistical information to the hospital. An accumulation of such vital statistics helps show the community the many types of services the hospital renders.

5. Provides valuable information in court should there be a lawsuit concerning the patient's nursing or medical care, or both. Thus, the *time* something occurred becomes as vital as what specifically occurred.

6. Serves as a source of information for medical and nursing students.

Taking all of these purposes into account, remember that the information on the patient's chart is there to assist only those people directly concerned with his care. The nurse handles and works with charts perhaps more than any other person. It is her responsibility to see that patients' charts are protected from those who might have no authority to know about or even share such information. All chart information is considered confidential and, as such, is used in the best interests of patients. The hospital chart is the property of the hospital. The medical record in a physician's office belongs to the physician.

Contents of the Chart

Each hospital provides the type of sheets or records used in its charts. While the forms used may vary from hospital to hospital, certain basic information must be available in each chart. This includes:

1. A personal and medical history.
2. A report of physical examination findings.
3. A report of any tests performed, i.e., laboratory, diagnostic.
4. Physician's order sheet.
5. Nursing care notes.
6. Physician's progress report.
7. A final diagnosis.
8. Autopsy findings (if done).

Nursing Care Notes

The term *nursing care notes* as it is used here refers to that part of the patient's chart where the nurse records all (meaningful) action she carries out and her observations while doing so. The sheet itself varies in design and content from one hospital to another, but space is provided to show drugs given, treatments carried out, temperature, pulse, respiration, blood pressure results, and for written comments pertinent to anything noteworthy (drugs, treatments, diet, personal hygiene, elimination, sleep, frame of mind, etc.).

Meaningful, accurate nursing notes are valuable because they show the physician what has been done for the patient and what the observed results were. They are valuable to the nursing team and to the charge nurse too, because specific observations are a source of information useful in planning and changing nursing care. In fact, from one shift to another (day to evening to night) this record of activities and results may be the best source of information available.

It stands to reason that it is wasteful to write non-essential, long accounts of what was done, seen, and said. Time and space do not permit word extravagance. Therefore, one learns through practice to state accurately and briefly all noteworthy observations. Record-

ing noteworthy information means putting down those observations which show change (any change) in the patient's condition. The physician is interested in the patient's progress or lack of it. He wants to know if what he orders is producing desired or undesired results.

As you begin to develop skill in recording action and observation, think of the nursing care notes as a running account of the important-to-know facts which represent patient progress (or lack of it). Consider too, that your observations could be used as legal evidence in the event of court action.

There is a difference of opinion about the value or the use made of the observations recorded by the nurse. This comes about when notes include unnecessary or useless comments. *A necessary comment is one that tells something that needs to be known;* a test for this is to ask yourself, "Would it be beneficial to the patient's well-being if the physician or the nursing staff knew such and such?" You may need to confer with the team leader or the charge nurse to help you answer this question. As you learn more about various patients' conditions and their complaints, your observational skills will continue to improve; meanwhile, remember that writing worthful nursing notes takes much practice. The following *general guidelines for charting* will help you get started:

1. Print all notes in legible form.
2. Record the exact time, care, treatments, and observations that were carried out.
3. Chart *after* a performance; charting is signed by the person who performed the task.
4. Capitalize, punctuate, and spell correctly; consult a dictionary, if necessary.
5. Draw a line through an error; *never erase.*
6. Use standard abbreviations (See Appendix I).
7. Record any signs of change that denote a departure from normal; report such promptly.
8. Use meaningful statements, avoiding vague or all-inclusive remarks such as "a poor night." Tell what was poor about it by using descriptive words (e.g., awake, complaining of sleeplessness, etc.).

Nursing in the home also requires record keeping which shows all essential measures provided and pertinent observations. The form used should suit the purpose of the physician; this means the nurse should inquire about it.

ADMISSION OF THE PATIENT

Going to the hospital to receive care is an accepted procedure in this country and in many others. This does not mean that the patients are "fear free," however. Patients and their families have many uncertainties about hospitalization. This is one reason why the admission procedure should be as pleasant and considerate an experience as possible for the patient and his family.

Arrival of the Patient

Admission procedures vary from hospital to hospital. In most they are handled by an admitting officer or clerk. This person may be the first hospital representative the patient meets; his impression of how he was handled will influence his reaction to the whole hospital experience. Certain basic information about each patient must be obtained, and this requires that many questions be asked. Sometimes the patient is unable to take an active part in the admission process because he is too young or his condition does not permit it. Parents, relatives, or close friends provide necessary information. Regardless of who participates, relationships start here and thrive best in a friendly atmosphere.

Meeting the Patient and His Family

First impressions are lasting. The person who meets the patient and takes him to his room or unit carries a special responsibility. If the patient feels he receives individual attention, this reassures him and the family. If the patient is not too ill, he should meet other patients in the room. In this way he is not apt to feel so strange or alone after his family leaves.

Whether the patient is young, middle-aged or old, male or female, he will have some concerns about his surroundings, what the family is doing, how they are getting along without him, and other things related to his family role.

Nurse-patient relationships start with admission. A sincere and considerate nurse reas-sures the patient far more than when the admission procedure is carried out as a matter-of-fact process that is merely intended to put the patient to bed.

Putting the Patient to Bed

When the admission office notifies the floor that a patient is to be admitted to a particular bed, the bed should be opened and made ready to receive the patient. Any necessary special equipment should be assembled. The unit should be given a final check for the usual articles found in the bedside table, and necessary linens.

Privacy is important to the patient and his family. It may be necessary to ask family members to step out into the hall while the patient undresses or is assisted by the nurse. Good judgment (sometimes called "common sense") helps the nurse do this in a helpful manner. Relatives respond more favorably to friendly, considerate requests. Relationships with family members play a part in nurse-patient relationships.

Observations

Observation begins when the nurse meets the patient. His general appearance and his remarks about how he feels should be carefully noted. Detailed observations follow. The "admission" temperature, pulse, and respiration are taken soon after the patient is in bed. One notices the condition of the skin, presence of any out-of-the-ordinary skin signs, pediculi (head or body lice), general appearance of patient, and any pertinent remarks (complaints). Be sure to get a urine specimen (if required) and provide a bath, if necessary and permitted.

Patients' conditions upon admission vary so much from one to another that it is unwise to suggest "a routine for admission." Seek direction from the charge nurse if you are unclear about how to proceed.

Care of Clothing and Valuables

In some hospitals the patient's clothes are stored in his room; in others it is necessary to make a written list of his wearing apparel and then take them to a large storage room where, with proper identification, they are kept until needed. Parents very often take a child's clothing home. Regardless of where clothing is kept, you need to remember that whatever the amount or condition of the clothing, all pieces must be accounted for. Nothing must be discarded or misplaced.

If the hospital regulations require that the clothing be removed from the room, this is explained to the patient. It can be upsetting to him to see his clothes taken away; tell him they are being cared for and will be available when he needs them.

Patients are encouraged to keep few, if any, valuables in their units. If a patient insists on keeping articles of value or large sums of money, this should be reported to the charge nurse. Hospitals provide space in the business office safe for storage of money and small articles of value such as jewelry. Special precautions should be taken to inform the patient of this service. Each hospital has its own procedure for handling valuables. Many require the nurse to make a notation on the chart regarding the care or disposition of the patient's clothing and valuables.

If the patient is willing, members of the family may take valuables home. This fact should be recorded. Items for daily care are kept in the bedside table. Personal items (pictures, religious materials, flowers, books, magazines, etc.) play a part in a patient's life too, and within reason, should be where he can use them.

Orientation of the Patient

Everything about a hospital can seem strange to a new patient. He has questions which he may or may not ask; there are many things he needs to know about his new surroundings. Nothing helps more to make a new patient feel secure than some understanding of what to expect. Mealtime, bedtime, daily care procedures, mail delivery, visitors' hours, physicians' visits, special treatments, and how to use the call system should be explained. The age and condition of the patient will influence the way this is done.

Admission nursing notes are charted. The form used and the extent of information required varies from one hospital to another. You should know what your charting responsibilities are when you admit a patient. Admission nursing notes can sometimes be very valuable during a lawsuit. What might seem

"routine" has a purpose; you have no authority to change or decrease the amount of information required by the hospital.

RESPONSIBILITIES OF THE NURSE DURING THE MEDICAL EXAMINATION

Purposes and procedures of the medical examination and the physician's role are discussed in Chapter 28.

Whether the examination is conducted in the hospital after admission, in a clinic, or in a physician's office before admission, the patient may have many uncertainties and even fears about the findings. The nurse can help allay some uneasiness by showing she understands his uneasiness. The physical examination may be started soon after admission to the hospital or several hours later. Whenever it starts, the nurse will need to inform the patient as simply as possible what he may expect. Fear of painful procedures is very often expressed by the patient as he anticipates his examination. Once he knows a little of what is to be done, he relaxes somewhat and finds it easier to cooperate during the process.

Preparation of the Patient

This begins when he undresses, puts on a hospital gown, and is put to bed. The admission temperature, pulse, and respiration should be charted immediately after they have been taken. A urine specimen is collected and sent to the laboratory; the patient's height and weight are determined if conditions permit.

If time permits, the routine laboratory work (complete blood count and urinalysis) is completed and attached to the chart.

Privacy is important and the nurse should assure the patient that she considers it important by seeing that privacy is provided. As routine as the medical examination may seem to be, each examination deals with an individual; it is not routine to him. Closing the door to the examination room, pulling the screens around the bed, and seeing that ample and adequate drapery linens are at hand and used are a nurse's responsibilities.

In large teaching hospitals patients are very frequently subjected to being "looked at" by medical and nursing personnel for learning purposes. The patient deserves an explanation and privacy regardless of what purposes these examinations serve. A nurse should be present to see that the patient is draped, provided privacy, and not embarrassed. Such visits can be upsetting to the patient unless care is taken to respect his feelings.

The examination may be conducted in the patient's unit or he may be moved to a special room for that purpose.

If, for some reason, a patient has to wait after you have readied him for the examination, he deserves an explanation. The need for this goes back to the point about "knowing what to expect."

Equipment and Articles Needed

When there is a special room for examinations the necessary equipment is usually at hand. However, it may save time to check the completeness of equipment beforehand. For bedside examinations the equipment is brought to the unit. Some hospitals have special trays set up for this purpose. Basic articles include: tongue blades, mouth wipes, paper towels, flashlight, stethoscope, sphygmomanometer, skin pencils, tape measure, percussion hammer, tuning fork, cotton balls, antiseptic solution, otoscope, safety pins, sterile gloves, and lubricant.

A bath blanket or sheet should be at hand for draping the patient. A face towel and emesis basin need to be available.

Assisting with Examination

The nurse is present for the entire examination of the female patient; for the male patient her presence may not be required. As the physician needs first one piece of equipment and then another, the nurse keeps them available. She helps the patient change positions, is careful to provide adequate draping, and provides for his safety as he shifts about. The nurse's concern is two-fold: (1) to be of assistance to the patient, and (2) to be of assistance to the physician.

The patient's chart is at hand because the physician may need to record information and refer to facts already charted or otherwise available (e.g., laboratory reports).

When the examination has been completed, the first concern of the nurse is to return the patient to his unit and see that he is comfortable. If the patient is examined in bed, the cover should be straightened, the back rest fixed, and the screens removed.

The equipment is cleaned and returned to its proper place. Some articles need to be sterilized, others disposed of. Replenishing the supply of tongue blades, paper towels, mouth wipes, and other such disposable items will help to have the equipment ready for the next examination.

POSITIONS FOR EXAMINATION TREATMENT, COMFORT

Placing the patient's body in certain positions makes it easier for the physician to examine certain parts of the body; some of these same positions are used while carrying out treatments and for rest and relaxation. Figure 34–7 shows six commonly used positions; the specific use of each is listed below.

1. *Lateral or Sims position* (either right or left side). To examine vagina or rectum; a good position for resting and sleeping. Drape patient to cover body except to expose anus and vaginal opening.

2. *Trendelenburg position.* Used in the operating room to displace intestines from the pelvis for pelvic surgery.

3. *Knee-chest position.* For therapeutic treatment of postpartum patients and for examination of vagina and rectum. Use two sheets (lengthwise) over body, separated so as to expose anus and vagina, and continue on to cover each leg.

4. *Jacknife position.* Used for rectal surgery.

5. *Dorsal recumbent position* (with knees flexed). For vaginal and rectal examinations. Drape body lengthwise with two sheets and so as to cover each leg and expose vaginal and rectal areas.

6. *Lithotomy position* (dorsal recumbent with feet in stirrups). Used for examination of cervix, vagina, bladder, rectum, and for surgery involving these parts. Drape as for dorsal recumbent position.

Other positions include *horizontal recumbent* (lying flat on back for examining neck,

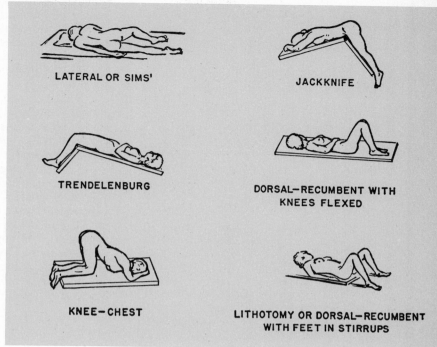

FIGURE 34–7 Positions: examination, treatment, comfort. (Frederick and Kinn: The Office Assistant in Medical Practice, 3rd ed.)

chest, abdomen, extremities), *prone* (lying on abdomen with head turned sidewise for examining back, spine, lower extremities), *Fowler* (back supported with elevated back rest and slight elevation of knee rest to relieve breathing difficulties and promote chest drainage).

REGIONS OF THE ABDOMEN

To specify the various regions of the abdomen, the physician uses the terms designated in Figures 34–8, 34–9 and 34–10. Knowledge of these general terms aids you in interpreting the physician's orders.

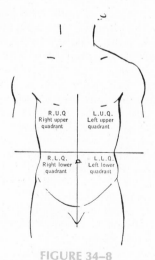

FIGURE 34–8

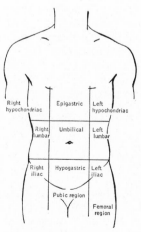

FIGURE 34–9

FIGURE 34–8   Quadrants of the abdomen. (Frederick and Kinn: The Office Assistant in Medical Practice, 3rd ed.)

FIGURE 34–9   Regions of the abdomen. (Frederick and Kinn: The Office Assistant in Medical Practice, 3rd ed.)

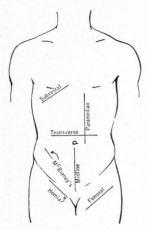

FIGURE 34–10 Abdominal incisions. (Frederick and Kinn: The Office Assistant in Medical Practice, 3rd ed.)

COLLECTING SPECIMENS

Today's storehouse of scientific knowledge provides the physician with many ways to "test" a person's state of health. He uses all types of devices to firm up a diagnosis. Among these devices are laboratory tests of body tissues, fluids, substances, secretions, and excretions to determine how normal or how abnormal they are.

To "run a test," the laboratory needs a specimen or a "sample" of the matter to be tested. Collecting some types of specimens is a nurse responsibility which calls for ability to follow directions with exactness and punctuality. Sometimes laboratory personnel come to the patient to get the specimen (e.g., blood). Sometimes the procedure for securing the specimen is a medical responsibility (e.g., spinal fluid). Here the nurse assists the physician. See Assisting with Some Diagnostic Tests in this chapter.

COMMONLY COLLECTED SPECIMENS

While each hospital or physician has instructions for collecting specimens, certain guidelines emphasize what should be kept in mind to insure accuracy insofar as your responsibilities are concerned:

1. Inform yourself of hospital or physician policies concerning the specimen to be collected, follow these policies and ask questions if you are unclear as to how to proceed.

2. Make certain of the type, time, and amount of specimen to be collected.

3. Notify patient, if appropriate.

4. Use proper containers; avoid overfilling.

5. Label specimen immediately, checking patient identification to insure correctness of name and location.

6. Send to laboratory at once, or store at proper temperature until sent.

7. Record the time, name of specimen, characteristics (color, appearance, etc.), and amount. Include any significant patient observations (objective or subjective).

8. Consult charge nurse (physician) when the situation is unusual or strange, such as if the patient is unable to void, unconscious or incontinent, is using drainage tubes for urine, or is menstruating. Also report if the specimen is accidentally "lost" (spilled, contaminated).

Urine

Review the color, specific gravity, and other characteristics of normal urine (Chapter 13). Urine specimens are examined for color, reaction, specific gravity, and presence of albumin, sugar, pus, blood, and casts. While it is not essential for the practical nurse to know the meaning of the laboratory findings, it is essential for her to follow directions very carefully when collecting the specimens. Several types of specimens are collected. (See Appendix III, Collection of Urine Specimens.)

1. *Clean single*. This may be called a routine specimen, collected upon admission and when otherwise ordered. Patients are instructed how and when it is to be collected. Collecting specimens from infants and incontinent patients requires special modifications.

2. *"Clean catch," "clean voided," "midstream," "sterile voided,"* and *"sterile."* The various names for this specimen furnish a clue that guides your action in collecting it. The clue words are *clean* and *sterile*. Because this type of specimen is often used to study the presence of foreign substance and microorganisms in the urine, the procedure points out how this urine should be collected to avoid "adding outside matter" to the urine.

3. *24-hour, single or cumulative.* Sometimes the physician wants to know the quantity and contents of urine eliminated during a

24-hour period. He is seeking diagnostic information about what the kidneys are eliminating and the amounts of what is eliminated.

4. *24-hour, fractional.* The key word "fractional" indicates that during a given 24-hour period, urine is collected and sent to the laboratory at specified times to determine the work of the kidneys during these intervals. The physician is able to compare the urine results from one period with another.

Stool or Feces

Feces are examined for such things as the presence of blood, pus, parasites, and worms, or to determine digestive disorders. The purpose of a test dictates the manner in which the specimen is collected and sent to the laboratory. Therefore, the nurse must be certain she knows the particular test to be done and the exact directions to follow. Proper labeling of the specimen tells the laboratory worker what needs to be done.

Sputum

Sputum is examined for microorganisms. Knowing which microorganisms are present aids the physician in prescribing drugs and treatments. The presence of some types of organisms alters the manner in which nursing care is provided (e.g., isolation of the patient).

Vomitus

Vomitus is examined for the presence of undigested food, blood, organisms, digestive juices, feces, and such. The physician often examines the contents of the stomach to track down pathological conditions of the stomach. When vomitus is not available (and often it is not), a tube is introduced into the stomach and contents are aspirated. One observation to make is the manner of vomiting. Was it ejected with force (projectile)? Did it occur unannounced without nausea? Did it occur at regular intervals (cyclic, periodic, or recurrent)? Did it seem to be uncontrollable?

ASSISTING WITH DIAGNOSTIC TESTS

In some instances the practical nurse assists with special diagnostic tests. This is a Role II activity which means you are a task performer assisting a physician or registered nurse in a given situation. It is necessary that you know what your responsibilities are in each situation.

To function intelligently in your assisting role, know (in general terms) the requirements of the test. You will be in a better position to appreciate the need for accuracy, punctuality, and essential precautions. Likewise, you will be able to ready the patient in a more intelligent manner. For example, if a patient is scheduled to have a basal metabolism test the next morning, all nursing personnel involved need to know that food and fluids are withheld after a certain period and that rest, quiet, and inactivity are necessary until the test is completed. Knowing that these things influence test results, you are in a better position to help the patient understand how he can cooperate.

The practical nurse is not expected to interpret test findings as such; her responsibility lies in helping with the procedure to ensure accurate results.

THE TRANSFER OF THE PATIENT IN THE HOSPITAL

For any one of several reasons a patient may be transferred from one unit to another or one floor to another within the hospital. When the move is from one floor or section to another, the admitting and business offices are notified. The charge nurse on the floor or section to which the patient is being moved is notified and preparations for his arrival are made. Notation of the move is made in the nursing notes; his chart and any medicine tickets accompany him. The patient is escorted on a stretcher, in a wheel chair, or on foot and he should be introduced to the new charge nurse. Personal belongings are accounted for and moved with him. Care should be taken to see that all belongings are moved safely.

DISCHARGE OF THE PATIENT FROM THE HOSPITAL

Leaving the hospital can be a happy experience, one mixed with uncertainty, or an

unhappy experience. Good nurse-patient relationships at the time of discharge can help the
patient leave with a warm, friendly feeling
about his hospitalization even though unpleasant things may have happened to him while
there.

Prior to his actually leaving, many things
are done. A discharge order is written by his
physician. If there is no order and a patient insists on leaving, he does so at his own risk. To
protect the hospital and physician, the patient
is required to sign a release slip. As a practical
nurse you may be responsible for seeing that it
is done. The business office, pharmacy, and
any other departments serving the patient are
notified of his departure. Arrangements for
paying the hospital bill may need to be discussed with the proper personnel.

Patient's needs and feelings vary when
dismissed from the hospital. Some need special living arrangements; others seem to prefer
the security the hospital provides rather than
go to new surroundings; but most patients are
eager to go home.

Personal Belongings

Every care should be taken to check with
the patient or his family to see that all clothing,
valuables, personal articles, flowers, and
plants are accounted for. Some hospitals
require that the patient or his family sign a slip
to show that all articles were in their possession upon discharge.

Closing the Patient's Chart

Nursing notes state the time of discharge
and how the patient left the floor (walking,
wheel chair, stretcher). The chart is removed
from its protective covering and prepared to
be sent to the medical record room. If responsible, you will need to familiarize yourself with
the process of closing the patient's chart in the
hospital where you are working.

SUMMARY

Observation of patients goes on all the time; it cuts across all nursing actions and measures. The ability to know what is important to
record and how to say it accurately and briefly is developed over years
of practice. It is best learned by following basic guidelines that apply to
any situation.

A nurse is an information gatherer. To do this effectively, personal
resources are trained to detect a patient's needs, his progress, or lack of
progress. The registered nurse is trained to detect more subtle needs
and signs of progress or lack of progress than is the practical nurse.
The practical nurse is trained to perform selected tasks and functions
with skill and accuracy (e.g., taking the blood pressure) so that what
she does renders accurate information. This type of responsibility does
not diminish the importance of the task, but rather it should emphasize
how essential it is to learn these skills well.

The patient's chart in the hospital provides the means to record
nurse observations. These observations serve the physician in making
his judgments, help the nursing staff plan patient care, and may be used
as evidence in court action; these are three good reasons why your observations should be accurate and complete enough to have meaning
for any legitimate purpose.

Observations, patient relationships, and communications are tied
together. A nurse cannot very well be observing a patient situation
without, in some way, interacting with the patient (or his family).

Signs and symptoms are objective or subjective. Objective information is gathered through one's capacity to look, listen, touch, smell,

and talk. Subjective information is gathered chiefly through one's capacity to listen, look, and question.

Regardless of where the nurse assists the patient or for what purpose, the patient's right to privacy must be respected. Likewise, he has a right to expect that his personal belongings will be kept intact and in safekeeping if removed from his presence. The nurse has responsibility to two persons while assisting with a medical examination: the patient and the physician.

Commonly used positions for examinations, treatment, or comfort include lateral or Sims', Trendelenburg, knee-chest, jackknife, dorsal recumbent, and lithotomy.

GUIDES FOR STUDY AND DISCUSSION

1. What does it mean to say a person is observant?
2. Why is observation considered a "key" to patient care?
3. As you understand it, what are your responsibilities for observation? Why is the practical nurse so important when it comes to observing patients?
4. Observations can be related to relationships and communications. How does this happen?
5. What personal capacities do you use when you observe?
6. In your opinion, what is meant by giving "full stop attention" during a patient conversation?
7. What is the difference between an objective symptom and a subjective symptom?
8. Why is it a good plan not to make written notes at the bedside? When should observations be reported/recorded?
9. What are the vital signs? Why do you suppose these signs are called vital?
10. What things might influence a body temperature reading?
11. Complete the following:

THE PULSE

Factor	What it is	Words to Describe
Rate		
Rhythm		
Quality		

12. What are the characteristics of normal urine?
13. Why does each patient have a chart? Who uses it? What kinds of information are available in it?
14. Be ready to discuss each of the eight guidelines for collecting specimens under **Commonly Collected Specimens.**

SUGGESTED SITUATIONS AND ACTIVITIES

1. Plan one or more of the following role-playing situations:
   a. Receiving a newly admitted patient.
   b. Answering some questions a patient has about being hospitalized.
   c. Helping a patient who is uneasy about his upcoming physical examination.
2. Set up a display of:
   a. All parts of the patient's chart.
   b. The various containers used for specimens.
3. Use the laboratory "doll" for practicing positioning of patients.

THE AMBULATORY PATIENT

OBJECTIVES FOR THE STUDENT: Be able to:

1. Explain who is the ambulatory patient.
2. Given the list of ten basic needs, make one meaningful statement about each and your responsibilities to this patient.
3. Describe four ways to promote ambulatory patient safety.
4. Name two things you can do to personalize care of this patient.

SUGGESTED STUDY VOCABULARY*

ambulation
independent
limitation
complication

chronic invalidism
state of dependency
convalescence
rehabilitation

dentures
posture
physical therapy
patient support

*Look for any terms you already know.

INTRODUCTION

This chapter introduces you to general nursing care by showing you how the *ten basic needs* can be used as a guide to nurse the ambulatory patient. Each need is described according to the ambulatory patient—his freedom and his ability to do things for himself.

The ambulatory patient is the "walking" patient. Ambulation means moving about; walking from the bed to a chair and back to bed is not ambulation, though it may lead to walking.

Ambulation makes the patient less dependent on the nurse for many things; he enjoys a degree of freedom which permits him some choice of activities not available to the bed patient.

In a way, this patient might be called the easiest type of patient to care for because he may be able to meet many of his basic needs with little assistance from the nurse.

Early ambulation after surgery is a special time in the life of the patient and the details of nursing care are discussed in Chapter 42.

WHO IS THE AMBULATORY PATIENT?

This patient may be of any age (except very young), male or female, and have one or more reasons for being under the physician's care. One thing these patients all have in common is they are not confined to a bed; they are allowed to walk about. Beyond that, many differences appear due to age, general physical condition, frame of mind, limitations (due to poor vision, slowness in movement, impaired hearing, unsteadiness on their feet, etc.), plus the reason for being under the physician's care.

Importance of Ambulation

It is a known fact that ambulation has physical and emotional benefits for any age group. The physician takes into account such things as age, type of illness or disorder, general physical and mental condition, any handicaps, and even the patient's self-determination when he decides whether or not a patient should be up and about.

Helping this patient to meet his daily living needs takes on more meaning for you when you understand some of the benefits of ambulation. These benefits can be grouped under two headings: *physical* and *emotional*. The patient derives physical benefits from improved functioning of the various body systems (e.g., circulatory, digestive, respiratory, musculoskeletal, and urinary). Walking improves muscle tone, appetite, and elimination. Blood circulation improves with exercise and so do sleep habits. Getting people on their feet prevents complications and chronic invalidism.

There are emotional benefits too. The patient who can walk senses a degree of independence in being able to do things for himself. Being able to walk about after bed confinement is an indication to him that he is getting better; this in itself can be very encouraging. In fact, he may consider himself as being well and attempt to act like it, doing too much for his own good.

One might think that without exception, every patient looks forward to going home. For most patients this is true; for them ambulation means being that much closer to returning to the family or home situation. However, keep in mind that *all* patients do not necessarily feel that way about it. Some resist ambulation because they dread the thought of leaving the security of the hospital for reasons that are real to them: fear of going back to work, not wanting to return to a former living arrangement, dread of going to a nursing home, living with relatives, or no home to go to. To them, the ability to walk represents the beginning of the time when they will no longer stay in the hospital and will have to make other plans.

You can do much to help the ambulatory patient. Most important is your capacity to understand and accept the fact that this person, though independent in many of his actions, needs attention and selected types of assistance (seasoned with good judgment) to handle his needs yet preserve his independence.

Planning the Nursing Care

The ambulatory patient needs a plan of nursing care as much as the bed patient does. How else can you be certain that he receives the proper attention? Just because he is on his feet does not mean he is on his own and can shift for himself.

The physician's orders (time limitations, extent of activity, etc.) determine any limitations for the patient. Plans for his care are based upon these orders and they influence the amount of time required, the time of day (or night) to do something, and the amount and extent of assistance you should give. The charge nurse should be consulted if there is any question about how much he may be permitted or encouraged to do for himself.

Nursing care means doing things with the patient as well as for him. This is especially true with the ambulatory patient. The nurse assists him to help himself. This may be an important part of his rehabilitation to more normal living activities. Success in helping the patient understand and carry out needed health practices depends upon the practical nurse, as well as the professional nurse.

One of the ways you can help the ambulatory patient is to encourage him to participate in activities he is permitted to do. Careful planning of his nursing care involves his actual participation in many ways. Some patients will want to do too much. You are responsible to see that a patient's activities are kept within the physician's orders for his care. Here again, sound judgment is an important factor in your success.

Some ambulatory patients need special treatments, various kinds of diversional activities, specific diets, assistance with some phases of daily care, or exceptional amounts of encouragement to overcome fear of moving about.

Practice (and assistance with planning) will soon teach you how to begin to fit the "pieces of this patient" together so that you will be able to outline a plan for his care according to his needs and state of dependency.

MEETING DAILY LIVING NEEDS

Personal Care and Hygiene

Daily grooming is as important to the ambulatory patient as to any other patient. Being clean, feeling well-groomed and appropriately dressed helps him to feel better. Some may need more encouragement to do this than others. For example, a particular patient may resist, be uninterested, or be slow to get involved. By showing interest in him and helping him plan how he can attend to his personal hygiene, it makes it easier for him to participate.

Most up-and-about patients will be able to take care of many or all of their personal care needs. They should be encouraged and expected to do this if their condition permits. Doing for themselves may be part of their convalescence and rehabilitation. The age, condition, and individual needs of the patient determine how much he does for himself and how much and what kind of assistance he should have.

BATH. The daily bath is for cleansing purposes. Most ambulatory patients will be able to take their own baths and enjoy doing so. The nurse has responsibility for this patient, however; he does not wander about without help or direction. She is familiar with his needs and personal hygiene habits and helps him to arrange a time, place, and materials with which to take his bath.

Not all ambulatory patients may need or wish to take a complete bath everyday. Mature judgment on your part in such a situation will be needed to avoid upsetting him. If a partial bath satisfies him and he is clean, little is gained if he feels guilty about it. See that he

has the materials he wants and assist him as needed.

The two types of so-called "complete baths" for this patient are a *tub bath* and a *shower bath*. Nursing action and responsibilities are very similar for both types. Safety is stressed and so is availability to give needed assistance.

BACK CARE. Upon first thought, one might believe that the ambulatory patient would have no need for back care. In some instances, this can be true, but not in every situation. A back rub is a valuable nursing measure, too little used today (Fig. 35–1). It requires easy-to-learn skills, few materials, and a bit of nurse willingness to carry it out. The benefits to the patient far exceed the time and materials to do it.

Why might an ambulatory patient benefit from a back rub? It relaxes tense back muscles; it lets the patient know his comfort is a concern of the nurse and at the same time observations can be made of condition of the skin.

As with any nursing measure, there may be medical reasons why a back rub would not be indicated and should not be given; this should be determined ahead of time. Certain body areas (extremities) are not rubbed; neither are edematous or painful parts.

Keep in mind that a backrub can be as comforting to an ambulatory patient who is

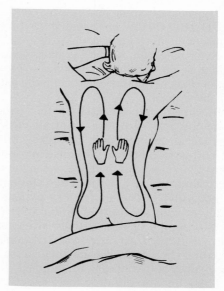

FIGURE 35–1 Hand movements for giving a back rub.

having difficulty going to sleep as to other types of patients with sleeplessness.

MOUTH AND TEETH. The patient may have a habit of brushing his teeth once, twice, or several times a day, or he may not feel that mouth care is important and will need encouragement to do it. Mouth care supplies (toothbrush, toothpaste or powder, mouthwash, if desired, and denture cup, if needed) are taken to the lavatory. In some instances you may need to help the patient.

HAIR. Most ambulatory patients will be able to care for their hair and should be encouraged to do so. For some you may need to arrange a convenient place and give them assistance. For the female patient, combing long hair and arranging it in a comfortable, attractive manner takes time. This should be provided; the patient should not feel hurried.

SHAMPOO. For the ambulatory patient who is in the hospital, nursing home, or at home ill for a long period of time, keeping the hair clean and manageable may be a needed nursing measure. Male patients experience less difficulty shampooing their hair than do female patients; they can usually manage this under the shower. Their problem may be getting a haircut. For the female patient the process may be handled under the shower or at the lavatory, but because her hair is longer she may require help. It is possible that the condition of either patient may be such that the nurse will have to assist.

Thorough washing and rinsing are necessary. Drafts should be avoided to prevent chilling. You may have to help dry the hair and comb it. Clean, attractive hair is part of good grooming. Some hospitals provide barber or beautician service to help the patient meet these needs.

SHAVING. Ambulatory male patients will do this for themselves if at all possible. When assistance is needed, the orderly or hospital barber is called. If for some reason the patient shaves at his bedside, he may need help to get necessary supplies and equipment.

DRESSING. The ambulatory patient will be fully or partially dressed, preferably in his own clothes. The family usually brings clean clothes as needed. At times when the ambulatory patient is dressed in hospital attire, pajamas, robe, and slippers are supplied. Properly fitting apparel not only feels better to the patient, it is safer.

In most cases the patient will want to and should dress himself. Clothing should be easy to put on and take off. Whenever possible, he should wear his own shoes. They provide better support than slippers and he is less likely to slip or fall. Being able to dress and undress with little or no help signifies independence for the patient. It may be one of the most important things he does for himself all day. He is to be helped if indicated (limited use of hands, arms, etc.), otherwise encouraged to do it for himself.

CLOTHING. The need for appropriate and adequate clothing may sometimes be a problem. Appropriate clothing would be garments which the patient can put on or remove easily. The family may take care of this or may not be available to help. In the latter instance, this should be called to the attention of the charge nurse.

Bed (the unoccupied, open bed)

When possible, make the bed while the patient is taking his bath so that you can be near at hand if needed. The bed linen should be completely removed even though some parts of it may be reused. The bed should be completely remade each day.

A bed which can be raised or lowered for patient and nurse convenience should be left in a position ready for the patient to use when it is finished.

Sleep and Rest

The up-and-about patient is not apt to rest so much as a bed patient during the day. However, he should not get overtired. This is especially true for the patient who has just been given walking privileges. Long afternoon rest or sleep periods, however, can interrupt night sleeping habits. This poses nursing care problems, and the patient should be helped to understand the need for some daytime rest and a good night's sleep as well. Nursing measures include attention to straightening and tightening the bed, giving a back rub, if possible, checking the room for proper ventilation, and giving any medications ordered.

Diet and Fluids

The physician orders the diet; see that the patient gets the right one. Observe the patient's appetite and note his likes and dislikes.

Mealtime interests many patients and this is particularly true of those who are up and about. If food is served in the room, there should be a clean, orderly place for eating. In some hospitals and nursing homes, the ambulatory patient goes to a dining room. Some dining rooms provide table service, and others serve cafeteria style. Patients with special dietary needs select foods with the help of the dietitian.

Good personal hygiene habits (washing hands before meals) should be observed. You may need to remind or help some patients do this; others will take care of it themselves. Encourage patients with dentures to use them if they tend not to.

As with any patient, fluid intake habits are observed. If the physician orders recording of fluid intake, the patient (if able) can be shown how to assist with this. The urinary output is usually measured, too, and if patients are too young or are unable to carry out this responsibility, the nurse assumes it.

Elimination

Walking helps the patient maintain or regain regular daily habits of elimination. Body movement and exercise stimulate bowel and bladder functions; habit and food-fluid intake influence frequency and amount of elimination.

Observing and recording information about elimination are essential (i.e., stool: amount, color, consistency, if required; urine: amount, color, etc.). Secure this information from the patient or by direct observation. Irregularities in elimination often require a physician's orders for treatment.

Body Alignment and Activity

Proper posture and exercise are beneficial to the ambulatory patient (improve muscle tone, body function and prevent deformities). Some patients need special treatments and exercise; they may go to the physical therapy department, or the therapist may work with them in their rooms. Find out the reason(s) for the treatment so that the patient's activities do not hinder his recovery and you understand what to do as well.

Walking with assistance for either a patient experiencing "first ambulation" or continued ambulation requires the attention and action of the nurse. The "assistance" in walking may be a person or some type of aid such as a walker, chair (two chairs), or cane.

Medical Treatment and Care

The practical nurse may be assigned to give all medications and treatments to the ambulatory patient, she may share this responsibility with other members of the nursing team, or the treatments may be so complex that either the registered nurse or the physician carries them out with or without the assistance of the LPN. Several facts should be kept in mind regarding medications and treatments for this type of patient.

1. Punctuality. Inform patient ahead of time when treatments and medicines will be given so that he is available.

2. Medication is not to be left unattended on bedside table. Nurse observes patient taking it.

3. Treatments (for any patient) are started and stopped as ordered. Be sure this patient knows the schedule (if possible) so there is no delay in carrying it out. Plan to give treatments other than at mealtime to avoid upsetting the patient or delaying his eating.

4. Observation of ambulatory patients' reaction to medications and treatments is as important as for bed patients. Recording significant observations should not be overlooked simply because the patient is up and about.

Environment

Provision for privacy and convenient arrangement of materials and equipment makes self-care easier and safer for the patient.

Slippery, litter-strewn floors are a real hazard for the ambulatory patient. Every precaution should be taken to make floors safe for walking. During the floor cleaning process, this patient should be sitting down or removed from the situation. Liquids, broken glass, shattered flowers, etc., should be removed from the floor immediately. This may mean that you will do this rather than risk waiting for some other worker to come and do it.

Ambulatory patients usually take care of environmental factors of light and heat or cold if they can. Be alert to the fact that, while they may wish to do this, they may need some help.

Emotional and Spiritual Support

Being up and about may be very helpful to the patient's frame of mind because he feels more sure of getting well or going home. It makes him independent in many ways and less apt to be upset or fearful about things that sometimes worry bed patients. On the other hand, a patient who is convalescing from a long or serious illness may have fear of walking. He may feel more comfortable and secure as a bed patient and not want to return home or to his family; to him walking may mean the time is soon at hand when he will leave the hospital. This patient will need encouragement to build up his feelings of adequacy or to allay his fears.

The up-and-about patient often visits with other ambulatory patients; he sees other patients who may be in greater need than he. When he is curious about other patients, answers to his questions should be tactful, but protective of other patients and their infirmities.

Patients satisfy their spiritual needs in many ways; some are visible means, others are not. The ambulatory patient may visit with his minister or the hospital chaplain in his room or go elsewhere (chapel, empty room) for more privacy. Special weekly prayer and worship services serve a real purpose for many patients.

Some patients discuss their spiritual needs freely, others do not. The nurse is there to listen and assist if she can. It is not her responsibility to change a patient's spiritual outlook or recommend one set of beliefs above another, whatever her own personal beliefs may be. You should accept him as a person and respect his right to carry out the habits of his religious practice.

Nursing care problems may arise because the patient is making, or is expected to make, adjustments—both emotional and physical. Whether, for example, he is up and about after a serious illness or is hospitalized for observation to determine the diagnosis of an ailment, he may find that being ambulatory has limitations which he has difficulty in accepting. Hospital routines may aggravate him. The nurse needs to appreciate the fact that he does not understand the functions of the hospital in the same way as she, so that when he goes about giving "expert" advice to other patients, he should be helped to understand why such routines are necessary.

Adjustments (timing, catering to likes, letting patient help make some decisions) in nursing care should be made when and where possible. This gives the patient a feeling of individuality, that the nurse is interested in him as a person and does not feel that he is "just another patient." While these facts may relate to all patients, the ambulatory patient may question more quickly or specifically the adjustments he is expected to make in his hospital living. For example, it may be difficult for him to accept the fact that he must be escorted to physical therapy or that certain daily observations are made concerning his elimination and eating habits. Often a simple explanation helps him understand.

Diversional and Rehabilitation Activities

For some ambulatory patients the hours may pass very slowly and there are those who have few if any visitors. When the possibility of going home is in the distant future, these patients need something to do to occupy their minds. Some will read, write letters, watch television, listen to the radio, do some kind of hand work, or visit with other patients. In large hospitals special recreation or diversional therapy departments help meet these needs. In nursing homes there is real need to provide diversional activities.

Conversation during the time you are making the bed or assisting the patient with some part of his care may help determine some of his interests or stimulate his interest in a new activity. You may have little or no time to help him with it except to get him started. Showing continued interest in his progress may encourage him to pursue it on his own for a long period of time.

Diversional activities must be planned in keeping with the patients' age and condition. Fatigue should be avoided; the patients' span of attention needs to be considered. Small children will tire of an activity sooner than adults. Some patients need to be encouraged to set their activity aside from time to time to avoid eyestrain or undue fatigue.

Rehabilitation is the act of restoring a person to full capacity or as close to former capacity as possible. It starts when illness starts. Everything done for and with a patient is done with the idea of restoring his body and mind to purposeful activity as soon as possible. Much of what you do as an LPN contributes to these rehabilitative efforts.

For some patients, a program of rehabilitation is a long process and proceeds according to a definite plan prescribed by the physician.

Some hospitals have physical therapy departments which help the patient re-establish the use of disabled parts. Sometimes a physician will order the patient to take certain exercises a definite number of times during the day. Observe to see that he carries them out.

Surgery or an accident may leave a patient with new adjustments to make concerning such things as bowel habits, eating habits, appliances to wear, or an entirely new orientation to caring for himself, such as in blindness or loss of a hand.

Rehabilitation is geared to both physical and emotional needs; many times they cannot be separated. Seek guidance from the physician or registered nurse when confronted with care problems that are beyond your knowledge and skill to handle.

SUMMARY

Ambulation is walking. The ambulatory patient needs the assistance of the nurse in many different ways. Provision must be made for his safety, comfort, and well-being even though he is up and about and fairly independent in his daily activity. Observation should not be overlooked simply because he is walking. The nurse makes his hospital experience more pleasant by making adjustments in keeping with his regular daily living habits insofar as his condition permits. The ambulatory patient, an interesting and challenging person, can be helped in many ways. Nursing homes provide many such opportunities.

GUIDES FOR STUDY AND DISCUSSION

1. What is ambulation? How is it helpful to the patient?
2. Under what circumstances might the ambulatory patient feel like a "forgotten" patient?
3. For each basic need, write down at least one thing you would/could do to assist this patient.
4. What things would you do to "ready" an elderly ambulatory patient for his noon meal to be served in his room? In a central dining room? What observations would you feel responsible for in each case?
5. Compare the situation in question four with that of a five-year-old ambulatory boy who was going to eat at a table with other young patients.
6. Safety is a recurring factor in *all* nursing action. Under each of the following headings list safety precautions you want to remember in caring for ambulatory patients:
   a. Environment.
   b. Personal hygiene.
   c. Medical treatment and care.
   d. Exercise and activity.
7. In your opinion, which of the ten basic needs might present the greatest challenge in caring for this patient. Be ready to support your decision in class.

SUGGESTED SITUATIONS AND ACTIVITIES

1. A young man age 25 has orders to ambulate in his recovery from a long illness. He seems anxious to get started. List (in order of priority) the actions you, his nurse, would take before, during, and following his beginning ambulation. Give a reason for each action you list.
2. Plan an inexpensive type of diversion for two elderly women who are roommates in a nursing home.
3. There are many similarities between the actions of the nurse assisting a patient who takes a tub bath and a patient who takes a shower. List as many of these similarities as you can. Next, list the differences in the actions of the nurse.

THE MILDLY ILL PATIENT

OBJECTIVES FOR THE STUDENT: Be able to:

1. Using the list of ten basic needs, describe at least five ways your nursing actions might differ between caring for the mildly ill patient and the ambulatory patient.
2. Give an example of a patient situation which shows how an adjustment(s) can be made to individualize nursing care.
3. Explain the role of cleanliness in the prevention of decubitus ulcers.
4. Describe four values of a cleansing bed bath to the patient.
5. Name two things you should be observing while giving a bed bath.
6. Identify ten factors which influence the assistance needed by the patient.

SUGGESTED STUDY VOCABULARY*

infirmity	senile	contraindicated
convalescence	incontinence	contractures
chronic	complication	muscle atrophy
therapeutic value	improvise	debris
fatigue	obese	continuity of care

*Look for any terms you already know.

INTRODUCTION

Mild illness is *a degree of infirmity;* it is something less severe and may be short or long-term. In this degree of infirmity, the patient requires some or complete bed rest for awhile, usually not too long.

The term "mildly ill" is an inexact term. It is difficult to be precise about the extent of variations found among patients who are neither ambulatory nor seriously ill. One could

liken this term to the color gray. Gray is not an exact color; it has many shades ranging from very light to very dark. So it is with mild illness; there are many variations which influence the type(s) and extent of assistance this patient requires from the nurse to meet his daily living needs.

This chapter tells how the 10 daily needs are met for the mildly ill patient. The purpose here is to show how the degree of illness and the state of dependency influence the types of assistance he needs; likewise, the purpose is to help you sense what it means to plan your role with a bed patient in mind. He needs some unique types of assistance from the nurse; examples of these are pointed out.

WHO IS THE MILDLY ILL PATIENT?

This patient may be of any age, male or female, and with one or more reasons for being under the physician's care. So far, this description is the same as for the ambulatory patient. The difference is that he requires more assistance from the nurse because he is not as independent as the "walking patient." At the beginning (at least) *this patient is usually a bed patient.*

The patient's condition (diagnosis, signs and symptoms, limitations, etc.) indicates to the physician what he must order for treatment and medical management. These orders, in turn, set the stage for nursing care.

Following are some of the factors which influence the type and kind of assistance the patient requires.

1. Physician's orders for such things as:
    a. Complete bed rest.
    b. Bathroom privileges and bed rest otherwise.
    c. Permitted to be up in a chair for certain periods of time.
    d. Side rails.
2. Something that limits his movability such as:
    a. Leg in traction.
    b. A cast on an extremity.
    c. Swollen, painful joints.
    d. Bandaged hands.
3. Limitations as to:
    a. Seeing.
    b. Hearing.
    c. Speaking.
    d. Swallowing.
4. Special diet, fluids, frequent feedings.
5. Special drugs and treatments.

As you can see, the mildly ill patient category includes a very wide range of sick people. Depending upon age, limitations, and such, this patient is going to need help with many aspects of his care. Very often he will be able to help himself, but judgment must be used in deciding how much he should do without your assistance.

MEETING DAILY LIVING NEEDS

The mildly ill patient's daily care can be fitted into the structure of the ten basic needs, too. As pointed out, this patient does not enjoy the extent of independence the ambulatory patient does. But for his own good he should not be denied the opportunity to help himself as permitted under his medical management. Translated into nursing action, this means that you render help to make it possible for the patient to do those things he is capable of doing and then step in and do what he cannot do.

Consider the fact that the mildly ill patient might have an extended period of convalescence or a long-term, chronic condition that raises questions of complications and possibly an unhappy attitude toward being sick so long.

PLANNING THE NURSING CARE

It is possible to develop a plan of care for the mildly ill patient which lets him know you take into account his uniqueness — his individuality. The plan will include the "exact" things (e.g., medical orders) and the "inexact" things (e.g., flexibility in relation to things without medical orders or time schedules). The patient senses this flexibility when your plan includes (when possible) his likes, dislikes, and his ways of doing things.

Plan his care to allow time for him to participate in a suitable manner. He may eat slowly and be upset when hurried. It may be important to him to clean his teeth or to drink a glass of warm water before breakfast. Any considerations which are within his prescribed orders for care should be provided if at all possible. This gives him a feeling of receiving individualized care and he has to make fewer adjustments. Each patient should experience some such feeling if he is not to look at his hospital stay as something he endures to enable the nurse to get her work done. This is an important aspect in nursing the mildly ill patient. Oftentimes he is well enough to want to do many things for himself and if this be the case, he appreciates being able to do them as he does when he is well.

Flexibility (making needed adjustments in nursing care plans) should be an active part of every nurse's ability. When flexibility is lacking the patient knows it. He could be justified in his feeling that *he* does all of the adjusting, when it should be a shared process. Both patient and nurse make adjustments when the best care is given.

Whether the patient is able to do much or little self-care is a matter the nurse considers in planning his care. The physician may want the patient to have some activity. As he improves, new orders are written for more self-care so that he gradually assumes self-direction in his recovery. Increased independence is a hopeful sign. The alert nurse makes the most of this fact as she gives him care. Encouragement from the nurse is all it takes for some patients to move toward independence.

Frequent patient contacts help the nurse to recognize his needs. Some may be minor; others will require the direction and supervision of the professional nurse.

To provide safe and intelligent care, you need to know about the patient's likes and dislikes, his illness, physician's orders for his care, nursing measures possible within the physician's orders, and what your role is in planning and providing this care. Is it Role I, Role II, or a combination of both? There should be no uncertainty in your mind about how much or to what extent the patient is permitted to do for himself. Any doubts or questions should be clarified *before* the patient is involved.

Observation, reporting, and charting are valuable here as with other patients. The physician can use this information to help determine how the patient's care is to be continued. Many facts about the activity of the mildly ill patient may not need to be recorded. Determine what is pertinent to report.

DAILY LIVING NEEDS

Personal Care and Hygiene

Being clean and well-groomed helps anyone to experience a feeling of well-being. From the onset of illness, mildly ill patients show varying degrees of interest in their personal hygiene. Life-long habits and what they are used to make some patients interested in their personal care; others are not. The very young would respond more to the manner in which it was done rather than resist the

process itself. The person who is senile may not be aware of actually what is happening, but may resist the process anyway.

For those patients who can assume some part of bathing, mouth care, hair, shaving, etc., nursing care plans should include their participation. In general, any of these patients feel better when clean; good personal care helps prevent complications and is rehabilitative.

BATH. If the patient is able, he should be permitted and even encouraged to take his own bath provided that it is within the physician's orders for his care. It may be taken in the tub, shower, or while the patient is in bed, depending upon his condition. A bath taken in bed by the patient, or given by the nurse, may be a *complete* or *partial* bath. A bath can be a fatiguing experience for the patient and there are times when it is better to give a partial rather than a complete bath.

While patient self-care is encouraged when feasible, there are many instances when the mildly ill patient needs to have his bath given by the nurse. Think, for example, of the patient who is unable to move, owing to a crippling condition of the musculoskeletal system, a severe stroke, or an accident that has left him paralyzed. Consider the very young patient who is not capable because of his age, if for no other reason. Then, at the other end of the life span, the aging process makes some persons irresponsible and unaccountable. For any of these patients and those who can help themselves, the cleansing bath is refreshing and relaxing. The warmth of the water, the washing and drying action, the back rub, the change of position are comfortable experiences and serve as a mild type of exercise.

The practical nurse soon learns that during the bath she can do much to promote good nurse-patient relationships. When the patient talks freely, show your interest by attentive listening and expression of acceptance of the patient as a person who has his own ideas. You may learn a great deal about the patient which will enable you to give him more individualized care and attention. On the other hand, the patient may be ill at ease, lonely and worried, or just quiet. Here again you will find it is not necessary to keep up a conversation throughout the process. There are many ways to help the patient overcome his uneasiness or loneliness. Providing privacy is one way. This indicates to the patient that the nurse respects his rights. The gentle yet thorough manner in which she gives the bath can leave him with a feeling of reliance on her ability. Acceptance can be shown by not being judgmental or threatening in word, deed, or manner.

Observation goes on throughout the bath. There is no better time during the day to notice any changes in the condition of the skin. presence of pressure and friction areas, or to listen to complaints of pain and discomfort or his expression of how he slept and the state of his appetite. Observe such things as limited motion in arms or legs, or difficult breathing, if they are present.

BACK AND SKIN CARE. Both take on particular meaning for the mildly ill person who is confined to his bed in a fairly fixed sort of way for long periods. This is especially true if he has no control over bowel and bladder elimination (incontinence). Back and skin care measures are restful and relieve weariness. They stimulate circulation to prevent pressure areas from persisting and eventually turning into decubitus ulcers (bedsores). The practical nurse who knows how and takes time to give back and skin care has learned a valuable lesson in patient care. Few nurse actions call forth more patients' comments of satisfaction than this one. More important, however, is the fact that a patient long confined to a bed without bedsores is a symbol of quality nursing care.

Nails should be cleaned, and filed or trimmed if necessary. A lotion or cream applied to the hands following the bath will help to keep them smooth and prevent chapping. The patient will take care of his hands and nails if he is able. At times you may need to encourage him to do this; it may be a health habit he has not practiced prior to his illness.

MOUTH AND TOOTH CARE. When patients have no mouth care equipment, discuss this with the charge nurse to find out what is available. Improvised materials may have to be used until other arrangements can be made. Bed patients need mouth and tooth care at least twice a day. The patient's condition, his habits and wishes may mean that this care will be given more frequently. Patients with dentures may have the habit of cleaning their teeth after every meal in their daily living. Such should be provided.

Certain conditions of the mouth or gums may require frequent cleansing and special care. For example, sore cracked lips need lubrication to promote healing.

Unusual appearance of the tongue should be called to the attention of the charge nurse or physician.

If a patient is able to clean and care for his mouth and teeth he will prefer to do this. The convenient arrangement of mouth care materials (toothbrush, toothpaste, emesis basin, glass of water, or mouthwash with drinking tube) on the bedside table or the overbed table is the responsibility of the nurse. The patient may need help to get started and carry on (you may put toothpaste on the brush, hold the curved basin, etc.). (Fig. 36–1).

Patients with dentures or removable bridgework require special attention. The first consideration should be the patient. He may be sensitive about the fact that he wears dentures. Some people want privacy when they remove them and are embarrassed if it is not provided; in fact, it may be the reason why they do not want to clean their teeth at all.

The nurse must clean the dentures if the patient is not able to do it himself; she asks the patient to remove and place them on a piece of clean gauze or mouth tissue. When dentures or bridgework are cleaned every precaution is used to avoid dropping them. They chip and crack easily and small pieces of bridgework can readily slip down the drain. If the patient does not prefer to replace his dentures after cleaning, they are placed where they will not be broken or lost—in the drawer of the bedside table or in plain sight, preferably covered with water in a denture cup, when stored. Patients should be encouraged to wear their dentures at all times, if possible.

HAIR. The bed patient looks and feels better when his hair is well groomed. This is usually a simple and easy matter for the male

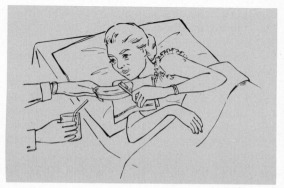

FIGURE 36–1 Assisting a patient with mouth care.

patient. The female patient needs more time and attention, especially when she has long hair. Lack of attention to the hair gives the patient a neglected look.

The female patient, especially sensitive about the appearance of her hair, may prefer to comb and arrange her hair and should be encouraged to do so, if able. Your responsibility, in this case, is to ready the environment so the patient can proceed.

One sign of getting well is when a patient begins to take an interest in his appearance. Provide time and encouragement for this need; permit him to proceed in an unhurried manner. Observe for undue fatigue.

Long hair is more comfortable for the patient when it is parted in the middle, from front to back, and braided or arranged on either side.

Matted, curly hair needs daily care to keep it comfortable and attractive. Careful combing and braiding usually keep it in good condition.

If hair needs to be cut, secure the patient's written permission first. If a barber is available, he is sought at the patient's (or family's) request.

SHAVING. The mildly ill male bed patient may or may not be able to shave himself. If he is able, his materials are assembled and arranged for his convenience. An overbed table with a mirror makes the most convenient arrangement.

For the patient who needs assistance, it is provided in one of several ways: by a family member or a friend, by a barber or the hospital orderly or a nurse.

DRESSING. For comfort and convenience of care, pajama tops or a short gown are worn, especially if the abdomen, buttocks, and lower extremities need special attention or treatment. When possible, the patient should wear his own apparel.

Bed jackets are usually worn by women patients to protect their shoulders.

Unless a patient is helpless or his activity restricted, he will dress himself or be encouraged to do so. Usually little help is needed unless the patient is fatigued, has limited motion, is too young, or it is otherwise contraindicated.

Some patients enjoy having a choice in the matter of what they wear and when. During the day they may wish to wear their own apparel and at night sleep in a hospital gown.

When patients have no personal bed apparel, use hospital gowns; some prefer them anyway.

The hospital gown is usually about hip length, opened full length in the back and easy to put on or remove. The back is secured by tying attached tapes. It is possible to reverse the gown and wear the opening in the front.

Bed garments should be changed each day and more often if necessary. Clean, fresh clothing following the bath is refreshing and helps the patient feel well cared for and comfortable.

BED, OCCUPIED. Usually the most satisfactory time to change and remake the bed is following the morning bath and toilet care. Linen is changed as needed. However, the bed patient requires some clean linen daily if he is to feel refreshed. His bed not only feels cleaner and more comfortable, it has a better appearance as well. This may be one way to help him accept the fact that he has to spend another day in bed.

While making the occupied bed, these points about the patient should be kept in mind:

1. Conserve his energy as you work. Avoid jarring the bed and jerking linen to release it.

2. Tell patient how, when, and where to move to help you. Assist him if he needs it.

3. Protect his privacy by providing cover.

Rest and Sleep

The amount and kind of sleep and rest a patient gets depend a great deal upon the nursing care he receives. The mildly ill bed patient could require more types of nursing care in relation to rest and sleep than the ambulatory or seriously ill patient because the up-and-about patient could get exercise and thereby be tired enough to sleep, while the seriously ill may be too weak or be receiving many pain-relieving drugs which relax him.

The mildly ill patient may be recovering from a long serious illness that has changed his sleeping habits; he may be restless and anxious to get home. Being confined to the bed all or most of the day provides little exercise and much opportunity for several short naps. Nighttime may find him wakeful and upset because he can't sleep.

"Putting patients to bed" or preparing

them for sleep is truly a nursing responsibility which should *precede* the giving of any sleep medications.

Although there are many important things the nurse can do to help the patient rest and sleep, there is, in all probability, no one part of nursing care which can induce sleep or relax the patient in preparation for sleep like that of "putting the patient to bed" by giving him complete evening care. Patients remember the real comfort of the soothing back rub and bed linen that has been straightened and tightened. No satisfactory substitute has been found to replace this. When it is skillfully done, the patient can fall asleep during the process. The medication may follow preparations for sleep but does not precede or replace them.

Proper sleep and rest promote recovery. The mildly ill patient may need the attention of the nurse during the night if it is only to talk a bit when she makes rounds and finds him awake. Very often the suggestion of a glass of warm milk will be enough to change his endless train of thoughts and relax him enough to fall asleep. Careful observation during the night means that the nurse visits each patient's unit regularly. The fact that a patient may not call for the nurse does not necessarily mean that he is sleeping. Accurate observations can be made only upon regular patient visits. Good judgment in using a flashlight while making rounds, not awakening patients for a treatment, unless absolutely ordered around the clock, and quiet go far to permit sleep and rest. Record any meaningful observations which may be helpful to the physician in determining a patient's need for medications.

Factors related to rest and sleep are:
1. Quiet, well-ventilated room.
2. Lightweight, adequate covering.
3. Evening care with soothing back rub.
4. A clean, smooth, tight bottom sheet.
5. Measures and devices to control pain and discomfort.
6. Avoid disturbing sleep or rest unless absolutely necessary.
7. Plan for rest periods during the day.
8. Observe the effect of presence or absence of visitors.
9. Adjust care to respect patient's habits.
10. Respect spiritual habits and needs.
11. Sedatives specifically ordered by the physician are usually meant to be used only if needed and not as a "routine" for sleep.

Diet and Fluids

Adequate food and fluid intake is a necessary part of recovery from illness. As with all other patients, the physician orders the type of diet and specifies any restrictions of food or fluids.

For this patient who might be well enough to enjoy his meals, you can help him look forward to mealtime. Attention should be given to the following, whether he can feed himself or must be fed:
1. Plan nursing care and treatments to avoid mealtime.
2. Handwashing before meals.
3. Provide comfortable, convenient position.
4. Arrange over-bed or bedside table to hold tray conveniently for patient.
5. Prepare tray; remove covers from dishes, cut meat, butter bread, if necessary.
6. See that tray is complete, e.g., if allowed salt and pepper see that they are on the tray and that hot foods are hot and cold foods cold.
7. Allow time for finishing meal.
8. Be seated, if possible, when feeding patient.
9. Observations to be reported include references to appetite, amount eaten or not eaten.

Many mildly ill patients will be able and will want to feed themselves (Fig. 36-2). Some will have limitations (burns of hands,

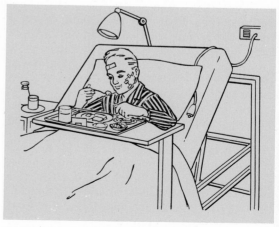

FIGURE 36-2 This patient is able to feed himself. Notice the convenient arrangement of his immediate environment.

fractures, paralysis) which will make it necessary to feed them.

Feeding patients requires patience. You should sit down and approach this task in a relaxed manner. If the patient cannot see, he should be told what is on his tray. Allow enough time between mouthfuls so that he can chew his food well. Small portions, spoon or fork about half full, are easier to handle. Variety feeding (offering different foods) is more interesting to him.

As patients with limited motion regain their health, feeding themselves may be a needed exercise. You can assist this patient in his recovery by encouraging him to feed himself. Allow ample time for the patient to do this. Feeding himself may be the one thing he does unassisted and he enjoys this feeling of independence.

As the patient improves, he may sit on the side of the bed or in a chair at the bedside while he eats. If in a wheelchair, he can go to the dining room to be with other patients if this service is available. Getting out of bed for the first few times could be planned to occur at mealtime, unless otherwise indicated.

Adequate fluid intake is necessary to proper body function. Any special orders for restricting or forcing ordinary or special fluids means that there is accurate measurement of all fluid intake and output.

Elimination

For the bed patient, lack of exercise plus the need to use a bedpan and urinal often changes daily habits of elimination. Many people have a daily bowel movement and some are concerned when this daily habit is interrupted. They are worried about this irregularity.

Observations and charting include the frequency and character (color, amount, consistency) of stools and urine.

As the patient uses the bedpan and the urinal the following practices should guide your actions:

1. Protect the patient's feelings. Be sure he has privacy to avoid embarrassment.

2. Provide for safety and comfort. Be sure the utensil (bedpan or urinal) is clean, dry, and free from rough edges. Pad the areas of the bedpan if the patient is thin, has bony prominences or pressure sores. A wet utensil leaves the bed and patient damp; a warm utensil is better than a cold one.

3. Position him for comfort. The helpless or heavy patient may need first to be turned on his side and then back onto the pan.

4. Remove the utensil(s) without delay. Few things disturb patients more than the helpless (and uncomfortable) feeling of being left on a bedpan too long. When this happens they feel the part of "the forgotten patient."

Body Alignment and Activity

The bed patient's position and movement are related to his comfort, prevention of fatigue and complications and, thus, to his recovery. Attention is given to the posture of the bed patient. Whether in bed for short or long periods of time, many patients lie on their backs or in one particular position most of the time. Encourage position change. This helps to prevent muscle strain, fatigue and pressure areas, and is restful to the patient.

Position change and body movements occur while the able bed patient bathes, eats, and dresses. Sometimes he needs encouragement to get this exercise.

The physician orders certain exercises when he is concerned about contracture, muscle atrophy, or joint stiffness; these are preventive and rehabilitative measures. Some patients may feel they are not able to carry out such specific exercises; in that event, the nurse helps them get started. She observes to see that they are done and encourages the patient as he progresses. Whenever special exercises are ordered, be sure you understand your responsibilities.

Sometimes these exercises are started while the patient is in bed, or he is moved to the physiotherapy department on a stretcher or in a wheel chair. Provide any special posture or position needed during this transportation. Between these treatments, the patient is to follow any directions for alignment, posture, and exercise; the nurse gives help as needed.

The physician writes the order for the patient to be out of bed. At first this may be for a very limited time and then gradually increased to full ambulation. Age, condition, and stage of recovery influence the length of time and amount of activity ordered. Learning to ambulate ranges from walking with assistance for a few first steps and then increasing the activity until the patient is able to walk about alone. Encouragement generally helps and provision for safety (support, properly fitting footwear, a floor clear of debris, etc.) is essential.

Medical Treatment and Care

The patient's illness condition determines his medical orders. They may include treatment measures to re-establish use of muscles or joints, relieve stiffness, or to regain use of an extremity. Orders may include medications to relieve pain, relax the patient, produce sleep, improve the appetite, prevent or check infections, improve the circulation of the blood, aid digestion, or eliminate constipation.

Whether the practical nurse gives the medications and treatments or not, she should inform herself about the purposes of them so that her observations are accurate and her plan of nursing care does not interfere with the giving or the effectiveness of them. For example, some treatments should be given before the bath is taken and the bed is changed. Evening treatments should be done before the patient is prepared for sleep. If the practical nurse is not taking care of the treatments and medications, she should know about them so she can plan her part of the care with the patient in mind. It seems inexcusable to follow sleep preparation with a treatment that would in any way disturb the patient. Likewise, it seems to be poor judgment to carry out a treatment measure which might soil or dampen the patient's bed right after it has been made for the day if this can be avoided. Painful treatments just before meals should also be avoided if at all possible.

Some medications have exact time requirements for administration. If a medicine is ordered to be given one half-hour before mealtime, the meal will have to be delayed if the medication is given late. This can cause the patient to eat or refuse to eat cold, unpalatable food.

If the mildly ill patient is in traction, movement and position of the patient must be considered when care is being given. The weights must *not* be removed, shifted, or loosened. The practical nurse assigned to care for such a patient is responsible for knowing (ask, if unsure) about any necessary precautions she must take during the bed bath, making the bed or doing any other care measures such as giving the patient an enema or treating a decubitus ulcer.

Get assistance to help move or lift a pa-

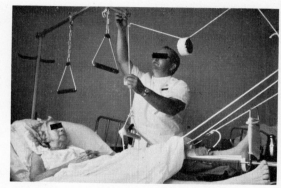

FIGURE 36–3 Adjustments to traction equipment are made by people who know how to do what should be done. (Courtesy of Palm Beach County Vocational School, Practical Nursing Program, West Palm Beach, Florida.)

tient if there is any question of safety. Special lifting devices are sometimes used. Be sure you understand what to do before you start (Fig. 36–3).

Environment

An observant nurse takes care of most environmental needs without the patient's asking. Additional bedding, proper ventilation, elimination of drafts, and convenient arrangement of needed articles such as signal light, water, reading material, and mouth wipes are some ways she provides for his comfort. She foresees or anticipates what his needs might be and asks him before he has to call her back and request her to do things for him.

Many things the nurse does for and with the patient during the course of a day have no orders written for them. These are the personal things he, when well, does for himself, so he especially appreciates the thoughtfulness and assistance.

Emotional and Spiritual

Many factors enter into the emotional well-being of the mildly ill patient. Some of these factors include:
1. Length of illness.
2. Whether or not he is getting better.
3. Degree of independence in self-help.
4. Visitors or lack of them.
5. Purposeful diversion.

People react as they do for a reason. You can help a patient's frame of mind by showing acceptance of him in your manner and willingness to help him. The practical nurse does not need to know all there is to know about behavior patterns of human beings to accept patients as they are. In fact, if you conduct yourself in a manner to "be well-received," as discussed in Chapter 3, chances are that the patient will know you accept him.

Patients have spiritual needs which are sometimes expressed more by what they do than by what they say. Observe and respect any such evidence. Seek guidance from the registered nurse or physician if you encounter a situation which seems beyond your understanding and role.

The practical nurse is most effective in helping to meet the total needs of her patient when she helps the patient obtain the kind of assistance he needs. She reports his needs so that people prepared to meet these needs are made available to him.

Adjustments

As the patient improves, his daily activities change. Self-help will be part of the rehabilitative process. Frequently patients need to be encouraged to make these self-help adjustments. If, for example, the nurse up to this time has been giving the patient his bath, and he has improved sufficiently to wash his own face, but hesitates, ways must be found to have him do this for himself. After the bathing materials are ready and at hand, prepare the washcloth for use, hand it to him (placing a towel close by) and ask him to wash his face while you leave to get an additional towel or for some other legitimate excuse.

Adjusting to the self-help role will be easy for some patients, more difficult for others. The same is true of the nurse. Some will guide their patients to self-help and others will do for their patients long after they should be doing for themselves.

The bed patient, even the one able to give partial self-care, must make many adjustments when he is ill. This is especially true for the hospitalized patient who is away from home, family, and familiar surroundings and routines; he may not know what to expect or how to act. First-time patients especially are apt to have mixed feelings about bathing or being bathed in bed, using a bedpan, taking care of

personal needs in a manner quite unfamiliar to them. Nurses, all too frequently, forget that these things call for adjustments by the patient and that they can be extremely helpful to him if they talk with him about what to expect and provide for convenience and privacy. The nurse's approach to the patient's adjustments should give him a feeling of being considered as a person.

Some patients may fail to see the need for doing things differently while hospitalized or even while sick at home. Very often the nurse, through patience and by careful explanation, can help them accept the reason(s) for such differences; sometimes a patient in the next bed helps, or the family helps him to adjust. On the other hand, these same people might hinder the adjustment. When you encounter patients having difficulty accepting their situation, consult with the charge nurse or physician to be sure you do nothing to delay the adjustment.

Many small, personal care variations or additions are possible and should be included without labeling the patient "difficult," "demanding," or "uncooperative."

Hospital "routines" may seem pretty unreasonable to some patients. Sometimes a simple explanation will help, such as answering the patient's questions about routines, special diets, the need for scheduling things at certain times, visiting hours, and the like. Avoid trying to teach or tell a patient something that needs explanation by the physician or the professional nurse; report the questions so that they may help the patient.

Careful observation and reporting are important to the other team members and the physician. Tomorrow's care can be influenced by today's observation.

Diversional Activities and Rehabilitation

Most patients, if not too uncomfortable and ill, will need some diversional activity. Reading is a popular pastime for many, almost a necessity for those who read a great deal when well. Listening to the radio, watching television, writing, visiting or doing some handicraft divert the patient's mind from his illness condition.

In some instances the physician orders specific exercise and treatments for rehabilitative purposes; they may start while the patient is in bed and continue after he becomes

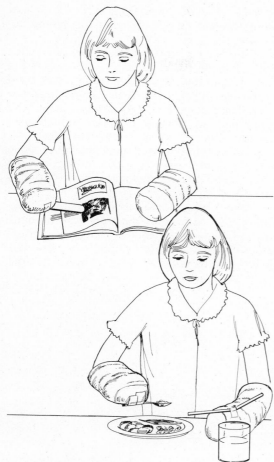

FIGURE 36–4 This shows how a patient can help himself when implements are taped to bandaged hands.

ambulatory. Everything that happens to a patient to assist him back to purposeful living according to his capacity to do so can be considered part of the rehabilitative process (Fig. 36–4).

SOME COMMON NURSING PROBLEMS OF THE MILDLY ILL PATIENT

Keeping the Bed Patient Comfortable

Normal living activity for the well person is a constant process of change in position and use of muscles. Being confined to a bed reduces muscle activity to a minimum, espe-

cially if the patient's condition permits little or no self-help. Patients prefer to lie on their backs and will remain in that position for long periods if not encouraged or helped to change. When permitted, his position should be changed regularly and be properly supported if he is confined to the bed. Whenever possible, the patient should do this by himself. Obese and helpless patients need assistance.

Here are some reasons for position change and proper support.

1. *Position change*
   a. Aids circulation.
   b. Relieves pressure areas.
   c. Reduces fatigue.
   d. Provides relaxation.
2. *Immobility causes:*
   a. Poor circulation.
   b. Loss of muscle tone.
   c. Joint stiffness.
   d. Pressure areas.
3. *Inadequate support contributes to:*
   a. Poor body alignment.
   b. Contractures.
   c. Fatigue.
   d. Aching muscles.
   e. Pressure areas.

Support and Comfort Devices

Pillows of all sizes, when properly used, help to provide real comfort for the bed patient. They support the body and provide change of position to avoid muscle pull and strain if used to maintain proper alignment of arms, legs and trunk (Fig. 36–5).

Improper use of pillows can cause dis-

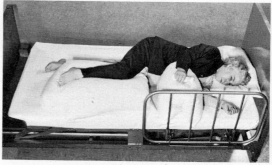

FIGURE 36–5 Pillow comfort. Notice the alignment of the right arm and right leg. There is no "pull" on the shoulder or upper arm muscles. The leg rests comfortably in a natural position. (A Handbook of Rehabilitative Nursing Techniques in Hemiplegia. Kenny Rehabilitation.)

comfort as well as poor body alignment. One of the most common examples of this is having too many pillows under the head. The head and neck are held forward at an uncomfortable angle and out of proper alignment with the spinal column. The shoulders need straight line support and too often do not get it when the patient is "over pillowed."

Foot rests aid comfort and prevent deformities; they prevent slipping down in bed and hold the bedding off the toes (preventing foot drop). Notice the several types of foot rests in Figure 36–6.

Cradles of various sizes are sometimes used to keep the top bedding from interfering with the feet and legs. Such equipment should be fastened to the bed (Fig. 36–6).

Sandbags of various sizes, when properly filled, can be used to hold a part of the body in position. Flexible, yet firm, they are placed along the part and fit up against it, giving full support.

Rubber air rings and *sponge rubber rings* are commonly used to relieve pressure from some part of the body. Caution should be used in not leaving the ring device in position too long. Hard-packed doughnuts of cotton and gauze may interfere with blood circulation to the area and do more harm than good. Air rings filled with too much air act in the same way. Pieces of sponge or foam rubber and the use of small pillows may be more helpful than ring comfort devices.

The *mattress* aids or limits patient comfort. It should support the weight of the body in good alignment (head, neck, back, and legs should be in line as the patient is lying down). A firm mattress with enough "give" to con-

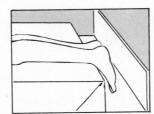
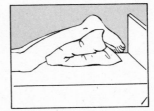

POSITION OF FEET WHEN LYING FACE DOWN, OR IN PRONE POSITION

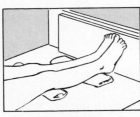
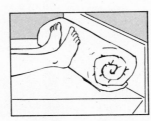
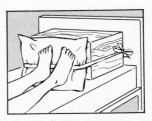

FOOT BOARD   BLANKET ROLL   PILLOW TIED TO BOX

PROVISION FOR SUPPORT OF FEET

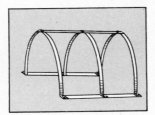
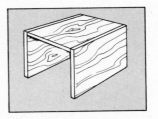

BED CRADLES, HOSPITAL AND IMPROVISED TYPE

FIGURE 36–6 Means for providing foot and leg comfort and preventing deformities such as foot drop.

form to body shape is the most comfortable. A plywood bed board (full size) placed between the springs and mattress helps to make a bed firm and level.

Whatever comfort measure is used, the nurse keeps several things in mind:

1. Maintain proper body alignment.
2. Relieve muscle pull and strain.
3. Avoid interference with circulation.
4. Provide clean equipment to avoid danger of reinfection from contaminated devices.
5. Frequent and regular change of position with proper support.

Skin Care and Prevention of Decubitus Ulcers

No other single fact points to negligent, inadequate nursing care more clearly than the presence of decubitus ulcers (pressure sores). Skin care is a nursing responsibility, one shared by every nurse giving care to the patient. Negligence by one nurse can undo the work of others.

A decubitus ulcer is a broken skin area caused by prolonged pressure on a part of the body of a bed patient. The places most likely to develop broken skin areas are over bony prominences (coccyx, elbows, heels, shoulder blades, hips) where the skin carries no large supply of blood to nourish the area and is apt to be moist. Once the skin is broken, infection sets in very readily and this sore or ulcer is difficult to heal, as well as being uncomfortable to the patient. Prevention is the best possible nursing treatment.

All pressure areas of the body are observed for discoloration. A bluish red or mottled skin is an indication of interference with blood circulation due to pressure. Bedding, bandages, casts, or lying too long in one position can create such areas. Body warmth and moisture from perspiration, urine, and other body discharges promote bed sores because soft moist skin is easy prey to bed linen wrinkles, objects such as crumbs, or restless moving about. It takes only a little pressure and friction to cause this skin to break.

Change of position is necessary to relieve pressure and to maintain proper circulation. If the skin ulcer is large the patient may be placed in a CircOlectric bed or on a Stryker frame to permit change of body tilt and thus relieve pressure. Use care in moving the patient off and on the bedpan (one with a smooth protected surface).

High protein, high vitamin diets are thought to be an added protection for patients subject to pressure sores.

Cleanliness is as important as any one factor in preventing decubitus ulcers. Effective nursing care provides for a clean, dry skin protected from undue pressure. This requires almost constant attention for some patients. After bathing and drying the skin thoroughly, the area is frequently rubbed with alcohol. This may be done several times a day. Sometimes a protective coating of cocoa butter or olive oil is applied to the skin to prevent urine and other discharges from irritating it. Body or talcum powder used sparingly helps to prevent friction. However, too much powder hardens into small particles and irritates the skin.

The hands, elbows, feet, and lips need special attention to keep them soft and free from chapping and friction burn. Skin lubricants such as cold cream are frequently used.

Weighing the Patient

Under certain conditions it may be necessary to weigh the patient. If he is able to get out of bed, the scale is brought to the bedside. For the patient who is unable to stand, it will be necessary to transport him in a wheel chair or on a stretcher to a large scale in the hospital.

The weight of the empty wheel chair or stretcher is subtracted from the total weight to determine the patient's weight.

Getting the Patient Out of Bed for the First Time

Preparation for getting a patient out of bed starts prior to actually doing it. If the patient has had a long or serious illness which has left him weakened, he may regain some muscle tone and strength by first practicing to pull himself up to a sitting position on the side of the bed for short periods of time. A chair to support his feet and legs helps to prevent fatigue. If a chair is not used, this position is called "dangling."

The pulse should be taken before, during, and following this procedure and when getting

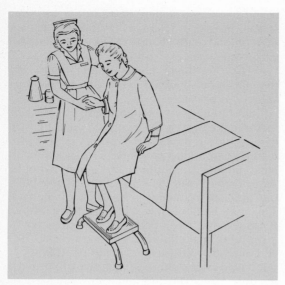

FIGURE 36–7 Slowly move patients to sitting position. Give support to assist a patient out of bed. Note use of firmly anchored foot stool if the bed cannot be lowered.

the patient out of bed. Your role is to assist the patient and observe safety precautions (foot stool, arm support, adequate clothing). See Figure 36–7.

Constipation

Illness frequently upsets normal bowel habits. Lack of normal amounts of exercise, the change in diet, the need for a change in fluid intake, and the abnormal position for having a bowel movement (the bedpan) all contribute to constipation. Lack of privacy may be another factor.

Because bowel habits vary from person to person, the nurse needs to determine each patient's habit. Some normally have a daily elimination (usually after a meal), others have them less often.

Patients frequently worry about a change in bowel habits and ask the nurse to give them something for their constipation. Observing and recording frequency, amount, color and character of stools will indicate to the physician whether or not medication or treatment such as use of an enema is indicated. Any type of bowel treatment needs a physician's order. One of the most frequently ordered treatments is the cleansing enema. (See Appendix III, Enemas.)

Another treatment to relieve constipation is the suppository, a small solid object shaped so it can be inserted into the rectum. Suppositories melt at body temperature and soften the feces, thus aiding in expulsion.

SUMMARY

"Mild illness" is an inexact term that refers to a degree of infirmity. This patient (of any age) may or may not be fairly independent in his self-help. It all depends upon how restricted he is by physician's orders, casts, traction, bandages, age, sight, etc. In a way, it takes more decisions to perform with responsibility in Role I in the care of this patient because there is apt to be the inclination to "do all" for him forgetting his need to do for himself. If judgment is lacking, he could be left alone to do too much.

Using the ten basic needs, it is possible to plan for and provide assistance to the patient who is neither ambulatory nor seriously ill. Many Role I tasks are performed by the LPN for this group of patients. The registered nurse renders initial and on-the-spot judgment which guides the LPN in providing this care.

The key word in maintaining good nurse-patient relationships is "flexibility." The mildly ill patient is apt to be less understanding of routines. Keep him (with his uniqueness) in mind when planning his care. Provide an environment suitable to his care; arrange it to help him be as independent as possible.

GUIDES FOR STUDY AND DISCUSSION

1. Why does a patient in bed require more assistance than an ambulatory patient?

2. In what way(s) does the challenge of caring for the ambulatory patient differ from that of the mildly ill patient?

3. What does it mean to be flexible and make adjustments in a nursing care plan?

4. Why is it necessary for a patient to move toward independence if possible?

5. How can one say that good personal care helps prevent complications and is rehabilitative?

6. Use Appendix III, Bathing, to find out how a complete bath differs from a partial bath.

7. Of what value(s) is a cleansing bath to the patient?

8. From the patient's standpoint, what should you keep in mind while making an occupied bed?

9. Why should preparation for sleep precede the giving of any sleep medication?

10. All manner of treatments are ordered. Why should you know about your patient's treatments even if you do not give them?

11. It is all too easy to label a patient "difficult" or "uncooperative." What are some things to keep in mind when a patient does not fit into hospital "routines"?

12. Under what circumstances would a mildly ill person need help to eat? read his mail? Who might give this assistance?

SUGGESTED SITUATION AND ACTIVITY

1. Using the 10 basic needs, develop a plan for carrying out this student learning experience. *Include all things you will be doing for and with this patient between 8:00 A.M. and 10:30 A.M.* Consider what you will do first, then next, etc. Be ready to discuss your plan and tell why you planned as you did. Make note of any nursing action(s) you are *not* responsible for at present.

Freddy Howick, age 21, has been hospitalized for 10 weeks recovering from a shattered right tibia. He has a pin inserted just below his right knee and the foot is suspended in a hammock type of arrangement. Because he developed foot drop during his hospitalization, the physician improvised an under-the-foot strap with ropes so Freddy could pull on the ropes and exercise his foot.

Freddy is a quiet, independent person who reads a great deal, talks little, and seldom asks for anything. The physician has ordered a regular diet, cleansing enema as needed, vitamin pills three times a day, out of bed on a stretcher or in a wheelchair with affected leg supported in an extended position twice a day, in the morning and afternoon.

A trapeze (attached to overbed frame) is available for Freddy's use. He is interested in keeping his arm muscles in good tone and in exercising his right foot.

CHAPTER 37

THE SERIOUSLY ILL PATIENT

OBJECTIVES FOR THE STUDENT: Be able to:

1. Using the list of ten basic needs, describe at least five ways your nursing actions might differ between caring for the seriously ill patient and the mildly ill patient.
2. Describe the term "seriously ill."
3. Give two examples of the LPN functioning in Role II.
4. Describe three nursing actions which provide proper skin care.
5. Name five things which contribute to this patient's rest and sleep.
6. Explain how a patient's state of dependency influences his need for assistance.
7. Describe four nursing actions which show consideration for this patient and/or the family.

SUGGESTED STUDY VOCABULARY*

malfunction	constipation	productive cough
axilla	fecal impaction	nonproductive cough
sordes	flatus	orthopnea
contraindicated	diarrhea	dyspnea
incontinence	oliguria	diaphoresis
anorexia	suppression of urine	restraints
intravenous	retention of urine	hemorrhage
hypodermoclysis	anuria	compassion
proctoclysis	distended bladder	aspiration
gastric gavage	obstruction	prognosis
	cyanosis	diagnosis

*Look for any terms you already know.

INTRODUCTION

Serious illness is an inexact term. In general, it means "the sickest patient." His disorder may have come on all at once or gradually. In great measure, nursing the seriously ill patient means providing measures to relieve symptoms and prevent complications, carrying out those medical and nursing actions necessary to preserve life and promote recovery.

The seriously ill patient has the same basic needs as any other patient, but due to his extreme dependence upon others, the manner in which they are met is different from the more independent patient. His body often needs assistance from machines and equipment in addition to skilled human hands to carry on its necessary functions. Everything done to and for this patient is done with the idea of conserving strength and aiding the body in regaining normal processes.

This chapter discusses unique problems associated with basic needs without including diseases to permit you to understand general dependence and your role (Role II) in directly assisting the registered nurse in caring for very ill patients.

The responsibilities of the LPN for the seriously ill patient have changed considerably. She is expected to give able assistance in Role II. To do this you will be responsible for some phases of patient care which include intelligent observations concerning patient reactions to therapy and safe practices with respect to equipment involved.

WHO IS THE SERIOUSLY ILL PATIENT?

The seriously ill patient may be of any age and his illness may be due to an accident, a disease, the malfunction of some part of the body, or a combination of these factors. Complications plague this patient because his body is less able to ward them off. He may or may not recover.

The term used in the hospital to designate the *very ill* patient will vary from one institution to another. Such terms as "the serious list" and "the critical list" are commonly used. Each term has a specific meaning in that institution. The physician usually designates when a patient is considered seriously or critically ill. In some hospitals, when a patient is placed on the "serious" or "critical" list, certain nursing care measures automatically become effective, such as more frequent readings of blood pressure, temperature, pulse, and respiration; rectal temperatures instead of oral; no visitors beyond a limited number of family members; special mouth and skin care; specific attention to keeping the patient dry and warm; and the need for adequate fluids and nourishment.

The Needs of the Seriously Ill

This patient's symptoms and the ability of his body to carry on vital processes dictate his medical treatment and nursing care.

The physician will, of course, prescribe the treatments and therapeutic measures specific for the patient's illness and needs.

Nursing care is oftentimes immediate and can demand almost continuous time and attention. Observation of the patient's vital signs and his response to any or all measures is a very important part of his nursing care. Sometimes astute observation by the nurse can mean the difference between continuing an ineffective measure and having the physician change it for something vital to recovery.

Many things a nurse does for a seriously ill patient have no specific orders written for them, such as special care of the mouth and nose, keeping the patient and his bed clean and dry, careful skin care and observation for pressure areas, a quiet environment, and thoughtful consideration for the patient in respect to his family.

Nursing this type of patient includes many measures of "prevention." Not only are therapeutic measures taken to control the symptoms present, but every precaution is used to prevent complications from arising which might be more serious than the original illness condition itself. "Nursing to cure" and "nursing to prevent" are of equal necessity.

Planning the Nursing Care

The seriously ill patient has the same basic needs as the ambulatory or mildly ill patient. He needs nourishment, sleep, rest, elimination, body cleanliness, and mouth and skin care. His environment takes on special meaning (quiet, convenient, safe, clean). The manner in which these and other basic needs are met varies from that of care for patients who are not so ill. In most instances the seriously ill patient will require nursing care given *to* and *for* him. It does not include any great amount of active patient participation. The seriousness (extent, nature) of his condition will indicate whether he is able or unable to do for himself.

Planning this type of care means that the patient's symptoms and problems must be known. Attention must be given to meeting his daily care requirements but undoubtedly many adjustments will be made in so doing. For instance, when temperature, pulse, and respiration are taken routinely twice a day for the ambulatory or mildly ill patient, it may be necessary to take the patient's temperature, pulse, and respiration, and even blood pressure readings, every two hours or more often. Machines which monitor vital signs provide a constant read-out.

The seriously ill patient may be extensively paralyzed, unconscious, or irrational. These conditions of infirmity dictate that more nursing time and even constant nursing attention may be required. The nurse takes this into consideration as she plans his care in relation to her other responsibilities. She may need to stay with the patient or check frequently to observe his condition.

More and more hospitals are providing certain areas for giving this type of constant, immediate care. It is commonly called the "intensive care unit." The seriously ill are brought together where their needs can be met more quickly and where close observation may mean the difference between recovery and death. This unit is furnished with all types of "life-sustaining" equipment and staffed by highly skilled personnel. The LPN functions in Role II, if employed here.

The recovery room is another example of an intensive care unit set up to sustain the patient right after surgery.

The seriousness of the patient's condition indicates the role of the registered nurse in planning, directing, doing and delegating nursing actions. In some instances she does not delegate any tasks to assistants because of the complexity of the measure and the knowledge it takes to render safe judgments. In fact, she may be the assistant to the physician who carries out the treatment and who uses the assistance of the LPN to help with some task(s).

Role II should become clear as you work with the seriously ill patients, performing selected tasks within your capabilities, directed by either the physician or the registered nurse.

MEETING DAILY LIVING NEEDS

For this patient, the emphasis in nursing care is to conserve his energy to help him fight his infirmity. He will need all manner of assistance in meeting his basic needs—some will come from equipment and the rest from medical and nursing personnel. The seriously ill patient is likely to be unable to do much for himself and is possibly unaware of his own requirements for recovery and the prevention of complications.

Personal Care and Hygiene

BATH. The bath is for cleansing and comfort purposes. The extent of the bath, the time it is given, and its frequency depend upon the patient's condition and his need for it.

Owing to the need to conserve energy, the bath may be only a partial one, giving attention to skin care that will keep him comfortable. If he is perspiring profusely, is incontinent, or has drainage difficult to control, gown and linen changes after cleansing the area are to be frequent enough to keep him dry and to eliminate odor.

When a full bath is necessary, caution is used to keep the patient warm and to use every means to prevent overfatigue. Two nurses may be needed, one to hold the patient in position while the other bathes the part. If the patient gets tired, the bath may have to be completed later. Throughout the procedure the nurse observes the patient closely (respirations, skin, color, etc.), and any evidence of negative reaction should prompt her to terminate the bath at once.

Skin care requires close attention to the axilla, the back, the buttocks, areas under the breasts, any folds of the abdomen, the inner aspects of the thighs, and the genitalia. Keep them clean and dry; use talcum powder in small amounts to prevent its caking and rolling off on to the bed. Heels and elbows need lotion to protect them from irritation.

The patient should not be expected to talk

unless he feels it necessary. The nurse communicates assurance to the patient through her manner and the skill she uses.

If an orderly is available to help bathe the male patient, he may help to finish his bath; if not, it is the responsibility of the nurse to do this for the patient who is unable to do it for himself.

CARE OF MOUTH AND TEETH. Prolonged elevation of temperature, forced mouth breathing, and insufficient fluid intake can cause an unpleasant odor on the breath and a serious, uncomfortable condition of the mouth, tongue, and lips. When a patient cannot cough or expectorate fluid or mucus, it forms a film over the teeth, gums, and tongue as it accumulates in the mouth; lips become dry, crusts form, and cracks develop. This condition is called *sordes*.

Mouth care (sometimes called "special mouth care") is a prevention and comfort measure repeated as often as necessary to keep the mouth clean and fresh-feeling. Various means (gauze swab, cotton applicator) are used to carefully clean the teeth, tongue and gums, and to avoid any injury.

It is not advisable to use dental powder or paste for the irrational or unconscious patient. There is danger of aspiration with serious results. Avoid asking him to take a drink of water if there is danger of choking and turn the patient's head to one side to permit any fluid to run out into a curved basin.

For infections of the mouth, the physician will order treatment. Observation (appearance) of the condition of the mouth should be reported when special treatments are charted.

Dentures are usually removed for comfort and safety of the very ill patient. They should be covered with water and put in a safe place to avoid loss or breakage. They should be close at hand, for, as the patient improves, one of his first requests will probably be for his dentures.

NOSE. Unless the anterior nares (tips of the nostrils) are kept clean and free from accumulation, crusts and cracks may form. These can be painful and can cause difficult breathing. Care of the nose is given during the bath and between baths as indicated. When the face is washed the tips of the nares and areas about them should be carefully washed and cleaned. Tepid water with little or no soap is usually all that is needed. A sparing amount of cold cream or petroleum jelly applied to skin surfaces around the nostrils keeps the skin smooth and free from irritation. Excessive nasal secretions or an infection in the nose may require orders for special medication and treatment (spray, drops, irrigation).

EYES. Very ill patients frequently spend long periods with their eyes closed. Secretions gather and crusts form on the edges of the lids. Gentle washing with clear, tepid water usually controls this condition. The washing strokes should be downward and outward away from the nose.

HAIR. Daily neglect of the hair soon poses real problems. It may be difficult to keep long hair combed and in good condition when the patient is very sick, restless, unconscious, or uncomfortable. Daily attention to the hair should not be done at such time or with such effort that it imposes upon the strength of the patient. Good judgment combined with the need to give the patient a well-cared-for feeling guides nursing action. This well-cared-for appearance is important to the family, too. It helps allay some fears they may have about the quality of care being given.

SHAVING. This also is something provided by the nurse if the patient is unable and no one is available to do it. If, for some reason, the patient is not to be shaved, the physician or the patient or both will specify it. Without such restriction, this is a daily need for most adult male patients. Appearance and comfort are important to them. It is a daily habit at home and, unless contraindicated, should be a part of their daily care during illness.

DRESSING. The hospital gown is desirable for this patient because it is (1) easy to put on and remove, (2) more comfortable for the patient, and (3) more convenient for the nurse and physician. Frequent gown changes are indicated where there are excessive perspiration, discharges, vomitus, and bowel and bladder incontinence.

BED. A *smooth, dry bed* aids the safety and comfort of the very ill patient whose skin can offer little resistance to moisture and bed linen wrinkles. Incontinence, profuse perspiration, or both necessitate frequent changes of bed linens. Moisture-proof drawsheets are used between the mattress and the bed linen under the hips and thighs. Moisture-proof material holds moisture above its surface and next to the patient's body, and while these materials are necessary to protect the mattress, the nurse needs to use additional precautions to see that the skin across the back and buttocks is kept dry and clean and that, if possible, there is frequent change of position.

The top bedding, lightweight but adequate for warmth and comfort, should be placed on the bed so that the upper edge extends up over the patient's shoulders. Patients too often remark that the top bedding is too short and that they feel chilly across the shoulders, especially at night.

Assistance may be needed while making the bed. If the patient is helpless or very large, have someone working with you at the opposite side of the bed. As the patient is turned or moved he will be supported and protected from falling out of bed.

The assistant should support the patient's shoulders and hips while the nurse makes her side of the bed. When complete, the patient is turned over to that side of the bed and supported while the bed is completed. If the bed has side rails and the nurse has no assistance, the side rail should be left up on the side of the bed opposite the side where the nurse is working. Some patients may be able to hold on to the side rail for support. *It is very important* that all equipment for such things as drainage or suction, oxygen, ropes and weights for traction, and the like be *left in place* and that they *continue to function* while the bath is given and the bed is made. The practical nurse who is expected to assist with patients, using special equipment and devices, has the responsibility of informing herself how to help *before* she attempts to give nursing care.

Rest and Sleep

Rest and sleep are vital to the recovery of the seriously ill patient. Many things contribute to this:

1. Physical comfort from adequate personal hygiene.
2. The presence of a calm, capable nurse.
3. Tone of voice and facial expression of the nurse.
4. Medications.
5. Quiet room.

Sleep habits during serious illness vary a great deal from normal sleep habits. A specific amount of sleep is essential to maintain health but even a greater amount is necessary to regain health. More sleep is needed to aid the recovery process and because body processes are slowed down. This patient may sleep more during the day than the night. The sleep pattern can be a continuous round of one- and two-hour naps with periods of wakefulness between. Seriously ill patients tire quickly, and if good rest conditions prevail, sleep may follow without effort. *Unless otherwise ordered, or indicated, a sleeping patient should not be disturbed.* Be sure you understand the physician's orders so that this principle is not violated unnecessarily.

Frequent visits during the night provide for close patient observation and reassurance if he is unable to make his needs known. The use of a night light will be reassuring to most seriously ill patients. It helps the nurse move about in the room without a flashlight.

Medications to prevent or relieve pain and to produce sleep are frequently ordered. They are extremely helpful but are no substitute for the nursing care which should precede giving sleep and rest medications.

Close observation (how does patient respond?) follows the giving of these medications. Even rational patients may become confused and restless. Side rails may be required to prevent the patient from falling; some hospitals have standing orders for their use. Keen observation of the patient's safety by the nurse can prompt side rails to be put on the patient's bed whether it is a standing order or not. Never leave a patient unattended if there is any reason to believe he might fall or hurt himself.

Diet and Fluids

If the seriously ill patient is able to take nourishment by mouth, plan time to feed him, unless there is a family member who can help; be seated and take sufficient time to do it unhurriedly (Fig. 37–1). Notice his appetite. Is he interested in nourishment? Must you urge him to eat or drink? Does he refuse anything? How much does he consume? Report any such meaningful observations.

In addition to the several basic points about the patient's diet and eating habits mentioned in the previous chapter, several adjustments may be necessary for the seriously ill patient:

1. Small and frequent feedings may be ordered instead of three regular meals.
2. Liquids may need to be offered with a spoon or through a drinking tube. Soup or tea may need to be placed in a small teapot or

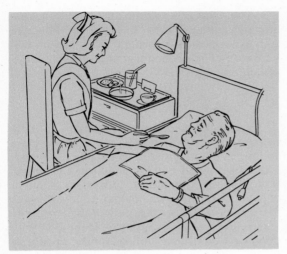

FIGURE 37–1 Nourishment time should be unhurried for this patient.

feeder and the spout placed to the patient's lips, being careful not to offer too much too fast. This method requires the least effort for the patient.

3. Use a spoon or small fork (salad fork) when utensils are needed.

4. Allow plenty of time for patient to chew and swallow, with time to rest between mouthfuls.

5. Remember the patient's likes and dislikes and include this information in his plan of care. He may refuse custard but accept Jello. If he does not like sugar in his tea, he should not have to tell every nurse every day. These occurrences can be avoided by the simple means of including these things in his plan for care. One patient said that he gave up the use of salt and pepper while hospitalized because he got so tired of asking for them.

6. Observations about the patient's appetite, the kind and amount of nourishment taken (or not taken), or any difficulties with swallowing or retaining food should be reported and charted.

Because body fluid balance is essential to recovery, orders relating to fluids are closely followed. When there is an order to increase or limit fluids it means that all fluids (water and beverages) must be recorded according to measure.

Appetites are usually poor (anorexia) during serious illness, making additional nourishment necessary. Fluids containing nourishment may be given by the vein (intravenous), subcutaneous tissues (hypodermoclysis), rectum (enema or proctoclysis), or by administering the substance directly into the stomach (gastric gavage).

Elimination

Special attention is paid to elimination (frequency, incontinence, character of stools, etc.) The absence or presence of certain factors is a medical index used for diagnostic and treatment purposes. Likewise, the elimination pattern dictates nursing action needed to keep the patient clean, dry, and comfortable.

BOWEL. Observations to notice and record:

1. Nature and consistency of stool (e.g., amount, color, form; presence of undigested food, mucus, blood, pus).

2. Frequency of bowel movements.

3. Patient discomfort.

4. Presence of flatus.

Lack of bowel movements for certain periods of time or dry, hard stools may indicate constipation. A more serious form of constipation, *fecal impaction*, requires special treatment to remove the feces.

Frequent and loose stools (diarrhea) coupled with incontinence require close attention to skin care and a clean, dry bed. This may occur while the patient is unconscious or paralyzed. When aware of it and yet unable to control it, the patient is bothered. The nurse's manner toward the problem should be one of acceptance and willingness to assist.

BLADDER. Observations to notice and record:

1. Time.

2. Amount.

3. Color.

4. Odor.

5. Presence of any blood, mucus.

6. Unusual appearance.

7. Painful, difficult urination.

During serious illness, it is a common practice to measure the exact amount of urinary output. Specimens, both single and 24-hour, are frequently ordered.

Involuntary urination (incontinence) takes close attention to keep the patient clean and dry. Frequent bathing and bed linen changes must be continued to prevent odor and decubitus ulcers, as well as provide patient comfort and well-being. In some cases of urinary incontinence, the physician orders the insertion of an indwelling or retention catheter. After the catheter has been inserted into the urethra, it is secured in place by fastening it to the thigh with adhesive tape; the end of the catheter is either clamped off or attached to a drainage bottle. Periodically the clamp is opened and the bladder drained; retention catheter drainage may be constant or periodic. It is checked often to insure proper functioning.

Serious illness often alters the amount of urine eliminated.

1. Diminished output (*oliguria*) may be due to limited fluid intake, loss of fluids due to vomiting, perspiration, diarrhea, fever, action of some drug, or obstruction.

2. No urine output (*anuria*) may be due to obstruction, failure of kidneys to form urine (*suppression*), or failure of bladder to empty (*retention*).

In case of retention the bladder is full and enlarged (distended) and can be seen and felt. While the patient may or may not complain of discomfort and pain, depending upon his condition, watch for signs of a full bladder. The inability to void and complaints or signs of a distended bladder should be reported at once. Every safe nursing effort should be made to help the patient void. Some of the most common measures include:

1. Use a warmed bedpan, provide privacy, and allow sufficient time for patient to relax.

2. Have patient sip small amounts of water or listen to running water.

3. Prevent chilling.

4. If condition permits, raise the back rest to bring patient to a sitting position.

5. Pour warm water slowly over the perineum. The amount of water should be measured first, if the exact amount of urine must be determined.

6. If condition permits, assist the patient to a sitting position on bedpan on the side of the bed with feet resting on a chair.

These measures can be used only when patient's conditions permit. Record any difficulties experienced by the patient and report at once if an untoward change occurs.

It is not uncommon for a physician to order a very ill patient to use a commode in the room to prevent the use of a catheter. Assist the patient to the commode and remain with him. Watch for signs of faintness, irregular breathing, or color and skin changes. Provide for privacy and protect from chilling.

The patient's care plan should include any measures used that have proved effective so that other nurses caring for this patient will be aware of his difficulties and possible ways of helping him.

Body Alignment and Activity

As a rule the seriously ill patient is likely to stay in one position most of the time unless encouraged and assisted to change. The restless or irrational patient would be an exception. Unless attention is given to frequent change of position, accompanied by support for proper posture, the patient will become very weary and uncomfortable and certain complications (i.e., contractures, decubitus ulcers, chest conditions) are likely to occur. There are many reasons why he hesitates to change position (pain, breathing difficulties, lack of energy). Give attention to his need for body alignment and position change. Prevent complications by providing support to body parts and a comfortable bed (see Figure 36–6).

MEDICAL TREATMENT AND CARE. Many times the treatment and care of the seriously ill patient are of an emergency nature. It is safe to say that whether of an emergency nature or to relieve symptoms and prevent complications, this patient requires considerable time and attention. Usually the physician has ordered several treatments, medications, or both. The LPN functions in Role II when special equipment and treatments are used. This means performing selected tasks either in the presence of or without the registered nurse. In every instance, you need to know what to look for and how to report your observations. For example, whether the nurse gives a medication by mouth or hypodermic or the physician gives the medication by intravenous injection, inform yourself as to what results are desired (or not) so you can observe accordingly.

Many types of equipment and treatment measures are used (i.e., oxygen therapy equipment, respirators, blood transfusion, and parenteral fluids apparatus, suction machines, traction and special beds). Precaution is used with any special equipment. Determine beforehand what to do and what not to do to insure patient safety and self-protection. Some equipment is "so special" it takes trained technicians to monitor and use it. If you have observation responsibilities, be sure you know what they are.

Environment

Time and attention usually make it necessary to have the very ill patient close to the nursing station, if possible. Many hospitals find that better care can be provided in intensive nursing units, as discussed previously.

The surroundings should be quiet, pleasant, and conducive to sleep and rest. Temperature and ventilation are controlled to prevent chilling, drafts, and odors. A low, but normal tone of voice is more acceptable to the patient. He is less apt to be suspicious of his condition if the nurse uses a soft, normal voice rather than a whisper. Any discussion of his condition, inside or just outside the room, must be done with caution. Even though the patient may appear to be asleep or unconscious, he may very well be aware of what has been said.

Essential equipment and supplies are kept on hand to save time because time can be in short supply when all at once some life-saving measure is necessary.

Emotional and Spiritual Care

While the physical needs of the very ill patient are many and complex, so may be his emotional needs. Many fears and worries can beset him (pain, paralysis, permanent helplessness, financial burdens, and death itself). The family fears and worries about the same things and, because they are often close at hand, they too need consideration. The nurse, expected to maintain desirable nurse-family relationships, will have to use good judgment in trying to meet their needs. The main thing is to show willingness to help and to relay their needs to others, if they are beyond your role and capabilities.

FAMILY CONCERN AND QUESTIONS. Family members often ask the nurse questions about the patient's prognosis and diagnosis. They are eager to know what "this test or that test showed" because they are apprehensive and are looking for hopeful signs of recovery.

While no question (simple or not) is ignored, do not hesitate to tell the patient or family member that the physician is the person who can best help them when the question is his to answer. This is not a matter of the nurse's "hiding behind" the physician to save her from such questions; this is the physician's responsibility. He is the person who is managing, determining, and directing the treatments, medications, and special care for the patient.

The nurse is the person who ministers to patient and family comfort. She helps them meet their needs, many times not by "doing" or "saying" herself, but by communicating their needs to others who are prepared to meet them.

On the other hand, some questions can and should be answered. Handle them in a manner of helpfulness. Offer assistance by showing awareness of need for food, rest, the use of a telephone, and a quiet place for family members to be alone if they are not able to be at the patient's bedside.

The practical nurse should look to the professional nurse for help and direction in learning how to handle questions with skill and understanding. Patients and family members have confidence in the nurse, practical or professional, who is reassuring yet sees that their particular needs are met by those authorized and responsible for doing so.

In cases of employment where the practical nurse is directly responsible to the physician, she would do well to err in asking for too much advice from him rather than too little. Decisions about what to tell patients and family members must be tempered with exceedingly good judgment if the practical nurse is to establish favorable nurse-patient, nurse-family, and nurse-physician relationships.

Religion is a part of living for many people. To some patients the presence of or visits from the minister, rabbi, or priest are comforting. Be ready and willing to assist in carrying out wishes in this respect. Under certain circumstances, you may need to contact the minister, priest, or rabbi directly. For certain ministrations by the clergy, special preparation in the room may be necessary. These needs are discussed in detail in Chapter 40.

At particular times of crisis or anxiety it is not uncommon for a patient to ask a nurse to pray for or with him. He has expressed a need for help and assistance that she cannot pass along to another. In a simple, quiet way this need can be met without imposing personal beliefs or emotions upon the patient.

Adjustments

The seriously ill patient often has to make radical physical and emotional adjustments; some do this better than others. When he resists certain procedures, such as being fed or forcing of fluids, using the bedpan or changing positions, it calls for real understanding and patience on the part of the nurse. Worry over his condition, whether he will be able to return to normal activity and his job, or fear of dying coupled with the burden of additional expense and his family's welfare may create some very difficult nursing care situations. The patient may not understand the seriousness of his condition and choose to carry on too much independent activity. He may not wish to face the seriousness of his illness and offer every kind of resistance to his care. In such instances seek appropriate assistance if needed.

Patients who have suffered serious accidents which might disfigure or cripple them frequently challenge the best in the physician and the nurse. The worry and anxieties such patients often have are understandable when one considers their problems. The nurse's manner should reveal that she accepts his feelings.

The patient who has been seriously ill for a long period of time may need help in adjusting to convalescence and rehabilitation. Many personal things which have been done by the nurse or family members will need to become his responsibility again. It is possible that he has come to like this dependence and attention, or to feel that he can never regain sound health and always have to use precaution. When this happens, the nurse and the doctor need to plan ways to return him to independence—ways the patient may be unaware of or find agreeable.

Diversional Activities and Rehabilitation

During the critical stage of illness one of the most important things to the patient is the presence of family members. They need to be encouraged not to tire or worry the patient by talking too long or expecting him to carry on a conversation. He may not say he is tired or that he would like to rest because he is glad to have his family with him, but he may need to rest nevertheless.

SOME COMMON NURSING PROBLEMS OF THE SERIOUSLY ILL PATIENT

In addition to the "whys" of skin care and the need for attention to the eyes, nose, and mouth, several other problems call for close observation and nursing action. These problems relate to respiratory difficulty, body temperature, appetite and digestion, moving the helpless patient, restricting patient movements, hemorrhage, shock, and pain.

PROBLEMS RELATED TO RESPIRATORY DIFFICULTY

Cyanosis is a blueness of the skin due to lack of oxygen in the blood. It is usually first apparent in the dusky blue color of the lips and finger tips. This sign should be reported immediately.

Cough is a noisy expulsion of air from the lungs. When the cough removes material from the respiratory tract, it is called *productive*. Some coughs have a harsh, dry sound and are *nonproductive*. Any type of cough is a sign of some type of respiratory irritation or difficulty and is reportable.

Very often this patient is too weak to handle nasal and mouth *secretions* in the usual manner. Sometimes the amount is increased and the character of the secretion changed. Suction or aspiration equipment may be necessary to keep the nose and throat free from mucus to aid breathing. Use care to avoid injury to the membranes and to prevent choking. Charting includes the frequency of this measure and the character of the material removed. Keeping the patient's head turned to one side will aid in drainage from the mouth and help to prevent aspiration of foreign material into the trachea.

Dyspnea is difficult or labored breathing. The patient may complain of a feeling of pressure in the chest and show signs of having difficulty getting enough air. Cyanosis frequently is present. The sensation of not being able to get enough air is frightening. The nostrils may be distended as the patient labors to get air; he may have an anxious look on his face.

Orthopnea means comfortable breathing only in an upright position. Two means to support the patient in an orthopneic position are (1) an elevated backrest, and (2) a forward sitting position using the overbed table (Fig. 37–2).

Pillows should be used to provide support for head, shoulders, and arms so that the patient uses as little energy as possible to maintain a comfortable position. Light weight, suitable bedding is needed.

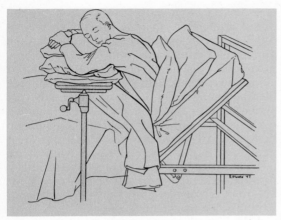

FIGURE 37–2 Use of the over-bed table to support patient who finds it more comfortable to be in a sitting position. Notice how pillows are placed for support. (Montag and Filson: Nursing Arts, 2nd ed.)

PROBLEMS RELATED TO BODY TEMPERATURE

PROVIDING WARMTH. Severe illness may slow down circulation and impair the heat regulating center of the body so that the patient complains of feeling cold, or you observe this as you touch and care for him. Additional warmth is necessary. This observation should be charted and reported. Extra blankets and warmer bed garments are provided without an order, but not a heating pad or hot water bottle. Heat source equipment must be ordered by the physician. Because there always is danger of burning a patient, extraordinary precaution should be used in filling hot water bottles with water of proper temperature.

Prolonged application of heating pads can produce burns. When this source of heat is ordered, be observant and use every precaution to prevent injury to the patient, either burns or some mishap with the electric cord or heating unit itself. Avoid getting the pad damp.

Charting the use of either the hot water bottle or electric heating pad includes the length of time applied and the area to which applied. The temperature of the water used in the hot water bottle is also charted. Some hospitals permit a hot water bottle to be placed at the feet without a physician's order; others do not. Almost every institution has specific regulations concerning the use of electric heating pads. It is important to *know* and *obey* the regulations.

DIAPHORESIS. This means profuse perspiration and very often is experienced at some stage of serious illness. Severe pain may produce a cold, clammy skin. A rapid drop in an elevated temperature often results in profuse perspiration. This sudden drop in temperature and its accompanying diaphoresis often leave the patient exhausted, and he may sleep for a long period of time. Whatever the cause, diaphoresis is uncomfortable to the patient and may result in chilling. The patient should have dry clothing and a dry bed as often as necessary to keep him comfortable. A warm bath is refreshing if the patient's condition permits. It aids circulation and, in turn, leaves the skin warmer. The room should be comfortable and the patient adequately covered during the bath to avoid chilling.

FEVER. The method for taking the temperature has been discussed earlier. For the very ill patient a rectal temperature is almost always taken unless contraindicated.

Serious illness generally upsets the body's normal metabolic processes, thus influencing normal heat production. Body temperature can decrease or it can increase; both are serious.

Hormone metabolic by-products are thought to be responsible for causing fever. As the temperature increases, the patient experiences headache, dizziness, and a tired feeling. Perspiration stops and the amount of moisture in exhaled air is reduced. The normal body cooling process is slowed down.

Nursing the patient with a high fever may include a tepid or cold sponge bath or an alcohol sponge bath, if ordered. The room should be warm to avoid chilling and all materials should be at hand before starting. The age of the patient can influence results—an elderly patient is apt not to respond as favorably as a child or young adult.

Observe for any indication of change of color or rate of respiration, of chilling, or other unfavorable signs; if present the treatment should be discontinued and the observations reported at once.

High temperatures and their treatment always require close observation. Each institution has regulations concerning the frequency for taking the temperature, pulse, and respiration in relation to any treatment for reducing fever.

PROBLEMS RELATED TO APPETITE AND DIGESTION

Poor appetite usually accompanies serious illness. Patients may have neither the energy nor the desire to eat. Because the body must have nourishment to mend itself, special diets (easy to chew and digest, high in special nutrients) are ordered in keeping with the illness. Additional fluids and food nutrients are frequently given by intravenous infusions because of the need for electrolyte balance. See Water and Body Fluids Chapter 6.

Plan sufficient time to feed this patient if he or a member of his family cannot do it; it should be an unhurried process.

Nausea and vomiting are two signs which frequently accompany serious illness. A clean emesis basin, mouth wipes, and a towel (to protect gown and bed) should be close at hand.

Observations recorded include time, character, amount of vomitus, and any complaints of nausea and gastric discomfort.

Vomiting is an obvious and distressing sign to the family; they become concerned about the patient's difficulty. If they can help you, let them; if not, provide for the patient in a careful way, showing your acceptance of the responsibility. Remove all evidence as soon as possible and attend to the patient's need to rinse his mouth and cleanse his face. If necessary, ventilate the room.

PROBLEMS RELATED TO MOVING THE HELPLESS PATIENT

Moving the patient up in bed may require two people, depending on his size and condition. Even then a moving sheet (placed under the patient) might be the safest way to do this. The same is true in turning a helpless patient from a back to a prone position. See that the patient's body is kept in proper alignment.

Getting this patient on and off the bedpan often requires two people. The patient may be (1) turned on his side and rolled back onto the pan, or (2) raised at the hips (lifted) and the pan slipped into place. Patients in body casts need body support as they are placed onto the bedpan.

Onto a stretcher and back to bed. When it is necessary to move this patient from his bed onto a stretcher, a moving sheet is very helpful. The size of the patient and strength of the nurses and attendants will determine how many will be needed. The stretcher is placed alongside the bed, with persons on either side holding and guiding the moving sheet as the patient, in proper alignment, is carefully pulled over onto the surface of the stretcher. The patient should be well covered so as to protect him from drafts and chilling as well as to prevent embarrassing exposure. The seriously ill patient should not be left on a stretcher for any unnecessary length of time regardless of why this change was necessary.

Making the occupied bed has been discussed previously. The very ill patient is apt to have some equipment in use—traction, intravenous fluids running, oxygen tent, casts, heat cradle, drainage. Proceed with making the bed without discontinuing the usefulness of any equipment. If uncertain what to do about equipment, find out *before* you start to make the bed.

PROBLEMS RELATED TO RESTRICTING A PATIENT'S MOVEMENTS

Restricting a patient's movements requires special equipment. For reasons of safety to the patient, his activity may need to be controlled. The use of *side rails* (one common measure) protects patients who are confused, disoriented, or unconscious. Sometimes older patients who appear to be getting along satisfactorily during the day become very confused at night, especially when sedatives are given. Small children have cribs to protect them. Whenever there is danger of a patient hurting himself from side rails, padding may be placed on the inside of the rail.

There are legal implications for the nurse who is negligent in the use or nonuse of side rails. Each institution has definite policies regarding this. One should be thoroughly familiar with all aspects of these policies. Falls due to negligence in the use of side rails occur all too often. Charting of observations and measures taken to protect the disoriented patient is essential.

Restraints are devices used to forcibly

confine a patient. Here again, become familiar with the policies controlling the use of such devices in the place of employment. The decision to place a patient in restraints should not be made by the nurse. Restraints are not applied without a physician's order or a hospital policy. In some areas they may not legally be used at any time.

Because patients "fight" restricted movement, it is very easy to injure the skin if restraints are improperly used or if they are made of hard substances like metal. The family (patient, too, if he understands) should be told why restraints are being used. Careful observation of skin (color, abrasions) under and around restraints should be made and charted.

PROBLEMS RELATED TO HEMORRHAGE

Hemorrhage (internal or external) is a serious problem. Internal hemorrhage occurs when blood escapes into a body cavity; the perforation of a gastric ulcer may release blood directly into the abdomen or into the stomach itself. Blood escapes through openings in arteries, veins or capillaries. Arterial hemorrhage is more difficult to stop. It is identified by the spurting of bright red blood. Pressure applied between the wound and the heart helps to control it. While hemorrhage from a vein is serious, it is usually easier to control because the blood is under less pressure; it flows in a steady manner and is apt to clot more quickly. This blood is not so bright red as arterial blood. Capillary hemorrhage is a slow oozing process. There is no pressure behind it and it simply fills up the wound.

Vomited blood means it has come from the stomach; it is usually clotted and darker due to the gastric juice. Blood from the lungs is brighter red and frothy in appearance. Stools can be bloody indicating hemorrhage in the lower tract. Black tarry stools suggest bleeding higher up in the digestive tract.

PROBLEMS RELATED TO SHOCK

Shock is an acute (critical) peripheral circulatory failure due to an interruption in the flow of blood. It should be treated at once so as to restore proper circulation. Prolonged shock can lead to death. Any blood loss should be replaced as rapidly as possible and every effort made to restore blood pressure and pulse rate to normal. Heat loss is avoided; the patient is kept as quiet as possible. The vital signs are clues to the patient's condition.

PROBLEMS RELATED TO PAIN

Pain, all too often, is a part of serious illness. The nurse is responsible for helping the patient bear the pain if it must continue; she provides nursing measures—treatments, medications, and support—to relieve it. Prevention of pain is the best treatment, if this is possible.

Patients have different ways of expressing their degree of discomfort. What might appear to the nurse to be a painful experience may draw little, if any, comment from one patient. On the other hand, another patient might complain bitterly of pain and there is no way for the nurse to know he has it except by what he says. The level or the point at which the sensation of pain is felt is called the *threshold*. People appear to vary in their pain thresholds.

Patients ask nurses many questions about their pain, such as "Why do I go on suffering like this?" "Why is this happening to me?" "Does this pain in my shoulder mean that I'm getting worse instead of better?" Many questions a nurse cannot, or should not, try to answer directly. If a question is one the physician should answer, call this to his attention. Do not feel hesitant to say to a patient or his family in response to a question which requires a direct answer from the physician. "I'm sorry but I cannot give as satisfactory an answer to your question as Dr. Smith. Would you like to talk with him about it?"

Many times a patient in pain is reaching out for something besides a pain medication. A nurse can help him by showing kindness, consideration, and compassion. She can communicate so much with a nod of encouragement or an extra pat on the arm. Compassion means "to suffer with." In nursing, compassion should give the patient the feeling that he is not alone in his suffering, that the nurse is sensitive to his needs, and her actions should tell him so. This will be reassuring to him and he will have confidence in her ability to give him care.

Some patients need diversion; they need to think about things other than their pain and discomfort. The nurse who can find ways to do this is helping the patient more than she realizes. The answer to such a problem may be as simple as a bowl of goldfish on the bedside table or a bird feeder on a window sill.

Nursing patients in pain requires more than a hypodermic or a pain pill; it takes compassion expressed through thoughtful acts for which there is no procedure or physician's order.

SUMMARY

The term "serious illness," in general, refers to the sickest type of patient. Some hospitals call it "critical," meaning that the needs of life-giving processes are pressing or crucial. This patient is highly dependent upon assistance of a skilled nature. The focus on all nursing care is to conserve the patient's energy, prevent complications from arising, and promote recovery.

Nursing the seriously ill patient involves much more than meeting his personal care and hygiene needs (as important as they are). Serious illness disrupts normal body processes and vital signs. Consequently the patient is often assisted by machines, equipment, and personnel expert in observation and providing needed care. The basis of this care is to conserve patient energy, aid and restore body processes and prevent complications. All of this must be accompanied by consideration for the person—the patient and family members.

When the practical nurse performs selected tasks in nursing the seriously ill patient, she is in Role II, assisting under direct supervision or with specific directions. The responsibility to perform *safely* belongs to the practical nurse in each case. She must be certain she understands *what* and *how* she is to perform *before* beginning because her contribution can be only as safe as her knowledge of what she is doing.

GUIDES FOR STUDY AND DISCUSSION

1. Skin care is a continuing nursing problem with seriously ill patients. List the precautions the nurse should take in doing the following:
   a. Bathing the patient.
   b. Caring for a patient who has bowel and bladder incontinence.
   c. Protecting pressure areas.
2. What care measures are used for a patient with sordes?
3. What things can a nurse do to help family members of a very ill patient?
4. What nursing measures can be used to:
   a. Prevent foot drop.
   b. Provide for good body alignment.
   c. Position a patient comfortably.
   d. Assist the patient with eating.
5. In what ways is the seriously ill patient like an ambulatory patient? A mildly ill bed patient? What is different about the way his basic needs are met?
6. Machines and various equipment are often used with or attached to this patient. What must you do to provide for safety if you are involved in his care?
7. What does it mean to say, "Nursing to cure and nursing to prevent are of equal necessity"?

SUGGESTED SITUATION AND ACTIVITY

Visit *one* of the following hospital areas—intensive care unit, recovery room, or a medical-surgical floor—to:
1. See how many Role II activities you can identify.
2. List the various pieces of equipment used to aid the patients.
3. Complete the following and add more problems if you can:

Seriously Ill: Problems and Nursing Action		
Problem	Describe it	Action/Observations
cyanosis		
dyspnea		
orthopnea		
diaphoresis		
incontinence		
anorexia		

THE PATIENT WITH LONG-TERM ILLNESS

OBJECTIVES FOR THE STUDENT: Be able to:

1. Distinguish between long-term illness and chronic illness.
2. Identify two ways to promote general rehabilitation of this patient.
3. State the goal of rehabilitation when a physical impairment is present.
4. Explain why taking medicine may become a problem.
5. Describe nursing action which provides safety for: disorientation, blindness, deafness, and skin care.
6. Give two reasons why this patient must become involved in self-care if possible.

SUGGESTED STUDY VOCABULARY*

disability
handicap
degenerative
incurable
cripple

custodial
impairment
therapeutic
hemiplegia
hemiplegic
amputee

addiction
food nutrients
disfigurement
disorientation
impaired vision
impaired hearing

*Look for terms you already know.

INTRODUCTION

Long-term illness has no respect for age; it occurs anywhere along the span of life. The tendency is to associate "that which lingers on" with elderly adults, but this is not necessarily true. Small children and youths are afflicted with diseases or disorders that linger on, just as adults are.

Actually, the lengthiness of an infirmity creates a challenge for the nurse. Helping this patient is a very satisfying experience when viewed in terms of his daily living needs and his state of dependence or independence.

There is no doubt that the patient with long-term and chronic illness has his unique nursing care problems. Meeting his daily needs calls for inventiveness and skill on the nurse's part in devising ways to involve him. You will soon recognize that your skill in managing the patient's attitude will be one of your most helpful tools.

This chapter includes the daily problems of long-term illness using the ten basic needs structure to point out *what* and *how* adaptations are made to accommodate the patient and to involve him in his care.

ATTITUDES TOWARD LONG-TERM ILLNESS

The label long-term illness somehow became a catch-all because the terms *chronic* and *long-term* are used one for the other. For example, either term is used in reference to the elderly patient's condition to designate any disease or disorder which is not acute and does not include a quick recovery period. The fact is these two terms are related, because both mean that a long period of time is involved, but they differ too.

Chronic illness includes all disabilities or deviations from normal which have certain (one or more) characteristics such as permanency, "left over" disability, noncorrectable body changes, special training needed for rehabilitation or a long period of nursing care.*

Long-term illness refers to those persons suffering from chronic diseases or impairments who require a prolonged period of care, that is, who are likely to need or who have received care for a continuous period of at least 30 days in a general hospital, or care for a continuous period of more than three months in another institution or at home, such care including medical supervision, assistance, or both, in achieving a higher level of self-care and independence.†

Labels Reflect Attitudes

The use of certain terms (labels) to describe a patient or an illness of long duration

can reflect the understanding and attitudes of the user (nurse, patient, family, community). Often some of these terms, such as "incurable," affect the attitude of the patient toward his condition and the type of care he might receive. He may consider his condition hopeless and feel that the nurse does too.

Terms carry messages. In the minds of the public (and patient) certain words are labels which signify or mean something less—often much less—than perfect or normal. Family members sense hopelessness and helplessness when a label is carelessly used by health personnel. You can help to remove or prevent some of these feelings by using terms that sound the *least* negative or hopeless.

Following is a list of commonly used words to study and discuss in relation to how, if at all, they should be used in discussion of patient care or in other conversation:

Invalid—not well and strong, one disabled by illness or infirmity.

Disability—lack of physical or mental fitness. This may be permanent or temporary, partial or total.

Handicap—a physical or mental condition that renders success more difficult. One may be born with it (congenital) or acquire it after birth.

Degenerative—a condition of marked decline or sinking to a state below normal.

Incurable—disease beyond cure, one for which there is no remedy.

Cripple—one who limps, creeps, or halts, as from loss of a limb; a partially disabled person.

Custodial—this word relates to guardianship or keeper. In relation to patient care it is often used to denote a watchful or guarded existence for the patient. Here the emphasis is on providing the necessities of life and patient protection with little or no emphasis on cure or rehabilitation.

Impairment—a condition which lessens or limits function (physical or mental) below normal. It may be injury, damage, or deterioration due to disease.

Some of these words have a harsh, unpleasant, and even depressing meaning for patients and their families. The word "cripple" means less than whole—a disabled limb. No one likes or wants to be less than able and much less, if he is crippled, does he want to hear that label attached to his infirmity. Another such word is "incurable." This word is

---

*Public Health Service Publication No. 344, 1954; Care of Long-Term Patient—Source Book on Size and Characteristics of the Problem. G. St. J. Perrott, et al.
†*Ibid.*

very final. The patient and his family come to feel everything is futile; hope is gone and they know nothing can be done. This word sets such patients apart from those who can get well; it should have very limited use, if any.

Nurses too often use and misuse these terms. They, too, can develop attitudes and feelings about patients who are "incurable" or to whom they must give custodial care. These feelings can affect the quality of care provided. It takes enduring compassion and sensitivity to work day after day with patients who may not get well. All too soon the nurse finds herself feeling helpless except to provide for as many of the patient's physical comforts as possible.

Today's Efforts with Long-term Illness

The past two decades have brought a much needed change in attitudes toward chronic and long-term illness. Today health forces are vitally concerned with prevention and rehabilitation, as well as cure. Science is constantly looking for ways to prevent, as well as restore. Many new discoveries bring hope and assurance; the Salk vaccine for the prevention of poliomyelitis is one such example. Others include medical efforts to replace diseased organs with nondiseased organs called transplants, or to replace a defective part of an organ with a man-made part, as is done in heart surgery.

Prevention to avoid illness, prevention to avoid further disability, and genuine efforts to restore a patient to former or highest possible capacity (rehabilitation) are now a part of all health care. Improved health habits—care of teeth, better nutrition, regular physical examinations, and medical supervision of early remedial health care—are taught and practiced today. Today's emphasis is on the individual's right to have fullest use of his capacities and lead a productive life.

Early detection of chronic disorders now sends more patients to the hospital or clinic for treatment.

The *attitude* among health workers is that something besides "custodial" care is necessary for such patients and so *new* and *varied therapy programs* are constantly appearing. The results are gratifying and often thrilling to observe and share. Sir William Osler said, "The way to live a long life is to contract a chronic disease—and take care of it."

Who is the Patient with Long-term Illness?

Long-term illness is found among all age groups and both sexes. (See Fig. 38–1). The patient might be ambulatory or mildly ill in bed. It is not too likely that he would remain in a serious condition too long, but this is a possibility. He is found in general hospitals, special hospitals, nursing homes, and clinics or outpatient departments as well as at home. If one were to single out an age group which seems to have more than its share of chronic and

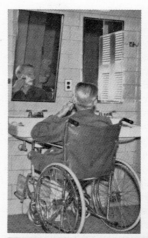
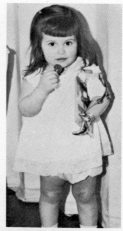
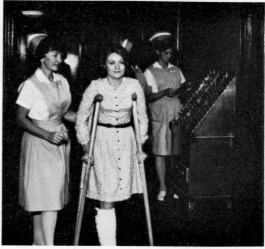

FIGURE 38–1 Long-term conditions affect all age groups. 1, Wohl: Long-term Illness. 2, Marlow: Textbook of Pediatric Nursing, 2nd ed., 3, Courtesy of Santa Fe Community College Practical Nursing Program, Gainesville, Florida. Photographer, Henry DeLoach.

long-term illness, it would be the oldest adult group. People are living longer; hence this group is larger than it has been in the past and continues to grow. About eight out of every 10 elderly adults have one or more disorders that require attention.

This patient has the same basic living needs as others; the challenge comes in assisting him in a manner that directs his attention to self-help and as much independence as his age and condition permit. Certain problems are apt to accompany any chronic and long-term illness; these are pointed out following the discussion of the daily living needs.

Rehabilitation

The word "rehabilitate" has such meanings as restore, put back, re-establish, return, and make whole. Webster says to rehabilitate is "to restore to former capacity." In medical language it means "making whole" (to the greatest possible degree) a person who is ill or impaired to a limiting extent. The patient is returned to his highest capacity to take care of himself or is returned to work with his highest possible skill.

Wherever you encounter patients, you encounter people who need to be restored and re-established. This process starts when the disorder brings the patient to the attention of the physician and therapy begins. Rehabilitation is not so narrow as to include only a readjustment to an artificial hand or leg, or to limited motion due to severe burns. Rehabilitation has many faces; it includes restoring body and mind, attitudes and feelings, spirit, and the desire to live with a purpose. All nursing action should support these goals.

There is a more specific meaning given to rehabilitation when a physical impairment is involved. The goal is to re-establish the use of the body part as much as possible and to help the patient make needed adjustments (learn new ways to do things or relearn old ways) so he can live as safely and independently as possible. Some people are never able to be safely independent; that is, they continue to require certain types of assistance in moving about or handling things.

Long-term illness creates many needs for rehabilitation. The list of chronic conditions is long; some of the more commonly mentioned ones are impairments of the back, limbs and trunk; palsy and paralysis due to stroke; vascular lesions affecting the central nervous system; heart disease; arthritis and rheumatism; diabetes; and senility. All these patients need to be helped (Fig. 38–2). The amount and type of help varies with age and condition. The heartening thing is that they can be helped. As a member of the health team, the

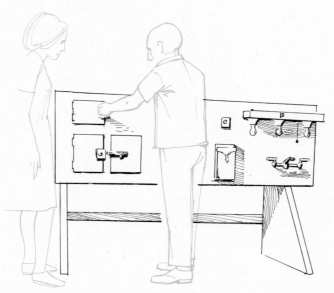

FIGURE 38–2   This patient is relearning household activities—opening latches, pushing switches, turning faucets on an "activities of daily living board" in the occupational therapy department.

practical nurse plays a part in restoring patients to usefulness. The most valuable asset in this respect is proper attitude toward rehabilitation. Recognize, from the start, that time and patience are involved and so is hopefulness. Watch for small improvements; these encourage the patient and the nurse, too.

All special types of activities and exercises are therapies ordered by the physician. The nursing team cooperates with other departments (e.g., physical therapy, occupational therapy) to see that the patient's needs are met. Be alert to the various measures being used to rehabilitate the patient to avoid a careless act which would undo the efforts of the physician and the various therapy departments. The patient's involvement in his self-care must support the therapeutic plan for rehabilitation.

A word of caution. Physicians may order such things as a range of motion exercises and self-assistive activities, be certain that you are *instructed as to any limitations* and *how to proceed* to avoid injury to the patient. What appears to be a simple matter of letting a patient do something for himself could be harmful if his mental capacities are limited even though muscular abilities seem normal.

MEETING DAILY LIVING NEEDS

A close companion to physical disability is attitude or outlook. The nurse notices the contrast between the patient's outlook with short-term, rapid recovery and the patient's outlook with a slow, drawn-out recovery or the absence of it.

The patient, as well as his family, is very apt to become discouraged when favorable results come slowly. He often leans upon the nurse for encouragement, and you will do well to help him sense his small successes. Accept the idea that assisting this patient requires considerable ability on your part to provide timely and appropriate kinds of encouragement in view of the fact that noticeable daily improvement is not to be expected.

Nursing this patient very often means doing things *with* rather than for him. All nursing efforts are directed toward maintaining or restoring the best possible state of health, both physical and mental.

Prevention and *restoration* of optimal capacity are stressed in relation to the care of any patient. However, long-term illness or disorder claims its share of attention for preventive and restorative measures because if any patient needs opportunity to participate in self-assistive activities, this patient does. It is therapeutic for him to be involved; the reasons are cited throughout this chapter.

Making this, or any, patient dependent upon the nurse when he is capable and should be doing things for himself is not considered effective nursing care because it delays the fullest possible recovery. Basic nursing skills and abilities focus on the patient's ability to participate in every way possible; this shows regard for his right to enjoy independent action even if it takes longer and causes you to make adjustments.

The physician determines and directs the extent of self-assistive activity. Let the patient know why he is involved; he is more apt to accept such information from the nurse who, herself, appreciates the true need for it.

To begin with, *this patient needs to learn how to assist himself.* You can help teach him. It is amazing how expert he can become in spite of limitations; strange as it may seem, the nurse can learn from the self-assisting patient who has mastered the art of meeting many of his daily living needs. For example, a patient hospitalized for a period of time with tuberculosis is taught how to manage himself, his environment, and his responsibilities to others. If observed "in action" either ambulatory or in bed, one sees how capably he manages self-assistive activities. With well-planned guidance (teaching) and selected assistance he generally meets his daily living needs very well.

Family relationships show. Every contact the nurse has with the family reflects her attitude (good or poor) toward them and the patient. Many times family members wish to talk with the nurse, the physician, or both. Relate such information to the charge nurse or the physician, depending on the circumstances.

FACTORS IN PLANNING NURSING CARE

Many things help to shape the care plan. Some essentials include the knowledge of:
1. The nature of the disorder.

2. The degree of dependence or independence in self-assistive activities.

3. Special rehabilitative activities ordered.

4. Diet, treatments, and medicines.

This information enables you to plan and carry out patient-focused nursing action alone or with other personnel.

Any plan for patient care should include consideration for him as a person. Know about his likes, dislikes, and habits of hygiene and daily living so that, wherever possible, adjustments in his care can be made to make him as comfortable and satisfied as possible. Some of these flexibilities help patients to accept their stay in the hospital or in a bed at home more wholeheartedly.

Because this patient may be doing many things for himself, he should not be denied individual attention or become a "routine" patient in the mind of the nurse. Receiving attention and feeling useful are therapeutic. The nurse who is skilled in caring for this patient is always challenged in finding ways to promote his independence safely and effectively.

Personal Care and Hygiene

Taking care of his own personal hygiene needs is something the patient finds satisfying and is often anxious to do. Experiencing even small successes in bathing, mouth care, shaving, and attention to nails and hair may be the most important first step in rehabilitation. Guidance in how much and how fast should come from the physician or registered nurse.

THE BATH. The patient's limitations (condition, ability) dictate how much he can do in taking his own bath, whether it be a shower, tub, or bed bath—partial or complete. He may need considerable assistance; it is hoped that he will become more self-assistive as he is taught how he can safely proceed, if his capacities warrant this. In any event, permit him to feel unhurried; allow time for him to cope with his tasks.

SKIN CARE. You will recall that older people tend to have drier skin. Since bathing removes natural oil, creams or lotions should be used to lubricate the skin, and the number of full baths should be limited (every second or third day) for the elderly or any other patient with dry skin. Talcum is used sparingly, if at all. Alcohol dries the skin. The idea is to keep the skin clean and dry, but also to keep it pliable and free from cracks.

If the patient is in bed, there are two other important facts to keep in mind about skin care:

1. Prevent pressure areas from forming because they lead to decubitus ulcers. Change patient's position to keep him off the reddened area until it returns to a natural color.

2. Avoid injury to the skin from faulty equipment, a cast or brace and from foreign objects in the bed.

Any special devices or appliances which need to be applied or removed will necessarily slow up the bathing process. If capable, the patient should be permitted to manage for himself. In fact, some patients might have helpful suggestions to offer about making the bathing arrangements more useful in self-assistance. Notice the tilted bathroom mirror for the wheelchair patient in Figure 38–1.

Patients who seem uninterested in personal hygiene, or who are lax in following through, need encouragement. See that materials and equipment are available. Mention these patients' improved appearance and help them feel important to themselves.

DRESSING. When possible, this patient will be out of bed and dressed. Also, when possible, he should dress himself. If the patient is a hemiplegic, he is trained to dress himself, providing that loose-fitting, easy-to-fasten clothing is available. This training is part of his rehabilitation.

Allow plenty of time for self-dressing; see that the patient is secure in his balance, sits when necessary, and has your support, too, when needed.

Regular habits of bathing, shampooing the hair, caring for the nails and teeth, and wearing clean clothing should be encouraged. Show interest in his appearance and regard for his likes and dislikes in personal grooming. *How* something is done may not be nearly so important as the fact that it *is* done, providing that it is done safely and is necessary for the patient. Keep him as independent as possible, for this is more satisfying than continued dependence.

Rest and Sleep

The long-term illness patient may present some nursing care problems when it comes to sleep and rest. Giving medications for this purpose should not be the one and only nursing answer. As a general rule, up-and-about patients get sufficient exercise to promote natural sleep. Short naps, or none at all, may help the patient to sleep at night, but avoid overtiring him in this process. A smooth, tight bed, a well-ventilated quiet room, and complete evening care (back rub included) go far toward inducing sleep.

One danger in long-term illness is the possible addiction to sleep-producing drugs. The same may be true of pain-relieving drugs. This is not to say that drugs are not and should not be used. However, they are not substitutes for good nursing care—one is important to the other.

Diet and Fluids

While the daily dietary requirements for the long-term patient may be essentially the same as for the well person, modifications in quantity and kinds of food nutrients are usually needed. In fact, the illness may have started because of a nutritional deficiency or a malfunctioning gland which upset proper utilization of food.

The physician's concern is to provide for nutrients which heal and repair tissue, build body resistance, improve muscle strength, and make up for any deficiencies. Inadequate nourishment invites complications.

The long-term patient has leisure time to think about food and develop definite likes or dislikes. This may present a nursing problem that will require some imagination in order that nutritious meals appeal to his appetite. Help him to understand how certain foods are beneficial to him; involve him in selecting his foods, if possible. Serve the food in an attractive manner to make eating a pleasant experience rather than something to complain about.

Patients with disabilities (hands, arms) usually can be taught to feed themselves, and should be allowed the time it will take them without being hurried (Fig. 38–3). The sightless patient, determined to eat by himself, needs special attention to the location and identity of food on the tray. Liquids may be put in a feeder or small teapot with a spout.

Eating in groups is practiced in some institutions. When a patient is able, he should be encouraged to eat with the group.

When special diets and restrictions are ordered, the patient should be helped to understand why they are needed, if possible.

Elimination

Proper diet, sufficient fluids, and exercise help to promote regular bowel and bladder habits. Problems in relation to elimination include incontinence of bowel and bladder, constipation, and urinary tract infection. Good personal hygiene habits (skin care, proper use of toilet paper, and a clean dry bed) help to prevent urinary tract infection. Proper skin care and clean dry clothing are essential for patients with incontinence. Whenever possible, the long-term bed patient uses the toilet or a commode chair to promote natural bowel and bladder elimination.

This patient can come to worry about his bowels to an extraordinary degree. Help him to maintain his normal bowel habits. Be available to escort him to the bathroom; encourage intake of fluids and roughage, as well as exercise; encourage his pattern of regularity; provide privacy. Problems with constipation may require special orders regarding medicine, diet, and treatments.

Body Alignment and Activity

In this respect the patient's needs will be influenced by whether he is ambulatory, in a wheel chair, or confined to his bed. Observe the patient's posture and body alignment in various positions to prevent or overcome restricted movements.

Prevention of deformities, such as foot drop, contractures, and wrist drop, is a nursing responsibility. Long-term illness patients need watchful attention if they are not to recover from one illness to find that they have developed some limitation which could have been avoided. This is especially true of a bed patient with a condition that limits his motion. Turn him frequently, providing comfortable support to limbs, arms and back. Be sure to get instructions *before* doing any arm or leg exercises.

Medical Treatment and Care

This patient may be quite familiar with his illness and care. At times the nurse may be confronted with such a patient's wanting to alter this care or even prescribe for himself.

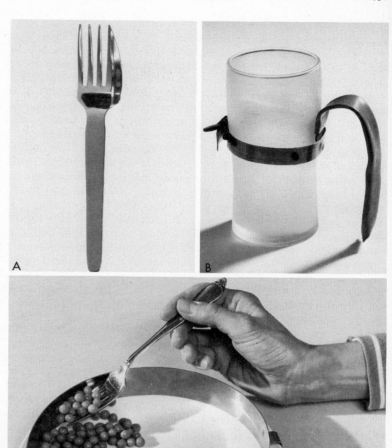

FIGURE 38–3 Adaptive devices to help the one-handed patient feed himself. (Stryker: Rehabilitative Aspects of Acute and Chronic Nursing Care.)

Some may be on no medications but insist they should be; others may, from time to time, refuse to take them. The same basic precautions are used in preparing and administering medicines to this patient as to others.

If the patient insists upon taking medicine he has been taking at home, the physician needs to determine the course of action. The same is true with any treatments he has been taking at home that must be continued in the hospital. Maintain your relationship with the patient by getting informed so that you will know how to function without unduly upsetting him.

Environment

The home, a private room in the hospital, a bed in a hospital ward or a nursing home may be the patient's "world." He may be close to patients with similar problems or surrounded by short-term or critically ill patients. These facts influence his well-being and adjustments. Some patients insist on being at home surrounded by family and familiar things; for others this is impossible.

The long-term patient has need to be as happy as possible with his surroundings. There is also need for him to have necessary equipment or special furniture conveniently located. If the patient is ambulatory, special care is taken to remove hazards and prevent accidents. To promote safety, floors need to be clean, dry, and nonslippery. Throw rugs are potential enemies of the person who is unsteady on his feet or has poor vision. Handrails along walls (hall, bathtub), trapeze arrangements above bed or toilet seat, and brakes or blocks to make chairs or beds stationary are some ways to adjust or equip the environment. While this patient should be encouraged to help himself when possible, precaution should be taken to provide for his safety and well-being.

Personal belongings can be especially important to this patient. He may want to keep such things as pictures, cards, books, and handicrafts close at hand. The nurse should appreciate his need to have his own things nearby and not interfere with his surroundings except to see that they are clean and in reasonable order.

Emotional and Spiritual Care

Emotional problems are difficult for the best trained personnel to handle at times; you can be of assistance if you know *how* to help. First realize that these needs are as important as the patient's physical needs. For example, he may easily become discouraged and lose interest in himself and his surroundings. One can easily understand how a patient might need much encouragement if he had an impairment which required a long, expensive hospitalization, caused loss of income, and created a radical change of plans for the future. Some conditions cause embarrassment as well as discouragement. For example, it could be disheartening to know that one has to wear a colostomy bag or use an artificial limb or some other prosthesis such as an artificial eye or hand. Some patients have real difficulty accepting such changes and living with them. They resent help and lose interest in themselves, and sometimes in living.

In all probability, some of the greatest emotional needs and adjustments arise with the patient who has had some change in the appearance of his face, head, or hands. Disfigurement caused by severe burns of the head or the hands is one example; facial surgery necessitated by cancer is another. Care of such a patient requires great emotional strength on the part of the nurse and the patient's family. Her actions should never imply that she is upset by his appearance or considers his care distasteful.

Your natural manner of acceptance can influence the patient's outlook; it can help him accept his feelings about himself and his condition. Try to help him to be as independent as possible. Expect him to do (and want to do) things for himself, because it is essential for him not to develop the habit of unnecessary dependence. If the physician orders that the patient do certain things for himself, his care is planned with this in mind.

Although the nurse should encourage the patient and give him the feeling of being useful and needed, she cannot give him the most help or have an effective desirable relationship with the patient if she permits herself to become personally involved with the patient and his problems.

The long-term illness patient may have regular visits by his minister, priest, or rabbi. In the home the practical nurse might be the one to make these arrangements. In the hospital there usually are policies or practices the nurse follows in securing this help for the patient. Her purpose should not be to change his religious beliefs, but rather to be of whatever assistance she can in seeing that his spiritual needs are met as he requests. Respect for another's right to his own beliefs is one way to show regard for the individual.

Adjustments

Chronic and long-term illness with or without a disability or complication may require a special way of living for a long time or perhaps the rest of the patient's life. Thus physical and mental adjustments are sometimes difficult to accept and make. This is especially true when the illness has a direct bearing or influence on the patient's physical activity, his family and social relationships, his work and way of life (e.g., a person who has lost his sight).

Acceptance by the patient of his infirmity or limitation is necessary to effective rehabilitation. The physician informs the patient and family of his condition and prognosis. He plans the treatment and rehabilitation. The nurse and the family can assist the patient in helping him to accept and understand. Their feeling of acceptance should be obvious to him. In turn, he may be less resentful and insecure if he finds that family members accept him as they always have rather than as someone who is now different or queer. To understand and accept the patient is far better than to pity him. Self-pity is an obstacle to recovery and to a return to purposeful living. The patient needs to return to as much independence as he can as rapidly as he is able. He needs to be encouraged to make his own decisions early, to spread his interests beyond his illness, and to think in terms of getting back to "normal" living. If he is treated normally, he is much more apt to adjust normally.

It is not always easy to encourage patients to look forward to a return to home or work. This may be one of the most difficult nursing care problems you and team members face with this patient—one of lack of courage. It requires unending patience and a thorough knowledge of how the patient can be helped. Here the physician will direct the approach and guide members of the team who try to help rehabilitate the patient.

Diversional Activities and Rehabilitation

It is understandable that the long-term illness patient can be discouraged, bored, and even lonely. For these reasons he may not respond very readily to the idea of diversional activities. While he may need interest in other things, people, and events, he can easily become too interested in his own difficulties. It is important that he direct some of his attention away from himself. In fact, his diversional activities may well be a part of his planned program of rehabilitation. Specially trained people such as vocational, physical, occupational, and recreational therapists aid in patient rehabilitation in some hospitals. Children have the services of teachers who help them keep up with their classwork.

Nursing homes need more planned diversional activities for patients. Of all daily living needs, it appears that this one receives the least attention most of the time. There is no better way to help these patients experience a little joy and sense a little accomplishment and satisfaction than to provide some interest-catching thing to do (Fig. 38–4).

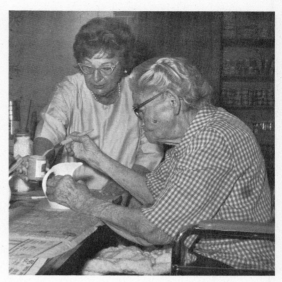

FIGURE 38–4 This 97-year-old person is "up" and purposefully occupied. (Courtesy of Jewish Home for the Aged, Miami, Florida in cooperation with Lindsey Hopkins Education Center, Practical Nursing Program, Miami, Florida.)

This particular need is something practical nurses can do something about. You can generate interest in all manner of simple but creative activities. In a sense, one is limited only by his imagination when it comes to providing for this daily living need. Find out what interests the patient. What did he do for diversion when he was well? What does this suggest now that he is living with a long-term or chronic disability? What community resources are available to help meet this need? This problem is an unmet challenge in our society, especially in relation to our disabled elderly adults.

SOME COMMON NURSING PROBLEMS IN LONG-TERM ILLNESS

Disabilities Which Complicate Nursing Care

While the following factors may make for needed adjustments in caring for all types of patients, the long-term illness patient may need more understanding during his prolonged infirmity. Adjustments will include time, convenience and safety of environment, and teaching the patient how to do for himself.

Impaired vision or blindness is always a handicap, but if newly acquired, the patient requires much help and support. He will need to relearn some things or make adjustments in doing them. For example, daily care which he has perhaps been doing for himself for years will present new problems. Familiarity with the location of objects will be necessary. More time should be planned for his care if he is to learn to do things for himself.

Impaired hearing or deafness, especially if newly acquired, requires many adjustments too. When addressing the hard-of-hearing patient, face him so that he can see lip movement. Writing rather than speaking may be necessary if the impairment is severe and the patient can read. Acceptance and understanding can be communicated through actions and facial expressions, as well as by speaking or writing.

If patients with either of these disabilities are receiving special therapy to aid in their rehabilitation, inform yourself about the treatment.

Disorientation is the loss of normal bearings, or a state of mental confusion as to identity, time, or place. This condition can come and go, be permanent or temporary. In the presence of a disoriented patient, remember to talk with him in normal tone and manner of conversation at all times. It can be upsetting to a patient to know that he is not responsible for what he says, does, or hears. One main problem will be to safeguard the patient from wandering and from injury.

Limited motion can include loss, or partial loss, of the use of the arms and hands, legs, and feet. Amputation of a limb will necessarily limit motion, as will paralysis of some part of the body. The extent of the restriction will determine how much or how little a patient can do or be taught to do for himself. In many instances the functions of arms and legs return fully or partially through use and exercise. Eating, daily hygiene activities, and exercises provide opportunities for the nurse to help rehabilitate the patient if he is able and should be doing things for himself.

The patient with a cast, in traction, or using a special bed frame requires attention to his safety, body alignment, skin care, etc., and needs time enough to help himself within his limits.

Observation and recording of changes, improvements, and appearances are vital parts of the care for patients with disabilities. Charting should not be repetitious, unless called for.

Prevention of Accident and Injury

This patient may need more continuous instruction and observation, so that he does not take chances or unsafe short-cuts in self-assistance. Prevent falls, burns, infections, or accidents with equipment.

Prevention of Complications

Long-term bed confinement can produce loss of function and malformation of parts of the body unless proper posture and exercise are provided. Frequent change of position, exercises, foot boards, and good body alignment contribute to prevention.

Pressure sores (decubitus ulcers) have been discussed previously. The long-term illness bed patient is an easy victim without proper nursing care.

SUMMARY

Nursing the patient with long-term or chronic disabilities calls for adaptations in meeting his daily living needs. Self-assistance is stressed when this is within the patient's capabilities; he must be encouraged to be as independent as possible for his own well-being.

Long-term illness lends itself to some complications if the patient is confined to the bed. Good skin care, frequent position changes, body support and proper alignment, a dry, smooth, comfortable bed and close observation are some of the main factors to keep in mind to avoid complications.

A point to emphasize is this patient's continuing need for diversion. Young, old, or middle-aged, he will find that time can hang heavy and be worrisome. Diversion is helpful to one's outlook whether well or ill; but somehow illness magnifies the need for it.

Use all appropriate means to promote rehabilitation. Treat these patients not as different or special people, but as people like yourself who have need for purposeful living. This outlook on your part will furnish you with more tolerance and fellow-feeling; it will be helpful to the patient in overcoming discouragement, fear, and boredom.

GUIDES FOR STUDY AND DISCUSSION

1. What is the difference in meaning between chronic illness and long-term illness?

2. Why must a nurse be careful in using words which label this patient?

3. What does it mean to say: "It takes enduring compassion to work with patients who might not get well"?

4. In terms of the patient, what is included in his general rehabilitation? Who is involved? What may make it difficult?

5. When a physical impairment is involved, what is the goal of rehabilitation?

6. Why must this patient become involved in self-care? What are some things you can do to make him more independent?

7. How can this patient benefit from eating with a group?

8. What problems might this patient encounter with respect to medications?

9. How can you demonstrate acceptance of an unpleasant/unsightly nursing situation?

10. Use this chart to help you organize the following:

PROBLEMS IN LONG-TERM ILLNESS	
Disabilities/Complications	Nursing Action/Observations

SUGGESTED SITUATIONS AND ACTIVITIES

1. Assume that you are employed in a nursing home where there is no planned diversional activity. The patients are elderly, but for the most part they are up and about during the day. Plan some purposeful activities for morning and afternoon hours that would be inexpensive and varied enough to capture the interests of several patients. Think about where you could get materials to work with; consider how you are going to proceed to interest these patients.

2. Assume that you are faced with a similar situation in a facility caring for young children from five to ten years of age. What would you do? How would you proceed?

3. Plan a short skit around the following situation that can be role-played in class. A daughter has just overheard the patient, who shares the room with her fifty-year-old mother, tell a visitor that the mother never will be right again because she has an incurable disease. The daughter is upset because she thought her mother was going to recover; she turns to the LPN and in so many words says, "Tell me it isn't so." Show how an LPN can be helpful within her role.

4. Locate a recent newspaper or magazine article that tells what some group (voluntary or official) is doing to help with some long-term illness problem.

CHAPTER 39

THE ELDERLY PATIENT

OBJECTIVES FOR THE STUDENT: Be able to:

1. List five general changes which may occur in an aging body.
2. Explain how each of the above changes could influence how this patient meets his basic needs.
3. Describe three nursing actions which show respect for this patient's individuality.
4. State two reasons why skin care may need special attention for the bed patient.
5. Name five disabilities or disorders commonly found among elderly patients.

SUGGESTED STUDY VOCABULARY*

gross body changes
ankylosis
contractures
hypertension
coccyx
arthritis

osteoarthritis
rheumatoid arthritis
cardiovascular diseases
diabetes
mental confusion
rehabilitation

supportive care
respiratory diseases
influenza
pneumonia
gastrointestinal disorder
genitourinary infections

*Look for any terms you already know.

INTRODUCTION

It will be helpful, at this point, to return to Chapter 21 and review the changes that occur in body structure and function of the elderly and the problems many of them face. Body changes play a part in the amount and kind of assistance an elderly person needs when he is sick. He brings his worries and problems with him, and he appreciates a nurse who understands him as a person as well as a patient.

Aging is a process common to all living things. It is sometimes called a "mysterious trend" because science does not exactly understand how it works; they do know what some of the changes in body structure and function are, but they are not sure how all of them come about.

The elderly patient represents the blend of changes which have been taking place throughout his life. In addition to the natural aging process, disease, disorders, accidents, malnutrition, defects since birth, and inherited weaknesses all may come to play a part in his present state of health. They show up as signs and symptoms needing medical and nursing care. The nursing care you give is made up of measures and actions to relieve and restore this patient; you assist him but you help him preserve his independence in every way possible. You provide for his safety and preserve his identity. In other words, there are no special treatments or peculiar things you do for the elderly patient. He has the same basic needs as any other patient; the secret of his care is to adapt or adjust your measures and actions to accommodate a person who has lived a long time and has had body tissue changes as well as a lifetime of habits.

There is medical reason to believe that people do not die of "old age," because healthy tissue does not wear out; it continues to function. Disease and disorder cause malfunction of tissue and it is this malfunction that causes death.

The purpose of this chapter is to show how body changes and the influence of disease and disorder create the need for nursing care adjustments and the need for paying special attention to certain aspects of this care.

ADJUSTMENT OF DAILY LIVING NEEDS

Factors which can influence the patient's needs are:

1. Diminished body power to restore and heal itself.
2. Diminished body power to move and maintain posture.
3. Slower adjustment to temperature (environment) changes.
4. Impairment in vision and hearing.
5. Changed eating habits.
6. Changed bowel and bladder functioning.
7. Altered sleeping habits.
8. Lack of interest in self and others.
9. Changed memory patterns.
10. Changed surroundings.
11. Retirement/loss of status.
12. Loss of mate.
13. Loss of authority to make own decisions.
14. Decreased income.
15. Loss of purpose in life.

Personal Hygiene

Hazard-free facilities prevent accidents. Safety features such as grab bars on walls near the tub, shower, and toilet, litter-free floors, and adequate lighting help prevent accidents.

Clothing should be easy to put on and take off; light-weight clothing is more comfortable. Devices to aid in dressing and grooming (e.g., slanted mirror for wheelchair patient, slanted foot stool) are useful. Pay attention to grooming. Care of the hair and nails, shaving the men, and providing cosmetics for the women are all important. Allow extra time to accomplish daily care and dressing. Encourage self-assistance, and recognize accomplishment of it, but don't fail to provide needed assistance to prevent feeling of neglect (see Fig. 39–1).

Skin needs careful attention. It is dry and its healing power is slower. Staying in one position too long and incontinence create problems in skin care.

Sleep and Rest

Some patients need a mid-day nap; observe nap habits to see if they upset the patient's night sleep. Early morning rising is common and could provide an opportunity for personal hygiene early in the day.

Provide good ventilation during sleep even though the oxygen intake is less, and safeguard the patient from falling out of bed or stumbling on his way to the bathroom.

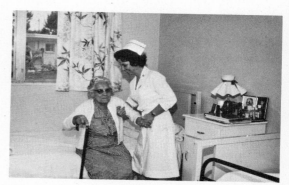

FIGURE 39–1 Dressed in her own clothes, this patient is being assisted to join the "activity group." (Courtesy of Santa Fe Community College Practical Nursing Program, Gainesville, Florida. Photographer: Henry DeLoach.)

Nutrition and Fluids

Helping the elderly patient meet this need may be a matter of thoughtfulness and observation as much as anything. Keep in mind that:

1. sense of taste is diminished.
2. energy may be in short supply.
3. dentures should be used (if possible).
4. encouragement may be needed.
5. food selection should be appropriate to ability to chew and swallow.
6. eating may be a slow process; allow time.
7. self-help is encouraged.
8. assistance is given as needed.

Sometimes it is difficult for the elderly patient to understand that he needs a balanced diet to help him regain his strength. Try to involve him in food selection and observe to see how much of his diet he eats. Watch between meal eating (e.g., whether empty calories or proper nourishment) practices.

Elimination

There may be a tendency to worry about bowel irregularity. Lack of exercise and roughage and reduced muscle tone alter bowel habits. Help patient to understand that "regularity" is an individual pattern that is aided by well balanced meals, adequate fluid intake and exercise. Persistent constipation is a medical matter.

Activity, Diversion and Rehabilitation

All patients, whether bedfast or ambulatory, require attention to maintain muscle tone, prevent contractures and abnormal immobility (a consolidated joint is called ankylosis), and to preserve independence. Avoid "doing for" if he can do for himself, but do provide proper positioning, turning, and range of motion exercises, especially for the bedfast patient. Be alert to ways to divert his attention and energies to something outside himself. He tends to detach himself from everyone around him; help him feel purposeful.

Environment

The key words are safety and convenience. Other factors are that it be pleasing to the eye and have some personal belongings in view or available. The patient's comfort may be his peace of mind with his belongings rather than "apple pie" order of the unit. Adjust it to his needs.

Allow sufficient time for doing what is to be done and permit as much independent action as possible.

Medical Care and Treatment

Often there is need to repeat instructions and explanations to gain the patient's cooperation and to reassure him. Attitudes may be inflexible; his memory may be limited. Permit the patient to help with care when possible (see Fig. 39–2). Be certain oral medicines are swallowed.

Physical changes in the body make it necessary to observe carefully timed treatments involving heat and cold, exercise, and positioning.

Emotional and Spiritual Needs

Show by work and deed that you do care about his well-being. The patient needs identity (use his name, not a nickname), self-respect, and a feeling of being important, of being wanted. He may feel he is a burden to the "busy" nurse, his family, or society. By your actions show him he is not.

A spiritual force, in the lives of many, is a source of inner strength that helps people to adjust and to be satisfied and happy. Show respect for his beliefs by listening, by leaving his religious materials where he wants them, and by escorting him to the chapel (or seeing that it is done) if this has meaning for him.

NURSING PROBLEMS COMMON TO THE ELDERLY

An elderly person can have almost any disease or disorder, but some conditions most frequently appear with old age just as some diseases are more commonly found among children; others among young or middle age adults. In other words, certain disorders occur more frequently in certain age groups.

What then is responsible for certain disorders and infirmity among elderly people? The "mysterious trend" called aging makes the body more susceptible to certain happenings because it seems to have less power per

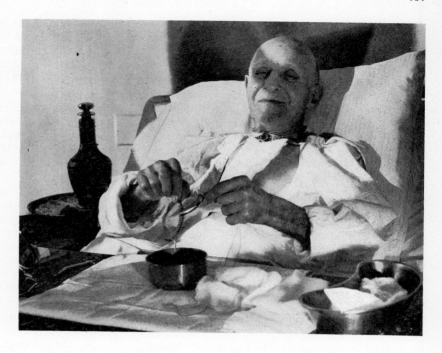

FIGURE 39–2 This 82-year-old man cares for his own tracheostomy tube. (Newton: Geriatric Nursing, The C. V. Mosby Co.)

cell to carry on than it once did (e.g., lack of muscle tone, bone tissue changes, special senses less acute, etc.). This trend produces signs of wear and tear, often leading to minor and/or major disabilities.

Eight out of ten elderly persons have one or more diseases or disabling conditions; the more common ones include:

1. **Arthritis**—inflammation of the joints; when it persists it becomes chronic such as: osteoarthritis, rheumatoid arthritis, and gouty arthritis.
   Chief characteristics: stiffness and pain after a night's sleep, painful, tender, and swollen joints.

2. **Cardiovascular diseases**—covering some twenty types of heart and blood vessel disorders (e.g., hypertension, diseased coronary artery, stroke and arteriosclerosis).
   Chief characteristics: with so many types only general considerations are included: under some circumstances (e.g., heart muscle damage) extreme limitation of activity with complete dependence for assistance in meeting basic needs; *stroke* patient with paralysis (without other disabling conditions) is directed toward self-caring activities in meeting his basic needs;

arteriosclerosis—a thickening of the walls (and loss of elasticity of the arteries, "hardening of the arteries," causes poor blood circulation, depending upon location of the thickening process there may be such symptoms as: cold/numb feet, lack of energy, shortness of breath, dizziness, headache, foot and leg cramps, loss of memory, etc.

3. **Cancer**—becomes more prevalent as people grow older. Chapter 43, *Patients With Cancer*, describes several types of cancer, positive attitudes toward it and general considerations regarding nourishment, appetite, purpose for living and self-caring activities. The elderly patient may need a generous amount of emotional support because he may feel he has lived his life and lost his purpose for living.

Impaired vision and impaired hearing get worse with age. Failing sight can be a much feared disability at any age, but for the elderly it can represent a loss of independence, which is frightening. The same could be said for the loss of hearing. One person out of 10 between the ages of 65 and 75 has some hearing impairment; the proportion is higher for persons older than that.

Diabetes affects one in 16 persons older than 60. It is a serious endocrine disorder that can be fatal. Early detection, medical management of diet, and insulin permit normal living. Problems for elderly people relate to foot and mouth care, staying on the proper diet, and taking insulin as ordered. Failing vision makes it difficult to prepare and self-administer insulin when the patient lives alone.

Acute Disorders

Acute illnesses (especially respiratory conditions) are frequently found among the elderly and often the cause of death for older people with chronic disorders. In addition to respiratory conditions (e.g., cold, influenza, pneumonia), acute disorders include gastrointestinal disorders, gallbladder difficulties, genitourinary infections, and infections of the skin. Even appendicitis is no respecter of age; the elderly have it, too. While relatively few of the so-called childhood diseases (e.g., mumps, measles, chickenpox) are seen among members of this group because there is a certain amount of immunity built up over the years, they do appear, often with serious results. A body invaded by a chronic disorder becomes easier prey for acute diseases and is less able to ward off infections.

ACCIDENTS. People over 65 have the highest death rate from accidents, except for children under one year of age. Most occur in the home (falls, burns, taking wrong medicines). For those already disabled, accidents multiply their difficulties, often leading to serious complications.

Attitude toward Prevention. Some uninformed persons think illness is bound to happen in old age; they argue that regular medical check-ups are an unnecessary expense and not as important as for younger people. One could return the argument that because the onset of many disorders in older people is slow and likely to go unnoticed, it is more important than ever to have regular medical examinations. Early detection and treatment arrest or "hold at arm's length" many chronic disorders, thus permitting the person to live and enjoy life.

Prevention is the aim of good medical care at any age. The elderly person should have a stake in good health the same as anyone else.

For the body with diminished power to heal and restore itself, complications are bound to occur more readily. This is why *care of the elderly patient includes all known nursing measures which prevent any complications, if at all possible*. In addition to this, it takes some insight into the problems that accompany doing the measures themselves.

Imagine, if you can, how painful joints limit a patient's desire to move, walk, turn, or be handled, or how a stroke that has paralyzed a part of the body or affected speech, memory, or judgment can discourage a person. Imagine how difficult it is to follow a strict diet after years of eating as you pleased. Imagine the difficulties encountered when vision or hearing is diminishing. The patient is hesitant about or openly objects to doing things or having them done for him.

Nursing these patients requires skill in knowing how to get them involved and interested in their own improvement. Imagination is one of the greatest assets a practical nurse can possess as she tries and tries again to bring the patient along the rehabilitation route, getting him to do and to participate. Several common problem areas are discussed to help you understand how to adapt your skills and approach to meeting his particular needs.

Nourishment and Intake

A common problem is disinterest in food and adequate fluid intake. It is not unusual for an elderly person to eat little because of what he calls poor appetite or because his dentures do not fit properly or he has few teeth. Because of these facts, the elderly patient needs to be observed for his food and fluid intake. Proper nourishment is one of his best defenses against complications. An adequate diet provides roughage, protective proteins, milk, and liquids, not empty carbohydrate calories. Help him to understand that an adequate diet need not be the most expensive diet.

Constipation

Self-medication and worry about bowel regularity are common in the elderly patient. He will ask for "something" for his bowels and be upset if he thinks his bowels have not functioned the way *he* thinks they should.

Keep two things in mind: 1. Observe the

frequency and character of stools. 2. Accept his concern and help him understand that bowel habits vary from person to person. For the unworried patient, you still have the responsibility of observing bowel habits and function.

Ambulation helps maintain normal bowel habits. For some patients, knowing this will help them to want to walk and get exercise.

Skin Care

While good skin care is a part of the care of any patient, it calls for special awareness when caring for the elderly.

The aging process reduces muscle tissue. Some of it is replaced by fatty tissue, but the loss of firm underlying muscle leaves the outer skin layers wrinkled and flabby. The skin is drier, less elastic, and less able to resist pressure and infections.

Keep the skin clean, dry, and lubricated as indicated by the physician. See that the bed is free of wrinkles and objects (e.g., food crumbs, talcum particles) to prevent pressure spots from forming over bony prominences (hips, coccyx, elbows, heels). Reposition patient frequently. Get him up in a chair regularly if permissible.

Mental Confusion

For some, this may come and go. Most often his confusion is associated with time and place, especially if he has just experienced a sudden change in surroundings. Chronic confusion is present in other instances; the patient continues to be disoriented at all times. In either case, extraordinary environmental safety precautions are used to protect the patient's welfare.

Incontinence of Bowel and Bladder

This problem frequently accompanies serious illness of the elderly. Skin care of the buttocks and genitalia is almost a constant nursing problem, and linens must be changed frequently. Many elderly patients are aware of their inability to control bowels and bladder and it is embarrassing to them. It should be of some comfort to them when the nurse displays no annoyance with this recurring problem and pays close attention to the need to be dry, clean, and as odor-free as possible.

Surgery for the Older Patient

The risk is greater for the elderly patient, but surgery is becoming increasingly safer for him. Newer types of anesthesia help, as do the measures taken to build up body resistance beforehand. Science has made great strides in determining how to maintain proper fluid balance in the cells and how to fortify the body through extra nourishment (fluids and blood transfusions). Electronic monitoring devices provide instantaneous information about the vital signs, alerting personnel to any changes as fast as they occur.

Some of the common types of surgery include: repair of fractured bones, removal of growths (tumors), eye surgery for cataracts and glaucoma, amputations, and surgical treatment of skin lesions.

Care for this patient includes the same basic nursing measures as for others, with the awareness that the body has less built-in power to restore itself and offer resistance. Knowing this, there needs to be close adherence to following all preventive aspects of care.

While the removal of any part of the body is a difficult experience for any person old enough to realize what has occurred, the elderly patient who has an extremity amputated, or has to use a tracheostomy tube or use a colostomy bag the rest of his life might find it easier to "give up" rather than adjust to such a change, unless rehabilitative efforts are at work from the start. Helping this patient to regain his courage and have an interest in rehabilitation efforts often requires continuing efforts on your part. Again, one's ability to imagine or devise ways to get him involved is a real asset.

PLANNING THE NURSING CARE

Keeping in mind the characteristics of older people, the nurse realizes that while the daily living needs are the same for everyone, regardless of age, she will need to make adjustments.

More Time and Convenient Environment

One such adjustment is in the amount of time needed for almost all activities, such as bathing, feeding, getting the patient up, treating him, and dressing him. His energy output is less and his disability can slow him that much more, therefore allow extra time for this patient to be self-assisting or for you to complete his care.

A convenient and safe environment is your responsibility, whether you are doing "all" for the patient or doing things with his help, or he is doing things for himself. Equipment should be conveniently located for his use and yours. If the patient is to get up, dress, move about, or be seated in a chair, he is to have help if he needs it.

Self-assistance and Routines

Making demands of the patient regarding what he should do for himself requires judgment and tact, and such demands must be within his prescribed medical orders. Furthermore, making demands of him regarding what you want to do can be equally upsetting. Who is to say that, while perhaps desirable, a complete bath is essential every day, or that, if it is to be given, it *has* to be given in the morning? An afternoon or evening bath can make a person just as clean and comfortable as one given in the morning. This may alter "the hospital routine," but it can be done. Likewise, it helps the patient's frame of mind if he feels he can share in making some decisions regarding himself.

Feeding patients takes time. Time and again the importance of adequate nutrition is mentioned. To get full benefit from a diet, it must be consumed. If it takes assistance to meet this need, provide it. Solicit the patient's participation openly or otherwise, by having him do all he can. Your presence should convey "unhurriedness." Be seated if possible and have the tray conveniently placed for both.

How does one talk with elderly patients? The same as with any other adult patients. Because some are repetitious and forgetful, certain questions will need answering more than once, certain things require discussion more than once. It does not help the patient to remind him of his forgetfulness or to treat him as a child; he does not consider himself a child, and resents this type of treatment. Your most valuable asset may be the ability to listen rather than talk in some situations.

Flexibility in Planning Nursing Care

An important quality for a nurse is flexibility (quick adjustability). This is demonstrated best when she shows some imagination in carrying out her care plan for the elderly patient. Cut-and-dried routines are abandoned in favor of small adjustments she can make to suit the patient and not be upset by this. Everyone has a right to his own feelings and wishes and in the elderly these may be more pronounced and exaggerated. It requires judgment and patience to know when a patient's demand is reasonable or possible to meet. Sometimes a small adjustment satisfies as well as a major one and alters the plan for care but little.

Factors in Planning Nursing Care

The *degree of illness* (how ill) influences the extent of assistance needed and the physician's written orders. If the patient's condition suggests to the physician the need for complex treatments (e.g., fluids, oxygen) quite naturally this influences the amount and type of assistance he needs from the nurse. More time is required to give proper skin and mouth care, to provide comfort measures, and to make more constant observations of the patient and the equipment being used.

Family is another factor. Members want to be near and they deserve consideration. While it is not possible to permit them to be present during every act of assistance to the patient (for the patient's good and theirs), when they are present they often observe the nurse's manner more than they do her skill in carrying out a procedure. They appreciate thoughtfulness in showing consideration for the patient, and a spark of humaneness, as much as or more than they do her perfection in handling equipment. Somehow they expect a nurse to know how to give a good cleansing bed bath, but when there is evidence that she does this with the patient in mind (safety, comfort, privacy) first and the procedure second, the family appreciates this. It can relieve their concern, at least in part.

The patient needs to *assist himself.* It may take longer, but the small feeling of independence is a big accomplishment for the patient who can do something for himself. For example, let us say a patient is able to feed himself if given enough time and if his food is in portions he can handle. His tray is served first, readied for him if he needs that help, and then picked up last. Provide needed assistance, arrange the environment, and encourage him to help; recognize his accomplishments afterwards. Throughout this action be mindful of the patient's limitations and safety.

Avoid *complications*. Complications or the onset of additional difficulties are more apt to occur in the elderly owing to less built-in resistance. For example, the elderly patient can develop contraction or shortening of muscles of the legs and arms sooner than the younger patient. This occurs when joints are stiff and motion or exercise is too limited. Deformity can result from his being too long in one position, pressure from bedding, poor body alignment, lack of movement and exercise of the part, and his resistance to moving, turning, or repositioning himself.

Pressure over bony prominences is the forerunner of the decubitus ulcer—an all-too-common occurrence in the elderly bedridden patient. The very best treatment for this complication is to prevent it from occurring. Watch for signs of redness and pressure.

Supportive Care

In addition to meeting the patient's physical needs, it is necessary to show the patient that he is accepted and acceptable. Listen to him, show respect for him, and reassure him by openly recognizing his participation in self-care. Things that make the patient feel calm and more confident are supportive.

Observation is a continuous process and a constant factor in providing care. During illness requiring frequent and careful observation, this should be carried out without being too apparent to the patient and his family. Change is more apt to be gradual in an older person, and it takes keen observation to detect slight differences; yet early detection may prevent serious complications. Recorded information should reflect any changes.

The need for rehabilitation is always present. Research shows that it is possible to help many patients regain usefulness. Patients long bedridden have been helped to get out of bed and resume some activities that they have not done in years. The attitude of the nurse has much to do with how honestly hopeful a patient can feel about rehabilitation. Know what is possible for a particular patient and be sincere in your efforts to help him, and answer his questions or see that he gets the answers. Most patients can spot the person who "talks" and says nothing; they soon have doubts about his sincerity or build up fears about such evasiveness.

SUMMARY

The aging process brings about slower body movements, lowered metabolism, slower circulation, and less flexibility in making adjustments. For the elderly patient, arrange time and materials so he may be as self-assistive as possible without feeling hurried. If you are helping him, see that he does not feel guilty about the time you spend with him. His basic needs are the same as those of any other patient; what is required are adjustments in carrying out nursing actions in line with his individual limitations, dependency, likes, and dislikes.

Special concerns for the elderly are good skin care, good elimination, exercise, body alignment, lessening of mental confusion, nourishment, diversion, dealing with incontinence of bowel and bladder, and emotional support.

The elderly patient must be encouraged to be active in as much of his own care as possible. This not only helps him retain his independence and identity, but he may want to do this as a matter of taking care of himself.

GUIDES FOR STUDY AND DISCUSSION

1. Aging changes the body. Use Chapter 21 to review the changes in tissue, physical appearance, and behavior in old age. Select any five changes and be ready to explain how each one could influence his need for assistance in meeting his daily living needs.

2. Listed on p. 465 are 15 factors which can influence how this patient's basic needs are met. See if you can describe one (or more) ways each factor might influence his nursing care.

3. What physical changes in the aged patient make it necessary to carefully time treatments (e.g., heat/cold, exercise and positioning)?

4. In your opinion, what are the most essential things to observe in caring for an elderly bed patient? Be ready to defend your answer.

5. Prepare a short written discussion on one of the following:
   1. Eating problems of the elderly patient.
   2. How to manage skin care problems of the incontinent elderly patient.
   3. How to help an elderly patient use his spare time.
   4. How to involve the elderly patient in self-care activities.

SUGGESTED SITUATION AND ACTIVITY

Select an elderly patient you are caring for and, using the 10 basic needs, list *any* adjustments you provide to make his care personalized or especially adapted to him. Describe any particular problem you met and what you did about it.

NURSING NEEDS OF THE DYING AND THE DEAD

OBJECTIVES FOR THE STUDENT: Be able to:

1. Give two examples which show how the nurse demonstrates respect for the feelings of the patient and the family.
2. Describe the signs of approaching death.
3. Explain what the patient's environment should provide.
4. Describe nursing actions which provide for patient comfort.
5. Formulate a rule which would guide an LPN with respect to witnessing a signature on a will.
6. Distinguish between nurse responsibilities for a body before and after a death certificate has been signed.

SUGGESTED STUDY VOCABULARY*

prognosis
respect
Cheyne-Stokes breathing
incontinence
diaphoresis

stertorous breathing
tact
reverence
nares
coma

consideration
dignity
religious customs
legal implications
mottled skin

*Look for any terms you already know.

INTRODUCTION

Life may end after long years as a result of an incurable illness; it may end at its beginning, or at any point, for any reason which makes it impossible for the body to sustain its vital processes. Death has always been a mystery to man, and life has always been something to preserve and cherish.

Humans experience the approaching cessation of life in many ways. It is fair to say that the termination of life is an entirely private

473

happening for each individual. For some it appears to be quiet and peaceful; others are extremely anxious, unquiet, and restless, and some seem to hold fast to the unwavering belief that life must continue. Whenever and however it happens, death causes feelings of genuine loss and deep loneliness to those who remain.

The nurse has unique responsibilities in caring for the patient who is incurably ill. These responsibilities are not easy to carry, but they must be met with poise, consideration, and helpfulness. Your presence and manner should convey the message of respect and reverence for life and for the dignity of each patient regardless of who he may be.

THE NURSE'S ROLE

Caring for the patient who is approaching death requires much from the nurse. In addition to the nursing measures needed to keep the patient physically comfortable, there are some other equally important considerations.

PRESENCE OF THE NURSE. Sometimes there is a tendency, in an effort to provide privacy, to seclude the dying patient and leave him quietly alone, except for frequent observations and needed care. We should remind ourselves, however, that the patient should not be alone. It is not unusual for him to ask that you stay, but this should be practiced whether or not it is requested. Remember, however, that the patient and family might want or prefer to spend time alone together.

MANNER OF THE NURSE. In carrying out all actions, nothing about the manner of the nurse should convey indifference, hopelessness, or the sense that nothing can be done to help the patient. Actions must express thoughtful understanding and an open respect for the feelings of the patient and the family. This type of expression (often not in words as much as in sensitive good judgment and appropriate behavior) is not a nursing procedure learned only for this type of happening; it is an expression that tells its own story as any care is being given.

ACTIVITIES OF THE NURSE. All activities are carried on in a manner of hopefulness. See that the patient's wishes are met and that he is as comfortable as possible. In doing this, avoid the appearance of attending to "routines." Observation is continuous and relates to changes in vital signs and to all manner of comfort measures.

Be ready to assist in getting the clergy if the patient or family ask your help. It would be poor judgment to bring this up without first having an indication that such help is wanted. The same would be true of making any other suggestion (e.g., calling a lawyer) which might indicate intrusion of a personal nature.

Protect the patient's rights by seeing that unwanted outsiders who might be seeking last-minute decisions (e.g., religion, money matters) are *not* allowed access to the patient. Be sure to seek help if this problem arises; find out what, if anything, should be charted.

The physician informs the patient and the family of the patient's condition. Only when requested by him should the nurse serve as direct source of such information. She should not place herself in the position of making judgments about the patient's prognosis. Neither should false statements be made about possible outcomes when direct questions are asked by the family or patient. The nurse has a responsibility to say that the physician is the person to ask, and she should offer to contact him or relay the message. Again, the manner in which this is done can make the difference between comfort or discomfort for the patient and his family.

Empathy, or entering into the feelings of the patient and family, can be communicated as much or more through manner as through words. In a quiet, thoughtful way, do those things for the patient which afford relief from pain, noise, and disturbing influences. Keep him clean, dry and odor-free, if this is a problem. Meanwhile, show every consideration for the needs of the family.

COMMON SIGNS OF APPROACHING DEATH

The signs of approaching death vary. The patient may be conscious to the end or may pass many hours in a state of coma. He may be alternately conscious and unconscious.

While each person dies in his own way, there are some signs which are more or less common as life ends. They include:

1. A change in the rate and rhythm of the pulse.

2. Excessive perspiration. The skin is very moist and pale or mottled.

3. Cold feet and hands, an evidence of slower blood circulation.

4. Mouth breathing as lower jaw drops when body muscles begin to relax and lose their tone. Cheyne-Stokes or stertorous breathing are other signs.

5. Inability to swallow. Breathing becomes noisy as mucus accumulates in the throat. Speech is labored and incoherent.

6. Vision diminishes, eyelids lower; the eyes lose their lustre, giving them a dull appearance as if coated with a film.

7. Ability to hear may be present until the end even if speech or facial expression is gone. This fact should be kept in mind when making any comments.

8. Pain, anguish, air hunger, fear, restlessness, peacefulness—any may be present.

PROVIDING NURSING CARE

The nurse serves two chief purposes as she cares for the dying patient: (1) her presence is reassuring, and (2) the care provided is comforting.

The patient may or may not be receiving assistance from equipment to aid breathing, to keep the heart beating, or otherwise to maintain vital processes. There are many such devices available today, and the serious decision of whether to continue or discontinue them in each instance rests with the physician. The use of such equipment with terminal patients raises questions about death and dying that are jointly being discussed by physicians, lawyers, the clergy, social scientists, and the public.

As for nursing the patient, care is taken to keep the patient as comfortable as possible. The family is quickly aware of the nurse who pays attention to the details of nursing care that give the patient a cared-for appearance and as much relief as possible from physical and mental suffering. Observations related to changes in any vital process (signs) are immediately reportable. The LPN may function in Role II, giving direct assistance to the registered nurse or physician (Fig. 40–1), or in Role I, depending upon the circumstances.

Questions raised by the family members should be answered with tact and good judg-

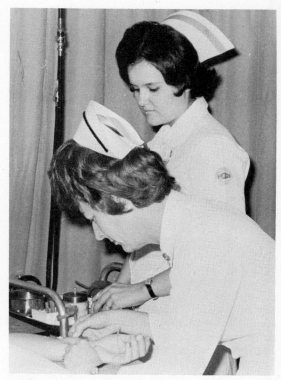

FIGURE 40–1 The LPN in Role II at this patient's bedside. (Courtesy of Pensacola Junior College Practical Nursing Program, Pensacola, Florida.)

ment. They are under stress and very often look to the nurse for support. However, the physician must be the person who gives or withholds information about the patient's condition.

Sometimes it may be more helpful to the patient (and family) to find a place where family members can be alone, at least periodically. Here again, each situation is judged on its own circumstances, and the physician or charge nurse may be the one to make the decision. Whatever the situation, your actions should be appropriate and in keeping with the circumstances.

The Environment

The patient's environment should provide quiet (not necessarily hushed) surroundings; provide for privacy. In a private room or the home this is more easily maintained than when other patients or individuals are close at hand. It may be necessary to move the patient to another room for reasons of privacy and to avoid upsetting other patients.

The room should have free circulation of air and natural light when possible. The air should be fresh and all odors removed.

Provide for reasonable quiet in the area outside the door. Normal activities are expected to continue but with regard and respect for this patient and his family.

Physical Comfort Measures

The slowing down of circulation usually produces a progressive cooling or coldness of the body moving from feet and legs upward to hands, arms, and nose. While the patient may have a steadily rising temperature he may feel cold. If he is conscious he may wish to have a hot water bottle placed at his feet or want additional bedding. Use lightweight blankets, when possible. The rising temperature accompanied by a feeling of cold makes some patients restless. Often they are not aware of this and it is difficult to quiet them.

Diaphoresis (excessive perspiration) is often present; this adds to the cold sensation and causes discomfort, too. Sponge the face with warm water and change linens, as needed. Bathing the patient may or may not be appropriate, depending upon the patient's general condition and hygiene needs.

Suction is often used to remove mucus from the mouth and throat. Nasal oxygen requires that attention be given to keeping the nares clean and lubricated. An indwelling catheter is checked, as for any patient, and observations are made of the amount and character of the urine or absence of it.

Special Observations and Nursing Care

Owing to the complete inability of the body to function properly, particular attention is paid to certain parts of the body:

The *eyes* should be wiped with moist cotton pledgets and dried to keep them free of crust forming discharges.

The *nares* are kept free from crust-forming discharges and are lubricated with mineral oil.

The *mouth* is kept clean and moist. Mouth breathing makes this a frequent treatment.

The *lips* are kept free of crust-forming material and are lubricated.

The *genitalia and anal region* are bathed as often as needed to avoid odor and, more important, to keep the skin clean, dry and nonirritated. Bladder and bowel incontinence commonly require ongoing attention. Any additional bed protection under the buttocks and over the genitalia should be provided and changed as needed.

A distended and full bladder is a painful experience which can be avoided. Observe the lower abdominal area to determine whether or not the bladder seems distended. Patient restlessness may be a sign of a painfully full urinary bladder. Supply the patient with a urinal or bedpan at frequent intervals. Observe the amount of urine and the time between voidings. Small amounts can be a clue that the bladder does not empty itself. Discuss this observation with the charge nurse or physician and chart your observations. Further measures might be required to give the patient needed comfort and relief.

As muscles lose their tone, additional support with pillows aids comfort. Changes in position are also necessary. Some patients breathe more easily when the head and shoulders are raised and supported. If the patient is conscious, he might be able to tell you which position is most comfortable; if not, observe facial expressions when any position change is made.

Fluids, Nourishment, Medications

Fluids and nourishment should be given as long as the patient can swallow. Many prefer ice chips or ice water. Very ill patients have difficulty drawing fluids through a drinking tube; a spoon, medicine dropper, or special feeder can be used.

The physician may choose to continue treatments and medications to the end or may discontinue some while retaining others. The nurse continues all medical orders as written. If for any reason they cannot be carried out, it should be reported at once.

Observations

Record all aspects of nursing care and observations, including visits by the physician, clergyman, lawyer, or other persons, other than family members, who might have reason to see the patient. Note the time of each such visit.

Temperature, pulse, and respiration may need to be, or are required to be, taken at definite intervals. If the patient's vital signs are monitored by electronic equipment, determine your responsibilities in this case.

Religious and Spiritual Needs

The patient approaching death may or may not wish to see a religious counselor. The family may seek or need assistance to locate the minister, priest, or rabbi. Every effort should be made to procure the clergyman while the patient is conscious. Sometimes time does not permit this. If at all possible, be familiar with the patient's beliefs and his wishes. The hospital chaplain may help or know what should be done. In hospitals without a chaplain local clergy may be consulted.

Different religious faiths vary in the way the dying patient's needs are met. Each has meaning and spiritual strength for its followers. The nurse needs to be aware that while the patient may follow beliefs unlike her own, his wishes are respected and every effort made to meet them. Protestants, Catholics, Jews, and other groups each have their own manner of ministering to a patient approaching death. The hospital may have special equipment available for this purpose; ask the charge nurse how to proceed unless you are familiar with hospital policy and provisions.

Make whatever preparation is required. A clean bedside table covered with a white cloth is useful in most instances. The clergyman usually brings materials with him; ask him if he needs other items. Record the time of his visit on the chart.

Usually the patient and his religious counselor will wish to be alone or with the family. A screened, quiet place is needed.

If the family needs further help, find a quiet place for them to go with the priest, minister, or rabbi.

WHEN THE PATIENT EXPIRES

The nurse never pronounces a patient dead. The physician always does this. Signing of the death certificate by the physician is a legal requirement and necessary before the mortician may accept the body for burial preparations. The time that the patient apparently ceased to breathe is recorded. The physician is notified immediately. In the hospital it is reported to the nurse in charge. If the circumstances are such that considerable time will elapse before the doctor's arrival, the nurse should see that the body is in good alignment and natural in appearance. The eyelids should be closed. If difficulty is experienced, place a small piece of damp cotton on each. The body should be placed in a recumbent position with the head and shoulders slightly elevated to prevent discoloration of the face. Any dentures which have been removed should be cleansed and replaced immediately.

The care of the body after death certification by the physician is a nursing responsibility. Families will differ in the things they permit the nurse to do for the patient after death. Some religions do not permit early care by the nurse; the family attend their own dead. When you encounter such requests, report this to the charge nurse. She or the physician should be aware of the family's request and can guide your actions or involvement. There should be no misunderstanding about respect for their beliefs nor for any legal implications.

When the nurse is responsible for the care of the body of the deceased patient (after the family has departed), certain things must be done. A regular bath is given. The rectum and vagina are packed with cotton to prevent secretions or discharges from escaping. A double thickness pad should be brought up over the rectum, vagina, and meatus and held in place with a T binder or diaper. Any soiled dressings should be replaced with clean ones. Hair should be combed, nails cleaned and trimmed. Cover the body with a clean shroud.

The hospital usually requires identification attached to the wrist and to the shroud. Careful labeling is essential. Such information as name of hospital, patient's name, address, date and time of death is included.

The procedure for caring for the expired patient is quite similar from one hospital to another. However, you should ask to be certain that all responsibilities are fully carried out as there are laws controlling the removal of the body from the supervision of one agency (e.g., hospital, nursing home) to another (mortuary).

LEGAL ASPECTS AND RESPONSIBILITIES

Personal Belongings

The nurse is responsible for taking care of the personal belongings after the death of the patient. In the hospital these possessions should be listed and handled according to the requirements of that particular institution. No article in the unit, regardless of worth, should be discarded or destroyed. If family members are present and remove the possessions, the nurse should record this fact on the chart. In the event the hospital requires a statement signed to that effect, it will be the nurse's responsibility to get this done. Valuables kept in the hospital safe are usually handled through the business office. Regardless of regulations for handling the possessions of others, good judgment and caution are always necessary. Lawsuits sometimes occur when such property is lost or damaged.

The Patient's Will

Sometimes a person approaching death may ask to make or remake his will. The patient should be advised to use the services of an attorney if at all possible. Helping patients make wills is not a nursing function. In *emergencies* only is it at all advisable to give any such assistance. The practical nurse should report this request to the nurse in charge immediately. In the home the family will take care of this matter.

Witnesses to signatures on wills are required. In some states two, in others three, persons have to be present at the time the individual signs his will. Each witness then signs in the presence of the others. Witnessing a signature on a patient's will should be avoided by the nurse if possible; it is not a nursing responsibility. Most hospitals will assist patients if they need help. The business office usually has a procedure for this purpose. When a patient makes a will the chart should contain a statement giving the exact time and the apparent condition of patient.

SUMMARY

Nursing the patient who is approaching death requires more than technical skill and procedures. It takes understanding, good judgment, and sincere concern for the patient and the family. Hope accompanies life. All functions of the nurse are directed toward possible recovery. The physician informs the family and the patient (if requested) about the patient's condition. This is not a nursing responsibility. Questions regarding this should be handled truthfully and with tact, indicating willingness to relay these not-to-be answered questions to the appropriate persons.

The nurse is very important to the family at this time. She is alert to their needs and comforts as well as the patient's.

Special religious customs should never be neglected. It is far better to ask and be sure than to hesitate and neglect something which is of real spiritual concern to the patient or his family.

Nursing actions have legal and ethical significance. The nurse's role is one of giving support to the patient and family without entering into matters of a personal or family nature.

GUIDES FOR STUDY AND DISCUSSION

1. What are the physical signs of approaching death?
2. The patient's environment needs special consideration. What should be considered? How can you provide it?

3. What nursing measures are particularly needed by the dying patient? How can a nurse show consideration and respect for human life while carrying out her responsibilities?

4. Discuss ways the nurse can help family members.

5. Why should a nurse avoid witnessing a will, if at all possible?

6. What are the first nursing measures taken after respirations have ceased?

7. What are the nurse's responsibilities after the physician has pronounced the patient dead?

SUGGESTED SITUATIONS AND ACTIVITIES

1. There are legal responsibilities involved in caring for a patient prior to and following death. Through a panel presentation, show the role of the LPN in meeting these responsibilities.

2. A stranger insists on seeing and talking with the patient. You found him alone with the patient when you returned to the room. How would you handle this situation?

THE PATIENT IN SPECIFIC MEDICAL-SURGICAL SITUATIONS

Unit X serves two purposes: (1) to introduce you to general signs/symptoms of illness and appropriate nursing care; (2) to introduce you to the signs and symptoms of diseases/disorders common to the various body systems and specific nursing measures.

Chapter 41 describes some 30 different signs/symptoms of illness which occur time and again with illness after illness. Rather than repeat information about each sign/symptom with each disease, they are discussed here for ready reference.

Chapter 43 deals with cancer because this common disease invades any body system or tissue.

The remaining chapters discuss diseases according to body systems and accidents. Actually the content focuses not so much on disease as the signs and symptoms of diseases, their medical management and nursing care.

Factors you will need to keep in mind are the patient's age, the extent of his dependence/independence, the limitations put on him by his disorder and the type of person he is. Remember too that the physician's orders are specific and dictate an essential part of the patient's care so your action(s) must be knowledgeable if your help is to be effective.

The "medical-surgical" label given to patients includes those who are ambulatory, mildly ill, seriously ill, old, young, long-term, or have chronic disorders; so we are here discussing the same patients discussed in Unit IX.

CHAPTER 41

WHEN ILLNESS OCCURS: BODY RESPONSES AND NURSING CARE

TOPICAL HEADINGS

OBJECTIVES FOR THE STUDENT: Be able to:

1. Given a list of eight major factors which cause/contribute to illness, name one illness caused by each.
2. Describe three ways in which the body adjusts itself to stay within normal bounds.
3. Name the three purposes of treatment for illness.
4. Explain how you would proceed to find out what is expected of you in carrying out a new, strange medical order.
5. Given a list of 12 common signs and symptoms of illness, describe one usual nursing measure and pertinent observations for each.

SUGGESTED STUDY VOCABULARY

(See Suggested Situations and Activities, item number 1.)

INTRODUCTION

When illness or disorder strikes, the body reacts and tries to correct the situation or at least overcome it. It does this in a total way; the whole being (body and mind) is caught up in the difficulty and shows signs that things are not normal within. These tell-tale signals, called signs and symptoms, help the physician diagnose the ailment if possible and treat the patient. Nursing measures include carrying out the physician's orders plus doing things for and with the patient which do not depend on medical orders as such, but are included in the nursing care plan. An example would be giving the needed time and attention to the incontinent patient's buttocks, back, and pubic area to see that he is kept clean and his bed dry.

Review Chapters 27, 28, and 34 regarding general signs, symptoms, and observations.

WHEN ILLNESS OCCURS

Within normal range, a healthy body is in the process of constantly adjusting itself to the environment and renewing and restoring itself physically and mentally. Each body meets these adjustments in its own way.

Causes of Illness

Review the eight major factors which either help to cause or directly cause illness (see p. 276).

Very often more than one of these factors is involved to cause and aggravate the illness condition, as would be the case when an undernourished person fractured his leg and developed an infection.

When you stop to think about the many different things which can invade and influence the body, you wonder how the body remains within normal range as much as it does. But one of its greatest abilities is to constantly adjust or adapt itself to try to stay within normal boundaries.

To do this, the body uses its built-in weapons and self-adjusting mechanisms. Familiar examples are the ability of the skin to heal a scratch and the presence of an automatic cooling system—perspiration. Another example is the power of the body to produce and supply extra red blood cells to meet the body's demand for more oxygen when it is in short supply.

The healthy body has normal limits for temperature, the amount of body fluids and the nature of those fluids, nourishment, oxygen, sleep and rest, blood pressure, pulse, and respiration, to name a few. The internal environment, which has to do with fluid balance, must be maintained in a stable manner.

When something occurs to upset one or more of these "normal limits," the body displays certain distress signals which we know as signs and symptoms of illness. In other words, a healthy body has changed to a sick body.

The General Treatment of Illness

Treatment (therapy) of a patient is directed toward (1) cure if possible, (2) changing the progress of the illness and further disability, and (3) altering the condition to permit the patient to live as comfortably and actively as possible for as long as possible.

1. *Cure* is successful treatment. All sorts of means are used to cure a disease. They include:

a. Using *specific known means,* such as surgery to correct a structural defect, an antibiotic to destroy a specific microorganism, and a drug to replace a substance lacking in the body.

b. Helping the body use its own *built-in resources* to the best advantage. Bed rest, ambulation, diet and fluid regulation, medicine, and physical therapy are some examples of this assistance to the body.

2. *Changing the progress of an illness and preventing further disabling effects* are the goals sought when no cure is known or available. For example, an illness may come on fast and attack the body in a violent way, threatening and even taking life. The earlier the progress of the disease can be checked, the better are the chances for saving life and reducing unwanted disability when the disease itself is over. Meningitis (inflammation of the membranes between the skull and the brain) is such a disease; poliomyelitis is another.

3. *Altering the condition* to allow the patient to be as comfortable and active as possible for as long as possible has such well-known examples as arthritis, diabetes, multiple sclerosis, terminal cancer, and epilepsy.

If there is no known cure for a disease or disorder, therapy is supportive (helpful to both body and mind) to keep the body functioning in as normal a way as possible. As in the case of diabetes, diet control and insulin are two means used to help this patient live an active, comfortable life. The patient with generalized cancer who cannot get well receives therapy to relieve pain, additional nourishment and fluids to maintain body fluids, and any other measures needed to keep him comfortable as long as he continues to live.

From the previous discussion, you can see that therapy or treatment is directed toward certain goals. The combination of measures used for a particular patient is the result of the physician's judgment of the patient's medical needs. He bases his decisions on the evidence he has at hand and the therapies he has available.

Do not overlook the vital fact that in addition to the many therapies used, the patient's will to live influences his treatment, too. The nurse can be as important as anyone in helping the patient find reason to want to live.

General categories of treatments (therapies) include the following:

1. Bed rest and sleep.
2. Diets.
3. Fluid regulation.
4. Medicine.
5. Therapeutic and diagnostic measures.
6. Surgery.
7. Emergency care.
8. Special therapies: laser beam, x-ray, radiation, physical therapy, speech therapy, controlled atmosphere ("chambers").
9. Rehabilitative efforts.

General Nursing Care

The overall work of the nurse may be grouped under four headings for convenience of study. In real life, however, nurse action is an intermixing of these factors geared to the basic needs of the individual patient. The four headings are *(1) observations, (2) physical comfort and safety, (3) emotional comfort and well-being, and (4) measures and procedures ordered by the physician for the patient's medical management, as well as measures determined by the charge nurse for the patient's nursing management.*

Observation (fully discussed in Chapter 34) is a word that covers a multitude of skills and actions in nursing. Among the many skills you develop as an LPN, the ability to observe accurately and to report meaningfully will be one of your most valuable skills. You are a data gatherer; you gather *facts*. Chapter 34 points out how you use your different personal capacities (special senses, among other things) to gather these facts.

Once the facts have been gathered they must be recorded so that others can use them. The physician needs them to diagnose and treat the patient; the nursing team needs them to know the state of the patient's care and condition. Other personnel use them for their particular purposes. If observations are to be meaningful, they must be stated in specific terms; factual nursing notes speak for themselves. Whenever possible, state your notes in actual terms. For example, *when exact numbers are involved, use them* (time, the number of times something happened, readings for temperature and blood pressure, the respiration-pulse count, how long something lasted, and so on). *Quote the exact words of the patient when pertinent. Use descriptive words that have specific meaning.* For example, in describing patient behavior, these questions might be helpful: *What* did the patient say, ask about, do or not do? *When* was it said, asked about, done, or not done? *Where* did he say he hurt? You can furnish many specifics without cluttering up the record with vague generalities that indicate a judgment on your part. For instance, instead of recording "restless," specify *what* the patient was doing—turning and tossing, said he could not sleep, and so forth. Or instead of recording "seems confused" (this is a judgment), specify *what* the patient said or did.

The following guidelines will help you make specific remarks:

1. Location as it relates to patient's body. Use common terms for region, area, and quadrants. Review Figures 34–8 and 34–9.
2. Onset. Sudden or gradual? What time?
3. Duration. How long did it last?
4. Nature of. What was it like (in the words of the patient). What did you see, feel, hear?
5. Degree of. Use words of patient, if possible—"mild," "uncomfortable," "severe," or "unbearable." State it according to what you saw, heard or felt. Describe, using specific terms, such as "500 cc. bright red, streaked vomitus."
6. Appearance of site, part, patient. *What* did you see? Use words which tell how it looked, how big it was, and so on.

Physical comfort and safety takes into account such things as the patient's personal hygiene and grooming, the comfort of his bed (smooth, clean, dry, enough covers), proper lighting, good body alignment, and proper support. Physical comfort and safety also raises these types of questions: Is the patient as free from pain as possible? Has he had the right kinds and amounts of fluids and nourishment? Was his intake-output measured and recorded? Did he receive his treatment on time? Does his back need rubbing? Are there pressure areas that need attention? Are the side rails in position? Can he reach his light or call signal? Is he wearing safe footwear for walking? Does he need assistance to walk?

Emotional and spiritual needs of the patient may be present because illness always is an unwanted expense and a worrisome experience. When it strikes mothers or fathers of a family, many things besides the illness cause them to worry. Children left at home, mounting unpaid bills, fear of what the future holds as far as their condition is concerned, and an almost constant feeling of wanting to go home and back to work may keep them upset.

Patients need help to adjust to or accept their illness whether young, middle-aged, or old. In the hospital things are strange to them and they do not quite know what to expect, especially during their first experience as a patient. They need to know such things as when meals are served, the visiting hours, and when the physician is likely to make his visit. Very often little things bother the patient because hour-to-hour or daily activities are strange and different. Take time to explain hospital habits and show willingness to make any adjustments you can.

We know that when a person is sick, he is apt to behave differently from when he is well. He is uncomfortable physically and this fact distresses his thoughts and feelings. Illness takes a person out of the mainstream of living; it curtails or limits activity, changes plans, and, in general, upsets his way of life. Knowing this, you should accept the sick person as he is and show by action and word that you realize that the patient is uncomfortable or upset and may be even angry about the whole thing.

Sickness causes people (patient and family) to worry about the outcome. Is the illness serious? What causes it? Does one ever get over it? How will it influence what I can do when I go home? People look to the nurse (among others) for bits of confidence, good signs, and hope. Some come right out and ask specific questions; others keep their questions to themselves.

As a practical nurse, you can build up patient confidence by showing that you accept his behavior and respect his feelings. Listen to him. Pay attention to his expressions of fear, complaints, and plans for the future — or whatever he wants to talk about. Your presence and your attention may be reassuring and perhaps comforting to him. Offer to share his questions with someone who can give him more exact information than you can or should give.

Quite naturally the chief concern of any patient (if he can understand) is recovery. He may or may not say much about it, but the possibility of surgery or future limited activity can prey on his mind. Fear and worry about an impending operation are natural. Some may say they have no concern about it, but usually they do, even if the surgical procedure is to be done under local anesthesia. The fear of not really knowing what to expect and of feeling somewhat helpless about it can cause concern. The practical nurse who understands this never uses a matter-of-fact approach; she accepts the patient's concern and tries to help him understand that she is aware of how he feels and accepts his feelings.

Another patient who may be almost numb with fear is the person waiting to receive a report from certain tests or examinations — the patient who fears he may possibly have cancer, for example. Sometimes the fact that no one (nurses or physician) comes near for a while causes him to believe that they are postponing the visit because the report is unpleasant. Be aware of what is being done for your patient by other personnel; it will guide your actions and help you to understand why the patient is concerned. Stop by a little more frequently during that day and suggest something to divert attention if appropriate. Your presence indicates your interest. It is not always what you say that matters most; it may be the thoughtful way you do something.

Spiritual needs are expressed in different ways. Frequently during illness spiritual reassurance takes on a stronger meaning. This may be due in great measure to being faced with uncertainty and having the time to think about it. Patients who are facing surgery or being treated for a condition that cannot be cured are seeking hope and something to rely upon; often they find the greatest comfort in talking with their minister, priest, or rabbi.

Certain religious beliefs and rituals have been a part of some patients' lives for many years. Make it as easy as possible for these patients to continue these practices. When these beliefs interfere with planned medical care (e.g., refusing to take medication), the matter should be handled by the physician.

The bedside table may be used for keeping the Bible, prayer books, medals, or other meaningful religious material close at hand.

Wearing certain religious objects around the neck or pinned to the gown has real significance for some patients; the practice should not be questioned.

Faith is a personal thing; everyone has a right to his own. Helping a patient meet his spiritual needs means getting assistance for him if he wants it and respecting him for having a faith even though it may differ from one's own. Elderly patients often display considerable inner strength in facing problems and adjusting to circumstances.

MEASURES AND PROCEDURES. You can tell by reading the discussions of both the physical and the emotional and spiritual factors that they are part of what the doctor orders and what the nurse must do both with and without a written plan of action.

Much of what is done for and with a patient is determined by the physician's orders (specific treatments, medications, special types of care). However, much of what is done for and with the patient has no written medical order at all, as indicated by some of the questions raised under "physical comfort," discussed previously.

To give effective care, you do not need a history of the patient's pathology, but you do need to understand what the doctor's intentions are for that particular patient. This is especially true for the various measures you carry out or assist with. To say it another way, you do not need to know the many detailed causes of the patient's illness; this is a medical matter. You do need to know what the doctor has in mind to safely and effectively carry out or assist with the doctor's orders and the nursing care plan. Sometimes the measures are more complicated than you are able to cope with; they require more scientific knowledge than a practical nurse possesses. In this event, you may be a Role II task performer in the situation or not involved in it at all.

For the things you can safely do, *be sure you understand what is expected of you.* For instance, if the patient has an order for "bed rest," you should know what the doctor has in mind for this patient. How much or how little self-activity does he want the patient to have? In addition, what must you do for the patient? One further thought: How much do you need to know about the reason why the physician has ordered "bed rest"? Do you need to know the detailed nature of what went wrong in the patient's body? No, this is a medical matter.

You need to know what signs or symptoms to watch for; you also need to understand the purpose of the orders (bed rest, in this case) to guide your nursing action effectively and safely.

While you do learn how a good many common illnesses affect body tissues and throw the body off balance, and you do learn what leads to or causes many types of complications, your chief concern is to *know the purposes of the measures you carry out,* so that you can practice safely and the results of your work will contribute effectively to the patient's well-being. For example, if the patient's diagnosis is still under question and the physician orders a series of special tests that involve you, it is your responsibility to know what you must do or not do (e.g., withhold food and liquids for such and such a time, get such and such a specimen at a certain time) to help make this order as productive as possible.

PAIN

The reason for including several general signs/symptoms of illness at this point without reference to specific diseases/disorders is because they are so often general in nature and accompany so many different diseases/disorders. It saves repeating the same content from disease to disease. You will notice in the following chapters dealing with diseases/disorders of the various body systems that with each disease, specific signs/symptoms are included as well as particular medical and nursing care for each. Use this chapter for reference.

It has been called "the cry of an injured nerve" but this may not always be the case—such as the unbearable pain in the phantom limb of the amputee or the sense of pain far from the site of disease called referred pain.

Pain is a common response to illness; it protects the body by indicating that something is wrong. Pain is a stubborn word to define because it comes in so many forms or degrees. Everyone has experienced and reacted to the sensation called pain at some time or another. Everyone knows, too, that a "hurting" part of the body captures one's attention; the mind is on the pain, regardless of where in the body it is located. The site of the pain can be local, but at times the whole body reacts.

CAUSES. Some of the common main causes of pain include the following:

1. Tissue damage (e.g., laceration, bruise, burn).
2. Tissue pressure (e.g., extra fluid, tumor, distended urinary bladder).
3. Tissue invasion by disease or infection.
4. Tension on tissues.
5. Stretching of skin.
6. Contracting of muscles (spasm).
7. Fear, anxiousness.
8. Posture, position.
9. Referred to one part from another source.

SIGNS AND SYMPTOMS. **Signs.** Evidence of pain shows up in a variety of ways: a complaint by the patient, an outcry, groan or moan; specific facial expressions (a wince, frown, a look of anguish, tears); body posture or seeming to favor a part (e.g., leg) when in use.

Pain is a personal matter; some people are able to stand more than others. Some talk about their pain while others "grin and bear it." Other things that enter into whether there is evidence of pain or not include one's beliefs, faith, culture, location and type of pain. Age too can make a difference.

Then there is a person's pain threshold; pain threshold means the point at which a person first senses or feels pain. It varies greatly among people and for the same person at different times. Drugs, alcohol, massage and denying the pain make it easier to tolerate (raise the threshold). Anger, worry, fear, fatigue, and boredom may lower the threshold.

Loss of the ability to feel pain is a warning symptom too; the patient may undergo damaging body changes without being aware that anything is wrong.

CARE OF THE PATIENT. The cause of the pain dictates what must be done for the patient. The physician will try to determine why the patient is having pain. At the same time he will order measures such as medications, treatments, positioning, exercise, support, elevation, or immobility to relieve it. As mentioned previously, pain is a signal that something is wrong. If there is evidence (e.g., an open wound, a new operative site, burns, fractured bone) of the cause, this is one thing; if there is no evidence, the search continues.

NURSING CARE. An important part of the nursing care of the patient with pain is to make observations, both subjective and objective, and to record and report them.

Pain is hard to describe; the person experiencing it is the most expert even if his words seem vague and lack preciseness. When a patient complains of pain listen to him (take some action) because his pain is what he says it is even though he may have difficulty being specific about it. You learn how and what to listen for. Ask questions to help him describe it in his own words. The recording and reporting should be in the patient's words, and should not reflect your judgment or feelings.

The *subjective* observations to be determined are:

1. *Location* — general or local; specific or vague. It may be difficult for the patient to say where the pain is. The location of a superficial pain is more easily and accurately given than that of a deep pain. The patient may *say* where the pain is: "over my right eye," "in my left big toe," or he may say, "I hurt all over." He may often place his hand over the part or area when he tells you where his pain is. The patient may hesitate to mention his pain or be afraid to tell where it is because he fears it might be "something serious" and he will need surgery.

2. *Nature* — the character of pain may be described by the patient as aching, dull, gnawing, prickling, burning, stinging, stabbing, piercing, cutting, sharp, knife-like, sharp-shooting, pressing, throbbing, pulling, stretching, pounding, squeezing, boring, cramping, or crushing.

3. *Intensity or degree* — mild, moderate, or severe; this may change or alternate. According to the patient and his tolerance, he may describe his pain as being mild or may say, "I can't stand it." Some may not mention pain until it becomes so severe that they cry, vomit, or become unconscious.

4. *Onset* — how did it start? Suddenly or slowly? Examples: "The pain started right after I finished eating my breakfast." "The pain in my chest started when I turned on my right side."

5. *Duration* — how long has the patient had pain? Timing may be vague and it may be necessary to clock or time some pains. Examples: "I had this pain on and off all afternoon" (intermittent). "This pain hasn't let up all day" (constant).

6. *Patient's comments* — regarding his pain — such as: "That funny kind of sharp pain

in my right side quit, all at once, just like that" (abrupt absence of pain is important to note). "When I stay on my right side the pain isn't so bad." "That aching pain in my right shoulder is now gone and I've got a pain in the center of my chest, here under my breastbone, and it feels as if it is crushing me" (a change of location or intensity is important to note).

The *objective* observations include:

1. *Skin*—becomes pale, cool and moist when pain is severe and prolonged.

2. *Facial expression*—brows may be knitted, mouth drawn, teeth set, muscles drawn and tense; patient may grimace.

3. *Eyes*—may be closed tightly or open and have a startled or tense look; pupils may be dilated.

4. *Pulse*—rate may change (increase or decrease) with degree of intensity.

5. *Respirations*—increase in rate and change in character.

6. *Blood pressure*—changes may occur with intensity and duration of pain.

7. *Skeletal muscles*—may be tense or rigid.

8. *Gastric distress*—nausea may occur, with or without vomiting; anorexia or refusal to eat may occur.

9. *Physical activity and reactions*—patient may be very quiet, only moving when asked or necessary; may be very restless and unable to sleep; may be listless and fatigued; may progress from weakness to fatigue to fainting to prostration to unconsciousness. Note any change the patient takes in his posture or position, e.g., keeps knees flexed or drawn up to abdomen.

10. *Mental and emotional activity and reactions*—patient may cry, "suffer in silence," complain, talk a great deal, or become demanding (e.g., about having a medication, calling the physician); may lose interest in personal appearance or an activity (e.g., reading); may have certain reactions when visitors (or a certain visitor) come.

11. *Observations regarding nursing care*—Is the patient satisfied with the effects of his medication, more comfortable, quiet, resting or sleeping? Does he mention getting any relief? Following a nursing measure (e.g., changing a dressing, having an enema) is mention made of any change in the pain?

Sometimes a patient is asked to estimate his pain on a scale from one (none) to four (severe) to give some notion of the severity of it.

The nursing care of the patient with pain, in addition to observations, will depend upon a number of factors, such as the cause, the physician's orders as to what may or may not be done, and the patient himself.

Because of the nature of pain and its being a very personal matter, it is the responsibility of the nurse "to do something" to help prevent or relieve it. The nurse can give attention to the needs of the patient for physical and mental comfort, of course, depending upon the orders of the physician as to what may or may not be done. The nursing care of the patient will include:

1. *Control of the environment.* Provide privacy, quiet, and desirable temperature.

2. *Control of activity.* Provide a different physical or mental activity; prevent fatigue (being up too long, being in one position too long); protect against any undue effort which causes fear, worry, or anxiety.

3. *Reassurance.* Show acceptance and understanding of the patient and his pain with your actions and words, as well as with your time, attention, and presence, by listening to the patient, giving attention to details, answering his signal or requests promptly, anticipating and being thoughtful about meeting his needs, checking with him without waiting to be called, respecting any requests, likes, or dislikes, if possible, and, finally, by being careful to avoid trite and false remarks that have no meaning.

4. *Nursing measures.* Unless contraindicated or prevented by the physician's order they may include: giving a back rub, preventing retention of urine, changing patient's position, being careful to avoid jarring the bed, using some means to keep weight of top bedding off patient's feet, adjusting the back rest, etc.

5. *Physician's orders.* Medications may be ordered according to a specific schedule or when needed by the patient; patients often react differently about the need for a medication for pain (some will ask, some will refuse). Treatments vary widely but may include local or general applications of heat or cold some of which may be carried out by the nurse.

A new experimental approach to the relief of untreatable and unrelenting pain is called "behavior modification." The idea behind it is to help people with unrelieved pain change their attitude toward pain so they can pursue their daily living activities. The patient must want to change his way of life or the approach does not work. He is not pampered and his activity is increased; this therapy does not "reward" the patient by sympathizing with him, offering assistance or giving medicine. Family members must cooperate with the plan too, if the patient is to develop a positive attitude. As with any new approach, this one has its critics.

INFLAMMATION, INFECTION, AND THE PROCESS OF HEALING

Inflammation

Inflammation is the most general response to an irritation that the body possesses. The irritating factor (causative agent) may be something physical or chemical, or harmful bacteria. The causative agent sets the built-in defense mechanisms in motion to destroy or eliminate the agent itself.

PROCESS OF INFLAMMATION. The word inflame, meaning "to set on fire" or "to cause to redden," gives you some clue as to what inflammation might feel and look like. Actually, inflammation has five qualities which can be identified:

1. Swelling.
2. Pain and tenderness.
3. Redness.
4. Heat.
5. Loss of function.

The swelling is due to blood plasma and lymph gathered at the site of irritation. Pain results from the increased pressure on nerve endings as fluids gather. Redness comes from increased blood brought to the site. Heat is due to increased cell metabolism and accumulated acids; if the inflammation is localized, one can feel that it is warmer than the surrounding area. Loss of function comes when the irritating force overcomes the body force to fight back to such an extent that the part is immobilized and cannot function as it should.

LOCAL REACTIONS. The causative agent may be localized in one spot, as with a scratch on the forearm from a thorny blush. At the site of the scratch, in this instance, the skin has been torn open, some cells have been destroyed, and whatever organisms were at the site on the skin and the thorn are in the wound ready to multiply among the damaged cells; this adds to the original irritation (the scratch). The body reacts by releasing plasma through the local capillary walls to seal off or trap the infection, and brings additional white blood cells to the scene to engulf the organisms. Pus is formed from an accumulation of destroyed organisms, dead white blood cells, and plasma.

The local area is red, tender or painful, somewhat swollen, and feels warmer than the surrounding area.

It is possible for a body part to become inflamed from a physical means such as a bruise, or a chemical means such as a drug, with no harmful bacteria being present.

GENERAL OR SYSTEMIC REACTION. When a local reaction cannot be contained (sealed off) and the organisms destroyed on the spot, the lymph carries the organism, wastes, and toxic substances to the lymph nodes where they are ingested, if possible. An enlarged lymph node means that it is infected; this is called a secondary infection. Mumps (enlarged parotid glands) is an example; kernels in the axilla is another.

Some microorganisms pass through the lymph nodes and into the blood. If they do not multiply or damage the blood, but use it for a means of transportation, this condition is called *bacteremia*. However, if the organisms multiply in the blood and throw off toxins, it is known as *septicemia;* any part of the body may become another site of infection when this occurs.

Several organs and tissues (e.g., bone marrow, liver, spleen) screen out bacteria from the blood at a very high rate of speed, providing built-in mechanisms that very often prevent bacteremia from becoming septicemia.

Infection

An infection is the reaction of the body to invasion by harmful microorganisms and the toxins they produce. Not all infections are due to carelessness, but many are; one carelessly started infection is one too many. Not all infections are simply complications but are rather infectious diseases (e.g., scarlet fever, measles). See Chapter 54.

For our purposes here, consider an infection a complication or a second disease going on at the same time as the first one. The best way to fight this second disease is to prevent it. As a practical nurse, you can help do your part in prevention by using the utmost care in handwashing and handling of all sterile and contaminated materials, and by practicing strict aseptic techniques (medical and surgical) and good habits of patient unit "housekeeping." An infected wound may be a sign of *your* carelessness.

The Healing Process

The body makes every attempt possible to restore tissue damage. If the injured area is small and cell damage is slight, the area reestablishes itself (recuperates) with no sign of the past injury. When the injury is more severe, the area heals by cells replacing similar cells; underlying layers of tissue contribute to this cell replacement process in much the same way that skin is replaced as it is shed.

If there has been extensive damage and an amount of tissue is lost, the body fills the gap with connective or scar tissue, which holds the gap together, so to speak. Scar tissue is not working tissue. If part of an organ repairs itself with scar tissue, it means that that part of the organ does not function; thus the entire organ functions less well than it did before. However, a small "weak" spot might be strengthened by the scar tissue (e.g., the wall of a blood vessel). Scar tissue is not elastic and can interfere with surrounding organs.

Not all tissue can replace itself as it was; some examples are nerve tissue, muscle tissue, and liver cells.

Connective tissue grows faster than other types of tissue and this is why it often fills wounds first. *Keloid* is new, dense tissue that appears (and often reappears, if removed) in whitish ridges or nodules. *Adhesions* are fibrous bands which abnormally join body parts together (e.g., abdominal adhesions). Death of tissue is called *necrosis*. When a large area of tissue is denied nourishment, the cells die and are invaded by organisms. The result is putrefaction (foul smelling, decomposed tissue); this is called *gangrene*.

SIGNS AND SYMPTOMS. The local and systemic signs and symptoms of inflammation are:

1. Local—swelling, pain or tenderness, redness, heat, and loss of function.

2. Systemic—abnormal temperature, increased rate of pulse or respiration, headache, restlessness, listlessness, dry skin, flushed face, malaise, general aching, nausea, vomit-

ing, increased white blood cell count, altered body fluids (blood, spinal fluid, urine), and altered metabolism (especially the body's use of protein).

These last three signs would have meaning for the physician. Your concern is to help collect specimens or otherwise follow through on special orders.

CARE OF THE PATIENT. The extent of the body's reaction to inflammation and the over-all ability of the body to cope with it are major factors in dictating what should be the medical treatment and the nursing. Age makes a difference in the metabolic process; young to middle-aged people have higher metabolic rates than older adults. Therefore, the elderly might need certain types of medical assistance that others would not. In the very young, the inflammatory process might upset some functions if they are not yet too well established (e.g., heat regulation).

NURSING CARE. All specific measures are by the physician's orders. Observations are both subjective and objective and become more specific and constant as a reaction moves from local to general. (See the care of a patient with a fever.)

The practice of strict medical or surgical asepsis is important. If there is an open lesion, sterile techniques should be used with dressings or irrigations. Protection must be taken against injury and complications.

Bed rest is usually one means taken to provide adequate rest to the area or part, to help prevent movement or use of a part, and to promote sleep.

The affected part is often elevated with support (e.g., back rest, sling, pillows, or appliances); if it is an extremity, the entire part should be raised and supported.

Applications of heat or cold, both dry and moist forms, are often ordered, as well as medications. Fluids may be increased with the intake and output measured. The diet may be liquid or soft with an increase of calories and proteins.

The temperature, pulse, and respirations are taken regularly and frequently.

FEVER AND CHILLS

Fever

Fever is an abnormally high body temperature. An oral temperature of 37.5° C. (98.6°

F.) is considered the upper limit of normal temperature for a person resting.

The body temperature control center is located in the brain (hypothalamus). Under ordinary conditions of health, this center (sometimes called "the body's thermostat") holds the body within a degree or so of constant temperature range. Various conditions cause the "normal" temperature to go up and down slightly—sleep, rest, food, and exercise. See Figure 12–1.

Abnormal conditions influence the control center and permit body temperature to go above normal or below normal (subnormal). Figure 41–1 points out the range from the lower limit to the upper limit of survival. Young children are apt to "run a fever" sooner than other people because their control centers seem to be more easily influenced; for the same reason, a child's fever is apt to drop fast.

When a patient with a high fever starts to perspire, the temperature soon begins to drop; this sudden change is called the *crisis*. A slow, gradual drop in fever temperature is *lysis*.

KINDS OF FEVERS.   The most common kinds of fevers are:

1. *Continuous or constant fever.* The temperature remains high and about at the same level for days or weeks; the temperature varies no more than about one degree in a 24-hour day.

2. *Remittent fever.* The temperature rises and falls (fluctuates) during a day but does not fall to the normal level; the temperature varies about two degrees in a 24-hour day.

3. *Intermittent fever.* The temperature rises and falls during a day with alternating periods of high and low temperatures.

CAUSES OF FEVER.   Common causes of fever are:

1. Abnormalities in the brain—injury, edema, tumors.

2. Toxic substances that influence the body heat regulating center in the brain; diseases, especially infections; metabolic by-products; dehydration; vaccines.

SIGNS AND SYMPTOMS.   The signs and symptoms of fever vary with the onset and also as the fever increases and continues. They include the sensation of feeling warm, fatigue, thirst, headache and generalized aching, irritability, chilly sensation (a chill may precede the fever), convulsions (may occur in infants and young children), hot and dry or parched and scaly skin, flushed face, elevated temperature, increased rates of pulse and respirations, poor appetite, dehydration, coated tongue, cracked and sore lips and nares, and nausea or vomiting.

CARE OF THE PATIENT.   It is thought that a moderate temperature elevation (not above 104° F.) might be beneficial to the body in some ways, but there is no exact proof as yet. The body's metabolism rate is increased during fever, and this fact may help the body produce more immune bodies to combat microorganisms. The possibility that fever "within bounds" might be somewhat helpful may cause some physicians to let it run its course without trying to drop it too quickly. Excessively high temperatures (uncontrolled) can damage body tissues.

When a fever must be brought down, some or all of the following means might be ordered:

1. Sponge baths—with tepid water or half water and half alcohol.

2. Ice bags—applied to the head, axilla, and groin.

3. "Wet sheet"—the patient is covered with a sheet dampened with tepid water.

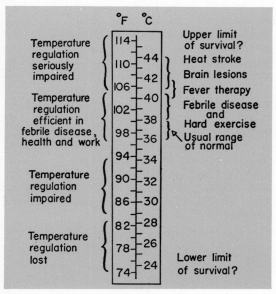

FIGURE 41–1   Body temperatures under different conditions. (From DuBois: Fever. Charles C Thomas Co.)

4. Enema—plain, cool water is generally used.

5. Lowered room temperature—an electric fan is sometimes used.

6. A hypothermia blanket—maintains body temperature within a specific range. Prevent shivering by adjusting bedding and patient clothing.

7. Medications—antipyretics to influence the heat-regulating center.

When following orders to reduce body temperatures, observe the exact duration required and note all patient reactions (subjective and objective). You may notice that orders might vary from patient to patient. Factors which influence this include age, the disease itself, and the general condition of the patient.

NURSING CARE. Bed rest is usually ordered for the patient with a fever to promote rest and sleep, although bathroom privileges may be permitted. The environment should be quiet, semi-dark, and cool (not cold).

A tepid sponge bath (if ordered) with a light back rub may be given for cleanliness and comfort. As perspiration increases the bath may need to be repeated. Care must be taken to avoid chilling the patient as well as to follow any specific directions (e.g., duration, temperature of solution, results to be obtained). The physician may order the use of an automatic temperature-control unit (blanket, mattress) to reduce the patient's temperature. Determine your responsibilities if you are involved in monitoring the use of a heating-cooling unit because of the differences in various models.

Careful observation of the patient is essential; any change should be reported at once. The temperature (usually rectal), pulse, and respirations should be taken frequently and as directed. The appearance and reactions of the patient should be watched when any means (treatment, medication) is used to lower the temperature.

A clean, dry, smooth bed helps to provide for the comfort of the patient; cover the patient lightly. The bed linen and the patient's gown will need to be changed often. Attention to oral hygiene is necessary with the teeth and mouth cleaned several times a day; apply a lubricant to the lips and nares.

Fluids are usually increased; those high in calories, protein, vitamin C, and certain minerals may be ordered in addition to water. Amounts are usually specified, with limitations and precautions taken for infants, children, and certain adults. Intake and output are to be measured and recorded.

Chills

Chills are a common companion of fever; they come about when the heat control center (the "thermostat") is suddenly changed from a normal to an abnormal temperature setting. While the overall body is catching up with the new temperature setting, chills occur. When the body temperature does catch up with the control center, the chills stop and fever is present.

SIGNS AND SYMPTOMS. The patient feels cold, he usually shivers or shakes, his teeth may chatter, and the bed may even shake if the chill is severe. He may become frightened. The muscles contract, hair on the skin elevates, and "goose pimples" appear. The lips are blue and the skin becomes pale and dry. The pulse and respirations increase in rates.

When a chill occurs notify the charge nurse or physician at once. Warmth should be provided to the body. Blankets are used to cover the body, and warmed bath blankets may be placed next to the skin. The use of hot water bottles or a heating pad requires an order from the physician.

Stay with the patient; your presence is reassuring. Note the exact time the chill started, if possible, and the time it ended to determine the length or duration of the chill. Take the temperature (rectal), pulse, and respirations when the chill starts, then every 10 to 15 minutes during the chill, and when the chill stops. Following the chill, take the temperature at least every hour, or as ordered, until stable.

Careful observations of the patient's appearance and reactions should be made. A few covers should be removed at a time to prevent too rapid cooling.

HEMORRHAGE

This is the escape of considerable blood from the blood vessels; it is continuous bleeding that reduces the volume of blood and, unless stopped, causes death. The blood may be bright red, spurting from an artery with each heart beat (arterial); it may be dark red, flowing continuously from a vein (venous) or oozing from a capillary.

In hemorrhage, the escaping blood may be visible, coming from a surface wound, incision, or body opening (external). When blood collects in the tissues in a tumor-like mass, it is called a *hematoma*. Internal hemorrhage means that blood is escaping within the body into a body cavity (e.g., peritoneal cavity).

CAUSES. Hemorrhage may be due to a number of causes such as injury (physical or chemical), wounds, incisions, a loosened or slipped ligature (surgical tie for a blood vessel), or hemophilia (delayed clotting of blood). The nature of a particular disorder may lead to hemorrhage (e.g., peptic ulcer, arterial aneurysms, varicose veins).

SIGNS AND SYMPTOMS. The signs and symptoms of hemorrhage, either external or internal, include pale, cold, moist skin; chilliness; a sudden or gradual drop in blood pressure; decreased temperature; increased pulse rate; increased rate of respirations; restlessness; fearfulness; thirst; ringing in the ears; seeing spots before the eyes; vomiting, possibly with force (the vomitus may show bright red blood, or may be black or the color of coffee grounds); black, tarry stool; brown to dark red urine; and general weakness or faintness, leading to unconsciousness, shock and death unless the bleeding is stopped and blood volume returned to normal. Not all these signs and symptoms occur at the same time; some occur as the hemorrhage continues and the body suffers blood volume loss.

CARE OF THE PATIENT. There are two things to do first in treating the patient who is having hemorrhage:

1. Stop the bleeding, if possible. Find the cause.

2. Replace lost blood.

Internal bleeding presents special problems, including locating the source, finding some means to stop it, and removing the accumulated blood to prevent further damage to surrounding organs. Sometimes internal pressure can be applied by inserting sterile packing, inflated (Foley) catheters, or balloons (e.g., uterus, mouth, nose, esophagus, penis). In other instances, a part might be irrigated (e.g., urinary bladder), immobilized, positioned, and supported a certain way to reduce

pressure—all to help the body seal off the bleeding area.

Continued uncontrolled bleeding may require emergency surgery to tie off the larger vessel or seal off small oozing vessels by cauterization, or both.

External bleeding may be more readily controlled because the source can be located. Direct action can be taken at once. Cold and direct pressure help blood to clot and seal off the ruptured vessel; of the two, direct pressure is applied with serile material being held firmly in place directly over the wound. In case of more severe arterial bleeding, pressure is applied between (close to) the wound and the heart. This action slows the flow of blood to allow clotting to take place. More is said about bleeding during or following surgery in the discussion of the operative patient in the next chapter.

Certain factors guide all action wherever hemorrhage occurs—at the roadside, at home, in the patient's unit, or in the operating room; it is an urgent situation, and becomes more so with the passing of time. The blood flow must be checked as soon as possible and the blood volume restored. If there is internal bleeding into body cavities, accumulated blood and clots must be removed to prevent further damage to surrounding organs.

NURSING CARE. Report, *at once,* any appearance of bleeding; notify the charge nurse or physician. Constant attention, must be given to the patient. Observe for and report any suspicion of change in the bleeding, such as the site, color, rate, or amount from any source; note all objective symptoms.

Save any evidence of bleeding: from bed linen, dressings, pads, body discharges, clots, or vomitus. Note the time, color, appearance, pain, and any change, frequency, or duration that may be pertinent to the evidence saved.

Take the temperature, pulse, respirations, and blood pressure frequently. Stay with the patient and reassure him. The environment should be kept quiet and the patient made as comfortable as possible. Excitement should be controlled and all evidence of bleeding removed from the bedside and room.

Every effort should be made to keep the patient quiet and still; maintain any body position that the physician has ordered for the patient.

Fluids and food are often withheld or restricted until the hemorrhage is controlled or further ordered. Applications of cold (e.g., ice bag, compresses) may be ordered to be applied over the site or region. Close observations must be maintained when transfusions or intravenous fluids are given; specific orders must be followed.

Quite often the family or friends may be near or present and they should be given helpful attention and appropriate reassurance.

SHOCK

Shock is a state of circulatory failure—a collapse of the circulatory system. The tissues of the body are denied sufficient circulating fluid and become progressively more damaged if the state of shock continues. The volume of circulating blood is reduced to a point where vital centers in the brain are denied sufficient oxygen and nutrients to carry on normal functions. As you recall, brain tissue cannot replace itself and it is fragile when it comes to lack of oxygen; therefore, a state of shock can soon seriously damage the brain. This and other tissue damage (e.g., to heart muscle) make shock very dangerous to the body; the more tissue damage, the faster the patient's condition worsens. Circulating blood volume must be restored as quickly as possible to prevent damage and possible death. The heart must have sufficient blood, with adequate blood components, to pump around the body if cells and tissues are not to die of starvation and lack of oxygen.

CAUSES. A state of shock occurs when the heart (for any one of a number of reasons) is unable to pump enough nourishing blood to body tissues. The reasons for this include a faulty heart muscle (cardiac shock); severe loss of blood (internal or external hemorrhage—hemorrhagic shock); escape of blood fluid through capillary walls into surrounding tissues (called "white hemorrhage"), caused by extreme fright, a terrifying experience or severe and prolonged pain; overall body antigen-antibody reaction (anaphylactic shock); severe plasma loss from obstruction in the veins leading to the heart, causing plasma to leak into surrounding tissues, or intestinal obstruction, causing plasma to leak through capillary walls into intestinal walls; starvation (low plasma protein); severe burns or anything else that damages great areas of the outer skin and provides an easy exit for plasma and lowered blood volume; and severe dehydration, which reduces blood volume.

SIGNS AND SYMPTOMS. Depending upon the cause, the onset of shock may be gradual or sudden in the appearance of the signs and symptoms.

If the onset is gradual, the patient senses that something is wrong and becomes irritable, or lethargic, uneasy or restless. He feels dizzy and thirsty, and may suffer nausea or vomiting. Other signs include a slight pulse increase, diminished urinary output, and slight drop in blood pressure.

As the state continues, the patient's pulse is feeble and rapid; his blood pressure drops; his breathing becomes shallow; his temperature lowers; his lips, ear lobes and fingernails may show cyanosis; and his skin becomes cold, clammy or colorless (pallor). He may become more anxious and restless if conscious, or mentally confused, or even unconscious.

If the onset is sudden and profound, all signs and symptoms can appear at once.

CARE OF THE PATIENT. The cause of the shock determines the treatment.

A state of shock can move rapidly from its beginning to seriousness and death if not treated at once. The chief and immediate concerns are to conserve all body energy and to position the patient correctly. The physician specifies the position (position is treatment). The airways are kept open, adequate ventilation is provided, and the patient is given a lightweight cover for warmth.

The physician should be notified at once in case of *any sign of possible shock*. The earlier the treatment, the safer the patient. The physician may use a drug to constrict peripheral blood vessels to try to increase blood pressure. If pain is severe, medication is generally given at once.

Thirst should not be treated by giving oral fluids unless ordered by the physician; they may cause vomiting. Fluid management is under the physician's orders.

NURSING CARE. Report at once any appearance of, or change in, the signs and symptoms of shock in a patient. Be especially alert when observing a patient who is predisposed to shock to help prevent it from occurring; stay with any patient in shock.

Keep the patient in a flat position until or unless directed otherwise; orders may be given to place or elevate the patient or the bed in a certain position.

Take the temperature, pulse, and respirations and the blood pressure at least every 15 minutes, or as directed.

Provide warmth with lightweight covers; omit any external heat unless ordered. Keep the patient quiet, provide for rest, prevent any unnecessary movement if possible, limit any personal care to use of bedpan or urinal or essential comfort measures, and reassure the patient by staying with him.

Control the environment. Keep it quiet and calm; limit the presence of family or friends but give attention and appropriate reassurance.

Give fluids by mouth only as directed; check frequently for urinary output—measure and observe urine; collect hourly specimens; record the time and amount; notify charge nurse or physician.

Assist with and maintain close observations when intravenous fluids or oxygen are used.

GASTRIC DISTRESS

Gastric distress means that the patient is experiencing one or more symptoms which indicate stomach malfunction owing to some disease or disorder of the stomach itself or related to some other body factors (e.g., drugs, emotions).

The signs and symptoms of gastric distress include *anorexia, nausea,* and *vomiting,* as well as pain and worry about the distress, belching, complaints about feeling pressure, and general concern about eating.

The physician may order special tests to aid in making the diagnosis, bed rest, special diet, medication, and parenteral fluids.

Anorexia means a lack of appetite. The loss of appetite is a signal that the body is rejecting the thought of food or the taste for food. The patient may tell you of his disinterest in food and you can observe it for yourself. Anorexia is relieved when the cause is determined and relieved; medications are often ordered specifically for this condition.

Nausea is a conscious sensation that the act of vomiting could occur. The impulse which signals this sensation comes from the brain (medulla); its site is close to or a part of the vomiting center. Impulses to the medulla

come from unusual motions (i.e., motion sickness), from the gastrointestinal tract, and from other brain sources.

The physician needs to know the cause of the nausea and to plan treatment accordingly. Medications may be ordered to control the nausea or vomiting center while further measures are taken to remove the cause. The patient will be kept quiet and provisions made for rest and sleep.

Vomiting is the act of the stomach ridding itself of its contents. Here too, as with nausea, the medulla receives the nerve impulse from almost any part of the gastrointestinal tract (usually the stomach and duodenum) that it is irritated and distended. In turn, the vomiting center sends a message via motor nerves to the diaphragm and abdominal muscles which contract (diaphragm downward) and actually squeeze the stomach. A reverse peristalsis takes place, forcing the stomach contents up through the esophagus and the mouth. A safety mechanism takes care to close the glottis over the trachea and lift the soft palate up so that it blocks the back of the nasal passages.

Vomiting can leave the patient weak and perspiring as well as dehydrated if it lasts very long. *Retching* is a sign that the muscular action is continuing after the stomach is empty, or it is an effort to vomit.

Other things which can cause vomiting are certain drugs (e.g., morphine, some digitalis preparations), rapidly changing motions, and offensive sights and odors, as well as some psychological reasons.

Types of vomiting are:

1. Cyclic or periodic—recurring at irregular intervals.

2. Dry—nausea with attempts to vomit; only gas is ejected.

3. Hysterical—vomiting accompanying hysteria.

4. During pregnancy—occurring especially in the early morning.

5. Projectile—when vomitus is ejected with force.

Fecal matter can be vomited when an intestinal obstruction is present, or sometimes with appendicitis.

Treatment centers around controlling the reverse peristaltic action, permitting rest and determining the cause, if unknown. It may include gastric suction, gastric lavage, gastric gavage, medications, and parenteral fluids.

Anorexia

SIGNS AND SYMPTOMS.   Subjective signs include the patient saying something like "I'm not hungry," or "I just don't feel like eating," or "My appetite is gone." Objective signs include the patient refusing his tray, turning his face from food, or eating very little or nothing.

NURSING CARE. To help prevent the development of anorexia, keep the environment clean, quiet, attractive, and comfortable. Keep the patient comfortable, clean, and relaxed, to give him a feeling of well-being.

Be alert to both subjective and objective signs and symptoms and notice what might stimulate or eliminate symptoms. Report and record specific, meaningful observations.

To prepare the patient for mealtime, give attention to his likes and dislikes, amounts, and time for eating. Encourage the patient to eat and assist him if necessary. Avoid the use of threats or undue concern with regard to food not eaten. Provide for and encourage adequate intake of fluids and also for regular and frequent oral hygiene.

Nausea

SIGNS AND SYMPTOMS.   The patient may react the same as mentioned previously for anorexia and may say something like, "I feel sick to my stomach." The patient may salivate excessively or perspire profusely, especially on the forehead and the lips. His face may be pale and his pulse may first increase, then decrease.

NURSING CARE. To prevent gagging or retching, keep the patient quiet and comfortable, and ask him to take deep breaths through his mouth. Encourage proper swallowing. Also prevent or try to eliminate the presence of unpleasant odors (e.g., food, smoke, feces, urine), sights (e.g., vomitus, bedpan, soiled dressings), or sounds (e.g., another patient in pain or gagging). Keep his unit clean, quiet, and well-ventilated. Prevent or avoid, if possible, anything that might suggest nausea. Provide fluids that are ordered and give sips or small amounts of water, ginger ale, or tea as tolerated and permitted.

Vomiting

SIGNS AND SYMPTOMS.   Nausea usually occurs before vomiting but not always. The patient appears pale, perspires, and may be dizzy. His pulse and respirations will increase, and he may experience a tingling sensation in his fingers or toes.

The patient may experience pain in the epigastric region before or with vomiting. Weakness and fatigue occur, especially with frequent or prolonged vomiting. The onset of projectile vomiting may be sudden with little or no warning; the stomach contents are ejected with force and at a distance, often several feet.

NURSING CARE. Assist the patient by holding a curved basin, supporting his head and shoulders, and wiping his lips. To prevent aspiration of vomitus, turn the patient's face to his side, and place his body in a side position, if possible.

Provide for oral hygiene by allowing patient to rinse or clean his mouth and teeth after each vomiting. Caution the patient about the use of the toothbrush to prevent gagging or stimulation to vomit. Keep the patient and his bed clean and dry; wash his face and hands and change his gown and bedding if necessary. Keep the environment free of the sight and odor of vomitus; remove, empty, and clean the container without delay and check the ventilation.

Stay with the patient and try to help him to relax and rest. You can do this by showing acceptance and understanding. Observe the time and amount, color, odor, consistency, presence of food, blood, and type of vomiting. Also observe the skin, pulse, and other vital signs. Save all or a portion of vomitus as a specimen for the charge nurse or physician to observe if unsure of your observations or if contents are suspicious or unusual in any way. Observe for signs and symptoms of thirst, decreased and concentrated urinary output, and constipation.

INTESTINAL DISTRESS

Many factors can cause the intestines (small and large) to malfunction, creating general or local distress; they include faulty chemical digestion, obstruction, infection, improper diet, dehydration, contaminated food, allergy, nervous tension, and the like.

Intestinal distress means that the patient is experiencing one or more symptoms of malfunction of the intestines or the result of a disorder elsewhere, as in the case of a person becoming dehydrated from a high fever and becoming constipated.

Three common distress signals of the intestinal tract are *diarrhea, constipation,* and *flatus.*

Diarrhea is the abnormal frequency of liquid stools. It is the result of fecal material moving too rapidly through the large intestine. Something—usually an infection of the lining of the large or even the small intestine (referred to as gastroenteritis)—irritates the lining of the bowel, causing it to secrete much more fluid than normal and become more active (increased peristalsis). These two stepped-up actions are thought of as the body's way of "washing out the infectious material" to protect itself.

Treatment includes measures to counteract the cause of irritation and to support the body in its efforts to overcome the hyperactivity in the bowel and the drain on body fluids and energy.

Constipation is the opposite of diarrhea; feces become hard and dry because they move too slowly through the large intestine. The slow peristaltic action allows the lining of the bowel to draw too much fluid from its contents. The result is an accumulation of hard, dry stool in the lower bowel.

Poor bowel habits are a common cause of constipation; other causes include obstructions, anomalies, loss of or weak muscle tone in the bowel, or a spasm in some portion of it.

A *fecal impaction* is an accumulation of putty-like, hardened feces in the rectum or sigmoid. Removal of this requires that the hardened feces be broken up by manual force, a procedure dangerous to the intestinal wall surrounding the impaction and one which should be carried out by the physician.

The treatment for constipation includes different types of enemas, medications, diet and fluid modifications, ambulation and exercises. The cause of the constipation determines the specific medical treatment.

Flatus is gas or air in the gastrointestinal tract; its presence causes discomfort and can be downright painful because it distends the stomach or the intestines. The presence of gas or air in the bowel makes the abdomen feel firm to the touch, not soft and pliable as it normally is.

This distention is called *flatulence* and treatment for it includes some means for expelling the gas or air (e.g., insertion of a rectal tube, body movement to encourage peristalsis, enema, position change, getting up to use bathroom instead of the bedpan).

Diarrhea

SIGNS AND SYMPTOMS. Feces are frequent, soft, watery, and loose. There is urgency in the need to defecate. The patient's abdomen may become distended, and he may experience pain that is generalized, gripping, and cramp-like. His urinary output decreases. As the patient's lips and mouth become dry, thirst occurs. There may be a slight increase in temperature and rate of pulse.

The anus and anal region become irritated and sensitive. Vomiting often occurs at the same time. Fatigue, weakness, and general malaise occur if diarrhea is excessive or prolonged.

NURSING CARE. Observe feces for color (clear, black, bright red, clay), consistency (all fluid, small pieces), foreign matter (old or fresh blood, worms, pus, mucus), and amount (measure if pertinent, or estimate). During defecation observe the time, force, presence of pain or flatus, expulsion of fluid or feces. Save a specimen if ordered or if it seems important for the charge nurse or physician to observe.

Maintain fluids as ordered; fluids are usually increased by mouth or parenterally, or there may be nothing by mouth. Fluid intake and output should be measured and recorded. Urinary output should be observed for time, amount, and color; save a specimen if ordered. Also maintain the diet as ordered; it is usually bland and non-irritating; provide a small amount at frequent intervals if tolerated better.

Keep the environment quiet, well-ventilated, and private. Provide quiet, usually with bed rest, and allow for the patient's ease and comfort in using the bedpan or toilet. Concerning personal hygiene, provide means for bathing the anal and perineal regions with warm, mild, soapy water after each episode; rinse well and pat dry. Apply a mild, emollient cream or ointment (on physician's order) to the anal region. Wash hands frequently and after each defecation. For general comfort, provide privacy and reassurance and keep the patient relaxed; show acceptance and understanding and keep the patient and bedding clean and dry. Place covered protectors under the buttocks. Give special attention to keep the skin clean and dry if fecal incontinence occurs.

Constipation

SIGNS AND SYMPTOMS. The feces are infrequent and hard, with dry stool or perhaps no stool for several days. The patient may experience painful straining before or with defecation. Headache, loss of appetite, and nausea may be present. The abdomen may be distended and the patient may feel bloated. Flatus may be present; large amounts may be passed by mouth or the rectum.

NURSING CARE. Observe feces for color, consistency, amount, and presence of foreign matter. At the time of defecation observe force, pain, presence of flatus, and presence or absence of stool. Observe and note complaints of the patient regarding general comfort, appetite, headache, and so forth.

See that the patient receives the diet that has been ordered, and encourage him to eat by stimulating his appetite if possible. Fluids are generally increased to a greater intake per day; warm fluids may be ordered.

To encourage the habit of regularity, see that the patient is provided with proper attention, privacy, adequate time, and prompt attention when he requests a bedpan or to go to the bathroom. Try to follow a plan for regular bowel elimination. Follow directions and practices to help *prevent* constipation by placing a bed patient on a bedpan in a near upright position, if permissible; encourage an ambulatory patient to use the toilet in the bathroom. Provide diet and fluids as ordered and use any appropriate means to help a patient relax. Provide any treatment or measure which may be ordered, such as rectal suppository, medication, enema (cleansing, emollient), or colonic irrigation.

Flatus

SIGNS AND SYMPTOMS. Flatus is accompanied by an uncomfortable, full, bloated feeling in the abdomen or rectum. The abdomen may appear swollen or distended and feel tense and hard upon palpation. The expulsion of flatus may be by mouth or by rectum, in small or large amounts, with some or no relief

attained. Often the patient is not able to expel any flatus and suffers from generalized, cramplike pains.

NURSING CARE. Observe for complaints and discomforts. When flatus is expelled, observe the results as to amount and patient comfort. See that orders for movement and activity are followed as directed or permitted; change the patient's position often, turning him from side to side, keeping his knees flexed. Encourage or assist the patient to sit on the side of the bed, to get out of bed into a chair, to walk, and to use the toilet in the bathroom.

See that the proper fluids and diet are administered as ordered. Usually iced fluids and chips are not permitted. Aid general comfort by providing means to help ensure comfort, relaxation, reassurance, and relief. Provide any treatment or measure which may be ordered, such as insertion of a rectal tube for certain periods of time, enema (carminative), application of heat to abdomen, medication, and gastric suction.

RESPIRATORY DISTRESS

Distress in the respiratory system shows itself in a variety of ways. A sign or symptom of respiratory distress can be local (cough) or generalized (cyanosis); it can greatly influence posture, anxiety, the ability to rest, and the general sense of well-being. Chapter 37 discusses dyspnea, cyanosis, orthopnea, and cough; that information is not repeated here except to restate definitions and to list some causes of each difficulty.

Dyspnea is difficult or labored breathing, sometimes called "air hunger." It is often accompanied by cyanosis and may be caused by:

1. The abnormal use of oxygen by body tissues.

2. The amount of effort it takes the respiratory muscles to perform their work.

3. The patient's frame of mind (emotional or neurogenic dyspnea).

Cyanosis is a blueness of the skin; it is a sign that the capillaries contain blood that has already lost its oxygen; in other words, the capillary blood lacks oxygen content. Cyanosis is a sure sign that there is some type of respiratory or circulatory difficulty somewhere in the body. The difficulty may be in the lungs themselves or in the performance of the heart; the cause may be a disease that affects the red blood cells or the blood vessels.

Orthopnea means comfortable breathing only in an upright position. This definition gives you some clue about the nursing measures needed to keep such a patient comfortable. The reason the orthopneic patient needs to sit upright is to aid an ailing heart; while in a sitting position, that heart has less work to do. Very soon after this type of patient lies down, he becomes dyspneic—has "air hunger." Consequently, this patient spends all, or almost all, of the time in an upright position—even sleeping. (See Fig. 37–2).

A *cough,* a noisy expulsion of air from the lungs, is an experience familiar to everyone. Whether productive or nonproductive, a cough is a sign of respiratory irritation and a reportable sign as far as patients are concerned.

The cough reflex (in the brain) is a safety mechanism; it takes only a slight irritation in the trachea to start one coughing. The sneeze reflex responds in the same way. Consequently, any foreign substance entering the air passages soon makes its presence known.

The term *expectoration* means coughing and spitting out materials from the lower air passageways; *expectorant* is the material coughed up.

SIGNS AND SYMPTOMS.   The patient may say things like, "I can't breathe," or "I can't get my breath," or "I'm so short of breath." Difficult breathing (dyspnea or orthopnea) and cyanosis may or may not be present. As respiration becomes more difficult and requires greater effort, the rate and depth increase and you will observe the chest and abdominal wall muscles being used ("heaving"). The patient often assumes a sitting or upright position with knees flexed in bed or in a chair—even to sleep.

The face of a person experiencing respiratory distress is drawn, with a pinched appearance and distressed expression. His lips, ear lobes, nail beds, and skin become dusky or have a bluish tinge. The skin itself is pale, cold, and blue; tingling sensations and pain may be present and dizziness or fainting may occur. The patient's reactions and mental responses may be slow and he may appear anxious, frightened, restless, and irritable. If the distress is severe or prolonged, weakness and fatigue occur.

NURSING CARE.   Observe subjective symptoms such as complaints, feelings, and the appearance of dizziness in the patient. Observe objective symptoms such as chest movements and depth and rate of respirations; note any sounds with breathing, the position assumed by the patient, the presence of cough (productive or nonproductive), the skin color and temperature, the facial appearance and expression, any mental and emotional reactions, and any changes in symptoms.

Use appropriate positions and measures as directed to keep airways open and to aid the comfort of the patient. *Sims' position* is generally used if the patient is unconscious since it aids saliva to drain from the mouth and helps to prevent the tongue from falling back and thus causing an obstruction. Change the patient's position from one side to the other with regularity, every two to three hours, or as directed.

Fowler's position is generally used if the patient is conscious; vary the patient's position or have the patient himself change; help him find the most comfortable position in which to rest or sleep. Help support his body and extremities for good alignment and comfort, and take the proper safety measures and precautions to prevent the patient from falling out of bed.

Movement and activity are usually restricted and complete bed rest is required in most conditions; help keep the patient quiet and prevent exertion. Ask him not to talk unless necessary, and try to anticipate and provide for his needs and comfort with as little effort on his part as possible. Place things within easy reach, feed him if appropriate, work slowly, and avoid tiring him. Provide for personal comfort, especially oral and mouth care, with regularity and according to treatments being used.

Provide or assist with treatments which may be ordered, such as artificial airway insertion, suction to the throat, postural drainage, local applications of cold, or inhalation therapy (oxygen or carbon dioxide, aerosal or steam).

Coughing

SIGNS AND SYMPTOMS.   Common types are short—shallow, dry, and nonproductive; deep—requiring effort, moist, and productive; and long—"spells" or paroxysmal attacks, ineffective and exhausting.

Pain may be present with coughing. An expectorant may or may not be present, may be clear or frothy, or may contain foreign materials such as blood, mucus, and pus. Blood expectorated may be bright red and frothy or dark in color. A lack of appetite often develops, and weakness, fatigue, or exhaustion may occur.

NURSING CARE.   Observe for type (with or without expectorant, moist or dry), sound (hacking, hard), effort (forced, shallow, deep), duration, pain, and the presence of sputum, blood, or other materials.

Keep the environment quiet for rest and sleep; regulate the temperature and ventilation to the patient's comfort (cool, moist air is often desired). Prevent sudden changes in temperature or drafts and prevent smoking by others (patients or visitors) in the room.

To further prevent the stimulation of coughing, discourage smoking by the patient (it may not be permitted by the physician), talking, and too warm covers or room temperature. Try to control or eliminate the presence of dust and lint in the room. Provide oral hygiene regularly and frequently, with special attention before mealtime if the cough is productive.

Encourage the patient to eat the proper diet and consume the necessary fluids, and make an effort to stimulate his appetite. Give consideration to his dietary wishes, if possible. Position the patient according to his needs and comfort; place him in an upright position in bed, or sitting in a chair if permitted, and use appropriate measures to provide for comfort and safety. If ordered, encourage and help place the patient who is coughing blood in a reclining position on his affected side, if known. Provide for general comfort and relaxation; try to anticipate his needs, and help the patient to exert himself as little as possible. Follow orders to collect sputum specimens, give medication or treatments, and give general or specific care.

URINARY DISTRESS

Distress in the urinary system may be from a kidney disorder, heart disease, metabolic malfunction, digestive problem, infection, or tumor, to mention only some of the many causes. The patient with urinary distress is subject to much discomfort, and sometimes to pain and embarrassment. Effective care requires a variety of nursing skills and much time in some cases.

Urinary incontinence, uncontrolled voiding, has been pointed out as a condition which requires constant attention if the skin involved is to be kept intact and the patient comfortable. Urinary incontinence is caused by the failure of the urethral sphincters to remain closed. For some reason, the sphincter muscle loses its tone and is unable to hold back the urine until the patient is ready to release it. Very often an indwelling catheter (Foley type) is ordered to control this problem.

Urinary retention means the holding back of urine in the bladder because of the inability to urinate. The cause of this inability may be trauma, swelling, injury to spinal nerves, infection, obstruction, tension, or anything that prevents the bladder from releasing the stored urine.

Retention with overflow means that the patient voids frequently in small amounts. The full bladder expels just enough urine to relieve the pressure; as it refills, a small amount is voided again. An indwelling catheter or catheterization may be ordered to help restore control.

Residual urine is that which remains when the bladder fails to completely empty itself. A urinary bladder that holds back urine in an abnormal manner can easily become infected because the urine left in the bladder is an excellent substance for growth of harmful bacteria. Medical treatment generally includes direct measures to empty the bladder as well as drugs to hold down infections.

Words you will hear and use to describe some common signs and symptoms of urinary distress are arranged in a manner to help you learn them:

1. *Uria*—the end of a word that tells something about urine.

2. *Dys*—painful (*dysuria* means painful urination).

3. *Olig*—little, scanty (*oliguria* means a small amount of urine).

4. *Poly*—many, much (*polyuria* means a large amount of urine).

5. *Hemat*—blood (*hematuria* means blood in urine).

6. *An*—absence of (*anuria* means no excretion of urine).

7. *Noct*—at night (*nocturia* means excessive urination at night).

Urinary Retention and Retention with Overflow

SIGNS AND SYMPTOMS The patient either is unable to void or voids small amounts frequently but does not empty his bladder. The desire or need to void occurs often and with urgency or difficulty; he feels generally uncomfortable and experiences pain with voiding. Anxiety and embarrassment are expressed. The bladder may be distended and feel firm.

NURSING CARE. Observe, record, and report the inability to void, frequency and time of voidings, and whether voiding is accompanied by urgent need or absence of any need to void. Record whether small amounts (30 to 50 cc.) are voided at one time, or every one or two hours; also record if large amounts or more than usual (300 to 500 cc.) are voided. Observe any difficulty and strain required to void. A burning sensation or pain may be present before, during, or after voiding. Notice the appearance, color, and odor, along with the presence of a foreign substance, such as blood (bright red or dusky brown) or white cloudy materials.

Save a specimen if so ordered. Watch for signs of patient dehydration and comfort before and after voiding. Movement and activity are usually encouraged and provided, if possible. Change or have the patient change position often, if in bed. Encourage walking, if ambulatory, and assist or ask him to walk to bathroom.

Here are some nursing measures to help the patient void:

1. Provide privacy with a drape, screen, and closed door and leave the patient alone.

2. Provide a warmed bedpan or urinal.

3. Use extreme patience and allow sufficient time.

4. Offer the patient small amounts of water to drink.

5. Provide the sound of water running by opening a water faucet or pouring water from one pitcher to another.

6. Have the patient hold his fingertips in a basin of warm water.

7. Pour warm water slowly over the perineum; measure the amount of water used if the output of urine is to be measured. This method may be contraindicated for some patients.

8. Provide as comfortable and natural a position as possible. Raise the backrest to bring the patient to an upright or a sitting position, or assist him to the toilet in the bathroom, if permissible.

9. Provide the patient with the opportunity to void at a regular time. Determine if he has voided and when; check voidings with regular frequency; place the bedpan or urinal (or have the patient go to the toilet) at his regular time.

10. Give prompt attention and assistance when the patient has a desire or need to void. Bring a bedpan or urinal or assist him to the toilet without delay.

Make sure that diet and fluids are provided as directed, since intake of fluids is usually encouraged and increased, often with a minimum amount ordered. Measure intake and output when required.

Provide for personal care and support by giving reassurance and showing acceptance of the patient's difficulty. Provide time and patience with daily care and hygiene. Limit fluids in the evening or at bedtime if contraindicated and have the patient void before bedtime if voiding during the night is a problem.

Urinary Incontinence

SIGNS AND SYMPTOMS. Since the patient is unable to control voidings, urine flows or may dribble from the bladder, even without the patient's knowledge.

NURSING CARE. Specific care and attention include the following:

1. Keeping the patient and bed clean and dry. Inspect regularly and give immediate care as soon as the patient or bed becomes wet. Bathe and change linen as necessary, and use a plastic mattress protector and drawsheet.

2. Preventing skin irritation, infection, and the development of decubitus ulcers. Keep bottom bedding tight, smooth, clean, and dry. Place soft, absorbent material under the patient's perineum and buttocks. Wash the perineum and buttocks with warm, mild soapy water and rinse and dry well with regular frequency during day and night. Use an absorbent powder or alcohol instead of a lotion or cream. Apply a medicated or antiseptic ointment or powder only upon the order of the physician. Change or have the patient change his position often; inspect his skin and watch closely for any signs of skin problems. Note the presence of any odor. Observe and report the condition of his skin.

3. Helping to re-establish control over voiding. Bring the bedpan or urinal or assist the patient to walk to the toilet at frequent, regular intervals, or without delay when requested.

4. Giving fluids as ordered. The type and amount are often specified and controlled.

5. Keeping the environment clean, well-ventilated, and free from odor.

There are several nursing procedures you may provide, assist with, or maintain as directed or ordered, such as:

1. Application of heat. A warm hot water bottle is placed over the lower abdomen or a sitz bath is given at a specified time.

2. Catheterization of the urinary bladder.

3. Irrigation or instillation of the urinary bladder.

4. Retention or insertion of an indwelling catheter.

5. Care of the perineal area.

FLUID BALANCE AND IMBALANCE

To understand what signs and symptoms show up when the fluids in the body are out of balance, one needs to be aware of the role fluids play in the body under normal circumstances.

Chapters 6 and 25 discuss the body's need for water and how it serves the cells and tissues. It will be helpful to review that discussion.

The Importance of Body Fluids

More than one half of the body is fluid. Children have a greater fluid volume than adults and obese people have the lowest fluid volume. The amount is not exact, nor does it remain constant. Factors which influence the volume of fluid in a healthy body at any given time are the weather, exercise, body temperature, and water sources.

Body fluids are chiefly water, but they also contain oxygen, glucose, amino acids, fatty materials and tiny particles of chemical substances called *electrolytes* which are vital to proper cell and tissue activity. Examples of some of these all-important electrolytes are potassium, bicarbonate, sulfate, magnesium, phosphate, sodium, and chloride. *Electrolytes*

must be present in proper amounts and strengths in body fluids to cause cells and tissues to function properly. The presence of proper amounts and strengths of electrolytes is called *electrolyte balance.*

Where is all this body fluid found? About two thirds of it is located inside the trillions of body cells and is called *intracellular fluid.* The remaining one-third of body fluid is located in spaces outside the cells; this "out-of-the-cell" fluid is called *extracellular fluid.* Extracellular fluid is in constant motion in the body owing to blood circulation and lymph movement in the tissue spaces. In a sense it is in the transportation business.

Extracellular fluid and its movement provide a watery climate or internal environment for all cells to live in. As long as this internal environment stays in balance (proper amounts of water, oxygen, food nutrients, and electrolytes), cells live, grow, and carry on their special functions. When one or more of these essential substances are not present in the right amounts (too much or too little), the internal environment is off balance and cells and tissues do not function as they should. These hampered working conditions for the cells and tissues create various signs, symptoms, or distress signals.

Intracellular fluid and extracellular fluid differ in their respective make-up; they must, if cells are to function properly. For instance, the fluid inside a cell contains less sodium (salt) than the fluid that surrounds it. This difference, plus a good many others, is what makes it possible for the passage of substances in and out of cells even though each cell is covered by a cell wall. When the right amounts of all needed electrolytes are present within the cell and the right amounts of all needed electrolytes are present in the fluid surrounding the cell, there is an *electrolyte balance.* This very important balance concerns the physician when treating patients.

To maintain a constant internal environment, all tissues and organs help. For example, food nutrients come from the work of the digestive system, which passes them along to the blood through the villi in the small intestine; the lungs supply oxygen; the kidney filtering system provides the right amounts and strengths of the electrolyte substances. An internal environment that remains constant and in proper balance is called *homeostasis.*

Fluid balance is essential to life and

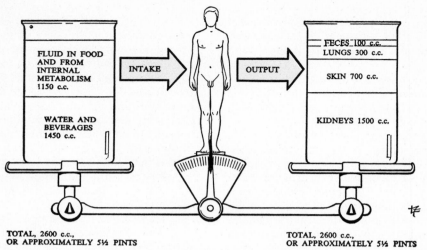

FIGURE 41–2   Fluid balance of the body. This diagram shows the sources and the quantity of fluids required by the average, moderately active man, and how these fluids are eliminated. (Miller and Burt: Good Health, 3rd Ed.)

health; imbalances cause illness and death if severe enough or if they go on for too long a time. Study Figure 41–2 and notice from what sources the body takes in fluid (intake) and how it throws it off (output) to keep the amount of body fluid in balance.

Now let us consider an internal environment that is *not* in proper balance. If some tissue or organ did not contribute what it should, or used up more of something than it should, the internal environment would not remain constant. Knowing that cells need a balanced environment to live, grow, and function properly, they will then be distressed. The body will show indications (signs or symptoms) that something is wrong. These include general weakness, flabby and weak muscles and possibly spasms. Headache may occur. Gastrointestinal symptoms may appear—nausea, vomiting, abdominal cramps, diarrhea, anorexia, or constipation. Convulsion and coma may occur, followed by shock and death. Urinary output is reduced to poor or none. Apprehension may be present, along with complaints of numbness and tingling of the nose, ears, toes, and fingertips.

The whole matter of how fluids serve body cells is under constant study by scientists; it is a very complicated process and much remains to be found out. As stated previously, cells communicate with each other; one cell might reject or refuse to use some substance available in the internal environment while the next one accepts it through

its cell wall. Scientists are trying to find out why this happens; if and when they do, such knowledge may help to diagnose and perhaps treat some illnesses.

As an LPN giving patient care, your knowledge of the body's need for a constant internal environment will help you appreciate why you must carry out certain tasks accurately and observe signs and symptoms carefully. Think for a moment about each of these medical orders and try to imagine what you should be concerned with as you carry them out:

1. Measure intake and output.
2. Force fluids.
3. Limit fluids to 500 cc.
4. No salt shaker on patient's tray.
5. Low sodium diet.

This general knowledge of fluid balance will help guide your nursing action in such things as being concerned about and reporting that a patient has not voided all day, that a patient keeps saying he seems so thirsty all of the time, or that a patient's skin feels very dry and his lips are parched and cracked. You will recognize that puffiness under the eyes, and swollen fingers, legs, and ankles are signs of faulty fluid balance.

Dehydration

To dehydrate something means to remove the fluid from it. For example, instant mashed potatoes and instant coffee are forms of dehydrated food, and they become tasty and edible when fluid is added. In relation to the body, dehydration means that both body cells and tissue spaces have lost some fluid. As a result, they do not possess the "water climate" they need to carry on their functions in a normal manner.

In Figure 41–2 one sees that this man's intake was about five and one-half pints of fluid and that his body excreted about five and one-half pints of fluid through the kidneys, skin, lungs, and feces. This is a balanced intake and output. Now imagine that something occurs in the body to make the kidneys excrete more urine than they should, to make the skin lose fluid faster than it does ordinarily, or to make the bowels expel loose watery stools instead of soft, formed stools; any extra output, over and above the intake, must come from the body's fluid supply. The body pulls fluid from the extracellular spaces, and they in turn pull fluid from within the cells. This process produces dehydration.

Some other ways to produce dehydration are through hemorrhage, sweating, fever, drugs, and starvation.

Treatment is directed toward replacing body fluids—not just water, but whatever is needed to put the body back into fluid balance—as soon as possible so that cells can live, grow, and carry on their functions. The route of administration (depending on the type of fluid and the condition of the patient) may be directly into the tissues, by way of the blood, or by mouth. Whichever additives (e.g., electrolytes, glucose, amino acids) are needed to replace those lost or changed are added to the water. This is called replacement therapy. As an LPN you will have responsibilities for observing patients who are receiving parenteral fluids; it is essential to these patients that they receive the fluids exactly as ordered. Observation should be regular and frequent to be sure that the fluid is being absorbed by the body.

Dehydration is a serious condition. You will notice under the signs and symptoms and the nursing care discussion that dehydrated patients require careful observation and meticulous nursing care.

SIGNS AND SYMPTOMS. The skin appears hot, dry, flushed and flabby. Muscles have poor tone (atonic), and eyeballs appear to be sunken. The patient's appetite decreases and may be lost entirely. A feeling of thirst is usually present.

The patient's lips appear dry, parched, and cracked and his tongue dry and coated. Since his temperature is elevated, he will show signs of fever. His pulse and respirations change and his blood pressure falls. A recent loss of weight may be very marked.

Urinary output decreases and may become scanty with signs of oliguria present. The patient's urine may appear dark and concentrated. Constipation develops. His breath may have a sweet odor. His mental state shows signs of confusion, irritability, lethargy, stupor, and delirium. He may have convulsions or appear comatose, and shock can develop.

NURSING CARE. Note, record, and report all observations. Note early signs of dehydration and report them promptly, especially if the patient is an infant, child, or elderly person. Watch for developing signs (any change of degree in, or a new sign) of prolonged or extreme dehydration, as well as any complaints of the patient.

Observe the patient's appetite and watch his food tray for any restrictions which may be ordered; encourage him to eat all of a special diet that has been ordered, and record as required. His temperature, pulse, respirations, and blood pressure should be taken regularly as ordered; take these more often if changes appear. Check the patient's weight as directed and under the same conditions (e.g., same time of day, same scales, same amount of clothing). Check and measure the patient's voiding accurately.

Follow these directions for care of fluid intake and output.

1. Know if fluids are ordered or specified as to the amount to be encouraged or taken.

2. Encourage fluid intake, unless otherwise ordered; make an effort to provide fluids according to the patient's likes. You may give fluids in sips or in smaller amounts at more frequent intervals, rather than larger amounts at a time. Remind and assist the patient to take fluids regularly. Keep fresh fluids in supply and within convenient reach of the patient; furnish ice chips only if ordered.

3. Inform and caution the patient about measuring and recording all fluid intake and output, if he is able to do so.

4. Make accurate measurements of *all* fluid intake and output; also make observations as to type, kind, and route of fluids.

5. Note time and amount of output of urine, vomitus, drainage bottles, and gastric suction aspirations. Obtain directions on how

to note, estimate, and describe the amount of perspiration, of drainage and of aspirations from a wound or body orifice. Note the amount and describe the color, contents, and odor of any diarrhea.

Provide personal hygiene as often as necessary. Protect the patient's skin and make sure that it and the patient's bed are kept clean and dry. Change or have the patient change his position frequently. Use a lubricating, emollient cream on his skin, especially on the lips. Take special precautions to protect him against injury, e.g., burns. Provide oral hygiene and mouth care several times a day; have the patient use mouthwash frequently. Make sure to give attention to any necessary and appropriate physical and mental comfort and support.

Provide, maintain, and assist with any treatments which may be ordered, such as parenteral fluids, proctocylsis, and gastric gavage.

Edema

Edema means that there is excess fluid in the spaces between the cells; the fluid is trapped there. In this fluid are valuable electrolytes which, because they are trapped, are of no use to the body. Edematous tissues are swollen because the fluid fills and stretches the tissue spaces. The condition can cause discomfort and pain, and may immobilize the part (e.g., leg, hand). Pitting edema is present when you can see the imprint of fingertips on the surface after pressing down on the edematous area; these "pits" may remain visible for quite a while.

The purpose of the treatment for edema is to correct the imbalance of fluid pressure that forced the excess fluids into the space to begin with. Drugs (diuretics) are used, salt intake may be reduced, the swollen part may be elevated, and for some causes of edema in the lower extremities, elastic (supportive) stockings may be used. Be sure that you understand *how* the physician wants a part elevated before you try to carry out such an order.

SIGNS AND SYMPTOMS.   The presence of edema is often noted first in the ankles, feet, or around the eyes; it may be noted in the sacral area and buttocks for bed patients and may develop into pitting edema. The abdomen may become distended and cramps may appear. Muscular weakness is present and apathy, lassitude, and headache usually appear.

Respirations increase in depth and rate and are difficult, the pulse is slow and irregular, and the blood pressure is decreased and unstable. A recent and sudden weight gain may be quite marked. Urinary output decreases and becomes scanty to the point of oliguria. The breath may have a sweetish odor or one of urine. The patient may not be able to talk and may be unaware of his surroundings; confusion and irritation may develop.

NURSING CARE.   Note where edema is located, when it is present or absent, and if there is pitting. Inspect the patient's feet, ankles, lower legs, buttocks, and the area around the eyes at different times of day, and note any increase or decrease in edema with change in position. Also note the presence and location of edema with activity, e.g., getting out of bed sitting in a chair, after walking, after getting into bed, and after sleeping.

Watch for any new symptoms or a change in the symptoms of tissue edema. Note the complaints of the patient and know what observations and symptoms to be alert for with any particular patient, especially an infant, child, or elderly person. Check temperature, pulse respirations, and blood pressure as well as weight, diet, and urination as described for dehydration.

Follow these directions for care of fluid intake and output:

1. Know specifications of amount, time, and inclusion of certain fluids or foods in the diet. Consult the charge nurse for directions of the exact amount (in cc.) if it is not stated in the physician's order.

2. Inform and caution the patient about measuring and recording all fluid intake and output, if he is able to do so.

3. Explain to the patient with "limited" or "withheld" fluids how and when fluids may be taken.

4. Use various ways to provide limited fluids with accuracy; regulate the amount taken at one time by asking the patient to drink only a certain amount within a period of time, or remove the water pitcher or glass from the bedside.

5. Make accurate observations of all fluid intake and output, including time, amount, type, kind, and route. Pay particular attention to a specifically ordered observation. Report at once if the amount of urine is greatly reduced or increased.

Provide personal and oral hygiene with regular frequency. Give attention to and observe the condition of the skin, especially in the sacral area, buttocks, heels, or other edematous parts. Observe for any signs of redness, irritation, or decubitus ulcer. Keep skin clean and dry and use a lubricating type of cream; protect skin against pressure, burns, and other injury.

Change the patient's position regularly and frequently; ask him to turn from one side to the other frequently. Know if special attention should be given to encourage and promote movement and activity; have a bed patient change position, using a trapeze bar and side rails to help him move himself about. Elevate and support an edematous, dependent body part (foot, lower leg) as ordered. Provide necessary and appropriate means for quiet relaxation, rest, sleep, and reassurance. Provide, maintain, or assist with any treatments or measures which may have been ordered, such as supportive stockings, elevation of the dependent body part, or administration of oxygen.

CEREBRAL AND NEUROLOGIC DISTRESS

Unconsciousness

The human mind can be altered so that it fails to respond in the usual way. Unconsciousness is the term used to describe a state when a person does not respond to anything except very severe pain; it is also called *deep coma*. Semicoma, stupor, and somnolence are terms used for lesser stages or levels of unconsciousness.

CAUSES. The many causes of unconsciousness include the following:

1. Effect of a drug (e.g., alcohol).
2. Upset in the physiology of the brain (hypoglycemia).
3. Edema.
4. Stroke (cerebral vascular accident).
5. Increased pressure within the skull.
6. Anesthesia.
7. Destruction of vital brain centers.

CARE OF THE PATIENT. How much or how little an unconscious patient responds actually does not influence his state of dependency; this patient is *entirely* dependent upon medical and nursing skill to meet his needs.

An immediate and constant need is to provide an open airway. This means that the patient must be observed closely. Mucus col-

lecting in the nose and throat needs to be suctioned; it is easy to see that if unconsciousness persists, the repeated act of suctioning can irritate these linings or even damage to point of bleeding, causing them to swell and creating further breathing difficulty.

Mouth tissues dry out from mouth breathing; this points up the need for careful and continued attention to the condition of the tissues. The physician may or may not write an order for this; it is an obvious need calling for nurse attention.

An unconscious patient cannot swallow; therefore fluids are given by parenteral means and by tube feedings. The amount given at a time is usually small to avoid overloading the stomach, which might cause vomiting. The physician orders the type and amount of feeding.

Bowel elimination is often irregular, ranging from diarrhea to constipation to fecal impaction.

The patient's eyes need attention; the pupils may vary in size, and this condition may change from time to time; report such changes. Sometimes the eyes are open, sometimes closed or partially so. The eyeball will become dry when the eye is open constantly, and this can be harmful to the cornea. The physician may order an irrigation or eye drops to prevent this; he may also order an eye patch to protect the eye.

Because the patient's muscles are flaccid and there is little or no body movement, the patient should be turned and his body parts exercised, unless his condition does not permit it. Skin care becomes a very important need for this patient because he does not move, has incontinence, and his skin tissues are poorly nourished.

SIGNS AND SYMPTOMS. The patient's muscles are flaccid and he shows no body movement and no reflexes. He is unaware of anything. Mouth breathing is present and respirations may be noisy. His pupils may vary in size. He is incontinent, and has constipation or diarrhea. His temperature fluctuates. His skin may be mottled and dry and show signs of dehydration.

NURSING CARE. Follow these directions for careful *observation*:

1. Note the response of the patient to noise, light, touch, and movement when giving personal care, changing the bed linen, turning the patient, speaking to him, or turning on a bright light.

2. Describe any response (verbal and nonverbal) of the patient *in detail and with exactness*. Avoid making an interpretation by using such words as confused, unaware, or disoriented in recording on his chart.

3. Note a marked increase or decrease in symptoms or the appearance of a new symptom and complication.

4. Know any specific observations to be made which may be specified by the physician's order or directed by the charge nurse.

5. Watch for signs of dehydration.

To maintain a proper *environment*—control temperature, ventilation, noise, order and appearance—follow these steps:

1. Keep the temperature of the room at about 70° F., or slightly warmer for comfort, especially for a young child or elderly person.

2. Keep the room as quiet as possible; control the presence and number of visitors. Avoid talking, especially loud, unnecessary, or inappropriate talking. Use a soft, normal tone of speaking to the patient and visitors. Prevent any discussion or conversation regarding the patient at the bedside or in his room by leaving the room and closing the door.

3. Keep the bedside unit and room clean, in order, and free from odors.

4. Adjust the light in the room according to the patient's condition by using a normal or dim light; avoid a sudden change in degree or amount of light.

To make certain of adequate and safe maintenance of *air passages* with positioning and suctioning:

1. Prevent the patient's tongue from falling to the back of his mouth and causing asphyxiation. Place the patient on his side or abdomen with his face turned to the side and down; elevate the head of the bed slightly only on order of the physician; prevent the patient from being placed (or allowed to remain) on his back unless necessary and then stay with him.

2. Use a small, firm pillow under his head only if required; usually no pillow is used.

3. Keep nasal passages and mouth clear of secretions and mucus; know if the physician's orders permit the use of swabs or suction to cleanse the nasal passages (after certain surgery and types of injury neither is used). Use suction carefully (as specifically directed) to avoid irritation and damage to tissues.

4. *Stay at the bedside* and give constant attention if there is vomiting or if there is likely to be vomiting; prevent aspiration of vomitus.

To make sure that the patient maintains the proper *position:*

1. Turn him to change his position frequently; plan a schedule for routine turning at specified intervals, e.g., every hour, or every two hours.

2. Obtain help and use a "turning sheet" to move or turn the patient; know how to assist or direct the turning of a patient who is using a Stryker frame or the CircOlectric bed.

3. Provide and maintain proper body alignment and support when turning and placing the patient in position; use firm, plastic covered pillows to support his body parts; prevent foot drop and wrist drop with proper position of feet and hands (Fig. 41–3).

4. Follow orders and directions for assisting and giving exercises to body parts; know which parts are to be exercised, the type and frequency of exercise or motion, and any special care or precautions to take, e.g., preventing strain on joints.

Take the *temperature (rectal), pulse, respirations, and blood pressure* as ordered, or directed. Note changes and report promptly.

To allow for *personal care:*

1. Keep bedding clean and dry; make certain the bottom sheet is tight and smooth; adjust top bedding to keep it loose over the body. Avoid sudden, jarring, and unnecessary handling or movements when changing the bed.

2. Give complete and partial baths daily and as frequently as needed; use slow, gentle, careful movements when washing and drying the patient.

3. Keep the hair brushed and combed and free of snarls; braid the hair, if possible; obtain a physician's order to give a shampoo about every two weeks.

4. Give mouth care several times a day, as often as needed; apply a lubricant to the lips; keep dentures removed and safely stored until the patient is fully conscious.

5. Inspect the condition of the eyes several times a day; follow orders for care to the eyes; watch for signs of irritation and dryness.

6. Observe bowel eliminations for frequency and type (diarrhea, constipation); follow orders for giving an enema.

7. Keep the nails short and clean; rub the hands and feet gently and keep them lubricated.

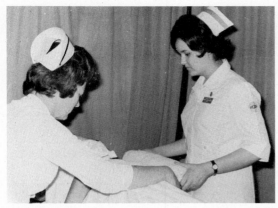

FIGURE 41–3 The unconscious patient needs to be turned frequently. Do this at regular intervals. Here the LPN is placing a firmly rolled pillow to the back as the registered nurse positions the patient. (Courtesy of Pensacola Community College, Practical Nursing Program, Pensacola, Florida.)

8. Pad side rails and keep them in place except when at the bedside giving care.

To provide for *skin care:*

1. Examine skin and pressure areas at the time of turning the patient and give care to his skin; keep the skin clean, dry, and lubricated.

2. Use a lubricating cream or lotion and powder, not alcohol lotion.

3. Rub the skin gently and briefly.

4. Provide the time, care, and attention necessary if the patient is incontinent of urine or feces.

5. Observe the color of the skin and the amount of muscle tone.

Give meticulous nursing care to prevent (1) *complications,* such as sordes, decubitus ulcers, infections, matted hair, foot or wrist drop, contractures, constipation or impaction, blindness, and dehydration; or (2) *accidents,* such as burns, falling out of bed, asphyxiation, dislocation or sprain to joints.

Provide, maintain, or assist with any treatments or measures which may be ordered, such as an enema, shampoo, perineal care, eye irrigation or drops, air-pressure mattress, sponge rubber or sheepskin under bony prominences, suction, indwelling catheter, parenteral fluids, oxygen, or tracheostomy.

Convulsion

A convulsion is a violent, uncontrollable (involuntary) contraction or series of contrac- tions of the muscles; sometimes it is called a seizure or spasm. Children are apt to have them more often than adults.

CAUSES.   Causes vary according to the type of convulsion. An *acute* convulsion is caused by high fever, intracranial pressure, toxicity due to certain drugs, metabolic or nu- tritional deficiency, brain edema, or brain tumor. *Chronic* convulsions are caused by epi- lepsy (hereditary or from previous brain dam- age), hysteria, lack of calcium, hyperinsulin- ism, hypothyroidism, certain liver disorders, migraine, or uremia.

CARE OF THE PATIENT.   The cause of the convulsion may or may not be known; convulsions may occur with a good many dif- ferent diseases and disorders.

The immediate needs of the patient are to protect him from choking, biting his tongue, and otherwise injuring himself. The nursing care, including essential observations, de- scribes in detail how to protect and observe this patient.

SIGNS AND SYMPTOMS.   At the *begin- ning of a seizure,* the patient may experience an aura or warning, such as a form of light, sound, or odor. An abnormal sensation in a certain place or part of the body may be noted, followed by a twitch. As the seizure becomes generalized, the patient becomes unconscious. A patient may, however, cry out suddenly, fall to the floor or ground, and become uncon- scious at once. Involuntary muscle contrac- tions are evident; at first the entire body is rigid and stiff, but then rhythmic jerky move- ments follow, and gradually these movements become slower and slower and stop.

During the seizure, the jaws are clenched tightly and quickly. The face is at first very pale, then bluish-purple ("black in the face") for a few moments until breathing becomes normal. Respirations may be absent (apnea) or of a snoring type (stertor) for a few seconds, after which normal breathing resumes. Exces- sive secretions that are frothy or foamy flow from the mouth ("foaming at the mouth"). In- continence of urine or feces may occur. Signs of consciousness usually return in about three minutes; the patient makes awkward move- ments, attempts to talk or cry out, and seems confused.

Following the seizure, headache often occurs and the patient experiences extreme fa- tigue. His body and clothing are moist from perspiration. The patient appears drowsy and often sleeps for several hours. Emotional and behavioral changes occur, for the patient feels confused, unaware of his actions or surroundings, does not remember the attack, and feels embarrassed.

NURSING CARE. Observe the patient and the seizure, and report and record as completely and accurately as possible the following:

1. The length of time the seizure lasted (exact time in minutes).

2. Part(s) of the body where the seizure started and parts that became involved.

3. Muscle response—describe contractions of muscles.

4. Respirations—rate and character.

5. Skin—color of face and presence or absence of diaphoresis.

6. Eyes—appearance of pupils; deviations, such as eyes turned up, down, or to either side.

7. Secretions—presence, amount and appearance, from mouth or nose.

8. Consciousness—apparent stage or degree; partial or complete loss.

9. Incontinence—if any (urine or feces).

10. Observations following seizure—subjective and objective.

11. Occurrence of any apparent injury.

12. Actions of the patient, especially before and after the seizure.

Give attention and care to the patient *at once;* stay calm; know what to do and what not to do; *stay* with the patient.

To protect the patient from injury:

1. Respond immediately to any signs of a beginning attack which may be noted first by the patient, yourself, or another patient or person.

2. Stay with the patient—whether he is ambulatory or in bed.

3. Prevent the ambulatory patient from falling; help him into bed if possible, or lower him to the floor gently.

4. Clear the bed of objects if the patient is in bed; lower or remove bedside rails; move the bedside table away from the bed.

5. Place a padded wedge quickly between the back teeth before the teeth become clenched. Do not use force to insert the wedge or put your fingers into the patient's mouth; use a wedge of hard rubber, two tongue blades wrapped and held together with adhesive tape, or a clean, folded washcloth.

6. Place a pillow or soft folded material under the patient's head; stand a pillow against the head of the bed if the patient is in bed. Support the patient's head against and between your thighs, just above the knees, if the patient is lying on the floor.

7. Loosen or remove any tight clothing.

8. Turn the patient's head to the side.

9. Do not try to hold or restrain the patient's movements.

10. Do not move the patient until seizure is ended, unless in or near some harmful location or equipment.

11. Obtain help if possible and needed, e.g., have a co-worker put on the patient's call signal, bring the charge nurse, provide privacy, stand on opposite side of bed, and so on.

12. Protect the privacy of the patient; ask any and all onlookers to leave; have someone screen you and the patient.

Show understanding and reassurance to the patient when the seizure has ended and the patient is conscious. Provide the necessary personal care and then quiet conditions for the patient to sleep.

Take the following precautions to provide for the care and safety of the patient if it is known upon admission that the patient has had or is likely to have a convulsion:

1. Place suitable mouth wedges at his bedside.

2. Pad sides of a crib or bedside rails.

3. Make certain the bed and mattress have suitable and adequate protectors.

4. Keep objects which may harm the patient removed from the bed, e.g., a hard toy.

5. Know if any equipment is to be kept at bedside and used, e.g., suction aspirator, oxygen, etc.

6. Know if and when any procedure or measure is to be used, e.g., tepid sponge bath.

7. Prevent, if possible, any known factors which might bring about a convulsion in a particular patient.

8. Know about the frequency and type of seizure that the patient has had, or may have.

9. Ask the charge nurse or physician about extra or special precautions to be taken, care to be given, or observations to be made.

Fainting (Syncope)

Fainting is the temporary loss of consciousness caused by excessive dilation of close-to-the-surface blood vessels, causing "blood pools" and reducing cardiac output. This state can lead to shock and death if the patient remains upright.

CAUSES.   Fainting can be the result of:

1. Side effect of some drug(s).

2. Assuming an upright position too quickly after being inactive in bed for a period of time.

3. Emotional factors and experiences.

4. Overexertion.

5. Standing too long without moving and becoming too warm or fatigued.

6. Hunger.

7. Intense, prolonged pain.

CARE OF THE PATIENT.   Fainting presents an emergency situation, and immediate care of this is described under nursing care. Some points are also made about how to help prevent fainting; they provide you with some facts which are useful in any patient situation.

SIGNS AND SYMPTOMS.   The patient may have no dizziness or some dizziness, and may say such things as, "I feel light-headed," or "I feel a little faint." His pulse rate increases and his face may appear pale (pallor) at onset.

NURSING CARE.   Observations to be made, recorded, and reported are:

1. Note both subjective and objective signs and symptoms.

2. Note and describe the patient's activity at the time (e.g., upon getting out of bed).

3. Take pulse, noting rate and character.

Help *prevent* fainting by:

1. Avoiding those factors and conditions which promote fainting, if possible, especially for those patients who are likely to faint easily and frequently, e.g., overexertion and fatigue, prolonged or extreme pain, and bathing for too long in water that is too warm.

2. Informing the patient what to do, and what not to do, if dizziness or a feeling of faintness occurs. Tell the patient to lie down on the bed or the floor, or sit down in a chair and lean over with his head on or between his knees for a few moments until the sensation leaves, and to call for assistance.

3. Assisting the patient to a horizontal position on the bed or the floor, or to sit in a chair. Stand in front of patient and push his head and shoulders low between his knees; prevent falling; loosen tight clothing, especially about the neck, chest, and waist; note the color of his face and take his pulse.

4. Cautioning patients against certain activities and movements.

5. Knowing if the patient is susceptible to fainting (easily and frequently), and having him avoid those movements and activities as well as any factors which are known or likely to produce fainting (e.g., standing motionless for a long period of time, sitting for a long time with pressure against the popliteal space, remaining in the dorsal recumbent position in bed, moving too quickly to an upright position to sit or stand, taking a bath in too warm or hot water, or staying in a very warm bath too long, and straining to have a bowel movement).

SUMMARY

The body has the ability to adjust itself in many ways in order to keep itself functioning within "normal bounds." Illness occurs when body functions get out of bounds and the body fights back, calling attention to itself with distress signals (commonly known as signs and symptoms).

The eight major factors which cause or contribute to illness are microorganisms, body deformities and abnormal functions, improper nourishment, trauma due to accidents, poisons and poisoning, housing, heat and cold, and heredity. One or more of these factors may be present during illness.

Therapy is treatment; it is directed toward cure, toward helping the body use its own built-in resources to the best advantage, toward changing the progress of an illness and preventing further disabling effects, and toward altering the illness condition in order to allow the patient to be as comfortable and active as possible for as long as possible.

Nursing measures and nurse action are geared to an individual who is responding to a condition of illness. These measures are a mixture of observations, physical comfort and safety factors, emotional comfort and well-being factors, measures and procedures ordered by the physician for the patient's medical management, and any other measures determined by the charge nurse or team leader as necessary to patient well-being.

Signs and symptoms of illness involve the whole body, some more widely than others. They dictate medical management and nursing care. There is a striking thing about signs and symptoms: they occur with one disease condition after another.

GUIDES FOR STUDY AND DISCUSSION

1. What is therapy? Why is it directed toward certain goals?

2. What does it mean to say a person's "will to live" can influence his recovery?

3. To be healthy, the body must maintain normal limits of such functions as fluid balance and temperature. What are some other functions which must operate within normal limits? For each function named, list a term which indicates dysfunction.

4. In general, *the work of the nurse consists of a combination of four areas of responsibility*. Complete the following for your own reference.

Responsible For	Facts to Remember
1. Observing 2. Providing physical comfort and safety. 3. Providing emotional comfort and well-being 4. Carrying out medical orders and nursing measures	

5. Why can the loss of ability to feel pain be dangerous to the patient?

6. What things about fever make it necessary to pay special attention to personal hygiene?

7. Why take a rectal temperature during a chill?

8. During shock, what should be the position of the patient until special orders are given?

9. What is the difference between retching and vomiting?

10. Why is the importance of skin care stressed with so many signs and symptoms in this chapter?

11. What is meant by fluid balance?

SUGGESTED SITUATIONS AND ACTIVITIES

1. This chapter contains many new and old vocabulary words you will be using and reusing. Prepare your own list; check it to see how it compares with lists made by classmates. Practice spelling words; learn to describe them in your own words.

2. Select one sign or symptom discussed in this chapter and assemble materials you will need to demonstrate in class one or more nursing measures to help a patient with this sign or symptom. Be prepared to explain what you are doing and why.

CHAPTER 42

INTRODUCTION TO MEDICAL-SURGICAL NURSING

TOPICAL HEADINGS

Introduction
Meaning of Medical-
   Surgical
Clinical Services,
   Specialties, and Ac-
   commodations
Surgical and Medical
   Asepsis

The Patient Before
   and After Surgery
Early Ambulation,
   Convalescence, and
   Preparation for
   Leaving the Hos-
   pital

Special Treatments
   and Measures
Who Is the Medical-
   Surgical Patient?
Summary
Guides for Study
   and Discussion
Suggested Situations
   and Activities

OBJECTIVES FOR THE STUDENT: Be able to:

1. Tell who is the medical-surgical patient.
2. Give four examples of ways patients are housed in a hospital.
3. Compare surgical aseptic technique with medical aseptic technique to show how they differ.
4. Explain how asepsis can be practiced in nursing care to reduce the chance of cross-infection.
5. Given a list of eleven rules that guide action in sterile technique, write one reason for each rule.
6. Describe the needs of the patient being prepared for surgery.
7. Describe the needs of the patient immediately following surgery.
8. Given a list of common treatments and measures, state one nursing responsibility for each.

SUGGESTED STUDY VOCABULARY*

asepsis
microorganisms
surgical asepsis
medical asepsis
sterile technique
contaminated
cross-infection
surgery

isolation technique
abrasions
infectious disease
secretions
terminal disinfection
parenteral fluids
operative site
anesthesia

wound healing
catheterization
distention of the bladder
early ambulation
stasis
convalescence
combustion
suction
nasogastric tube

*Look for any terms you already know.

INTRODUCTION

By this time you have heard of the medical-surgical patient. Do you know who he is or why he has this label? The label medical-surgical is used to classify patients perhaps for convenience and identity as much as anything else.

Patients with a medical or surgical label include all age groups, with many different illnesses and in varying states of dependency and independency. In fact, the bulk of the patients in any general hospital fit into the medical-surgical category. Other categories are pediatrics, small medical-surgical patients, maternity, mothers and newborns, and psychiatry, the category for mental patients. The hospital accommodates the medical-surgical patient in a variety of general and special ways as pointed out in this chapter.

Many things happen in the life of the medical-surgical patient as different personnel treat him and provide for his special needs. Some treatments and measures are very complex, requiring the knowledge and skills of specially trained persons; some require special equipment, special facilities, and special abilities. Other treatments and measures include many you are already familiar with and have been using in meeting the needs of patients.

As you can see from reading the topical headings, this chapter includes a variety of topics which might, at first glance, seem to be a collection of unrelated factors. However, they all relate to the medical-surgical patient, explaining what is done for him, where he goes or is taken to have these things done, what services and facilities are available to meet his special needs, and how you are involved in his care. The last topic identifies the medical-surgical patient as the same patient you may have been caring for while learning about the needs of the ambulatory, the mildly ill, the seriously ill, the long-term, and the dying patient, because he can be any one of these patients.

MEANING OF MEDICAL-SURGICAL

The medical profession is made up of physicians trained to practice medicine in one of a vast number of special fields or in a general way. The person trained to treat patients in an "all systems approach" or a general way is said to be in general practice and is called a general practitioner. The person trained to treat patients with a disease or disorder related to a particular part or function of the body, or trained in a particular therapy, is called a specialist. The list of specialties is long and continues to grow as knowledge of human anatomy and physiology and the causes of illness grows. Some of the main specialties are surgery, orthopedics, urology, obstetrics, gynecology, ophthalmology, otolaryngology, dermatology, neurology, psychiatry, pediatrics, gerontology, anesthesiology, internal medicine, cardiology, hematology, and radiology. Two newer ones are space medicine and environmental medicine.

An old definition of the work of a physician is "to cure sometimes, to relieve often, to comfort always." This is still true, but the physician has more to work with—more to cure with and more ways to relieve the patient. There is still need for a great measure of *comfort always* in caring for the many patients who have incurable diseases and conditions which seem to defy relief giving measures. Medical science is concerned with prevention, restoration, rehabilitation, and finding out more about the structure and function of the body to promote health and to effect new cures. Surgery is a special branch of medicine which treats disease or disorder by operative procedures.

The term "medical-surgical" is used to designate a broad group of patients. To someone unfamiliar with the many specialties within the practice of medicine, this broad label can be confusing. Actually, a medical patient is one who is treated by means other than surgery. When surgery is performed on a medical patient, he is called a surgical patient. It is entirely possible after the body has mended that this same patient may be called a medical patient again.

The medical patient who does not need surgery may be treated by a specialist trained to treat patients with his particular disorder. For instance, the patient with a skin eruption may be under the care of a dermatologist—a physician with special training in diseases and disorders of the skin, or the patient with heart disease may be under the care of a cardiologist—a physician with special training in diseases of the heart. The cardiologist, in turn, may determine that his patient needs heart surgery, and this treatment requires the skills of a physician trained in the techniques of cardiac surgery. When thought of in this manner, surgery becomes a therapy. It is a very highly specialized branch of medicine which has many specialties and specialists within itself.

CLINICAL SERVICES, SPECIALTIES, AND ACCOMMODATIONS

Hospitals are arranged to accommodate patients in a variety of ways. The size of the hospital and the purpose often influence how patients are clustered or located. Other factors which control patient placement to a certain extent are the rules and regulations of outside agencies (e.g., the State Board of Health, accrediting groups).

The small hospital is apt to have areas called "medical floors" or "surgical floors," or "medical-surgical floors." Here are located the medical-surgical patients without regard to specialties. However, even with this general grouping of medical-surgical patients it is likely that a portion of one of these "floors" may be designated to accommodate a particular group of patients, such as orthopedic patients. In that case, the area is likely to be called the orthopedic floor, wing, area, or ward.

The large hospital most often has many definite areas set aside to accommodate a variety of different "specialties" (e.g., urology, orthopedics, gynecology, and cardiology).

Another accommodation for patients is set up according to age (e.g., pediatrics, geriatrics) or according to a condition that must be set apart to protect that patient from the hazards of possible cross-infection, namely the obstetric patients, the newborn, and the burn patient.

Still another type of accommodation which is becoming increasingly more popular is the area staffed and equipped to specifically meet the needs of patients who are dependent upon special life-sustaining skills and equipment in a guarded environment. The staff is made up of personnel who are "specialists" in caring for patients needing this equipment. Examples of these areas are the recovery room and the intensive care unit (called ICU).

See Figure 42–1. Some hospitals and community facilities have carried the idea of patient dependence and independence several steps beyond the recovery room and the intensive care unit. The provisions are geared to the patient's needs and this concept is called *progressive patient care*. For instance, after the operative patient has regained consciousness and no longer needs to stay in the recovery room, he is moved to a part of the hospital called the *intermediate care unit*. The patient remains there, receiving the types of assistance he needs, until he is ambulatory and capable of self-care under supervision with the types of assistance he needs. Then he is moved to *a self-care unit*; here the ambulatory patient is given a full share of attention geared to his daily living needs and his degree of independence.

If the patient's condition worsens, he is moved back to the area which can best meet his needs; if critical, he is moved to the intensive care unit (not back to the recovery room, which is for new operative patients only).

To relieve hospitals of increasing patient loads, there are other care facilities in the community if the patient cannot be cared for at home. One is the extended care facility; it is equipped to help a patient through his conva-

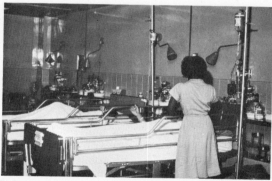

FIGURE 42–1 The recovery room is equipped to meet the immediate needs of the patient after surgery. Here the word "recovery" means regaining consciousness from a general anesthetic, having the vital signs return to more normal ranges, and getting over the initial effects of a local anesthetic. There is close observation for hemorrhage, shock, or other untoward results before returning the patient to his own room The LPN functions in Role II in the recovery room. (Courtesy of Santa Fe Junior College Practical Nursing Program. Gainesville, Florida. Photographer, Henry DeLoach.)

lescence. Another is the nursing home, which provides care for patients (chiefly elderly patients) with long-term and chronic conditions, although elderliness is not always a requirement for admission.

Patient accommodations can be thought of from another angle, too—by the number of patients in a room. Examples are the private room, the semi-private room (with a roommate), or the multiple bed accommodation called a "ward," designated by the number of beds in the room, as a "four-bed ward."

There are differences of opinion about mixing medical patients and surgical patients in multiple-bed accommodations. Practices vary from hospital to hospital. Then, too, there are the very real problems of placing patients due to the lack of beds, according to the patient's wishes, or according to the physician's recommendations in relation to the needs of the patient, or the ability of the patient to pay for a certain type of accommodation.

SURGICAL AND MEDICAL ASEPSIS

The word "asepsis" means the absence of any matter which causes putrefaction or decay—in other words, the absence of microorganisms which cause the decay. Microorganisms are present in the air and on dust, hands, clothing, and hair—on all objects; for an object to be free of these organisms it must be sterilized. Things that cannot be sterilized harbor organisms; they transport them. This includes people as well as air and objects. In a hospital, this fact of transporting harmful microorganisms is a serious matter. It is not enough to handle sterile equipment properly, important as that is. Personnel must use methods which prevent infection or reduce the chance for spreading infection to an absolute minimum. They must follow the rules very conscientiously if patients and personnel are to find the hospital a safe place. The rules amount to a great number of *safety practices, commonly called aseptic technique.* In special places such as the operating room or the newborn nursery, or when changing certain types of dressings or inserting a catheter, there is a strict set of practices called sterile technique or *surgical asepsis.* In special places such as

the unit of a patient who has an infection or an infectious disease, there is a strict set of practices called *medical asepsis.* You will need to know the basic rules or guidelines for each of these two types of asepsis.

It has been about one hundred years since the germ theory of disease became firmly established; during this time it has been known that microorganisms cause disease and are responsible for infections. Until the germ theory of disease was established, the physician considered the presence of pus in a wound as a normal part of the healing process.

Infection is still present in hospitals today. Of late there has been a steady increase in the number of cases of infection among hospital patients. There are many reasons why this is true. For one thing, studies show that the increase started after the "wonder drugs" were introduced. It is possible that personnel started to depend upon these drugs to do their work for them and developed poor aseptic habits. Then too, in time, organisms built up resistance to the drugs. People have come to think that "a shot of penicillin" is the answer; they even tell the physician they think that is what they need. The fact remains that the fight against infections is more real today than in the past. If the hospital is to be a safe place for patients and personnel, personnel must practice aseptic techniques accordingly. Two factors must be considered: (1) The knowledge of the germ theory of disease must guide actions; this means developing and using suitable methods and techniques. (2) The germ theory must be practiced all the time. The spread of disease makes no allowance for careless, halfway techniques. As a practical nurse you are as responsible for your convictions and safe practices as is any other member of the team. Chemicals and "wonder drugs" are not safe substitutes for safe action.

Surgical Asepsis

The idea behind surgical asepsis is to hold to an absolute minimum the chances for infection in a wound or the chances for introducing microorganisms into a wound or body cavity. To say it another way, the idea is to do every reasonable thing to *prevent microorganisms from having entrance to a wound or body cavity.* To prevent this entrance means that certain rules must be strictly followed; these rules guide action and every action has a purpose;

that purpose is to prevent contamination. Sterile objects must remain sterile, free from organisms, until used. If these rules are not followed and a break in technique occurs, there is contamination.

Here are the rules that guide action in practicing sterile technique:

1. *Start with clean hands.* The scrubbing technique in the operating room is a special process; on the floors the process is one of thorough scrubbing and rinsing (see Handwashing Technique in Appendix III).

2. Handle sterile equipment only with sterile equipment (forceps, sterile gloves) or in such way as to keep sterile the part or portion that will come in contact with the patient.

3. Establish a sterile field (area) for receiving all sterile equipment and supplies from other sources.

4. Keep the field sterile; the surface underneath must be *dry*; do not reach over or across it.

5. Open sterile packages with one thought in mind: the inside of the wrapper and contents must not be touched by any unsterile object.

6. Avoid opening sterile packages until ready to use the contents; exposure to air or unnecessary handling increases the possibility of contamination.

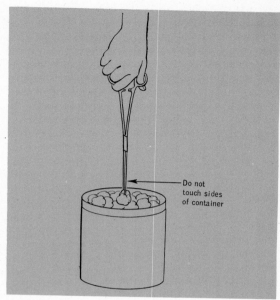

FIGURE 42-3 Hold lifting forceps downward to prevent antiseptic solution from running onto unsterile portion and then back onto sterile portion; do not permit the sterile portion to touch any unsterile object. (Sutton: Bedside Nursing Techniques, 2nd Ed.)

7. Use sterile lifting forceps according to the rules. Notice in Figure 42-2 the two rules to follow in removing forceps from the container of antiseptic solution. Notice in Figure 42-3 that the forceps are held downward and the sterile portion of the forceps (if it is to remain sterile) must not touch the side of the container when removing an object. The object itself is dropped on the sterile field, and the forceps do not touch anything else if it is to be returned to the antiseptic solution. Replace lifting forceps in the container with antiseptic solution without touching the sterile portion to the edge of the container.

8. Do not remove a sterile object from a sterile container with anything but a sterile instrument.

9. Open the sterile container according to the rules. Lift the cover by the handle, holding the cover downward. If the cover must be placed rather than held, place it so that the handle is next to the table; in this way the cover edges are up and away from a contaminated surface. Replace the container cover as soon as the sterile object has been removed.

10. Discard, as contaminated, any sterile equipment and supplies coming in contact with any unsterile object or any instruments

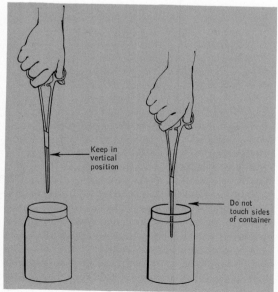

FIGURE 42-2 Two rules to guide action when removing or lifting forceps from a container of antiseptic solution. (Sutton: Bedside Nursing Techniques, 2nd Ed.)

and equipment used in directly treating a patient.

11. *Finish with clean hands.* The last thing to do is thoroughly wash your hands.

These rules are used to guide your action when you open *any* sterile package to use yourself or to assist a physician, a registered nurse, or another LPN. The rules apply to handling *any* sterile equipment or material for any purpose, and they apply when setting up a sterile field for *any* purpose.

Washing your hands before, during if necessary, and after carrying out any measure should be as much a habit as answering to your own name. Applying these rules in a strict manner at all times expresses your conviction that you do, in fact, believe the germ theory of disease—so much so that if you break technique you discard the contaminated equipment or materials and start over whether anyone is watching or not.

Medical Asepsis

The idea behind medical asepsis is to prevent the transfer of microorganisms (infection) by confining them within the source area. To say it another way, the idea is to do every reasonable thing *to prevent microorganisms from leaving an area.* To prevent this escape, so that other patients and personnel are safe, certain rules must be strictly followed; these rules guide action, and every action has a purpose—that purpose is to hold to an absolute minimum the chances of spreading infection.

Microorganisms have no power to move by themselves; if they get moved, something or somebody provides the transportation. By practicing medical asepsis (confining infection to its source), the chances of transporting organisms are held to a minimum.

The rules of medical asepsis apply in two ways in the hospital (the first is no less strict than the second, although it does not require the same equipment owing to the nature of the circumstances):

1. In all general nursing care.
2. In a unit where a patient has an infection or infectious disease.

ASEPSIS IN GENERAL NURSING CARE. One way to make nursing care safe is to protect patients and personnel from cross-infection. Some of the ways you practice this are:

1. Washing hands before, during, and after working with a patient.
2. Keeping your hands free of cuts and abrasions, with the nails trimmed and clean.
3. Removing and handling soiled linen in such a way that soiled portions are to the inside and are not permitted to come in contact with the uniform.
4. Disposing of all soiled dressings and discharges promptly and safely; this may mean wrapping them in paper first.
5. Keeping the patient's unit utensils and the bedside table clean.
6. Keeping equipment clean while in use and cleaning it thoroughly between uses from one patient to another.

ASEPSIS IN A UNIT WHERE A PATIENT HAS AN INFECTION OR AN INFECTIOUS DISEASE. It seems easier to impress upon personnel that they should practice stricter medical asepsis when a patient has meningitis, diptheria, typhoid fever or some other serious infectious disease than when the infection is in the form of boils or a wound infection. Actually, this is part of the difficulty in the increasing spread of hospital infections; personnel do not take the germ theory of disease as seriously at one time as another.

The group of safety precautions for confining harmful organisms to the area of source is called *isolation technique.* To isolate means to set apart or separate from. Therefore, *isolation technique is made up of a series of actions which are intended to set apart the source of infection, to keep it confined to the area, and to keep it from infecting personnel and being transported to other patients.*

Some of the steps in the isolation technique include the following:

1. To set the nurse apart from the patient requires the nurse to cover her uniform with a gown—a large, loose, coverall with short or long sleeves. The open back ties in place at the back of the neck and at the waist, with strings which cross at the back and tie in front. This garment is now made and used in a disposable form, as well as in the reusable form. It is either discarded for disposal or left within the patient's unit if it is to be reused. Putting on and removing a gown requires special handling to ensure that the wearer's clothing is protected at all times.

2. Another item which sets the nurse apart is a mask worn to protect her from the

coughs, sneezes, and air droplets of the patient. In some instances the patient wears the mask, such as when he is being transported to another area. There are differences of opinion about personnel wearing a mask. When a mask gets damp, it is a suitable place for organisms to grow and should be discarded. Masks are not reused; a clean one must be worn each time you enter a patient's unit. (Some surgeons do not talk any more than is necessary when performing an operation, in order to keep the mask dry; they do this to protect the patient.)

3. Hand care and handwashing also help to set the nurse and patient apart. The nurse's hands should be soft and free from cuts and abrasions. Broken skin serves as a portal of entry for organisms. Hand lotion will help to keep the skin smooth and free from cracks and chapping. Thorough handwashing must be practiced before, during, and after contact with the patient to reduce to an absolute minimum the chance of transporting organisms from one patient to one's self or to another patient or person.

4. Patient secretions (from eyes, nose, or throat) and excretions (feces, urine) are disposed of in the manner prescribed by the board of health or by hospital policy. These body discharges may require special handling in some instances (e.g., a typhoid fever patient's stools when sewage disposal is inadequate).

5. Any utensils, equipment, food, and personal possessions which are brought into the unit are considered contaminated, and must remain there or be handled with precautionary measures according to hospital policy. The use of disposable equipment makes it easier and safer to carry out medical asepsis.

6. Terminal disinfection is the cleaning of the unit after the patient leaves. Equipment is washed thoroughly and boiled (if possible) for at least 10 minutes or sterilized (if possible) in an autoclave to make it safe for use again.

A comparison of surgical asepsis and medical asepsis may help you understand their differences and guide your action in each situation. The idea behind the one is the opposite of the other. In surgical asepsis all action taken is *to prevent infection from reaching a wound* or body cavity. In medical asepsis all action taken is *to prevent infection from leaving its source.*

THE PATIENT BEFORE AND AFTER SURGERY

Surgery is a highly specialized branch of medicine which treats a patient by operative procedure. Everything about the operating room environment is closely controlled to reduce to an absolute minimum the chances for wound infection.

Hand scrubbing is a timed technique carried out in such a way as to help control contamination. Special clothing is worn, sometimes including shoe coverings. Hair is covered, and personnel admitted are limited to those who have a purpose for being there. Personnel who have colds or harbor any type of infection (in nose or throat, boils) are not allowed to work. The immediate area where the surgery is performed undergoes special preparation; so does the patient when he arrives there.

All precautions are only as good or safe as the personnel who carry them out. It is one thing to know and believe in the germ theory of disease, and it is another thing to practice surgical asepsis in a way that proves that you believe it.

Preoperative Nursing Care

Preparation of the patient going to surgery takes place ahead of time unless it is an emergency situation; in that case the patient is moved directly to the operating area. Besides *emergency* surgery, there are such categories as *elective* (something done when convenient, such as repair of burn scars), *required* (something that needs attention and is planned for ahead of time, such as removal of bunions or tonsils), and *urgent* (something that needs attention as soon as possible, such as bleeding from the uterus, stomach, or intestine).

THE PATIENT'S FRAME OF MIND. In situations other than an emergency, one part of the patient's preparation may have been taking form since he knew or suspected that he needed surgery; that part is his frame of mind about it (his mental and emotional feelings). The prospect of surgery causes a person to wonder and often to be fearful about what is involved and how it will come out. It is a stressful time for the patient, whether he talks about it or not. It is natural for a person to show concern under such circumstances; he is influenced very much by the personnel who are involved in readying him for his operation. His remarks indicate his concerns and furnish clues for helping him: "I don't know why they had to come here and take a sample of my blood; they must think I am going to bleed a lot and want to be ready." "I wish the operation could be today so it would be over with." "Will I feel anything during the operation?" "Why are you shaving such a large area? The doctor told me the scar would be small."

One of the main things that helps the patient and his family at this time is his confidence in his physician or surgeon and all other personnel involved. It is a known fact that secure feelings help the patient to more fully benefit from the preoperative medications; he goes to surgery in a better condition to receive the anesthetic. Your manner contributes to this feeling of confidence. Every contact you have with the patient should help him to feel that he is among people who are concerned about his welfare. One way to do this is to pay attention to the details of his care in such a way as to indicate interest in him as an individual.

PERMISSION TO PERFORM SURGERY. In almost all cases, this is a written permit signed by the patient (unless he is a minor or unable) or else by a family member or guardian. The hospital has a special form for this purpose, and under certain circumstances it may be your responsibility to see that this form is signed and witnessed. Such permission is necessary because a person does not have to have surgery unless he so chooses. Performing surgery without the consent of the patient can be grounds for a lawsuit against the surgeon.

If a patient, or his guardian, refuses to sign the permit, report this to the charge nurse. No patient should be prepared for surgery or sent to the operating room without a signed surgical permission. When any exception is made to this rule, it must be the decision of the surgeon.

PHYSICAL EXAMINATION. The family physician may have completed this examination in his office or in the patient's home prior to admission to the hospital. However, it may be done in the hospital. See Chapter 28, The Medical Examination.

If the medical-surgical patient has been in the hospital prior to the decision to perform surgery, much information will already be available on his chart. The physician or surgeon often seeks last-minute information and laboratory findings to determine the patient's immediate condition and his fitness for surgery. For example, evidence of a respiratory infection would postpone the operation unless it was an emergency.

PREOPERATIVE ORDERS. The preoperative patient's needs include some special preparations which are ordered by the physician. These written orders, called preoperative orders, list the things that must be done before surgery is performed, in order to reduce the risk of complications during surgery and following it; they also make the patient more comfortable, especially when he understands why they are carried out and that a variety of personnel are involved.

Following is a list of things needing attention (not always all of them); many of these items are included in the preoperative orders:

1. *Food and fluid intake by mouth* will be ordered stopped at some time before the operation. The order generally reads; nothing by mouth after such and such a time. The patient's stomach should be empty when he goes to the operating room. It is a nursing responsibility to see that orders for nothing by mouth are strictly observed. A sign to that effect should be fastened to the bed or placed on the bedside table to remind personnel and the patient, if necessary.

2. *Additional parenteral fluids*, blood, or plasma may be ordered to improve the body's fluid and electrolyte balance and thus aid the patient's resistance to operative and postoperative complications. In fact, the fluids may be running while the patient is enroute to the operating room.

3. *A complete bath*, in bed or otherwise, depending upon the patient's condition, should precede skin preparation of the operative site. Special care should be taken to see that the skin (cosmetics removed), nails (polish removed), ears, hair, elbows, knees, heels, and umbilicus are clean. Nothing is more disturbing to operating room personnel than to discover inadequate personal cleanliness; it is a direct reflection on the patient's nursing care unless he was taken directly there upon admission.

For the female patient with long hair who may be confined to bed for considerable time following surgery, a special effort should be made to see that her hair is clean and arranged in braids.

Mouth care should be thorough, and if the patient wears dentures he should be told the evening before that they will be safely stored in his room when he goes to surgery. Special care is used to keep dentures in a safe place, but they should be visible so that they are not mistaken for something else and broken or lost.

4. *Valuables* such as money and jewelry are the responsibility of the family or are deposited with the hospital business office. The method for handling valuables varies from hospital to hospital; it is important to know how it is done at each place of employment. It is an unsafe practice to leave them unattended in the bedside table.

5. *Preparation of the operative site* means making it as free as possible from contaminating material and over a much wider area than just the place where the incision will be made. This often means shaving a large area. The person shaving the area must know the location and the extent of it. When you are responsible and have any doubts, ask the charge nurse or the physician to mark it off or specifically indicate the area. Figure 42–4 illustrates the extent of areas shaved.

Shaving should be thorough and all hairs on the area removed. A sharp razor and good light are essential. It may be necessary to go over the area two or three times to remove all signs of hair. Hair makes the removal of adhesive tape a painful process when dressings are changed.

6. *A cleansing enema* is ordered to empty the colon and rectum. For abdominal surgery this is essential, but it is given generally to prevent incontinence during the operation.

7. *A urine specimen* is usually ordered (a delay in getting this may mean a delay in surgery). Other tests may be ordered (e.g., blood count, bleeding time).

8. Taking the *temperature, pulse,* and *respirations* is a regular part of preoperative care. Any elevation of temperature is of concern to the surgeon and should be reported at once.

9. *Medications are ordered.* Most often there are two times for giving the patient medicine. A sleep medication is given the evening before surgery to enable the patient to relax and sleep well and a "preoperative medicine" is given about an hour or so before surgery (the exact time is specified). The purpose of the preoperative medication is usually two-

fold; to relax the patient, relieve his anxiety, and make it easier to administer the anesthetic; and to control secretions in the mouth and throat. This is one reason patients complain of dry mouth and lips after surgery.

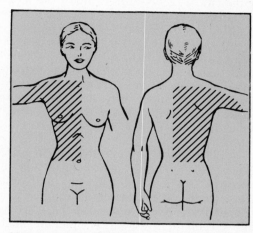

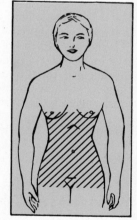 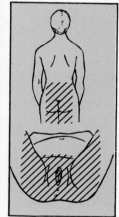

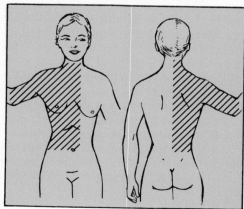

FIGURE 42–4 Preparation of several operative sites.

Commonly used preoperative drugs include morphine, scopolamine, and Demerol, among others.

Finish all preoperative measures *before* the preoperative medicine is given to enable the patient to receive full benefit from it. He should be as undisturbed as possible and not permitted out of bed after the drug is given.

FINAL PREPARATIONS. Patient care the morning of surgery should be well planned. The patient is usually called for or taken to the operating room 20 or 30 minutes before his scheduled operation. Any final preparation should be completed *before* the preoperative medication is given, and that should be given *on time*.

A clean gown is put on the patient; some hospitals also require special head and leg coverings. All jewelry, hair pins and ornaments, dentures, eyeglasses, hearing aids, or artificial body parts (e.g., artificial eye) are removed and safely stored. The patient should void before going to surgery; his bladder should be empty.

Identification of the patient is essential so that there is *no* error in his therapy. Each hospital has some means (tag or bracelet around the wrist) for doing this. Some provide it upon admission; others have tags to be filled out and tied to the person before he leaves his room for surgery.

When the above preparations are finished, the preoperative medication is given and the patient rests until he is taken to surgery.

THE PATIENT'S CHART. *All* treatment should be recorded with accuracy and the chart checked for completeness. The permission for surgery and the most recent laboratory reports should be attached. The chart either accompanies the patient or is picked up at a designated time. The nursing notes, laboratory reports, and any other information, e.g., x-rays, are important to the surgeon. He needs to know the patient's immediate condition and what has been done for him.

TRANSFER TO THE OPERATING ROOM. The patient, transported on a stretcher or in his own bed, is usually moved to the operating room by the attendant. Sufficient covering during this time protects the patient from drafts.

The nurse in charge of the operating room assumes charge of the patient upon his arrival. He should not be left unattended on the stretcher or bed because medications have made him sleepy and not responsible. The person bringing the patient to the operating room stays with him and retains the chart until some member of the operating room staff assumes direct responsibility.

Family members do not go to the operating room except by special permission. Conveniences for their well-being should be called to their attention if they are unfamiliar with regulations and surroundings. They should be told about how long it will be before the patient returns. If he is going to the recovery room, it will be longer than if he is brought directly back to his room.

SURGERY: INJURY BY CONSENT

Surgery is planned invasion of the body with the intent to cure, to reconstruct, diagnose or relieve symptoms; the surgeon(s) must have the consent of the person (or someone legally responsible) before the process begins.

The act of surgery disrupts body processes and causes body healing powers to come to the rescue of the injured tissues. It causes increased endocrine activity and influences metabolic processes — slowing some while increasing others. In its defense, the body conserves fluid (related to amount of blood lost), reduces urinary output and slows intestinal peristalsis.

Wound Healing

The injured area must have a newly created blood supply to bring nutrients for new cell formation and for power to rid the site of harmful organisms, dead cells, etc.

Wounds may heal by the following means:

1. Primary (by intention) — a clean cut wound closed by sutures or tightly bridged by adhesive bandage permitting no gaps. The scar will be slight.

2. Secondary (by granulation) — a gap between edges to be filled in by new tissue from the bottom and the sides. The scar will be more pronounced if excessive tissue needs to be replaced (e.g., wound infection, traumatic injury).

3. Tertiary — helping secondary healing by bringing wound edges together.

The pulses and temperature might be

slightly elevated as wound healing gets underway.

Postoperative Nursing Care

The type of anesthesia received by the patient determines many things about his postoperative care. Orders are written on the chart and accompany the patient.

Minor surgery usually involves a *local anesthetic*. The part to be operated is injected with a substance to deaden all local sensation. The excision of an ingrown toenail or the removal of a small skin tumor are examples. Some surgical treatments of the eyes or nose are performed under local anesthesia. Special nursing care for specific conditions is required, but many patients having minor surgery are returned directly to their rooms. Observation for bleeding is important for any postoperative patient. Orders for pain medication, diet, and any specific treatments are written on the chart in the operating room and accompany the patient.

Spinal anesthesia may be used for surgery of the abdomen. It is not used for surgery of the upper part of the body because it would paralyze the diaphragm. It consists of injecting an anesthetizing solution into a specific part of the spinal structure in the lumbar area of the back.

The patient may be awake during the operation but does not feel pain. He will be relaxed, sleepy, and without anxiety owing to his preoperative medication, but he is able to hear conversation; his eyes are usually covered and every care is used in talking so that he is not upset by what he hears.

The patient lies flat for several hours following surgery to prevent a headache if possible. If you assist with this patient's care, inform yourself of any special precautions relating to turning, using hot water bottles, observing respirations and pulse.

Orders for diet, fluids, and medications are specified.

Two complaints often noted after spinal anesthesia are headache and backache; they may continue for some time.

A *general anesthetic* puts the patient to sleep (unconsciousness). There are two common methods:

1. Inhaling vapors of certain gases or liquids. A mask is used over the mouth and nose or a tube is inserted into the trachea, the latter serving as an airway and providing for direct suction of accumulated secretions.

Some of the common types of gases and liquid include: ether (liquid), ethylene (gas), nitrous oxide (gas), cyclopropane (gas), and vinyl ether (gas). Oxygen is usually given along with the anesthetic.

2. Intravenous method. Certain anesthetizing drugs are introduced directly into the blood stream by vein. Pentothal is frequently used. The patient rapidly loses consciousness and recovers it the same way unless he has had a large dose of the drug.

Any patient who has had a general anesthetic requires specific and exacting nursing care immediately following surgery.

Most hospitals have a recovery room for meeting this patient's needs until he regains consciousness and seems to need less constant attention.

The recovery room, preferably close to the operating room, is equipped with beds, suction devices, oxygen, fluids, drugs, and every device to ensure proper recovery from a general anesthetic. Until the patient regains consciousness and his pulse, respiration, and blood pressure return to normal range, he needs close attention to his immediate needs.

Respiration and ability to breathe should be of first and continuous concern. The patient's head is turned to the side to allow for drainage of secretions (mucus, blood, emesis). A rubber nasal catheter attached to a suction device is gently inserted into the nasal passages to remove secretions and keep the airway free. Aspiration (breathing in) of emesis, blood, or the like can be a very dangerous thing. Observation for bleeding is almost continuous. Dressings are checked for bleeding as well as the area of the bed directly under the patient's body. It is possible for hemorrhage to occur without too much evidence on the dressings if the patient's position is such that the blood collects on the bed beneath him.

Intravenous fluid flow is checked, as are drainage tubes or other equipment attached to the patient.

Temperature, pulse, respiration, and blood pressure are taken and recorded frequently. Specific regulations govern the frequency of observations and recording.

Nursing the new operative patient in the recovery room requires keen observation, a knowledge of what to look for, the use of complex equipment, and extremely good judgment in observing the patient's vital signs and providing for his immediate needs. The practical nurse functions in Role II in carrying out selected tasks.

In the event there is no recovery room, any necessary equipment is taken to the patient's unit. His bed is prepared so that it is easy to remove him from the stretcher to the bed and cover him. The procedure for making the bed for the postoperative patient varies but it always provides for protection of the patient and the mattress. Bath blankets are used for additional warmth in some instances. They replace or cover the regular sheets.

Mouth wipes, tongue blades, emesis basin, suction equipment, and equipment to hold bottles of intravenous fluids are among the usual items ready for the patient's return.

Immediate observations include the following:

1. Check pulse and respirations.
2. See that air passages are open.
3. See if the patient is awake.
4. Check for bleeding.
5. Check the rate and flow of intravenous fluids.
6. See if drainage tubes are in place and in working order.
7. Keep the patient flat unless otherwise indicated.

If the patient is not awake, *stay with him;* his ability to breathe must be watched *until he is conscious* and until he is able to recognize his need for assistance if something should occur to hamper his breathing.

Unless contraindicated, the patient's position should be changed from time to time and parts of the body (back, knees, legs, arms) supported with pillows for comfort.

Turning the patient and getting him to cough and breathe deeply help to avert respiratory complications. Close attention is paid to urinary output. Offering the bedpan or urinal regularly may be sufficient to help reestablish regularity without catheterization. Frequently the inability to void is due to tenseness and a fear of being unable to do so because of not being used to a bedpan or urinal. The physician's orders may include getting the patient out of bed for this purpose. The patient's inability to void should be reported. Distention of the bladder is an unnecessary and uncomfortable condition.

Orders for medications, fluids, diet, positioning, voiding, ambulation, and special treatments are on the chart.

Sufficient fluid intake should be encouraged and observed. A special order to push fluids means that the fluids should be available to the patient and that he should be encouraged to take them.

Movement in bed is helpful to a patient in many ways unless his condition indicates otherwise. Body alignment and support are important factors in his comfort and well-being.

EARLY AMBULATION

This means getting the patient out of bed relatively soon after surgery; it has many direct patient benefits.

Early ambulation decreases complications. Being up and in a normal position helps body functions to return to normal. Circulation is improved, muscle tone returns, and healing is promoted; stasis (standing still) of blood and other body fluids is prevented. Clots in the veins of the lower extremities are a common complication and it is felt that improved circulation helps to prevent this. Digestive and elimination processes are improved also. Patients are not so apt to have gas pains or difficulty in voiding and having bowel movements. While fatigue should be avoided, the exercise of moving about helps to promote sleep.

When the patient is to sit on the edge of the bed, walk to a chair, and sit down or walk down the hall is determined by the physician. It may be much sooner than some patients feel they are ready, and they need reassurance that it is helpful to move about.

Planning Nursing Care

Getting a patient up, especially for the first time, requires planning and observation. Older patients and those with casts and other impeding conditions require more time and assistance. They should not feel hurried and you should plan how you are going to manage them before you start.

The patient's reaction, color, pulse, and respiration are observed closely. Any change in condition is an indication that the patient should be returned to bed and the observations reported.

Moving about in bed and out allows the patient to be more independent. Self-care, totally or in part, is possible and should be encouraged. In planning his self-care, equipment should be available and sufficient time allowed for him to use it. Dressings may need to be changed, and appetite, intake, urinary output, and elimination need to be observed as well as the condition of his operative site.

CONVALESCENCE

While early ambulation is an accepted practice and many patients go home soon after an operation, some medical-surgical patients must remain in the hospital for convalescence and rehabilitation.

When convalescence is slow, the patient has periods of discouragement. You can help him to understand that time is essential to his recovery and encourage him to carry on as many daily activities as he is able. A feeling of independence is an important factor in convalescence and rehabilitation.

Special treatments, exercises, and diversion are a planned part of recovery. The treatments and exercises have written orders; diversion may not, but it is essential during a long convalescence. Show interest in his need for diversions by making suggestions or commenting on those he does pursue.

The family will be informed by the physician about the patient's progress but will have questions to ask the nurse as well. You may need to direct some of these questions to the nurse in charge, but some you can answer yourself. The important thing is to use good judgment in trying to help family members.

LEAVING THE HOSPITAL

Getting ready to leave the hospital may seem like an easy thing for a patient. It is, when he and the family are not burdened with an unpaid hospital bill, an uncertain health future for the patient, or the proper means for his care. While it is not the responsibility of the practical nurse to solve such problems, any undue patient or family concern should be noted and reported. If they need help to understand how some of these needs can be met, the hospital (physician, nurse, social service department, business office, and dietary department) can provide this assistance.

Plans for Home and Follow-up Care

The patient's needs determine what care must follow.

Some conditions require daily attention. For example, the patient who has had a colostomy needs help to know how to handle his daily hygiene habits, his diet, and his feelings about his condition. This training should start long before he leaves the hospital so that he and the family know what to expect when the patient goes home. You may not be responsible for any such training, but your understanding and encouragement will help the patient and the family to make necessary adjustments. Another example is the patient who has had an amputation. The family needs to know how to accept the patient back into the family circle, how to help him maintain his fullest independence mentally and physically. Help for the patient actually starts before surgery and continues through his entire hospitalization. Mention is made of these two examples because you, while not responsible for this planned care, as a team member should support all such efforts. This means you need to understand the general plan of approach to each patient's care.

The physician may order special drugs, equipment, or both, to be used at home. Sometimes this is available for purchase from the hospital; when it is not, directions for purchase should be given if needed.

Follow-up care in the physician's office or outpatient clinics or by the public health nurse will be explained by the physician. The patient may have questions he hesitates to ask him and waits to ask the nurse. This may be a practical nurse, and you should not hesitate to seek help for him if you cannot or should not try to answer them. See Chapter 34, Patient Discharge.

SPECIAL TREATMENTS AND MEASURES

The physician has a variety of therapies and measures he uses to help him diagnose and treat the patient; new ones are being added every day. The practical nurse is not always involved in these therapies, but if your patient is, you need to be aware of what is happening to him.

INHALATION THERAPY

The word inhalation indicates that treatment is by way of the lungs. The most common example is providing the patient with extra *oxygen*. Another common example is the administration of air or oxygen laden with *water* vapor (croup tent or vaporizer). Others include *antibiotics* in compressed air called aerosols, a water-detergent mixture requiring special equipment (Alevaire), and bronchodilator drugs inhaled for relief of breathing distress (e.g., in asthma or emphysema).

The Bird respirator is a device used to force air (oxygen) under pressure into the lungs. This is a type of positive pressure mask.

Inhalation therapy is a specialized type of treatment requiring the services of specially trained persons called inhalation therapists. The therapist administers the prescribed treatment and is responsible for checking the patient and the equipment being used.

Oxygen Therapy

PURPOSE OF OXYGEN THERAPY. The therapeutic use of oxygen is for one main purpose—to provide more oxygen to the body having an oxygen need. The cause of this need may be one of several things; obstruction in the respiratory tract, poor blood circulation, asphyxiation, and so forth. The body needs a certain amount of oxygen to function adequately; when something occurs to prevent proper amounts of oxygen from being available throughout the body, a higher concentration of it by oxygen tent, nasal catheter, or mask helps the body to meet this need.

ADMINISTRATION OF OXYGEN. To safely administer the proper concentration and pressure of oxygen requires certain skills and background knowledge. The inhalation therapist is trained to do this and to observe the patient's reactions in carrying out the treatment ordered by the physician.

The practical nurse gives nursing care to patients receiving oxygen and must be aware of any signs of respiratory distress, such as cyanosis, anoxia, or dyspnea. In addition, several other factors concerning the patient's safety and comfort should be mentioned.

1. When a cylinder of oxygen is at the bedside, it should be strapped to the head of the bed to prevent its falling and thus avoid injury to the patient, others, or the equipment.

2. When oxygen is being used, *no smoking* should be allowed. Oxygen supports combustion and is dangerous to use in the presence of any spark or flame. Visitors as well as the patient need to know the importance of this regulation, and NO SMOKING signs should be placed for all to see; even then frequent reminders may be necessary.

3. Electrical appliances should not be used; a spark might result in an explosion. A hand bell is used instead of the usual call bell.

4. Cotton rather than wool blankets are used for patient warmth.

5. All oil or grease is kept away from the regulating equipment and away from the patient's unit.

6. When an oxygen tent is used, every precaution must be taken to tuck in the top of the tent under the mattress. The bottom of the tent is enfolded in the top sheet which is tucked under the side of the mattress. A rubber sheet is placed over that portion of the mattress covered by the tent to avoid the escape of oxygen into the mattress.

7. Be familiar with the proper amount of oxygen each patient should be receiving, observe for proper readings during each patient contact.

8. Patients receiving oxygen will need many things done for them to conserve their energy.

9. Patient comfort includes such things as meticulous care of the skin around the nose and face where a nasal catheter has been inserted and then taped to the face; it should be taped to the cheek rather than the forehead to prevent pressure within the nostril.

Some patients do not like the feeling of being enclosed in an oxygen tent; they feel that they are too set apart from others and thus may not be able to make their needs known. You can help them by explaining how they can summon assistance. It is reassuring to them, too, if their care is thorough and attention is given to the details of their comfort. Frequent checking with the patient also helps.

PARENTERAL FLUIDS

The most commonly used means for giving a patient additional fluids other than by mouth is through a vein directly into the blood. This is called *intravenous infusion*. The physician uses this therapy to replace lost body fluids and reestablish fluid and electrolyte balance as well as to administer drugs and nourishment. Whatever the fluid and the substances added to it, the physician writes the order and in many instances starts the therapy. As for the LPN starting intravenous infusions, the question of legality should be determined *first*. There seems to be little or no evidence that it is a legal practice at this time. It can be her responsibility to observe the rate of flow and to see that the fluids do not enter the tissues at the needle site. Be sure that the arm or leg (receiving the fluid) remains immobilized so that the needle does not move out of its location in the vein. Another practical nursing responsibility might be to help keep track of the amount of fluid the patient is to receive within a given length of time, if this has been prescribed. The system for keeping track should be worked out by the nursing team.

Patients receiving parenteral fluids usually are required to remain in fairly fixed positions for hours. The site of the injection influences how much mobility, if any, can be allowed. Children and infants in particular present problems; they are not easily confined and do not understand the reasons for it; the same is true for a confused patient.

Pertinent observations are recorded; time required, amount, type of fluid, any additives, urinary output, and untoward signs, such as shortness of breath, which might indicate pulmonary edema and the infiltration of local tissues. You will not be responsible for recording the amount and the kind of fluid; the person who starts the infusion is.

Blood and blood derivative transfusions are considered medical uses of blood (i.e., treatments). The important first step, of course, is to cross-match blood so that the patient receives a blood type compatible with his, in order to avoid the serious result of a toxic reaction which can cause death.

One serious problem is screening donor blood for hepatitis virus. Many hundreds of deaths each year are caused by hepatitis (liver disorder) from blood transfusions. The Food and Drug Administration has started to regulate the screening of blood donors and testing for hepatitis virus at all federally regulated collection centers.

A subcutaneous infusion is the administration of fluids under the skin. Sites for this are the lateral aspects of the thighs, the axilla, and the back. Because some solutions irritate subcutaneous tissues, they cannot be administered this way.

Parenteral fluid therapy is so common and requires such definite skills to administer that teams of personnel are specially trained to do this in many hospitals. They not only learn how to start the process, but have the knowledge to make critical observations regarding the patient's reactions. As an LPN, you also observe the patient while with him and are responsible for reporting any untoward signs or symptoms at once. Your observations are as important as any other team member. In fact, in some instances, you may be asked to remain with the patient for the purpose of watching for specific reactions; this is another example of Role II function.

SUCTION

Suction is not a therapy; it is a measure used to suck or aspirate unwanted fluids and secretions from body cavities or openings. The sucking action is created by an electric machine or by hand with a syringe of some type.

The practical nurse uses suction mainly to keep the patient's mouth and nose free of fluids and mucus to maintain a clear air passage. The chief things to remember about nasal or mouth suction are the following:

1. A syringe or catheter used in the nose is *not* also used in the mouth.

2. Each type of suction machine is designed to be operated in a certain way for desired results. Familiarize yourself with the equipment *before* using it. The directions are usually right on the machine.

3. For patient comfort and safety to nasal and mouth tissues: (a) Observe the catheter markings for insertion to avoid overinserting it. (b) Insert the catheter *before* turning on the suction; use a rolling or turning motion as you withdraw it, thus avoiding a pull on the tissues. If you must turn on the machine before inserting the catheter, *be sure it is pinched off* so that there is no suction during insertion. (c) Listen during the process; if the catheter becomes clogged, remove it and flush it out.

4. Record the time, amount, and character of secretions (color, consistency) and any patient reactions.

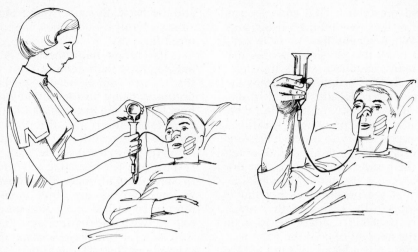

FIGURE 42–5   Left, the nurse is shown pouring the tube feeding into an Asepto syringe, which is being used as a funnel. The tube is kinked while the syringe is being filled. Right, the feeding is permitted to flow through the tube by gravity. Before the syringe is empty, more of the feeding will be added. The patient is encouraged to help with the procedure.

TUBE FEEDINGS (NASOGASTRIC TUBE)

Before going on, return to Figure 11–4 and notice the area within the circle. This shows where the air route crosses the food route. It is essential that the person inserting a tube into a patient's stomach understand the very real danger of getting the tube into the lungs by mistake.

Feeding a patient through a tube means that for some reason he is unable to take food by mouth (Fig. 42–5). The Levin tube is passed through a nostril, into the pharynx, and down the esophagus into the stomach (Fig. 42–6). The proper length for insertion may or may not be marked on the outside of the tube. The tube is secured in place by taping it to the cheek (to avoid pull against the nostrils) after it has been determined that the lower end is in the stomach. One way to determine this is to place the outside end of the tube in water; if bubbles appear, *do not* proceed to feed the patient; the tube in all probability is in the lungs. In fact, one should check this possibility before each feeding in case the tube has moved since the last feeding.

The physician orders the diet, stating the amount and time for each feeding; the patient assists when possible.

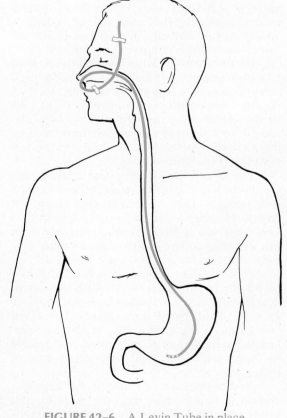

FIGURE 42–6   A Levin Tube in place.

POSTURAL DRAINAGE

In postural drainage, the patient is placed in a position with his head lower than the part to be drained so that gravity can help remove the unwanted secretions. This measure is carried out according to the physician's order (type of position, how often, how long). Sometimes the patient's bed can be adjusted to the desired position, but not always. Be sure you understand how the patient is to be positioned, how long, and how frequently. Every possible means to make the patient comfortable should be used during this procedure; even then, some patients (especially the elderly) cannot tolerate a "severe" position without becoming faint and dizzy; the danger is that the patient may fall. Encourage the positioned patient to help the drainage process by coughing and taking deep breaths.

RADIATION THERAPY

Radiation therapy is used to destroy the growth and reproduction of body cells. It is a treatment used to discourage the growth of cancerous cells in body tissue.

The therapeutic use of radioactive materials is hazardous to the therapist as well as to the patient if the control and use of these materials are not accurately carried out. This makes it a highly specialized type of therapy handled only by persons skilled in the use and control of the equipment as well as a knowledge of tissue reaction to the treatment.

Patients may experience what is called radiation sickness (diarrhea, vomiting, nausea, loss of appetite, fluid and electrolyte imbalance in severe cases) and are apt to show signs of being under stress and emotional strain. The nurse needs to recognize this and to accept the patient's behavior as it is.

DIAGNOSTIC TESTS

Today the physician has a great many diagnostic tests he can use if there is a clinical laboratory at hand equipped to handle them. He uses test findings to diagnose the patient's condition and prescribe needed treatment.

It is not the purpose of this brief discussion to single out any but the more commonly used tests with which you may be involved.

The practical nurse has the responsibility to collect some types of specimens and to assist in the collection of some others, depending on the situation. Some tests are carried out entirely by the physician. You need to know what type of specimen the physician seeks. You do not have to interpret laboratory findings.

Four body discharges commonly used for diagnostic tests which often involve the practical nurse are urine, feces, sputum, and vomitus.

The main thing to remember in collecting a specimen is to follow the procedure carefully to secure the best possible results. The laboratory is limited in its effectiveness if the specimen is questionable. The patient bears additional expense when tests have to be repeated.

Patients sometimes become upset when they are told that the physician has ordered a test. They wonder what it is for, how much it costs, and if it will hurt; they also become tired as the result of experiencing certain tests. Show that you understand their concern, and if a patient needs an explanation concerning a test that you cannot give or should not try to give, let the charge nurse or the physician know about the problem. When you are in a position to explain what you are going to do, use simple explanations, especially with children or people who speak another language.

WHO IS THE MEDICAL-SURGICAL PATIENT?

By now, it should be clear that the medical-surgical patient may be of any age—old, young, or in between—and that he can be a bed or ambulatory patient. He may be critically or mildly ill. His illness may require a long recovery period; or it may never be cured but only held under control; or the patient may be made comfortable until life ceases.

The medical-surgical patient may actually be a medical patient who has had surgery and has returned to being a medical patient again. By now, too, you are aware that each patient experiencing the various diseases and disorders discussed in the following chapters brings with him his basic living needs. The plan for his care involves these basic needs. You are required to make special adaptations to meet his particular needs at a given time. These adaptations are influenced by the severity of the disease as well as by the signs and symptoms it produces. In addition to these factors, the adaptations you make will be influenced by how much or how little a patient can do for himself.

Certain factors influence the nursing care plan for any medical-surgical patient and the meeting of his individual needs. These include:

1. Age.
2. The disease or disorder and its severity.
3. The signs and symptoms of illness present.
4. The physician's orders for medical treatment.
5. The degree to which a patient can or cannot participate in self-care.
6. The patient's attitude toward his illness and his will to live.

SUMMARY

Labeling a patient "medical" or "surgical" tells little about his particular nursing needs. The kind of assistance a patient needs is influenced by age, disease or disorder, degree of severity, the physician's orders, signs and symptoms present, ability to participate in self-care, and the patient's attitude toward illness.

Patients categorized as medical-surgical include those in all age groups, even though young patients may be set apart in a special hospital area known as the pediatric area and the elderly patients grouped in a geriatric area. The hospital accommodates patients in a variety of ways according to age groups, illness, need for specialized equipment, degree of illness, and need to be protected from infection.

Today's hospital is equipped to provide a wide variety of special services and therapeutic measures involving complicated equipment and procedures. Personnel other than nurses are trained to carry out many of these services; many deal directly with patients and their well-being. This requires teamwork on the part of everyone doing things for and with patients.

If the hospital is to be a safe place for patients and personnel, personnel must develop and use suitable techniques with respect to the germ theory of disease and have conviction about practicing accordingly.

Surgical asepsis is action taken to prevent infection from reaching a wound or body cavity. Medical asepsis is action taken to prevent infection from leaving its source.

A medical-surgical patient's disease is not nursed; the patient is nursed because he has a disease or disorder that has disabled him with its signs and symptoms.

Knowing what is done to treat signs/symptoms and to provide appropriate nursing care is more important for the LPN than being able to recite the names, etiology and pathology of long lists of diseases.

GUIDES FOR STUDY AND DISCUSSION

1. Who is the medical-surgical patient? How is he sometimes "housed" in the hospital?

2. In medicine there is the general practitioner and the specialist. As you understand it, what is the difference?

3. If your hospital is close by, find out how many different patient areas there are (by name), how many special therapy/treatment areas, and what other service areas are there.

4. What is asepsis? What does handwashing have to do with it? In giving nursing care, when should you wash your hands?

5. What is surgical asepsis? What is medical asepsis? To which asepsis is isolation technique related?

6. What is meant by the term "sterile technique"? Be ready to discuss the eleven rules described in this chapter that caution you about safe sterile technique practice.

7. How can you help the preoperative patient and his family feel confident that he is in good hands?

8. What is the patient's state of dependency in the recovery room? What is done to meet his immediate needs? How can suffocation and strangulation of this patient be prevented?

SUGGESTED SITUATIONS AND ACTIVITIES

1. Following is a chart to help you summarize the chief precautions/responsibilities you will have with respect to some common treatments and measures. Duplicate the chart in your notebook, allowing plenty of room to include your remarks.

Treatment-Measure	LPN Responsibilities
Inhalation Therapy	
oxygen	
water vapor	
water-detergent mixture	
antibiotics	
Bird respirator	
Parenteral Fluids	
intravenous infusion	
blood transfusion	
subcutaneous infusion	
Suction	
Tube Feedings	
Levin tube	
Postural Drainage	
Radiation Therapy	
Diagnostic Tests	
urine	
feces	
sputum	
vomitus	

CHAPTER 43

PATIENTS WITH CANCER

TOPICAL HEADINGS

Introduction
What Is Cancer?
How Prevalent Is
    Cancer?

Present-Day Treat-
    ments and Outlook
Attitudes Toward
    Cancer
Types of Cancer

Summary
Guides for Study and
    Discussion
Suggested Situations
    and Activities

OBJECTIVES FOR THE STUDENT: Be able to:

1. Give two reasons why a diagnosis of cancer raises fear in the minds of a patient and his family.
2. Name three factors in the treatment of cancer that represent hopefulness.
3. Explain the terms neoplasm and neoplastic cell.
4. Compare the growth pattern of the normal cell with the neoplastic cell.
5. List the types of health workers who make up the cancer team today.
6. Name the two essential factors in a favorable prognosis.
7. List the seven danger signals which require early medical advice.
8. Describe one way a practical nurse can show the cancer patient that she has a positive attitude toward his condition.
9. Name three therapies used for treating cancer patients.

SUGGESTED STUDY VOCABULARY*

neoplasm
neoplastic cell
mitosis
metastasis

prognosis
mastectomy
biopsy
leukemia

anemia
carcinoma
melanoma
sarcoma
dyspepsia

*Look for any terms you already know.

INTRODUCTION

Perhaps no diagnosis stirs a patient and his family more than the diagnosis of cancer. The person's mind jumps to the conclusion of early death preceded by severe pain and suffering. Such attitudes create endless fear and anxiety for the patient and his family.

The purpose of this chapter is twofold. The first is to point out what cancer is and is not, how prevalent it is, therapies being used, and what attitudes health workers and patients too often have toward it. The second is to point out some common types of cancer, some common signs and symptoms, and some specific nursing problems associated with patient care.

Cancer may attack any type of body tissue. It has no respect for body systems and attacks all of them, although not with the same frequency.

Review Chapter 6 and study the normal cell, with its orderly manner of working and reproducing itself. This review will help you compare normal cell activity with the abnormal activity of the cancer cell.

WHAT IS CANCER?

One might start answering this question by saying what cancer is not. It is not inherited as such in humans; however, there may be a hereditary tendency toward it. Cancer is not contagious. It is neither a hopeless nor an untreatable problem. Cancer is not caused by bruises, and it does not lead to early death in *every* patient.

You will recall from Chapter 6 that under ordinary, normal body conditions, cell division is a very orderly process. A normal cell subdivides in a predictable manner, which in turn controls cell population. How this process works is not understood.

Cancer is the name given to cell growth that seems to run away with itself, without regard for the normal cells growing around it. Cancer cells seem to thrive in their own independent way quite apart from the checks and balances which control the orderly mitosis of normal cells.

Two terms frequently used to mean cancer are *neoplasm* and *neoplastic*. Neoplasm means a new tissue mass (tumor). Neoplastic cell means a lively-growing cell responsible for producing the tumor. Not all neoplastic cells grow at the same rate; in fact, some may grow no faster than normal cells.

For some time it was felt that neoplastic growth started from the uncontrolled growth of one "wild" cell and spread from that point; but it is now apparent that neoplastic cells may appear in various locations in an area and organ and produce patches of cancer, seemingly at the same time.

One characteristic of neoplastic cells is their ability to invade or attack tissue. Some types invade tissues more readily than others. Cancer cells seem to be able to quickly enter or penetrate normal cells and tissues and disrupt their functions. This disruption ac-

CANCER SPREADS BY SEVERAL ROUTES

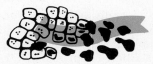

1. By direct extension into neighboring tissue

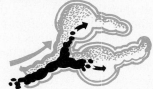

2. By permeation along lymphatic vessels

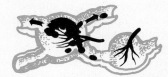

3. By embolism via lymphatic vessels to the lymph nodes

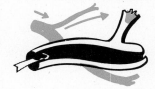

4. By embolism via blood vessels

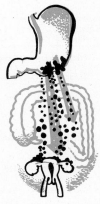

5. By diffusion within a body cavity

FIGURE 43–1 Cancer spreads by several routes. (A Cancer Source Book for Nurses, American Cancer Society, Inc.)

counts for some of the signs and symptoms of the disease. For example, when normal nerve coverings are invaded, pain can result; when blood vessel walls are invaded, hemorrhage can result.

Cancer is really a "family" term for a disease which behaves in a variety of ways in different body tissues and has special names when it does. Some neoplastic cell behavior is strange. Its growth pattern cannot always be predicted. Medical scientists are trying to determine why neoplastic cells grow as they do. What causes the uncontrolled cell population to behave as it does is the subject of much research. At present it seems that the endocrine system plays an important role; certain endocrine factors seem to be related to cancer of the breast, prostate gland, and thyroid gland.

The spread of cancer is known as *metastasis*; the disease appears in one location, then another location, and so forth. Neoplastic cells can enter the blood and lymphatics and spread the disease in this manner as well as by direct cell invasion. Metastasis of cancer is not thoroughly understood as yet. See Figure 43–1 and notice the several ways cancer spreads.

New tissue masses or tumors that are not cancerous are called *benign*; they do not tend to spread elsewhere, but may do so. However, a benign tumor may become large enough to cause local pressure, pain, obstruction, or displacement of surrounding tissues and organs, even if it remains noncancerous.

HOW PREVALENT IS CANCER?

Cancer ranks second as a cause of death among all people in this country. Cancer has no respect for age; it occurs among all age groups, but it becomes more prevalent as people grow older.

Some types of cancer are more common than others. For example, among all types, cancer of the breast in middle-aged women is the most common and is the leading cause of death in that group. Lung cancer is on the increase among both men and women. Research is concerned with trying to determine what direct influence cigarette smoking, smog, and other air pollutants have on this increase.

Table 43–1 shows the most frequent

TABLE 43–1. MORTALITY, FIVE LEADING CANCER SITES, AGE GROUPS AND SEX

	All Ages Male	Female	Under 15 Male	Female	Age 15-34 Male	Female	Age 35-54 Male	Female	Age 55-74 Male	Female	Age 75 and Over Male	Female
1	Lung	Breast	Leukemia	Leukemia	Leukemia	Breast	Lung	Breast	Lung	Breast	Prostate	Colon, Rectum
	45,383	27,985	1,107	856	695	459	8,365	8,617	29,479	13,328	8,893	8,652
2	Colon, Rectum	Colon, Rectum	Brain	Brain	Hodgkin's Disease	Leukemia	Colon, Rectum	Uterus	Colon, Rectum	Colon, Rectum	Lung	Breast
	21,041	22,472	520	387	476	435	2,404	3,641	11,508	10,929	7,363	5,576
3	Prostate	Uterus	Lympho-sarcoma, etc.	Kidney	Brain	Uterus	Pancreas	Colon, Rectum	Prostate	Uterus	Colon, Rectum	Stomach
	16,345	13,143	179	126	360	351	1,443	2,711	7,160	6,503	6,947	2,855
4	Stomach	Ovary	Bone	Bone	Testis, etc.	Hodgkin's Disease	Brain	Lung	Pancreas	Ovary	Stomach	Uterus
	10,396	9,168	105	94	349	318	1,303	2,464	5,702	4,972	3,520	2,639
5	Pancreas	Lung	Kidney	Lympho-sarcoma, etc.	Lympho-sarcoma, etc.	Brain	Stomach	Ovary	Stomach	Lung	Pancreas	Pancreas
	9,696	9,024	82	75	275	246	1,289	2,457	5,516	4,712	2,495	2,549

Source: Vital Statistics of the United States, 1967

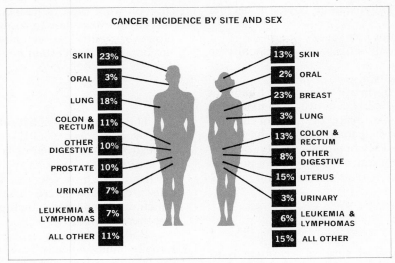

CANCER INCIDENCE BY SITE AND SEX

	Male		Female	
SKIN	23%		13%	SKIN
ORAL	3%		2%	ORAL
LUNG	18%		23%	BREAST
COLON & RECTUM	11%		3%	LUNG
OTHER DIGESTIVE	10%		13%	COLON & RECTUM
PROSTATE	10%		8%	OTHER DIGESTIVE
URINARY	7%		15%	UTERUS
LEUKEMIA & LYMPHOMAS	7%		3%	URINARY
ALL OTHER	11%		6%	LEUKEMIA & LYMPHOMAS
			15%	ALL OTHER

FIGURE 43–2 Cancer incidence by site and sex. (Prepared by Epidemiology and Statistics Department of the American Cancer Society.)

types of cancer by age. Notice what is common among children, adolescents, and adults. Compare the sites (organs) affected in children under 15 years with those of people over 75.

Figure 43–2 points up the prevalence of fatal cancer in body organs by sex. Compare the incidence rates between males and females for the various parts of the body.

PRESENT-DAY TREATMENTS AND OUTLOOK

Surgery was once the chief treatment for cancer patients. The surgeon would perform extensive (radical)surgery to try to completely remove the diseased tissue, hopeful that "all" was removed and that the patient would recover. This is no longer the case. Instead of just the surgeon fighting the disease, a team approach is becoming more common. The medical specialist and the medical x-ray specialist join the surgeon in a long-range effort to treat and cure this patient. Treatment is continuous. The patient is watched to see if, or to what extent, treatment is beneficial, or whether treatment should be changed, increased or decreased. Other members of the enlarged team are the skilled nurse, the social service worker, the official and voluntary health agencies, and the research laboratories.

Cancer is treatable, and most patients benefit from treatment. The benefits may be complete cure, long-term arrest giving the patient long-term well-being, or symptom relief for patients with rapidly worsening conditions.

The word cure is used with hesitation when treating a cancer patient because it takes time to tell whether surgery or cobalt or drugs or a combination of these treatments does cure the patient. It is generally felt that if there is no recurrence within a five-year period the patient may be considered cured.

Efforts are made to urge patients not to seek quack remedies for quick cancer cures. Despite such warning, many patients do.

Early detection and prompt, proper treatment have always been essential factors in a favorable prognosis. The absence of any treatment leads to fatality. The federal government is trying to bring detection and treatment services closer to the people. Also, it is spending large amounts of money to find a cure(s). The National Cancer Act of 1971 provides for more than 1.5 billion dollars (over a three year period) for finding cancer causes and a cure(s).

The American Cancer Society lists the following *seven danger signals* to help people realize the need to seek medical advice early:

1. Any unusual bleeding or discharge.

2. A lump or thickening in the breast or elsewhere.

3. A sore that does not heal.

4. Persistent change in bowel or bladder habits.

5. Persistent hoarseness or cough.

6. Persistent indigestion or difficulty in swallowing.

7. Change in a wart or mole.

The three forms of acceptable treatment are surgery, radiation, and drugs. In using one or more of these forms, the patient and his family must be helped to feel hopeful rather than hopeless. This requires honesty, sympathy, and encouragement on the part of persons who share in the patient's medical and nursing care.

Surgical Treatment

The purpose of surgical treatment is to remove the local growth, including marginal normal tissue and area lymph nodes. This "wide area" excision of tissue is called radical surgery (e.g., radical mastectomy) (see Fig. 43–3).

The decision to perform surgery is sometimes a difficult one for the surgeon and the patient. Factors to be considered include the patient's age, general condition, will to live, evidence of type and extent of cancer, and disfigurement or disability which may result. If the surgeon feels that surgery will give the patient a reasonable chance of cancer arrest, he is likely to urge this treatment.

A *biopsy* or examination of a tissue sample taken from the patient indicates to the surgeon what type of neoplastic cells are involved; this helps him to know what to expect. However, until he actually performs the surgery, he is not certain how widespread the disease might be.

Radiation Treatment

The purpose of radiation treatment is to destroy all neoplastic cells. It is impossible not to destroy some normal cells in the process; the location of the cancer, whether or not it is localized, and how sensitive the local normal cells are to radioactive materials are factors which determine how much normal cell damage there will be.

Radiation therapy is used externally, internally, and topically. Sources for internal use include radioactive substances inserted in a body cavity (e.g., uterus) and those administered orally which seek and locate in a particular type of tissue (e.g., radioactive iodine localizes in the thyroid gland).

Topical use of radioactive material means concentrating a source of radioactive matter, such as inserting radium needles or seeds into a tumor. This method is used to strike directly at the neoplastic cells without harm (or with minimum harm) to surrounding normal cells.

Examples of radioactive drugs are:

1. *Radioactive gold* (radio-gold colloid)—used for intracavity injections.

2. *Radioactive iodine* (Radiocaps)—given orally.

3. *Radioactive phosphorus* (Sodium Radiophosphate, Phosphotope)—given orally, intravenously, and topically.

The dosage of any of these drugs is adjusted for each individual patient; he is observed for signs of toxicity.

Drug Therapy

Radioactive drugs are discussed in the preceding paragraphs. At present, no drug has been found to cure cancer. Many drugs are used to control pain (analgesics); as a rule, narcotics are not used for pain early in a patient's illness owing to their habit-forming nature. Analgesics commonly used include aspirin, Empirin, codeine, methadone, Demerol, morphine, Pantopon, Dilaudid, and Metopon hydrochloride.

Chemotherapy has become an estab-

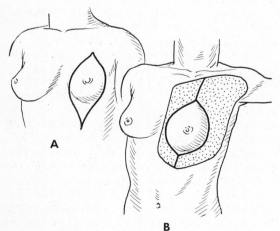

FIGURE 43–3 Incisions for a simple (*A*) and radical (*B*) mastectomy.

lished part of cancer treatment, and the list of such drugs is long and changes as new ones are discovered. Each patient must be observed closely to note any unwanted side effects. The physician often uses the laboratory to check for possible side effects. Overuse of a treatment may lead to severe toxicity which can cause death. Signs of toxicity vary, but some of the signs include sores in the mouth, nausea, vomiting, diarrhea, and skin rashes.

One type of chemotherapy involves the use of hormones, including estrogens and androgens. Adrenal hormones, such as ACTH and cortisone, are also used.

Other forms of chemotherapy include the use of nitrogen mustards, Myleran, Leukeran, and other cell-poisoning drugs. *Antimetabolites* are drugs used, in combination with other drugs, to treat such diseases as acute leukemia; they do not cure the disease but often produce remissions.

New drugs for cancer treatment appear at a rapid rate; some have a proven value (for some types of cancer) while others do not. Serious side effects often accompany various drug therapies and require supportive therapy (i.e., antibiotics to reduce the frequency of infection).

Vitamin supplements and other drugs are often used. Large doses of vitamin supplements are almost always ordered. In addition, iron (ferrous sulfate) is commonly ordered along with ascorbic acid if anemia is present. Appetite boosters (e.g., alcohol) may be ordered before meals.

Immunotherapy

Work is underway to stimulate a patient's own immunity against cancer, possibly by transferring immunity from immunized donors or by the use of a vaccine.

Nonspecific Treatments

NUTRITION. Nourishment may have to be provided by tube feeding if the mouth tissues are edematous or are being treated by radiation, or if the normal food route to the stomach is otherwise interrupted. The patient must consume a nutritious diet, one fortified with body-building nutrients to offset the heavy demands made upon body tissues in the case of the patient with a rapidly worsening condition. The convalescent patient should have extra-nourishing foods to help the body regain strength.

A poor appetite (anorexia) is a problem calling for unusual efforts to serve attractive meals, favorite foods, and small portions; large servings discourage a person who has little or no desire to eat. In-between meal nourishment can be offered to boost the nutritional intake.

EMOTIONAL SUPPORT. As mentioned previously, a diagnosis of cancer stirs the patient and his family to feelings of fear and hopelessness. There is a constant need to support this patient by listening to his concerns, paying attention to the details of his care so that he does not feel by-passed, bearing a presence that is positive, sympathetic, and understanding, and being available. It is difficult to say what crosses a patient's mind if and when he is able to contemplate his condition; in all likelihood he wants to know that someone is available and interested in him and his condition.

ATTITUDES TOWARD CANCER

The fact that there is no known or positive cure for cancer should not prevent health team members from taking a positive attitude toward patient care. It is a known fact that many patients are cured and many live long, active years. For those patients who have a rapidly worsening condition, their symptoms can be relieved more effectively than in the past; they can be more comfortable. This fact should guide effective nursing action in a positive rather than a negative way. If the patient can experience some sense of well-being, he can find some purpose for living, and the quality of his survival improves. Part of this purpose is found in the positive way health team members help him do it. Their attitudes and relationships with the patient must reflect a living-for-today spirit, a hopeful climate that helps the patient and his family realize that he is receiving care rather than neglect or hurried nursing that indicates no hope.

Three words which can guide action are *honesty, sympathy* and *encouragement*. The physician must decide what the patient and his family are to be told; other team members should honestly support his approach. No one should have to be reminded to be sympathetic or encouraging. The patient needs to feel these qualities in every contact he has with nursing and other personnel. Nothing about nurse-to-patient contact should leave the patient with a feeling of neglect, of being uncared for, or that his plight is hopeless.

Team members can help the patient and his family to believe that he can be independent, involved in self-care, and productive for a longer time than was thought possible in the past. This outlook helps the patient to live with a purpose and maintain his will to live.

TYPES OF CANCER

As mentioned previously, cancer may start in or spread to any type of body tissue. There are special names for the many types of cancer cells, but each type has some distinguishing features about it (e.g., its place of origin, its behavior) which help the physician make a diagnosis and start appropriate treatment.

Three major types of cancer are:

1. *Carcinomas*—they invade the skin, the lining of body cavities, organs, and glandular tissues (e.g., breast, prostate). Organs and systems involved include the mouth, respiratory system, digestive system, genitourinary system, breast, brain and central nervous system, and skin.

2. *Sarcomas*—they invade bones, cartilage, fat, and nerves.

3. *Leukemias*—they invade blood-forming tissues, causing overpopulation of immature white cells.

The term *lymphoma* is a general term applied to a cancerous disorder of the lymphoid tissue (e.g., Hodgkin's disease).

The following sections include general information about the common types of cancer, treatments and nursing care. Keep in mind that the patient with cancer is concerned about the outcome, if he is capable of understanding. Therefore, it is essential for you to have a positive attitude toward assisting the patient in meeting his daily living needs. He needs to feel that his situation is hopeful rather than hopeless.

CARCINOMA

Skin Cancer

Two types of skin conditions which may lead to cancer are dark, mole-like pigmented areas and horny, dry patches of skin of the elderly (senile keratosis).

Early signs to watch for include:

1. A sore that does not heal or increases in size; the outer edges of the sore often are raised and waxy looking.

2. A wart or mole that increases in size and appearance. Dark moles need close attention and early treatment if changes occur.

A *melanoma* is a dark, mole-like cancer most frequently found on the feet, palms, head, neck, and genitalia. It is removed surgically, including a large surrounding area; surgery may include removal of lymph nodes if the cancer has spread.

Skin cancer from senile keratosis may require surgical removal with skin grafts or plastic surgery. Radiation therapy may also be used.

Skin cancer is a common type of cancer and is the most easily cured. Treatment may take place in the physician's office or on an out-patient basis. The main thing to remember is that treatment should be carried out in the proper way by approved means, and not by persons who claim fast, positive cure.

Cancer of the Mouth

The prognosis is usually not very hopeful if it is recurrent and advanced, especially if the tongue is involved. It is difficult to treat, and care must be taken to avoid mouth infection.

Cancer of the oral cavity is generally very painful; the patient experiences difficulty swallowing and in some instances breathing (depending on the location of the cancer). This can make him apprehensive.

Treatment may include mouth irrigations, sedatives, narcotics, radiation therapy (e.g., radium seeds), and tracheostomy. To provide adequate nourishment and fluids, tube feedings and intravenous therapy may be used.

Because the patient with advanced cancer of the oral cavity may suffer from intense pain, you must understand his need for attention and emotional support. Meticulous mouth care is required, as well as general comfort measures. Be prepared to take time to assist this patient.

Cancer of the Breast

This is the most common cause of death among women in the middle years. The chances for cure are better when breast cancer is detected early and treated properly and immediately.

Regular periodic breast inspection should be carried out by the physician (if possible) or by self-examination (Fig. 43–4). Be able to explain this examination procedure to patients and use it for your own self-examination. Examination of the breasts by x-ray is called *mammography*.

At present there is no answer to a possible relationship between the use of an oral contraceptive ("the pill") and breast cancer.

Surgical removal of a breast is called *mastectomy* (Fig. 43–3); when additional muscle tissue and axillary lymph nodes are removed it is known as a *radical mastectomy*.

The prognosis is uncertain after a radical mastectomy; the extent of metastasis and involvement of lymph nodes at the time of surgery have a great deal to do with the successful removal of all cancer tissue. It is usually not safe to consider a cure complete until about five years after surgery; the survival rate after five years is gradually increasing. While metastasis is usually slow, cancer does spread to the lungs, the other breast, the brain, and the skeleton if not removed in time.

The thought of cancer and the loss of a breast is a frightening experience for a woman. This is understandable, and it will help this patient to relieve some tension and anxiety if she can talk about her fears. Praise the patient for getting surgical attention and not postponing

BREAST SELF-EXAMINATION

1

Sit or stand in front of your mirror, with your arms relaxed at your sides, and examine your breasts carefully for any changes in size and shape. Look for any puckering or dimpling of the skin, and for any discharge or change in the nipples.

2

Raise both your arms over your head, and look for exactly the same things. See if there's been any change since you last examined your breasts.

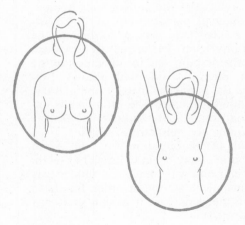

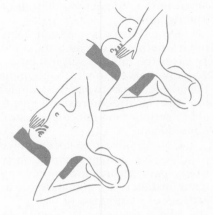

3

Lie down on your bed, put a pillow or a bath towel under your left shoulder, and your left hand under your head. (From this Step through Step 8, you should feel for a lump or thickening.) With the fingers of your right hand held together flat, press gently but firmly with small circular motions to feel the inner, upper quarter of your left breast, starting at your breastbone and going outward toward the nipple line. Also feel the area around the nipple.

4

With the same gentle pressure, feel the lower inner part of your breast. Incidentally, in this area you will feel a ridge of firm tissue or flesh. Don't be alarmed. This is perfectly normal.

FIGURE 43–4   Breast self-examination. (The American Cancer Society and The Nursing Clinics of North America.)

it. Sometimes a breast lump is not malignant. To know this is a great relief; but until the surgeon examines the removed tissue, he cannot be certain.

The removal of a breast and the fact that its removal detracts from a normal body appearance is of real concern to a woman. Very natural-looking artificial breasts (prostheses) are widely used today to help this patient feel more comfortable because her outward appearance is unchanged.

POSTOPERATIVE CARE. The type of care depends upon whether the tumor was benign or malignant and if it resulted in a radical mastectomy.

The patient with a radical mastectomy will return to her room with massive, tight dressings, and a closed drainage system which usually remains in place for about five days before it is removed. Pressure dressings are then used, and are changed daily or more often if needed, even after the patient goes home.

The medical management of this postoperative patient may vary according to the individual physician, but usually the medical orders on the first day call for elevation of the arm on the operative side with pillows. Following this the patient is usually ambulatory, and no pillows are used. She often needs encouragement to ambulate and use her arm.

Returning to self-care activities is a planned part of rehabilitation. Find out if and when the patient may begin to brush her teeth, comb her hair and wash her face. Under certain circumstances a written order for these activities is needed (e.g., if a skin graft has been performed).

Special arm exercises are ordered; they may include exercising both arms to help maintain proper posture and alignment. Here again, determine what types of exercise the physician wants the patient to have, and where and when she is to have them. The idea behind the exercise is to reestablish the use of the arm on the affected side as soon as possible. Using it aids in maintaining normal circulation to the part and reducing the amount and extent of edema which may result from interruption of the lymph flow in the axilla. Using the arm also helps the patient "get back to normal," and this can be very encouraging to her. Arm exercises are prescribed for the patient at home, too. Many homemaking activities contribute to this rehabilitation.

Radiation therapy may be a part of follow-up treatment; so might the use of hormone manipulation and chemotherapy.

Cancer of the Stomach

Cancer of the stomach is one of the most frequent types of malignancy. Too often by the time it is detected it has progressed to an incurable state. When it is detected early with no metastasis, surgical treatment is often successful. While cancer can develop in any part of the stomach, the pyloric region is most often affected; an early symptom may be an obstruction of the opening between the stomach and the small intestine causing dyspepsia and gastric distention. Appetite is very poor and there is severe weight loss.

The tumor may infiltrate the tissues, causing slow bleeding and anemia; it may perforate a large blood vessel and produce fatal hemorrhage or perforate the stomach wall and likewise be fatal.

Symptoms of stomach cancer vary. Pain and gastric distress appear early. A person who has persistent gastric distress should not camouflage the symptoms by taking a variety of medicines on his own; cancer of the stomach is often found too late for this very reason. Vomiting of great amounts of foul material which may be blood-tinged is common in obstruction. The patient loses weight rapidly, is weak and anemic.

X-rays (GI series) show deformity of the stomach: sometimes the tumor mass can be felt. Miniature camera-scopes are being used to take pictures of the inside of the stomach. The small picture-taking device is shifted about in the stomach so that all areas can be photographed.

Surgery may or may not help, depending upon whether or not metastasis has occurred. In cases too late for surgical cure, the patient actually starves to death. Sometimes an artificial opening between the stomach and small intestine (gastroenterostomy) is provided to aid in getting food into the intestine to supply nourishment.

Comfort measures include medication for pain. As the patient's condition worsens, he needs pain medication more frequently. In many instances this condition is a long, slow process of wasting away.

The patient and the family depend upon the nurse in many ways for support and reassurance even though the family, and perhaps

cannot be used in sufficient strength to help without damaging surrounding tissues.

Surgical treatment consists of removal of the lung (total pneumonectomy); by evidence of its high mortality rate, it is a serious risk but there is a possible chance of cure. The survival rate beyond five years is very low (about one in 20) because the disease is difficult to diagnose. It progresses slowly, and by the time definite signs or symptoms are apparent the condition may be inoperable; approximately seven out of ten cases are inoperable upon diagnosis.

Symptoms may include a wheezing, productive cough; blood-streaked sputum, a low-grade fever, weight loss, and pain may likewise be present.

Cancer of the lung may originate there, or the lesion may result from a metastasis of a lesion in some other part of the body.

BONE TUMORS

Some tumors of bone start there (primary) and are very difficult to diagnose and treat, but most bone tumors are metastatic from a primary source some place else in the body.

Metastasis makes itself known by pain, pathologic fracture or is discovered on x-rays. Contrary to what may be supposed, bone metastasis may not follow a rapid course of deterioration. Depending on the primary site, a patient may live many productive years.

Medical management varies depending upon whether the tumor is of primary or metastatic origin and from which part of the body it spread. In some instances (breast, prostate, thyroid cancer) treatment is by manipulating the hormonal environment, further surgery and radiation therapy.

Non-narcotic drugs for the relief of pain are usually ordered as long as possible due to the generally slow progress of the cancer.

In addition to meeting the general nursing needs of this patient, there may be special requirements related to diagnostic laboratory work. Pre- and postoperative care include the same nursing measures as for other patients.

The patient may be very anxious, and his daily comfort measures become very important to him. Observe the patient's needs; do something to help keep him as comfortable as possible. Report increased insistence upon pain medication.

If the patient is able to understand, he has the same fears and uncertainties as any patient who feels or knows that recovery is impossible. The need is to keep him independent by some self-care as long as possible. At certain ages or times, diversional activities absorb attention. Some patients will manage their own means of diversion, while others, especially children, need help.

LEUKEMIA

Leukemia is a disease which causes the body to overproduce white blood cells (leukocytes). Not only are the numbers of leukocytes increased, these cells are immature and do not function as do mature white blood cells in fighting body infections. This disease may be acute or chronic.

Leukemia occurs in all age groups and is increasing. Among children under age fifteen, it is the leading cause of death, as it is for males in the 15 to 34 year age group. Death from leukemia is increasing among people over 60.

Intensive research on child-patients with acute leukemia is producing some "exciting advances." Through treatment at a specialized cancer center it is possible for a young patient to have a chance to live out a normal life; an unheard of happening a few years ago. The use of chemotherapy (highly active anti-cancer drugs) with other treatments has made this progress possible. The problems with chemotherapy are many despite the progress afforded. Normal cells can get killed along with cancer cells; natural immunity defenses of the body can be upset, creating the hazard of infection, and there is toxicity. The cause of leukemia is not known at present. Some causative factors being studied include heredity, infection, viruses, unruly cancer-cell activity, and overexposure to radiation.

The signs and symptoms of leukemia include fever, chills, anemia, pallor, bleeding (in the nose, mouth, or vagina), fatigue, and a feeling of fullness in the abdomen. Treatment includes chemotherapy, the selected use of irradiation, and measures to relieve symptoms (e.g., blood transfusions, antibiotics, analgesics), as well as meticulous mouth and skin care. Extreme care is used to prevent infections; sometimes it is essential to control the entire immediate environment.

SUMMARY

Cancer ranks second as a cause of death among all people in this country. Some types of cancer are increasing; others are decreasing. While the cause of cancer is not known as yet, it is known that early detection and proper, prompt treatment influence a favorable prognosis.

There is more reason to be hopeful about cancer than in the past because detection techniques and treatments are improving. Patients are experiencing longer survival periods and are freer of pain and disability. Research is showing us that many ideas of the past are not necessarily true; this in itself raises hope for health workers and patients alike.

Health workers need to have positive attitudes toward patients with cancer. The patient and family need the support that comes from workers who find purpose in rendering assistance to this patient.

The daily care measures needed by patients with cancer are not new measures; patients with other diseases need the same care. What could be new is the attitude of the nurse toward the patient's future well-being. It should be positive and portray hopefulness.

GUIDES FOR STUDY AND DISCUSSION

1. In your opinion, why is the federal government putting so much time and money into cancer research?

2. What do the terms neoplasm and neoplastic mean? Compare the activities of a neoplastic cell with the activities of a normal cell.

3. What is hopeful about cancer? Why are people so fearful when this is their diagnosis? How might this influence their nursing needs?

4. What types of workers are involved in the cancer problem today? How does the practical nurse fit into this group?

5. A favorable prognosis is influenced by two essential factors. What are they? Why do some persons pay little or no attention to these factors?

6. What does it mean to say that a nurse needs a positive attitude toward the patient with cancer? How can such an attitude be gained?

7. Identify three special nursing needs the cancer patient might have. Be ready to discuss them.

8. How many different therapies for cancer treatment can you name? Why are they apt to be used in combination(s)?

9. Why can treatment of pain become a problem?

SUGGESTED SITUATIONS AND ACTIVITIES

1. Scientists are seeking answers to questions about cancer. Watch the daily news media for a period of time and see if any new findings are reported. Share your news items with classmates.

2. Select a patient (of any age) who has a diagnosis of cancer. If possible, provide his nursing care for several days. Make a list of any adjustments or adaptations necessary to meet his daily living needs. See if you can identify a nursing care problem which was different from that of any other patient you have ever cared for.

PATIENTS WITH MUSCULOSKELETAL DISORDERS

OBJECTIVES FOR THE STUDENT: Be able to:

1. Explain the term "limited movement" as it relates to the orthopedic patient.
2. Name five signs/symptoms commonly associated with rheumatoid diseases.
3. Describe two nursing actions intended to prevent deformity.
4. Defend the statement—strict medical asepsis must be observed in caring for a draining wound.
5. Explain the need for special emphasis on skin care for the orthopedic patient.
6. Identify eight nursing responsibilities with respect to caring for a patient in a cast.
7. Describe three ways a patient may be immobilized.
8. Tell how patient immobility influences his need for assistance by giving three examples.

SUGGESTED STUDY VOCABULARY*

arthritis
rheumatism
localized
systemic
aspirate
exudate
osteomyelitis
sinus
fistula
rickets
closed reduction

osteoporosis
muscular dystrophy
trauma
wound
strain
sprain
dislocation
devitalized tissue
fracture
open reduction
Stryker frame

paralysis
paraplegia
hemiplegia
quadriplegia
congenital deformity
orthopedic
scurvy
hereditary
necrosis
abscess
purulent
gouty arthritis

*Look for any terms you already know.

INTRODUCTION

The work of the musculoskeletal system is to hold the body in position(s), produce movement, and perform endless tasks. So when something happens to the bones, joints and muscles, body movement and performance are hampered; motion is limited to a lesser or greater degree depending upon the location and the extent of the disorder. The limitation may be minimal and not prevent a person from carrying on and attending to his own needs; on the other hand, the extent of limitation may be so great as to hospitalize the patient on a special type of bed, with assistance from a respirator to breathe and paralysis in all extremities. Between these two extremes are many degrees of limited motion, temporary and permanent.

The extent of the patient's loss of movement influences his state of dependency or independency and consequently dictates many things about his need for assistance. Keep this thought in mind as you plan your nursing care for these patients and for patients who have limited motion for some other reason.

The list of conditions which affect the muscles, bones, and joints is long and varied; this chapter includes a representative group of the common ones. As you study them make note of how often the symptoms of pain, swelling, tenderness, and restricted movement are mentioned.

DISEASES AND DISORDERS

Rheumatoid Diseases

This group of diseases includes two well-known joint and muscle disorders—arthritis and rheumatism. It doesn't help one to sort out the differences between rheumatism and arthritis when these two terms are commonly used interchangeably. In this country, the term arthritis is often used as a family term to include rheumatism; in Great Britain it is the other way around.

Rheumatism is actually any one of a vast number of conditions related to the musculoskeletal system when pain and stiffness are present. The group of rheumatoid diseases includes about 100 different disorders.

When joints are inflamed, painful, and stiff, the condition is called *arthritis*. How-ever, the tissues related to the joints (e.g., tendons, tendon sheaths, nerves, muscles, bursae, etc.) can become painful and stiff without involving the joint (called nonarticular rheumatism). When both joints and connective tissues are involved throughout the body it is known as *rheumatoid arthritis*. This shows you how closely related they are and how difficult it is to separate them.

Arthritis occurs in many forms but basically two pathological changes affect the joints: (1) inflammation accompanied by exudates and/or local growth and (2) degenerative tissue changes. These changes vary but may be present in any joint. The arthritic process may be in an acute or in a chronic form but an acute form can become chronic. Likewise the chronic form may flare up into an acute state.

The cause(s) is known for some types of arthritics (e.g., when associated with staphylococcus organisms) and for others it is not (e.g., rheumatoid arthritis).

In general, arthritic joints are painful and stiff. They are tender to touch and even slight pressure and movement cause pain. More detailed discussion also follows under **Infections of joints and bones**.

Rheumatoid arthritis (atrophic arthritis) is a "whole body" or constitutional disease with inflammatory changes in the connective tissues. The inflammation (of the synovial membrane) is chronic and causes irreversible damage to the joint covering and the associated cartilage; they change to roughened and scar tissue. It usually continues in cycles of severe episodes and remissions.

More women than men have rheumatoid arthritis; it strikes the young adult (average age of onset 35) but it can start in older and elderly adults.

Despite the fact that great efforts have been made to establish a cause, the cause of rheumatoid arthritis remains unknown and it continues to be a most disabling disease.

While all/any connective tissue may be involved, target areas are the joints of the hands, arms, feet, legs, and hips.

SIGNS AND SYMPTOMS. No two patients necessarily follow the same course of disease onset or development; this often makes early diagnosis somewhat puzzling. However, some early symptoms can include poor appetite, fatigue and weakness, weight loss, and tingling or numbness of the hands and feet.

Onset may be gradual with stiffness and pain in one or a few joints; swelling follows. With an acute onset many joints may swell and be painful; chills and fever are apt to be present. No matter how it starts, sooner or later the cycles of severe episodes and remissions are established.

In general, the signs and symptoms are swelling of the joints (especially hands, fingers, knees), joint deformity and immobility (ankylosis).

Pain varies and is usually helped with heat, rest and analgesics. Stiffness is almost always present (most pronounced upon getting up in the morning). The neck and shoulders may ache and be tender to pressure. Skin over the affected joints usually feels warm and becomes shiny.

Other symptoms may include some weight loss and fatigue, some temperature elevation, tingling or numbness of hands and feet, irritability and some loss of mobility.

MEDICAL TREATMENT AND NURSING CARE. Medical treatment is directed toward (1) rest; (2) relief of pain; (3) maintaining joint function; (4) use of orthopedic devices and principles to prevent and correct deformities; and (5) correcting any faulty health factors.

Rest. This patient needs a generous amount of rest—often 10 or 12 hours out of the 24. However, staying in bed all of the time contributes to ankylosis and loss of muscle tone.

Pain. The drug of choice seems to be salicylates (aspirin, sodium salicylates). In some instances codeine may be used too, but is generally avoided on a constant basis.

Heat and Exercise. A combination of these two treatments is considered essential. Heat may be applied locally (e.g., infared lamp, hot towels) or to the entire body (e.g., hot tub bath, hot pack, steam cabinet). The use of massage is questioned by some. The idea behind a program of exercise is to maintain muscle tone and useful joint movement, if possible.

Prevention/Correction of Deformities by Orthopedic Treatment. The bed should be flat with only one pillow. Avoid putting a pillow under painful knees to prevent flexion deformity. A foot board helps prevent foot drop.

Splints and half-shell molds (plaster/plastic) are often used with developing deformities (remove for exercise and physical therapy). Surgical corrections of deformed and ankylosed joints are often carried out.

Correcting Faulty Health Factors. *Diet* is usually dictated by the general nutritional state of the patient. If undernourished and underweight such things as a high caloric, high protein diet plus vitamins and minerals are ordered. An obese patient may be placed on a reducing diet. *Anemia*, if present, does not always respond favorably to such treatments as iron therapy, folic acid, vitamin B_{12} and blood transfusions.

Emotional reactions of the patient need the understanding and support of personnel and family. One way to encourage him in his long treatment is to be sure he knows what his condition is and why certain treatments are used; this is the physician's responsibility but he will expect nursing personnel to support his honest efforts to maintain positive relationships with the patient.

This patient is easily discouraged with his lengthy therapy and becomes irritable, often becoming angry without reason. Allow plenty of time for his personal care activities as movements are painful. Avoid overtiring the patient but try to involve him in self-care in so far as possible. He may even prefer this because then he can move at his own speed and be more independent.

Comfort measures include: (1) Warmth of bath water, back rub lotion, nurse's hands. (2) Light weight covering. (3) Avoiding pressure on painful joints by careful use of hands; support when moving extremities; use a bed cradle to hold off pressure of bed linens. (4) Allow patient to turn and position himself; support proper body alignment to prevent deformities.

Infections of Joints and Bones

Arthritis can be caused by specific infectious organisms. The causing organism may be identified through laboratory procedures which help make the treatment as specific as possible.

Some of these conditions include: *gonococcal arthritis* associated with genital gonorrhea; *tuberculous arthritis* which may involve any body joint but common targets are the hip, spine, and knee; *arthritis of rheumatic fever* usually leaving no permanent bone damage; *arthritis of rubella*—a short term complication of German measles.

Suppurative arthritis is a pus-forming condition most commonly caused by streptococcus, staphylococcus, pneumococcus and meningococcus microorganisms. An open or penetrating wound may be the gateway for the organisms or they may be brought by the blood as a complication in bacteremia (bacteria in the blood).

SIGNS AND SYMPTOMS. The joint cavity fills with exudates which cause the swelling, inflammation and severe pain. Chills and fever may occur.

MEDICAL TREATMENT AND NURSING CARE. The purulent exudates are withdrawn (aspirated) and the causative organism identified. Appropriate drugs (specific chemotherapy) are used and a drain inserted if necessary.

A draining wound requires specific nurse actions: (1) strict medical asepsis. (2) frequent dressing changes. (3) attention to skin care around the area. (4) observe the amount and character of drainage and the appearance of the area.

Osteomyelitis is a localized infection in bone due to the presence of pus-forming organisms; they may come from an open sore, penetrating wound, compound fracture, open surgery or by way of the blood stream and be acute or chronic.

Common sites include long bones in children and in adults the pelvis and vertebra.

SIGNS AND SYMPTOMS. Some of the signs and symptoms include a usually abrupt onset, starting with a chill; high fever; intense pain, aggravated by the movement of a part; tenderness (sometimes swelling) at the site of infection; and a draining abscess, an infectious exudate coming from pus forming within the bone. The abscess may break through or the physician may make several holes to promote drainage, relieve pressure, and treat the area.

MEDICAL TREATMENT AND NURSING CARE. In acute osteomyelitis, the physician determines the organism by laboratory tests (e.g., blood culture) and plans the antibiotic therapy accordingly.

It should be mentioned that chronic bone infection which started before the discovery of antibiotics is seldom cured or helped by this therapy. These patients require surgery to remove the abscesses, dead bone, and chronic sinuses.

Pus confined within the bone cavity is very painful; the bone does not stretch as the exudate accumulates and thus pressure builds up within. Drainage may be natural, such as when the bone gives way and the soft tissues open up, releasing the pus and causing an open abscess. One complication to be avoided, if at all possible, is development of the draining abscess into an abnormal drainage channel called a *sinus or fistula*. Drainage may be established by surgically drilling holes into the area to release the pus. In either event, antibiotics are usually put directly into the wound by some type of irrigation. The wound may be aspirated and the body part held in a good wound-drainage position. Traction, splints, or partial casts are often used to maintain drainage and promote comfort by preventing movement.

As mentioned earlier the nursing care of a draining wound requires several essential actions on the part of the nurse. See suppurative arthritis.

This patient has severe pain, which is especially aggravated by movement, so the manner in which he moves or is moved should be cautious and unhurried. Support must be provided along the infected limb (pillows, sandbags, splint) to immobilize it. Avoid jarring the bed and see that it is positioned so that other persons do not jar it as well. The patient is apt to hold his limb in a position of least strain regardless of body alignment; because he is confined for a long time, deformities can occur if body alignment is not watched.

Young or otherwise, these patients need diversional outlets; they become discouraged and restless with their long-term illness. This is a continuing problem, especially with children. Get them involved in as many self-help activities as possible, and see that they have opportunity to do some meaningful things to absorb their attention and their time.

Metabolic Diseases of Bone and Joints

Osteoporosis is a condition whereby bone tissue decreases because of some faulty way the bone uses minerals to maintain its normal composition. It could be called the "absence of a normal quantity of bone," or a decrease in bone mass. Under normal conditions the formation of new bone tissue and the resorption of old tissue occur at the same rate, thus the components of the bone stay in balance.

When the rate of resorption exceeds formation, the bone mass is less; this is called osteoporosis.

The condition (not disease) called osteoporosis is somehow related to faulty protein metabolism, body hormone disturbances, following menopause, the aging process and disuse. It is not yet known why bone resorption exceeds bone formation.

The abnormal composition of bone in osteoporosis can produce "hidden" fractures and contribute to known fractures. For example, an x-ray may reveal the fracture of a vertebra or a hip that had been unknown because pain was absent or slight; the discomfort had been slight or there was general weakness but it was overlooked. Elderly people (especially) should have a medical examination if use of the back or hips causes fatigue or discomfort because a "hidden" fracture continues to deteriorate with use.

MEDICAL TREATMENT AND NURSING CARE. The factors that cause osteoporosis dictate the patient's treatment. He needs to be mobile and to have as much exercise as possible. A high protein diet is ordered. Hormones are given. If pain is present, analgesics (e.g., aspirin) are usually given rather than narcotics. Vitamins D and C are also given.

This patient, if hospitalized or in a nursing home, will probably have medical orders to move about unless otherwise prohibited. He can be involved in his self-care which provides exercise and helps him to retain as much independence as possible.

If the physician orders some type of spinal brace or back support to help relieve strain, the patient may need encouragement to wear it. In some instances surgery is required (e.g., to repair the fracture of the neck of the femur). Nursing care in this case is similar to that of the pre- and postoperative patient described in Chapter 42.

Other metabolic diseases of the bones include:

1. *Rickets* — a childhood disease caused by faulty metabolism of calcium and phosphorus due to the lack of vitamin D in the diet. The use of vitamin D fortified whole milk or evaporated milk has reduced the incidence of this bone deforming disease.
2. *Scurvy* — a disease caused by the lack of vitamin C in the diet for a long period of time causing gums to swell and bleed; teeth loosen and bones break easily. Joints are stiff and tender. Small hemorrhages occur under the skin because blood vessels become fragile. A diet which includes plenty of fruits and vegetables provides the necessary vitamin C.
3. *Gouty arthritis* — dates back to ancient history. Gout is a metabolic disease affecting the joints and kidneys caused by too much uric acid in body tissues. Gouty arthritis is the term used when the salt of uric acid forms in one or more joints causing inflammation and severe pain. Swelling results as fluids filter into the affected area to repair damaged cells. The dark reddish color of the inflamed joint(s) is caused by extra blood at the site. Untreated gouty arthritis can produce permanent damage and deformity; however, early and continued treatment can prevent that.

MEDICAL TREATMENT AND NURSING CARE. Treatment consists of a variety of drugs (e.g., ACTH, cortisone, colchicine, indomethacin, aspirin, combinations of drugs), rest (affected part), avoiding injury, surgery, and diet restrictions (low purine diet — omitting such foods as liver, kidneys, sardines, meat extracts, and gravies).

Muscular Dystrophy

This term applies to a group of muscle disorders that are marked by progressive weakness and wasting away of muscles. The condition is hereditary. One type appears in early childhood; the disability increases so rapidly that by puberty the child is unable to get about without a wheelchair. Another type appears at about puberty; it progresses more slowly and these patients are ambulatory until late in life.

SIGNS AND SYMPTOMS. Some of the signs and symptoms include contractures, beginning in the lower extremities, in which the feet are drawn downward and inward; restricted movements; weak muscles; and anxiousness about the worsening condition.

MEDICAL TREATMENT AND NURSING CARE. Many different therapies are used; there is no specific therapy because, as yet, nothing seems to halt the progress of the muscle weakness. Among the many types of drugs used are vitamins and hormones. The anxious patient often says that he feels better when a new drug is used because he becomes hopeful that some cure will be found; this well-being lasts but a few weeks.

Splints, braces, corrective orthopedic surgery, and carefully prescribed exercises represent some of the many physical efforts being made to prevent contractures and to keep patients mobile.

Because disuse and immobility increase the rate of deformity, these patients are kept ambulatory as long as possible. Likewise, they are encouraged to participate in all types of daily living activities, even to the extent that special equipment is designed to help them do this.

This patient should avoid any respiratory infection because weakened respiratory muscles reduce lung capacity; coughing is less effective in reducing mucus in the trachea, and there is always the possibility of obstruction. The rocking bed and respirator are used as lifesaving devices when respiratory muscles are weak.

INJURIES

Types of Trauma

The word *trauma* might be called a representative term because it includes any wound or injury to any part or organ of the body. It is usually thought of as being caused by some external force. While the focus here is on the muscles and bones, you must keep in mind that anything that causes any degree of muscle or bone damage also injures other body parts (e.g., nerves, circulation, soft tissues).

Accidents rank high among causes of crippling and death in this country. Almost half of the accidents causing death involve motor vehicles. Motor vehicle accident victims usually have multiple injuries (from traveling at high speed), involving many body systems including the muscles and bones.

Home injuries lead the danger list; power tools cause increasing injury to hands. Farm machinery injuries are increasing also, because farms are becoming more mechanized.

The discussion that follows will relate specifically to orthopedic trauma.

WOUNDS (OPEN AND CLOSED). A wound is an interruption of the "normal" external or internal tissues of the body caused by some type of physical force. In an *open wound* the external tissues have been "opened," exposing underlying or internal tissues to outside contamination. The opening may range from a gaping wound (wide-open) to a puncture wound, in which some pointed object pierces the skin and reaches into underlying tissue. In a *closed wound* the skin remains intact, but the underlying tissues are injured from the pressure of a blow, pinch, or squeeze of extraordinary force. As a rule, if the blow is severe, it damages bones, muscles, and tendons as well as producing a gaping wound. The degree of tissue injury ranges from slight bruises that produce muscle and bone tenderness, to extensive damage in which all underlying structures are torn apart and bones are fractured.

STRAINS AND SPRAINS. A *strain* is a painful condition, characterized by soreness or tenderness, caused by overuse or harmful use of a muscle or set of muscles. A *sprain* is a joint injury that interrupts or ruptures the ligaments; however, they remain intact with swelling, pain, and discoloration present owing to local hemorrhage. The joint cannot be used until the ligaments heal.

DISLOCATION. As the term implies, to dislocate means to move out of the usual position. Bones become dislocated. Notice the direction of the arrows in Figure 44–1, indicating from which direction the various bones have moved.

A dislocated bone means that surrounding supporting tissues have given way—either on their own or from external force—and the body has lost the effective use of that joint. In the case of a congenital deformity (discussed later in this chapter), a person lacks effective use of the joint from birth.

SIGNS AND SYMPTOMS. They include hemorrhage, in which blood may escape through an opening or into surrounding tissues; discoloration ("black and blue"); swelling; pain; and disuse of the part.

MEDICAL MANAGEMENT AND NURSING CARE. The *open wound* is cleansed and all devitalized tissue and foreign matter are surgically removed. The patient is given antitoxin to prevent tetanus, and aseptic measures are used along with drugs to prevent infection. If bones are broken (see Fractures), care is taken in handling and movement to avoid further trauma until the bone can be set.

Pain is a usual symptom in any trauma and ranges from mild to severe. Observation for shock, vital signs and blood pressure are

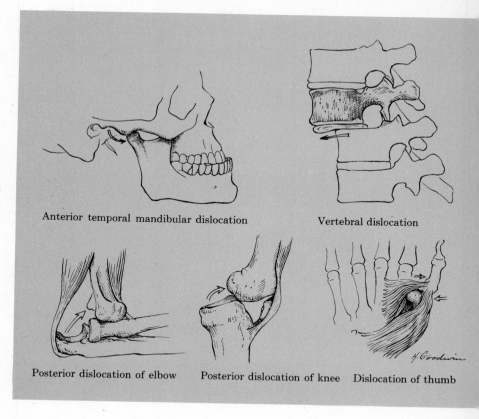

FIGURE 44–1 Various types of dislocations. (Dorland's Illustrated Medical Dictionary, 24th Ed.)

Anterior temporal mandibular dislocation

Vertebral dislocation

Posterior dislocation of elbow

Posterior dislocation of knee

Dislocation of thumb

made; fluids are usually given if the trauma is severe.

Nursing measures are planned according to the type, extent, and location of the wound, and the patient's age and size. The degree of injury, his dependency, and the stability of his condition together determine nursing action. In the beginning you may be functioning in Role II, carrying out assigned tasks; you may move into Role I as the patient's condition becomes more stable and his independence greater.

All medical and nursing measures are directed toward prevention of infection and deformities and toward restoring the patient to his fullest possible capacity.

Closed wounds usually require elevation and rest of the injured part. The patient has local and general discomfort, and treatment for pain is common. Observations include watching for shock, observing vital signs and blood pressure, and looking for swelling and skin discoloration at the site of the injury and for evidence of a cold, clammy skin or a chill.

Medical orders include administering drugs for pain, instructions for amount of movement and position, and other preventive therapy measures, as well as the specific diet, fluids, and the like.

Care of the injured patient—depending on the nature and extent of his wounds—can bring into play all sorts of medical orders and nursing measures. His particular signs and symptoms are treated, many types of preventive measures are used, dressings are changed, bones are set, special diets are ordered, and restorative treatment including special exercises and equipment may be needed. All these related factors are taken into account in assisting the patient to meet his daily living needs; adjustments in providing care and involving him in self-care are made according to his abilities and his medical orders.

Dislocated parts or strained muscles require some measure to hold the joint or muscles in position while the wound heals. Strapping is one method used for this purpose (Fig. 44–2).

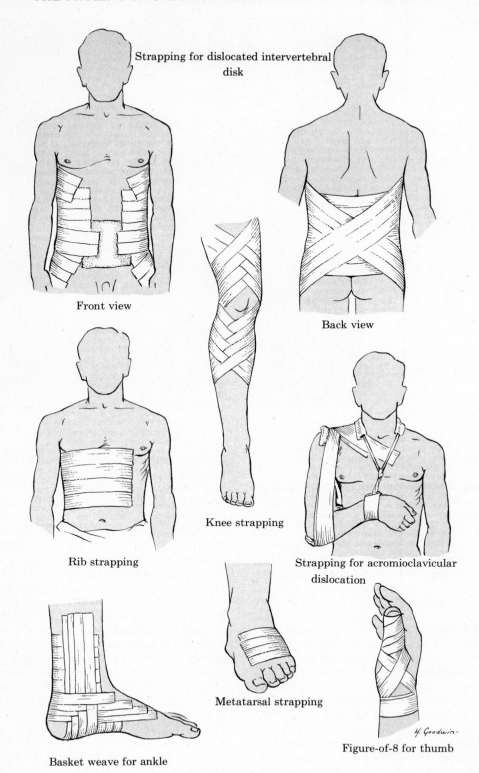

Strapping for dislocated intervertebral disk

Front view

Back view

Knee strapping

Rib strapping

Strapping for acromioclavicular dislocation

Metatarsal strapping

Basket weave for ankle

Figure-of-8 for thumb

H. Goodwin

FIGURE 44–2   Various types of strapping. (Dorland's Illustrated Medical Dictionary, 24th Ed.)

Sprains are usually treated with hot soaks, spraying or injecting an anesthetic, and strapping or minimal support. The physician tries to determine the extent of injuries (i.e., chipped bone, torn ligament) to provide necessary measures to prevent later complications or permanent joint weakness.

Fractures

Chapter 51, The Accident Victim, includes an illustration (Fig. 51–3) that shows the different ways in which bone can break. One example is the *partial* or *green-stick fracture*. This occurs in children because the normal growth of bone at early age makes it softer; there is less rigidity because there is less calcium. The older the patient, the more calcium and less bone marrow he has. Consequently in older patients there is a brittleness of bone not present in youth, and healing is slower. It should be pointed out that if a child's fracture involves the growth plate (epiphysis), treatment is not simple or short-term as a rule. The bone may stop growing, or as it grows it may have a deformed shape. Any infection following a fracture likewise may damage the growth plate and cause deformity to occur.

Notice also in Figure 51–3 that only one type of fracture breaks through the skin and produces an open wound; this is the *compound* or *open fracture*. The others are grouped under the term *simple* or *closed fractures*. The word simple may be misleading because a bone can suffer extreme damage without the skin breaking. For instance, note the illustrations of comminuted fracture, fracture of the neck of the femur, and impacted or compression fracture of a vertebra and see how these might cause all types of pain and immobility for the patient.

The nature, extent and location of the fracture, as well as the patient's age, influence many things about the patient's medical needs and nursing care.

SIGNS AND SYMPTOMS. Some of the signs and symptoms of fractures are pain, swelling, hemorrhage, discoloration, shock, nausea and vomiting, and nonalignment and disuse of the body part.

Following surgery to set the bone, observe the patient's vital signs and blood pressure and be on the lookout for hemorrhage, swelling, and pain.

MEDICAL MANAGEMENT AND NURSING CARE. The physician is concerned with prevention of further injury and infection. Steps are taken to realign the injured part and "fix" it in position to permit proper healing. X-rays help determine the exact location and extent of damage; later they are used to compare progress of the healing process.

Bones are realigned by one of two processes: (1) Closed reduction—accomplished without surgery. Traction is used over a period of time to pull and hold bone ends in proper position while they heal. Or, the ends are manipulated back into place and the part immobilized by cast, splint, or traction. Strapping may be used for fractured ribs. (2) Open reduction—accomplished with surgery. The surgeon fits the pieces together; if this is not possible or he sees the necessity for reinforcing the structure, metal plates, pins, and screws are used to hold fragments or replace parts. The repaired part is always immobilized by cast, traction, splints, or sandbags.

The open wound is an invitation to infection; therefore, the object of all care is to prevent infection from happening. The surgeon exercises every precaution to see that all hidden particles which entered the part under high pressure (e.g., a splinter of glass or metal) but left no telltale signs on the surface are removed. If not removed, these particles can cause infection; this is one reason why close observation of the local area and systemic signs—fever, pain, discoloration, and swelling—is necessary.

Other medical orders include drugs for pain and to prevent infection, special diet, fluids, and cathartics or enemas; in some instances a special bed is used. Early ambulation is common, too.

Nursing care for the immobilized patient is concerned with prevention, comfort, and restoration. Some of the needed measures require medical orders; others do not. When care is watchful, complications such as decubitus ulcers, bladder distention, constipation, contractures, and infections are held to a minimum, and can even be prevented from happening.

A patient requiring long-term care may or may not be able to do anything for himself. Any self-care within his limits should be encouraged. Keep the skin clean and dry; powder sparingly. Massage and protect pressure areas to prevent decubitus ulcers and other irritating discomforts.

The condition of the bed and bed linen has a great deal to do with patient comfort. A firm, well-supported mattress and a smooth, clean undersheet prevent skin wrinkles and ultimate pressure areas. A bed cradle prevents pressure of the upper bedding from falling upon extremities.

If the bed is a special frame, the purposes of bedmaking remain the same; it should be clean, firm, dry, smooth, and free from pressure sources. (See special frames under Spinal Injuries.)

Proper body alignment is maintained to prevent any deformity (i.e., foot drop). The correct use of pillows, foot boards, and sandbags aid proper body alignment and patient comfort.

Immobilization generally makes the digestive and elimination processes sluggish, thereby causing poor appetite. Effort should be made to make eating a pleasant, self-help experience as soon as the patient is able; you may need to use imagination to get some patients interested in eating—especially the young and the very elderly.

Exercise of movable body joints is necessary and should begin as soon as possible to prevent stiffness and impaired function. If able, the patient in traction should be taught to help move himself up in bed or use the trapeze and uninvolved leg to lift himself onto the bedpan.

The Patient in a Cast. A new plaster of Paris cast usually dries completely within a couple of days, but it needs protection while this is happening. Undue pressure (e.g., a hard surface) on the outside will create inside pressure against the patient's skin. Use a pillow(s) with a water proof covering to cradle the cast; this also elevates the part to help fight edema.

Nursing care includes:

1. Inspecting the edges for roughness and cutting into the tissues.
2. Noticing the color of the skin of extending part(s). It should appear the same as other body skin.
3. Touching extended part(s) to see if it is as warm as other body parts.
4. Looking for the presence of edema. Any indication of swelling, color change, or coldness of part(s) should be reported at once.
5. Being alert to odor coming from the edges of the cast. It is possible to smell the presence of any necrotic tissue.
6. Paying attention to the patient's complaints of pain and discomfort; if he mentions numbness or tingling, listen and do something about it. It is better to be over cautious than to run the risk of nerve and skin damage.
7. Inspecting to see that foreign objects are not "lost" between cast and the patient.
8. Protecting the cast from all moisture.
9. Devising ways to reach under the cast to relieve itching.
10. Helping the patient get answers to any questions regarding his cast, how long it will be on, and so on.

Turning the patient in a body cast requires two people. One supports the pelvis and the other supports the leg in the cast. Both work in unison to turn the patient on his side. Then one goes to the opposite side of the bed to help turn the patient onto his back.

The pull of traction must be maintained at all times if it is to be useful. Any adjustments of weights and cords are at the physician's direction; weights and cords must *not* otherwise be moved or changed. If you observe a change or shift in the pull of the traction, report this observation.

The immobilized patient is a long-term patient. His needs for emotional support are evident. One thing which is helpful is purposeful diversion. Enlist the family's help if this is practical or possible. Keep in mind that any type of self-care will be encouraging and diversional if his environment is conveniently arranged and adequate time is provided so that he can carry it out.

Spinal Column Injuries

A fracture almost anywhere along the spinal column may be serious enough to damage or sever the spinal cord, causing paralysis, the extent of which is dependent upon the location of the injured cord and nerve tracks. If injury occurs in certain locations, the patient has widespread disability and disorder. When this happens his life may depend upon a respirator; elimination may be severely impaired, requiring an indwelling catheter and bowel attention. The skin requires close observation to keep it intact and free from decubitus ulcers. Circulation is poor and muscles are useless or weak and flaccid. The term *paraplegia* means the loss of the use of lower extremities; *hemiplegia* refers to the loss of the use of an arm or leg on one side; *quadriplegia* means paralysis of all four limbs. The degree of dependency of the quadriplegic patient at any age is complete when so much disability is present.

Not all spinal fractures produce widespread, serious results. If the vertebrae collapse (as in osteoporosis) or the fracture does not involve the spinal cord or nerves, the patient has use of his limbs and vital processes continue unaided, but he is immobilized to some extent or other so that the column can heal properly.

Very often a fractured spine requires that the patient be immobilized on some type of bed or frame that will provide immobility and permit adequate nursing care and prevent pressure areas and decubitus ulcers. One example is the Stryker frame (Fig. 44–3). It permits a supine (face upward) position and a prone (face downward) position. Patient position changes are made every hour or so. Por-

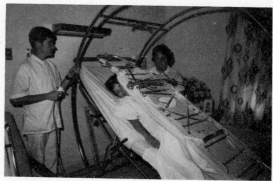

FIGURE 44–4 The CircOlectric bed with the patient ready for a position change. (Courtesy of Hillsborough County School of Practical Nursing and St. Joseph's Hospital, Tampa, Florida.)

tions of the canvas covering are removed for use of the bed pan and for the prone position (e.g., eating, reading). This frame can be managed by one nurse. Another special bed is the CircOlectric bed. As you can see in Figure 44–4 the patient is secured between an upper and a lower bed frame when his position is changed. It is powered by electricity and controlled by a switch.

MEDICAL TREATMENT AND NURSING CARE. Depending upon the location of the injury and the extent of nerve involvement, if any, the physician performs the reduction and immobilizes the patient. Immobility may be a surgical wiring of spinal bones in place until bone grafts can be done to provide a permanent fixation. Casts or braces (or both) are used to immobilize different regions of the spinal column. One commonly used device is Crutchfield tongs for providing traction in the cervical spine area (Fig. 44–5). The prongs are inserted into the skull and pull is exerted by weights on a rope.

Sometimes the physician splints, braces, or casts the body and permits the patient to ambulate at the earliest possible time; this helps other body systems to maintain normal functions.

In addition to proper bone alignment, treatment includes rehabilitation of muscles and improvement of general muscle tone. A high-protein, high-calorie, high-vitamin diet is usually required. An indwelling catheter may be needed at least at first, as well as regular enemas or cathartics.

Nursing care for the patient with a spinal injury is difficult and exacting, especially dur-

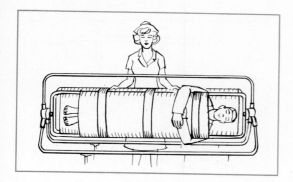

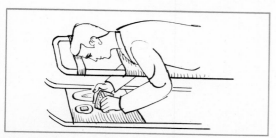

FIGURE 44–3 The Stryker frame is a "frame upon a frame" with the patient securely strapped in between the two canvas covered frames when he is being rotated for a position change. Following the change, the upper frame is removed. The patient may be on his back or lying face downward. (Sutton: Bedside Nursing Technique, 2nd ed.)

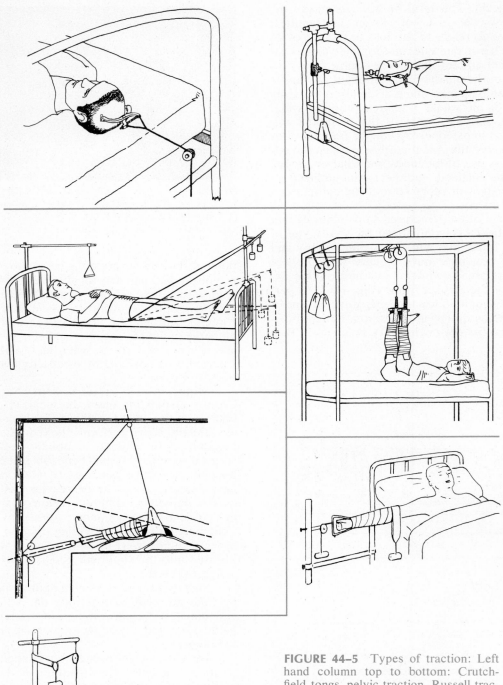

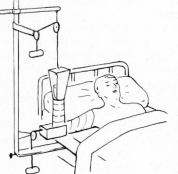

FIGURE 44–5 Types of traction: Left hand column top to bottom: Crutchfield tongs, pelvic traction, Russell traction, skin traction. Right hand column top to bottom: traction by halter, Buck's extension, skeletal traction device. (Miller and Keene: Encyclopedia and Dictionary of Medicine and Nursing.)

ing the first few days. Paralysis from injury to some part of the spinal cord may affect bladder and bowel elimination, thus necessitating special bladder drainage and irrigation treatments. Bowels do not move without regular enemas, at least for a while, and then need to be aided by a mild laxative and an increase in intake of fruit juice.

The appetite is usually poor and the patient is not too interested in a proper fluid or food intake despite the fact that a high-protein, high-calorie, high-vitamin diet with plenty of fluids is necessary. It is a challenge to interest these patients in eating.

Effective skin care is essential, including special attention to pressure areas and care of the buttocks and genitalia. The general idea is to keep the skin firm (tough) and dry. To avoid a dried-out skin, modest amounts of oil or lotion are used.

Whether the patient is in bed or ambulatory, observe the skin to see that there are no pressures exerted against it. A paralyzed part has no feeling, so the patient cannot tell if something is pressing against it.

It is easy for this patient to give up and decide that he never will be any better. Every effort should be made by all members of the team to help him maintain courage and a positive outlook. As soon as possible, he should begin to assist himself by getting involved with his daily living activities.

The special bed frames make it possible for the patient to feed himself, read, write, and do some types of hand work as well as manage many daily grooming activities.

CONGENITAL DEFORMITIES

A congenital deformity is one existing at and usually occurring before birth. Defects in bone structure and formation are responsible for such conditions as clubfoot, dislocation of the hip, and misshapen spinal columns.

Corrective devices are used to support proper position in young children with clubfoot. Surgery may be necessary for older children when the foot has become more fixed in the abnormal position.

A congenital dislocation of the hip means that for some reason the head of the femur is out of the acetabulum; it must be returned to proper position and held there until it is well-socketed and will remain so when the patient is no longer immobilized. This manipulation may or may not require surgery, but some form of body cast or splint is used in either case.

Curvature of the spine may or may not require immediate surgical treatment. Braces may provide temporary relief, but a spinal fusion before full growth is attained may be necessary to prevent permanent curvature.

Patients receiving corrective measures for bone deformities are immobilized in some manner or other depending upon the extent of correction required and the type of restricting device or method used.

Nursing care includes the same precautions and measures needed for other immobile patients. The special problems related to the newborn with congenital deformities are discussed in Chapter 53.

SUMMARY

A disability of the musculoskeletal system usually has a long duration; that is, the correction, the healing process, and the rehabilitative therapies generally take time. Some disabilities cannot be corrected at all. The patient often has to learn to readjust his living habits and use special equipment or conveniences in his self-care and daily living practices.

Some diseases or disorders of this system are hereditary, and some are present at birth. There is no known cause or cure for certain diseases or disorders; others show dramatic improvement with treatment. In general, treatment and nursing care are directed toward comfort, prevention of deformities, and a return to self-assistance to the fullest extent possible.

What you know about growth and development will be useful in nursing these patients because musculoskeletal disorders occur at all ages. The duration of most conditions and the length of time you will be working with these patients make it essential not only that you understand what is occurring in the body but also how age influences behavior.

These patients need your skills, but they need your understanding too.

GUIDES FOR STUDY AND DISCUSSION

1. Chapters 7 and 8 tell you how bones grow and age. They describe how muscles work with joints to render certain services to the body. Test yourself on chapter objectives and review the summaries and vocabulary.

2. What is the work of the musculoskeletal system?

3. Healthy people enjoy a wide range of body movements. The orthopedic patient often experiences some/much limited movement temporarily or permanently. Think of some examples of limited movement which would influence his nursing care.

4. What is the difference between arthritis and rheumatism?

5. Use this chart form in your notebook to organize your thoughts for this chapter. When you have completed it, notice how much similarity there is among signs and symptoms. What does this tell you?

Disease/disorder	Definition	Signs/Symptoms	Nursing care

6. What is a purulent wound? Do you use surgical or medical aseptic technique when changing dressings? Why? Be ready to defend each nursing action listed under the care of a draining wound.

7. When a joint is inflamed, swollen, painful, tender, and maybe discolored for whatever reason/diagnosis, how should this set of circumstances influence your nursing actions?

8. Why is proper skin care such a challenge in orthopedic nursing? How is it provided?

9. If a patient is on a Stryker frame, which of his ten basic needs will have to be met in other than regular ways?

10. When a patient is in a cast, much depends upon observant nursing care. What does the knowing nurse do?

11. Several things are stressed in the care of the orthopedic patient. Why self-care in so far as possible? prevention of deformities? rehabilitation? emotional support?

12. When caring for a patient in traction, what are your responsibilities?

13. For what reasons might patients be immobilized? What are some common means used for this purpose?

SUGGESTED SITUATIONS AND ACTIVITIES

1. Johnnie is a seven-year-old boy with a draining abscess on his lower right leg; the leg is immobilized with a half splint and positioned to promote drainage. He has been hospitalized for two weeks and is improving; it is difficult for him to stay positioned because he is restless. Make a list of ways in which he can be involved in his daily care. Think of ways to help him manage these activities in spite of the fact that you have two other patients who need much of your time.

2. Arrange a bulletin board display of materials from community agencies concerned with musculoskeletal disorders.

CHAPTER 45

PATIENTS WITH DIGESTIVE TRACT AND METABOLIC DISORDERS

TOPICAL HEADINGS

Introduction
Diseases and Disorders of the Digestive Tract

Diseases and Disorders Influencing Metabolism
Summary

Guides for Study and Discussion
Suggested Situations and Activities

OBJECTIVES FOR THE STUDENT: Be able to:

1. Explain how digestion and metabolism are related.
2. Describe three situations where taking nourishment might require something other than normal eating.
3. Differentiate between gastric analysis and gastrointestinal siphonage.
4. Give one example each of drainage by force and drainage without force.
5. Given a list of eight nursing responsibilities related to an irrigation treatment, defend each one.
6. Distinguish between a functional disorder and a physical disorder.
7. Describe five signs of gastrointestinal distress.
8. Explain why strict asepsis is observed in caring for a patient with acute viral hepatitis.
9. Describe three precautions the diabetic patient must observe.
10. Identify three postoperative nursing care problems of a cholecystectomy patient.

SUGGESTED STUDY VOCABULARY*

trauma
suture
inflammation
stomatitis
glossitis
esophagitis
gastritis
enteritis
peritonitis
adhesions
lumen
stricture
obstruction
distention

toxemia
pyogenic organism
toxicity
ascites
prognosis
malfunction
hypothyroidism
hyperthyroidism
metabolism
thyroxin
diabetes mellitus
hypoglycemia
glycosuria
polyuria
polyphagia

polydipsia
insulin shock
acidosis
varicose veins
jaundice
hepatitis
cirrhosis
cholelithiasis
cholecystitis
cholecystectomy
irrigation
pancreatitis
Addison's disease
intubation
peritoneal dialysis

*Look for any terms you already know.

INTRODUCTION

Whenever anything interferes with the normal structure and function of the alimentary canal, the body reacts in a great many different ways. As pointed out in Chapter 41, anorexia, nausea, vomiting, diarrhea, constipation, and flatus are common body reactions. You might add inflammation, pain, fever, hemorrhage, dehydration, electrolyte imbalance, anxiety, and restlessness. The list is longer, but these examples show how far-reaching digestive disturbances can be.

The cells must be able to receive proper nutrients, minerals, and chemical elements in the amounts needed if they are to carry on their metabolic activities. The work of the digestive system, of course, is to render food that is eaten into forms and substances that the cells can use.

This chapter is divided between digestion and metabolism for the convenience of study, but in real life these two processes go hand in hand. Remember that the digestive tract could not do effective work without support from the liver, gallbladder, pancreas, and even the thyroid gland. Notice in Table 11–1 the contributions made to digestion by pancreatic juice and by bile from the liver.

Thus, if something occurs in the pancreas or the liver to hinder their normal functions, chemical digestion becomes upset, just as it will if something goes wrong in the mouth, stomach, or intestines.

Review of the following will help round out your understanding: Chapters 11, 12, 26 (dietary requirements related to digestive and metabolic disorders) and 41.

DISEASES AND DISORDERS OF THE DIGESTIVE TRACT

The mouth and the esophagus are portals of entry for food to get to the stomach. Anything that causes chewing difficulty (e.g., fractured jaw, burns from acid, inflammation of the tongue) or swallowing difficulty (e.g., burns from acid, a foreign object in the esophagus, a tumor obstructing the esophagus) must be treated, along with the feeding or nourishment problem it might create.

CONDITIONS OF THE MOUTH

The tongue is a fairly good index to disorder elsewhere in the body. For example, if it is coated with a white, furry substance, it may indicate a low grade fever or mild dehydration. Dryness of the tongue, with a color ranging from white to dark brown, suggests dehydration. Scarlet fever and other "high fever" illnesses cause the tongue to become bright red and painfully sore, often called "strawberry tongue." *Glossitis* means inflammation of the tongue.

Tongue soreness and inflammation are treated locally (irrigations, local application of medicine, mouth washes) but steps are also taken to treat the original cause of the inflammation.

Feeding the patient with a severe mouth disability is often a matter of frequent and small high caloric liquid feeds through a straw. Frequent mouth washes and irrigations of normal saline may be ordered to keep the mouth and breath odorfree and to help prevent infections.

Injuries to the mouth range from mild (biting the tongue while chewing) to severe (lacerations of the tongue, cheek, and lips; broken teeth; fractured jaw). The traumatized tissues swell and cause discomfort. Wounds often require sutures which add to the feeling of mouth stiffness and immobility. Patients are concerned about disfigurement when there are sutures and wounds on the face. The less strain on sutures and healing wounds, the better the patient's chances are for minimal scarring.

Elevating the head (if allowed) helps to relieve swelling. Depending upon the location, amount, and extent of trauma and surgical repair, the patient is encouraged to keep his face and mouth as immobile as possible to permit healing.

Mouth Infections

Mouth tissues can become infected even if they are able to ward off organisms in normal daily contact with them.

PAROTITIS. The "itis" means that there is an inflammation—in this case, in the parotid glands located just below the ear on each side of the lower jaw. Parotitis is caused by an organism in the mouth that has found its way into the glands, perhaps because of poor oral hygiene. Another reason may be the patient's generally low resistance to infection. Mumps is an epidemic form of parotitis, a communicable disease discussed in Chapter 54.

Parotitis is a painful condition; there is local swelling on one or both sides. The treatment consists of antibiotics and meticulous oral hygiene. The swelling in the glands prevents the usual flow of saliva; in some instances the physician may recommend that the patient chew gum to help increase the flow of saliva. If the parotitis leads to an abscess, stones in the glands, or a chronic inflammatory condition, steps are taken to drain the abscess, remove the stones, or even remove the gland itself.

VINCENT'S ANGINA. This condition is commonly known as "trench mouth," coming from World War I days when it was so prevalent among soldiers. Vincent's angina is an infection of mouth tissues that produces ulcers with a grayish white appearance. The body can react with fever and local lymph nodes may become enlarged and tender.

Antibiotics usually clear up the condition but it can spread fast if it goes untreated. Mouthwashes (sodium perborate) are commonly used.

CANKER SORE. A canker sore is a common type of mouth inflammation of unknown cause. Some people have these sores often; others seldom do. They are painful and bothersome, but there is no specific cure. A canker sore runs its course in a few days and disappears.

STOMATITIS. Stomatitis is a term meaning inflammation of the mouth. As pointed out in Chapter 41, this inflammation is the body's reaction to a disorder somewhere in the body.

GINGIVITIS. Gingivitis means inflammation of the gums. Here again something is responsible for making the gums red, sore, and tender. It may be an ill-fitting removable bridge or a reaction to infection.

HERPES SIMPLEX. This condition is a cluster of small transparent blisters that are inflamed and usually itch or burn. When these are present on the skin of the face, lips, or membranes of the mouth, they are called *cold sores* or *fever blisters*. When present on the labia they are called herpes labialis. They come spontaneously, for no apparent reason, and within a week or two they "cure" themselves if untreated.

CONDITIONS OF THE ESOPHAGUS

The esophagus may become inflamed and infected, obstructed by some foreign object or abnormal growth, or burned by some corrosive agent (acid, detergent, lye); or it may be abnormal in its structure at birth or become so later on.

One of the chief nursing problems of patients experiencing a disorder of the esophagus is nourishment. The extent and type of disorder determine what therapy the physician will carry out. Surgery, called a gastrostomy, may be necessary to create an artificial opening in the stomach and thus feed the patient directly into the stomach. A Levin tube (Fig. 42–6) may have to be used to bypass the condition. In either event, the patient receives his liquid high caloric diet by artificial means (gavage). The nurse uses an Asepto syringe to introduce the feeding into the Levin tube, or the tube is inserted through the gastrostomy. Patients can be taught to assist with these measures if they are able to follow directions and their condition permits.

DIAGNOSTIC TESTS AND SPECIAL THERAPEUTIC MEASURES

A variety of tests, equipment, and procedures are available for diagnostic purposes. You will be involved with many of them to greater or lesser degrees. Some of the more common ones are included here.

Intubation means inserting a tube. Gastric intubation means a tube is inserted into the stomach/intestines by way of the mouth or by way of the nose (nasogastric.) See Figure 45–1.

A tube is inserted (usually by the physician) to remove contents for analysis, to relieve/prevent distention, or for tube feedings. *Gastric analysis* is when a sample of stomach contents is withdrawn (aspirated) with a syringe attached to the outer end of the tube. Food and fluids are withheld (usually eight hours) before the tube is passed. Specimens are placed in clearly identified containers. Sometimes a medication is ordered following the aspiration and another sample(s) withdrawn at a specified time(s).

Practical nurse responsibilities may include: (1) Instructing the patient about the

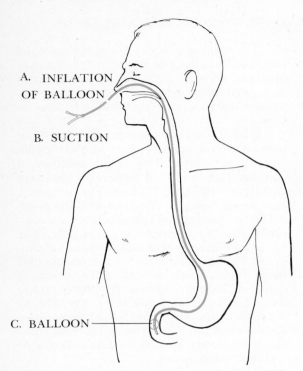

A. INFLATION
OF BALLOON

B. SUCTION

C. BALLOON

FIGURE 45–1 A Miller-Abbot tube in place. This tube has two parts to it and two openings. A, to inflate the balloon. B, to attach to the suction machine; this branch of the tube is labeled "suction" to avoid getting them mixed up.

need for "nothing by mouth" before the test and placing an appropriate sign to notify others. (2) Assembling the equipment for the test and arranging the patient's unit. (3) Participating in the process by assisting the physician, supporting the patient, and taking care of the specimen.

If the tube is left in place, the outer end is clamped off and taped to the patient's face (Fig. 45–2). It should not pull against the nares. Pay particular attention to skin care around the nose and keep the mouth and lips clean; mouth breathing tends to dry the lips and membranes. If the tube is removed, provide mouth care and ready the patient for eating unless otherwise indicated.

A tubeless method of gastric analysis consists of giving a drug by mouth (e.g., Diagnex Blue) and the urine is tested twice to determine the hydrochloric acid in the stomach. Follow all directions for withholding food and fluids and getting the needed specimens.

Gastrointestinal siphonage means drawing off contents from the stomach/intestines.

The reason may be to: remove swallowed poison, relieve/prevent distention, prevent nausea or vomiting, provide a continuous means of keeping the region empty to reduce peristalsis, secure specimens, or relieve a condition surrounding an obstruction.

Various types of tubes are used, depending on the region to be served and the purpose of the procedure.

Types of tubes (See *Drainage* for siphonage force) include: (1) Levin: single lumen rubber/plastic in common use (Fig. 42–6). (2) Miller-Abbot: see Figure 45–1. Double lumen used in the small intestines. (3) Abbot-Rawson: Double lumen with one (inner) end extending several inches beyond the other. Permits feeding and siphonage; used with gastric surgery. (4) Blakemore (Blakemore-Sengstaken): Triple lumen used to stop hemorrhage (esophagus, stomach, etc.) and for siphonage (Fig. 45–6). (5) Others: Rehfuss, Jutt, Cantor, Rectal.

Swallowing a tube is not the easiest thing a patient does; precautions should be taken to reassure him that by doing certain things it can be a much easier experience.

Passing a mouth/nose tube is an exacting procedure usually done by the physician or the registered nurse. The danger of getting the tube into the lung instead of the stomach is very real and is not considered a procedure for the LPN. However, you can help prepare the patient by telling him the tube will be moved along with each swallow and no faster. He will breathe through his mouth and the process will be slow to prevent gagging. He should know, too, that the doctor or nurse knows ahead of time just how far the tube will be inserted.

A rubber tube should be chilled first by placing it in chipped ice for a few minutes; a plastic tube is made more flexible by placing it in warm water.

Drainage. There are two main ways to remove accumulations from body cavities and tissues: (1) by a force that exerts suction; or (2) by drainage without suction.

1. Suction is a sucking up of fluid and gases to a partial vacuum; this vacuum may be created by a hand process (e.g., Hemovac, Asepto syringe), by an electric pump or machine (e.g., Gomco, Emerson) that is adjustable to various rates or pressure, by attachment to piped suction from a wall

outlet, or by creating a vacuum with a Wangensteen type set up. Suction is used with most tubes inserted into the gastrointestinal tract (one common exception is the rectal tube inserted in the anus).

2. Drainage without suction is usually associated with a surgical site; the drain is inserted as part of the surgical procedure and removed by the surgeon at a later time. Two common types of drains are: (1) the Penrose (Fig. 45–8); and (2) the T tube.

Whatever type of drainage is used, you will have responsibilities for observing the amount and character of drainage.

EXAMINATION BY LOOKING

The physician uses any number of tests, scopes and other pieces of equipment to diagnose gastrointestinal difficulties.

Tests

Gastrointestinal Series (GI Series). As the patient drinks barium sulfate (a chalky substance that outlines a part) the physician in the x-ray department watches it move down the esophagus into the stomach by using the fluoroscope. Also, x-ray pictures are taken then, again in six hours and in 24 hours (sometimes).

The stomach must be empty for the test so nothing can be taken by mouth after midnight and until after the 6 hour x-rays have been taken. If 24 hour x-ray pictures are needed be sure any ordered cathartic or enema is withheld until after these x-rays are taken.

Studying the colon (Barium enema). Here again, the physician in the x-ray department uses the fluoroscope (and takes x-ray pictures) while the patient receives a barium enema. The colon must be clear of any solid fecal material prior to the test. Preparation usually includes a cathartic (e.g., castor oil)

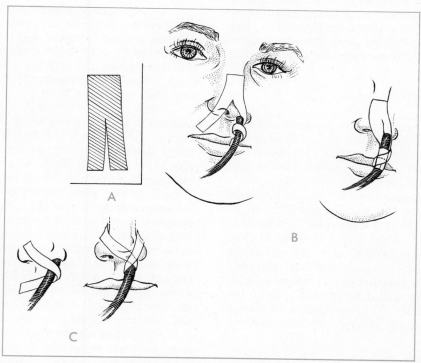

FIGURE 45–2 Ways to anchor a naso tube to the face. A, Split a length of adhesive tape. B, Attach the unsplit portion to the nose and wrap one of the split ends around the tube; wrap the other split end around the tube. C, Wrap a narrow strip of adhesive tape around the tube and attach ends to the nose. (Adapted from Dison, N. G.: An Atlas of Nursing Techniques, 2nd ed. The C. V. Mosby Co.)

the afternoon before and a clear liquid diet and cleansing enemas until there is no solid fecal matter in the return flow the day of the test.

Other Instruments for Looking

(1) Gastroscope—an instrument used to examine the interior of the stomach. *The stomach must be empty;* food and fluids are withheld at least eight hours before the test. It may even be necessary to do a gastric lavage; all stomach secretions are removed just prior to inserting the gastroscope.

Pre-examination medication is sometimes given as well as a local throat-pharynx spray anesthesia. Post-examination orders include nothing by mouth until the effects of the local anesthesia are gone to avoid drawing any foreign substance into the trachea.

(2) Protoscope—a lighted tube-like instrument used to examine the rectum by way of the anus. *The bowel must be free of fecal material.* Pre-examination orders include: (1) A cathartic the evening before; (2) liquid diet the day of examination; and (3) enemas until the return flow contains no solid fecal matter.

(3) Sigmoidoscope—a lighted tube-like instrument used to examine the sigmoid by way of the anus. Directions for preparing a patient for this procedure are the same as for a proctoscopy.

Irrigation

In medical terms this means washing a wound or a body cavity with a fluid under pressure. Irrigation is used to: (1) cleanse and medicate areas (wounds, cavities, etc.); and (2) keep drains open.

Almost any part of the body may be subject to irrigation. When it is ordered be sure to determine: (1) Why it is ordered. (2) What is to be irrigated. (3) When it is to be done. (4) The solution (kind, strength, and amount) to be used. (5) The technique to use (clean/sterile). (6) How much pressure to use (height of solution above the area determines the force behind the stream). (7) How irrigation solution is to be returned. (8) The equipment to use.

Colostomy Irrigation

A colostomy is an artificial bowel opening (temporary or permanent) brought to the surface of the abdomen for the purpose of bowel evacuation. A two-opening colostomy is called "double barrel"; the opening closest to food coming through the tract (proximal) is called the working end; the other opening (distal), closest to the anus, is non-working with respect to evacuation. See Appendix III, Colostomy, for details of irrigation.

Stool Specimens

The physician will order a stool specimen when he is seeking evidence of gastrointestinal difficulty, such as bleeding, disease-producing organisms (e.g., the typhoid fever organism) or the presence of pus, mucus, parasites, or undigested food. Determine ahead of time if certain precautions must be taken (e.g., time, amount, warm specimen) to ensure satisfactory laboratory results.

GASTRIC AND INTESTINAL DISORDERS

Emotions and Digestion

Appetite and digestion are closely related to emotions. Tension, fear, sorrow, and anxiety can and do interfere with the feeling of hunger, swallowing, and the normal process of digestion. Some persons seem to experience more difficulty than others. *Dyspepsia* means impaired digestion.

When a disorder shows no apparent changes in body tissue, it is called a *functional disorder*. However, it is true that certain functional disorders of the stomach can create changes in stomach tissue. Common signs or symptoms of functional disorder are belching, complaints of nausea, vomiting, tenderness in the epigastric area, and rapid heart beat. Psychogenic vomiting is seen in children more frequently than in adults. It is repeated vomiting which has no apparent physical reason for happening and is a means to call attention to oneself. For example, a small child may develop this technique when a new baby joins the family. There also may be deep-seated psychological reasons for vomiting.

Medical management of patients suffering from nervous dyspepsia is directed toward more regularity in sleep and slowing down the rate of tension-producing activities or eliminating them if possible. Sedatives may be necessary to help make such adjustments. Reassurance that the symptoms are functional and can be helped often relieves the fear of a possible physical disorder.

Gastritis

Gastritis is inflammation of the gastric mucosa. It may be short (acute) or long-term (chronic). Acute gastritis may result from eating some irritating food or from a surface infection of the lining of the stomach by some microorganism (as with measles). During the attack (which may disappear rapidly), there is formation of considerable mucus which is later vomited; the patient complains of tenderness and is unable to retain anything in his stomach.

Chronic gastritis may develop from numerous attacks of an acute nature. The exact cause is unknown, but all food substances which tend to irritate the gastric mucosa need to be eliminated from the diet. Some microorganisms infect the stomach lining and produce inflammation; there is marked increase in the mucoid secretion. The character of the gastric mucosa changes, as do the functions of the glands producing gastric juices.

The patient is bothered with epigastric distress, loses weight, has some nausea and vomiting, poor appetite, and complains of general weakness and fatigue. Mental depression is common; the patient worries about his condition. This disease is fifth in the cause of deaths for children from one to four years of age.

Diet should be bland, avoiding sharp spices or roughage. Medications are given to supplement vitamin and mineral intake, to "pep up" the appetite, and to control pain and discomfort.

Continued inflammation is observed for possible cancer. Hemorrhage may be a complication in some instances.

Peptic Ulcers

Peptic ulcers are lesions/craters in the mucous membrane of the lower esophagus, stomach, and the first portion of the small intestines (duodenum).

The cause is not easily understood, however, much is known about the development and course of the peptic ulcer. Opinions about cause vary, but there is general agreement that certain types of people are more likely to have peptic ulcers than others: they live with constant inner tension; work hard; are anxious; and worry. There is some question about a possible relationship between peptic ulcer and certain endocrine abnormalities. Eating habits and the state of emotions while eating seem to influence the condition. Hurried, irregular eating when upset, tired, or worried, seem to be predisposing factors. Other factors include: genetic influence, association with other diseases (e.g., pulmonary disease, rheumatoid arthritis) and the use of certain drugs.

Whatever the cause(s), there is increased gastric secretion and decreased mucous membrane resistance producing localized area(s) of mucosa unable to withstand the digestive action of gastric juice (hydrochloric acid); the membrane erodes and tissue is lost producing the ulcer or crater.

Peptic ulcer may be acute or chronic. In the acute stage healing is faster than in the chronic stage. Healing and activity may go on at the same time in an ulcer; healing is from below upward.

One of the greatest dangers in a chronic ulcer condition is hemorrhage; this can be severe and is often fatal. The walls of the stomach may be perforated by the same process that erodes the blood vessels and this causes another acute condition called peritonitis.

SIGNS AND SYMPTOMS. Most pronounced is the burning, gnawing, cramplike sensation (mild to severe pain) in the epigastric region, relieved by eating but returning later on. Pain usually occurs during the night, some one to four hours after retiring, depending upon when the person last ate; it is apt to be absent before breakfast. It is said that the pain is caused by hydrochloric acid lowering the pain threshold in the nerve endings in the ulcer.

Other signs/symptoms include belching and distress and changed bowel habits (constipation, flatulence, tarry stools).

The distress is periodic and may come and go for years (average 5 to 8 years). For many patients the recurrences become less frequent and the ulcer heals. Elderly patients are apt to have large craters subject to hemorrhage and perforation.

MEDICAL TREATMENT AND NURSING CARE. Treatment is geared to relieving epigastric pain, healing the ulcer, and preventing its return. This all takes time, as well as taking the patient's cooperation to live within the requirements for rest and food.

With tension a factor in producing peptic ulcers, it is easy to understand why a patient may be put on bed rest, away from his work so that he has an opportunity to relax. Drugs are given to help him relax and to relieve his distress (antacids).

If there is blood loss, transfusions may be ordered to help restore blood volume and energy.

One of the most important parts of treatment is diet. While there are differences of medical opinion about what the patient should eat, the tendency is to require frequent small feedings of food the patient likes and can tolerate. However, some physicians prescribe a four-stage diet, in which the patient moves from milk and cream to frequent small feedings of bland foods with milk and cream to a six-feeding routine of selected foods and finally a three-meal-a-day schedule, avoiding roughage and irritating foods. This diet is more fully discussed in Chapter 26. You will notice that the one factor these two therapies have in common is frequent small feedings.

It is a nursing responsibility to see that the patient receives and consumes his food as ordered, making note of any complaints or untoward signs. He often complains about the monotony of his diet and needs reassurance about the need to stay with it.

Good diversional activities in keeping with the need for rest and relaxation should be considered for patients who are restless or discouraged with diet and bed rest. Find out if there are any restrictions about the number or frequency of visitors or the extent of "work" activities the patient can or should do while hospitalized. For example, if his office calls him every day and discusses business with him, this should be reported. The physician may or may not permit it, depending on the circumstances.

If permitted, involve the patient in as many aspects of self-care as possible, but in so doing do not forget the necessity to observe his needs and reassure him with your frequent presence and help. If worry caused his ulcer, he could easily continue to worry if he is hospitalized with little or no personal attention.

Observation of stools (frequency, character, presence of flatulence) should be continued. If there is a question about the appearance of the stool, report it. Other necessary observations include belching, pain (time, location, patient's description, duration), and the amount and character of any vomitus.

SURGICAL TREATMENT. When there is uncontrolled hemorrhage, an obstruction that cannot be otherwise reduced, an acute perforation, or signs that the ulcer refuses to heal, it is usually treated surgically. The type and extent of surgery depends upon the age and condition of the patient, the location, and the extent or number of lesions. Sometimes both the stomach and duodenum are involved. Two terms used to identify removal of part of the stomach are *gastric resection* and *gastrectomy* (which may include the whole stomach). Again depending upon circumstances, the operation may include a new opening between the partial stomach and the jejunum, completely bypassing the duodenum; this is just one of a dozen different ways surgeons have of removing the diseased portion and joining together healthy tissue between the stomach and some part of the intestinal tract.

This surgical patient receives the same general postoperative care and observations as other patients. He will have a Levin tube in place and suction will be attached to keep the stomach free of fluids. The drainage should not contain any amount of bright red blood; this would indicate hemorrhage and should be reported immediately. It should be brownish-red at the beginning and gradually become yellowish-green.

The patient is usually quite uncomfortable for several days, with gastric suction and parenteral fluids (electrolyte and fluid balance are important to healing and recovery) being administered. Nothing is given by mouth for a period of time; this necessitates frequent and thorough mouth care to keep it clean and odor-free.

Another surgical treatment is called vagotomy. The vagus nerve stimulates gastric secretions and stomach activity. A vagotomy interrupts the work (nerve impulses) of the vagus nerve thereby reducing gastric secretions and stomach activity; it is sometimes done in combination with gastric surgery.

Enteritis

This is a long-term inflammatory disease of the small intestines—most common in young adults—that may or may not require surgery. It is caused by a nonspecific organism (i.e., streptococci, pneumococci) that infects the bowel lining, causing it to become painfully swollen and edematous. The swelling may close the lumen of the bowel and produce an obstruction. This condition may erode and perforate the bowel, causing abscesses. Draining the abscesses can lead to a fistula. Any of these complicating conditions in enteritis are serious and usually require surgery. If the diseased portion of the bowel can be removed, a colostomy may or may not be performed. However, many times enteritis must be treated medically. The age and general condition of the patient influence the physician's decision.

SIGNS AND SYMPTOMS. These include fever, diarrhea (frequent semi-solid stools containing mucus and pus), blood in stools, abdominal pain, dehydration, and weight loss.

MEDICAL TREATMENT AND NURSING CARE. As you can see from the signs and symptoms, the physician is concerned with treating the patient to maintain fluid and electrolyte balance and increase weight, as well as to find drugs that will clear up the infection medically. However, as stated previously, complicating conditions may require surgery.

Nursing care for this patient involves eating problems (because of abdominal pain after eating), skin care of the buttocks and anal region due to diarrhea, and helping the patient's outlook toward his long-term (often recurring) illness. In addition to the regular orders for his comfort and personal care, the practical nurse might be involved in some Role II tasks if the patient undergoes special therapeutic measures.

Irritable Colon

This is a group name for a variety of disturbances of the function of the colon related to emotional tension and nonspecific stress. The group includes: mucous colitis, spastic colon, unstable colon, and adaptive colitis.

Irritable colon is common, is said to account for more than one half of all gastrointestinal disorders and ranks with the common cold for frequent minor disability. It is associated with life stress situations and often disappears when the stress situation is gone.

SIGNS AND SYMPTOMS. Abdominal pain (mild to severe) is usually in the lower abdomen and is most often relieved by passage of feces and/or gas. Other colonic signs are constipation, flatulence, diarrhea and painful straining at stool (tenesmus), small stools with visible mucus or just mucus.

Anorexia, nausea, belching and sometimes vomiting indicate disturbance higher up in the GI tract. These symptoms may be accompanied by shortness of breath, palpitation, headache, fatigue, faintness and/or sighing respirations and hyperventilation. Usually not all symptoms are present, rather a few, but different from patient to patient.

The physician determines whether or not the signs/symptoms might be the result of some specific disorder (e.g., cancer of the colon, ulcerative colitis, gall bladder disease) before proceeding to treat the patient. Treatment may include psychotherapy, tranquilizers for insomnia, and drugs for diarrhea, though it usually does not respond to ordinary anti-diarrheal treatment.

Colitis

Inflammation of the colon is called colitis. It is caused by many different organisms and frequently is a long-term, chronic condition, similar in many ways to enteritis. It is very serious and may be fatal if it becomes ulcerative.

This inflammatory process, if not checked, involves all layers of the bowel wall and destroys large areas; extensive destruction includes the anus and surrounding tissues.

Patients (more frequently women than men) suffering from this disease often have a background of conflicting emotional factors and characteristic traits. They seem overly anxious about things (i.e., husband-wife relationships, family). Psychotherapy has been known to help some resolve their conflicts with subsequent improvement in the disease.

SIGNS AND SYMPTOMS. The disease runs a course of remissions and recurrences. First symptoms are flatulence and indigestion. Loose stools occur with increasing frequency. The appetite diminishes and the patient seems weak and worried. As the inflammation progresses, the loose stools turn to diarrhea of pus, blood, mucus, and feces. Abdominal cramps are present.

The patient suffers from malnutrition, anemia, and dehydration. This causes general exhaustion and the patient has many reasons to complain.

MEDICAL TREATMENT AND NURSING

CARE.   Body fluid and electrolyte balance is an essential part of treatment. The diet is highly caloric and high in protein, minerals, and vitamins, avoiding all foods that irritate the bowel. Drugs include medications to control diarrhea, relieve anxiety, control the inflammation, treat any open lesions, and avoid complications.

Nursing care involves meeting many mental as well as physical needs. Worry often prevents rest, and complete rest is essential.

Additional time is needed for daily care if open lesions need irrigation, treatment, and dressings changed. Because this patient is worried he may talk a great deal about himself, his condition, or his family. Questions about his progress should be handled by the physician. This does not mean that you do not reassure the patient and help him to relax. Everything about his care seems to be important to him. Well-planned, unhurried care helps to relieve worry; this patient needs confidence in his nurse and wants to feel that his needs are being met. It helps if he is able to be involved in self-care activities.

Congenital Malformations

As with any other part of the body there may be malformation of the intestine. Some malformations are apparent soon after birth and others may not become apparent for some years.

Possible malformations include enlargement of a segment of the bowel; outpouching of the intestinal wall (diverticulum); or the absence of the lumen (intestinal atresia) in some portion of the bowel. This latter condition needs immediate repair if the infant is to live. (See Chapter 53.)

Some malformations need early repair and usually respond well to surgery. In the instance of weakness in the wall with diverticula, these pouches may retain feces and set up an inflammation (diverticulitis) which can lead to perforation of the pocket and peritonitis; it may also obstruct the bowel. Resection of the diseased portion or, in some instances, a colostomy is the surgical treatment.

Medical Treatment and Nursing Care. Both are geared to relieving any signs or symptoms of intestinal distress and systemic reactions. If surgery is performed, regular postoperative care and observations are involved.

Appendicitis

Inflammation of the appendix is serious; it requires medical management instead of "home remedies" (hot water bottle, cathartics, enema).

The function of the appendix in the human being is thought to be of little importance; however, its possible contribution to the normal body is being studied. It extends from the cecum and has a narrow lumen which can easily accumulate feces or hard foreign substances passing through the bowel. Pyogenic organisms can set up an inflammation (more likely in children) which leads to a pus-forming infection, suppurative appendicitis. In young and middle-aged adults there is more apt to be an acute or chronic ulcerative infection which produces a thickening of the appendix and often leads to bothersome adhesions; it is also possible for this type of appendicitis to become suppurative.

SIGNS AND SYMPTOMS.   At the onset, which is sudden in acute appendicitis, cramping pains surrounding the umbilicus spread throughout the abdomen and quite soon localize in the right lower quadrant; this is accompanied by nausea and vomiting, usually some fever and no appetite. It should be reemphasized that cathartics, hot water bottles, and enemas should not be used. A ruptured appendix produces peritonitis.

An appendectomy is performed (usually an emergency operation) and, in case of abscess, peritonitis, or local fluid, drains are put in the wound. Without complications this patient has a short convalescence; he is usually ambulatory the day after surgery and back at school or the job in two or three weeks.

Hemorrhoids

When veins in the internal wall of the rectum or outside the anal sphincter dilate or outpouch, they form enlargements called *hemorrhoids* (Fig. 45–3). Man's upright position, prolonged sitting or standing, straining at stools, or a systemic condition producing pressure on the hemorrhoidal veins cause them to enlarge or outpouch (varicose veins).

Internal hemorrhoids cannot be seen without a proctoscopic examination unless they have protruded through the anus. They can become ulcerative masses, causing severe pain. Rectal bleeding may result.

INTERNAL HEMORRHOIDS

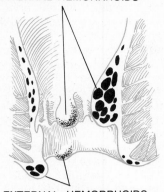

EXTERNAL HEMORRHOIDS

FIGURE 45–3   Hemorrhoids may be internal, external or a combination of both.

MEDICAL TREATMENT AND NURSING CARE. Treatment of internal hemorrhoids may or may not include surgery. If the inflamed tissue is not too extensive and not ulcerated and bleeding, suppositories may be ordered to shrink the tissues and bring relief. In severe cases (bleeding, protrusion, ulceration) surgical treatment or injection is needed. Surgical treatment is called a *hemorrhoidectomy*. Injecting the veins with chemicals is a hospital procedure also. Complications from injection therapy include severe hemorrhage and sloughing off of tissue which makes healing a very slow, painful process.

A patient is usually very uncomfortable after a hemorrhoidectomy. The surgical procedure may not be very involved, but the pain and soreness from pressure on the anal area can be very annoying.

A rubber ring under the buttocks may remove some pressure; lying on the abdomen may afford a comfortable change. The physician usually orders warm, wet compresses, analgesic ointments, or ice packs. Pain medications may also be ordered. Sitz baths afford relief from discomfort; they are usually ordered early in recovery and continued when the patient goes home.

Whether spontaneous or the result of an enema, bowel movements can be most painful. The patient should be attended during this time as he may become dizzy or faint from the pain.

Diet is planned to avoid constipation and straining the area during defecation.

External hemorrhoids are visible upon inspection. They can cause a burning, itching sensation and be very uncomfortable. The inflammation causes swelling and pain; this discomfort usually responds to a warm sitz bath unless the affected area is extensive. A simple surgical removal of the clot under local anesthesia affords relief.

Intestinal Obstruction

The lumen of the bowel is the passageway for the contents of the intestines. When anything occurs to obstruct this passageway, either partially or totally, it is called an *intestinal obstruction*. Figure 45–4 shows how a twisted bowel completely obstructs the passage of any material.

Some obstructions are termed mechanical and include such things as compression of the lumen due to tumors (see Cancer, Chapter 43) or adhesions; impacted feces; or a narrowing of the lumen due to strictures, foreign bodies, strangulated hernia, or a twisted bowel.

Some toxic and nervous conditions interfere with normal peristalsis and slow down or stop the movement of bowel content.

SIGNS AND SYMPTOMS. A bowel obstruction, regardless of cause, produces some general symptoms. When the lumen is

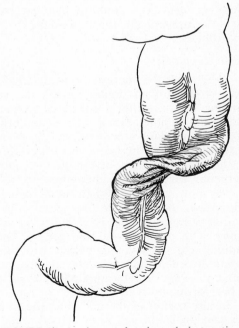

FIGURE 45–4   A complete bowel obstruction.

blocked, the intestine close to the obstruction sets up a reverse peristalsis; this finally results in moving fecal matter back to the stomach and then it is vomited.

Right above the point of complete obstruction, there is an accumulation of decaying fecal material whose bacterial toxins are rapidly absorbed by the blood, causing toxemia. Increased blood (hyperemia) and exudates are present at the site of inflammation. Death usually results within several hours.

The presence of fecal material in vomitus always indicates an intestinal obstruction. Other signs or symptoms include changed bowel habits (constipation or diarrhea), severe intermittent cramps, abdominal distention, dehydration (fluid imbalance due to diarrhea and vomiting), fever, and rapid pulse.

MEDICAL TREATMENT AND NURSING CARE. The object of treatment is to determine the cause and extent of obstruction and remove or reduce it as soon as possible. It may require emergency surgery. The patient cannot long survive if the obstruction is severely limiting the normal peristaltic action of the bowel. Fluids, food, and feces accumulate, and the bowel distends with increasing pressure. Circulation that is cut off produces gangrene, and perforation of the distended bowel causes peritonitis. One of the serious problems is dehydration and fluid and electrolyte imbalance. Food and fluids cannot be given by mouth because they cannot be handled properly in the intestine and only add to the distention problem.

Hernia (Inguinal)

A hernia is the abnormal protrusion of an organ or part of an organ through the surrounding structure that is supposed to house it. It should be noted that just about any organ or part can herniate or push through surrounding structures (e.g., in the newborn a congenital hernia in the diaphragm requires emergency surgery), but abdominal wall hernias are more common. When the hernial sac is removed, the defective abdominal wall is repaired surgically; this is called a *herniorrhaphy*. The patient's age and general body condition (e.g., very young, elderly with other chronic disorders such as a chronic cough or cardiac disorders), determine whether or not the herniorrhaphy is to be done.

In any region of the abdomen the intestines can push through a weakened area. It may be at the site of an operation (recent or otherwise), through a muscle area weakened from heavy lifting or severe coughing, or it may be present at birth.

Usually the contents of the pouch (hernial sac) can be pushed back by pressure. However, a portion or loop of the bowel sometimes adheres to the lining of the hernial sac; this is called an *irreducible or incarcerated hernia*. When the loop of the bowel is so constricted by the opening that there is some obstruction, it is termed a *strangulated hernia*.

MEDICAL TREATMENT AND NURSING CARE. When a herniorrhaphy is performed, the wound must heal well to make the repair successful. Early ambulation is an essential part of the healing process. The patient is usually permitted out of bed the day after surgery. Male patients are sometimes allowed to stand at the bed (with assistance) to void on the operative day. Patients may be hesitant about walking for fear of straining the incision. Walking, deep breathing, and self-care activities help prevent complications by reestablishing normal muscle tone and normal body processes. It helps the patient to have this explained to him. Arrange the environment so he does not have to lift, push, or pull any objects that would put a strain on the sutures. Make it possible for him to get in and out of bed without stretching abdominal muscles.

If the hernia repair is in the inguinal area, the male patient may experience some pain and swelling of the scrotum; some type of scrotal support or suspensory is usually provided for comfort.

Vomiting, coughing, and straining during defecation all put strain on the incision and should be avoided. A medication may be ordered to permit easy passage of soft stools. If vomiting and retching is present, a nasogastric tube with low pressure suction may be used for several days. Something might be ordered to control the coughing.

Diet is restored to food and fluids as soon as the patient can tolerate them. In some instances, the patient has nothing by mouth for a few days; parenteral fluids are given and the nasogastric tube is used.

Strict aseptic practices should be used to avoid any possibility of infection. Keep in mind that the object of all treatment and care is to promote good wound healing; an infection in the wound could seriously hamper this process.

Other Bowel and Abdominal Conditions

For a discussion of diarrhea, constipation, and flatulence, see Chapter 41.

INTUSSUSCEPTION. The telescoping of one segment of the bowel into another is called *intussusception*. It occurs in all age groups and causes obstruction. Venous congestion may lead to necrosis of tissue. Overdistention may lead to perforation and peritonitis.

As described previously under Obstruction, treatment to relieve this condition should be immediate.

PERITONITIS. Peritonitis, with either generalized or local walled-off pockets of pus, is an inflammation of the peritoneum. It is a dangerous condition and requires emergency measures if it is generalized. It is caused by pyogenic organisms reaching the peritoneal cavity by way of the blood or by some substance escaping into the cavity from a perforated bowel, gastric ulcer, or ruptured appendix. It spreads rapidly and paralyzes the bowel, producing high fever and toxicity.

Lifesaving measures are used in generalized peritonitis to reverse the state of toxicity; death soon follows if this cannot be accomplished.

ASCITES. Ascites, which accompanies many types of abdominal conditions, is an accumulation of clear yellow fluid in the peritoneal cavity. The abdomen is full and distended and responds with a dull sound when tapped or thumped. Fluid exudate is present from an infection, from faulty blood circulation, or from improper kidney or liver function. The condition is painless but distention causes discomfort. Ascites often recurs.

An abdominal paracentesis may be carried out to remove the fluid. Using a surgical procedure, a small abdominal incision is made to insert a cannula and a small drainage tube into the peritoneal cavity; the accumulated fluid drains off into a container. Observations include patient reactions and type and amount of fluid drained in a specified time.

ADHESIONS. Adhesions are fibrous bands or tissues attached to organs, holding them in abnormal positions. They can cause bowel obstructions. They are caused by surgery or as a result of blunt abdominal trauma or old peritoneal infection. Recurring adhesions create continuing, stubborn problems. One thing that has promoted prevention is the discontinued use of talcum powder on surgical gloves; the starch now used is wiped off before entering the abdominal cavity. Surgeons also have limited or discarded the practice of pouring therapeutic substances such as sulfanilamide powder into the abdomen.

DISEASES AND DISORDERS INFLUENCING METABOLISM

Chapter 12, The Process of Metabolism, points out how a living cell is a working cell, producing heat and energy for the body to carry on its activities. Heat and energy production in the cells is a complicated chemical process; it includes using food substances, storing these substances until needed, and ridding the cell of wastes. The rate of heat production is called metabolic rate.

Many glands and organs play a part in making it possible for cells to carry on the chemical process called metabolism. This section of the chapter discusses four glands or organs which can malfunction and upset the digestive process and cell metabolism.

MALFUNCTION OF THE THYROID GLAND

The thyroid gland is situated against the front of the trachea just below the larynx; it produces and stores a hormone that is released (in part) into the blood as the body demands it. The part that is released is called *thyroxin*. Thyroxin directly influences all cells by regulating the oxygen they use; thus it regulates metabolism because oxygen is needed to release energy from food nutrients in each cell. Any malfunction (too little thyroxin or too much) of the thyroid gland is felt in all cells, producing some generalized body signs or symptoms of disorder.

Hypothyroidism means that the thyroid gland is underworking, producing too little thyroxin, and causing cell oxygen use to be less than normal. Signs and symptoms of hypothyroidism include lowered metabolism rate, lowered blood pressure, overweight (even on low calorie intake), and the presence of a sluggish, tired feeling.

This condition usually responds favorably when additional, daily thyroid substitute is prescribed. The patient may need to continue taking this drug for years. Regular medical examinations should accompany the use of this substitute to see that body needs are met. Signs of overdose include nervousness, palpitation, rapid pulse, sleeplessness, dizziness, and excessive warmth.

Myxedema is another disorder resulting from lack of thyroid hormone. Adults with this condition have a dry, waxy type of facial swelling, especially noticeable about the lips and nose. Metabolic rate is far below normal. There are two types of myxedema:

1. Juvenile type—characterized by slow tooth development, obesity, coarse hair, and dry and slightly yellow skin; facial changes are not noticeable.

2. Adult type—characterized by coarse hair, dry and coarse skin, a face that appears puffy, and voice that is coarse.

Both groups respond to thyroid drug therapy; however, with the adult it takes time for facial changes to take place.

Hyperthyroidism (thyrotoxicosis) means that the thyroid gland is overworking; it secretes an excessive amount of thyroid hormone. This condition occurs in all age groups. Sometimes when it is present in adolescence, it disappears in time and reappears later or not at all. However, it seems more common after pregnancy and menopause. It is more prevalent among women than men.

SIGNS AND SYMPTOMS. The list includes: weakness of muscles and increased fatigue, weight loss, insomnia and tremor. Hair thins and nails become brittle; the skin is moist with excessive perspiration. The palms of the hands and the elbows may be red. Thirst and polyuria, abdominal cramps and frequent loose bowel movements may be present. Itching (pruritus) and hives may occur. The eyes may be prominent and lids puffy. Exertion usually produces palpitation and dyspnea. Irritability and restlessness accompany hyperthyroidism.

Diagnostic tests include: PBI, Protein-Bound Iodine—a blood test; sample taken before breakfast. Radioiodine Uptake-I[131] administered orally or IV and accumulation of the iodine in the thyroid measured with a scintillation probe; it can be an out patient procedure. Other tests are: TSH (thyrotropin test); B.E.I., Butanol Extractable Iodine—a blood test (sample taken before breakfast); and B.M.R., Basal Metabolism Rate—if used, generally in relation to other tests.

MEDICAL TREATMENT AND NURSING CARE. Treatment of hyperthyroidism varies as there seem to be differences of opinion about this therapy.

Radioactive iodine is used for some patients (over 25) under certain circumstances. Antithyroid drugs (for children), for long-term treatment, must be taken according to schedule to be effective; side effects may be skin rash, pruritus, and lowered leukocyte count, and hypothyroidism.

Treatment by surgery (thyroidectomy) is often used for children, young adults and others who may want faster relief, fear radioactive iodine treatment, have large goiters, or when cancer is suspected.

As pointed out, hyperthyroidism increases nervousness and restlessness. When a patient is being treated for a toxic thyroid condition, one of the most serious nursing problems is to see that the patient gets enough rest.

The bed should be as comfortable as possible to afford rest; it should be smooth and top bedding should be arranged for freedom of movement. Excessive perspiration may require frequent changes of the patient's bed linen and his gown.

Tremor of the hands may be embarrassing and aggravating; it may be necessary to help put toothpaste on brushes or pour water for the patient.

Effective nursing care takes into account that almost anything can irritate the patient and cause him to be upset, even talking about things that one normally takes in his stride. Family members need to understand that such irritability and nervousness are symptoms of his illness.

If surgery is indicated it cannot be done until the patient is less toxic and symptoms are under control. It may take a strict regimen of treatment at home as well as in the hospital before the patient is ready.

Preoperative orders are the usual ones; it is essential for the patient to sleep well the night before surgery. This may require heavier sedation than usual because the patient may be worried and anxious. The environment should be quiet to help promote sleep.

The postoperative position of the patient is very important before he awakens from the anesthesia and after. Until he responds from the anesthetic, the patient will be in some type of dorsal position with the head supported, slightly elevated, and turned to one side for drainage. Surgeons vary in the position requirements for the patient at this time. Observation of breathing with any accompanying sounds indicating presence of moisture (gurgling) requires immediate aspiration through the airway. This observation continues until the patient is awake. Dressings are inspected (along the sides and back) for bleeding.

Any increase in temperature or pulse rate or restlessness should be reported at once.

The bed is elevated some after the patient awakens; it is more comfortable because it reduces pull on the neck muscles and aids breathing.

Along with the close observation which is necessary for all postoperative patients, there should be careful watch for evidence of muscle twitching or complaint of numbness or tingling sensations in the extremities. This is a serious sign and needs prompt reporting.

Early ambulation and involvement in self-care are part of convalescence, which usually is short. In normal recovery, emotional aspects of the presurgical condition soon begin to disappear.

THE PANCREAS

Diabetes Mellitus

Diabetes mellitus (diabetes) is a chronic disorder concerned with faulty carbohydrate metabolism which in turn influences protein and fat metabolism, body electrolytes and water. It may control the rate at which the cell utilizes glucose. It is considered to be hereditary or to be somehow related to an inherited weakness which produces the disease. About four people out of every 100 develop some degree of diabetes in their lifetime. It ranks seventh among the leading causes of death in this country. Although this disease occurs in all age groups, two out of three diabetics are over 55 years of age.

The prognosis for diagnosed diabetics is better today because there are better means to detect it, better treatment since the discovery of insulin (1922), better understanding of diet regulations, better treatments for infections and complications following surgery, and a better informed public. Being overweight and having a family history of diabetes are factors frequently present when the disease is discovered.

Diabetes cannot be cured, but it can be controlled. The exact cause is unknown, and this makes prevention questionable. However, its apparent relationship with obesity and heredity should serve as a caution to avoid overweight and to seek signs of the disease periodically since early detection and control are important in achieving a favorable prognosis.

In the pancreas there are isolated groups of cells, called the islets of Langerhans, which produce the hormone *insulin*. These cells are unlike those of the rest of the pancreatic tissue. Diabetes is thought to be due to the inability of these cells to secrete a normal amount of insulin into the blood. There may be other unknown factors.

SIGNS AND SYMPTOMS. These include high blood sugar level (hyperglycemia), sugar in the urine (glycosuria), frequent and excessive urination (polyuria), excessive appetite (polyphagia), and excessive thirst (polydipsia). The patient exhibits signs of weight loss, fatigue, and general weakness. His tissues heal slowly, and tremor and poor vision are both present (especially in older patients).

Diagnostic tests include testing the urine for sugar and the blood for blood sugar levels.

Tests for determining sugar in the urine include Benedict's (commonly used and less expensive than some), Clinitest, Clinistix, and Testape among others. Urine is tested from single, fractional, and 24-hour specimens. A specimen of four ounces is sufficient for analysis purposes.

Blood sugar levels are an important index to the presence of diabetes. The blood sample is taken *before* the patient has had breakfast. Inform the patient that he is not to eat until the specimen has been obtained. Be sure that serving his breakfast tray is not overlooked following the procedure, if indicated.

MEDICAL TREATMENT AND NURSING CARE. Treatment cannot cure but it is aimed at (1) preventing ketosis—the accumulation of ketone bodies in body tissues and fluids (which result from incomplete burning of fatty acids due to faulty use or absence of carbohydrates); (2) preventing hyperglycemia—excess glucose in the blood; and (3) preventing complications.

The physician orders individual treatment after determining the amount of sugar in the urine, amount of sugar in the blood, and after assessing the general nutritional status and history of the patient.

Treatment may include one or more of the following: (1) oral antidiabetic drugs; (2) insulin; (3) diet regulation; and (4) exercise.

If diet regulation does not control the diabetes, drugs (oral or insulin injection) may be used. For some, insulin injection is the chief control. The amount and type of insulin is determined and reevaluated by the physician. See Table 31–16, Drugs Used for Endocrine Disorders, for types of insulin.

The patient needs to understand two main facts about taking insulin: (1) *drug measurement must be accurate.* (2) *drug must be taken on time.* The young patient sometimes rebels against taking it (does not take it, is aggressive or withdrawn). Older people with tremor, poor vision or both, may need special devices to control the dosage and injection. See Figure 30–5 for syringes. See Figure 45–5 for insulin administration and injection sites.

Diet Regulation. Some type of diet regulation is essential, but the tendency today is away from the so-called "diabetic diet." People with diabetes have the same nutritional

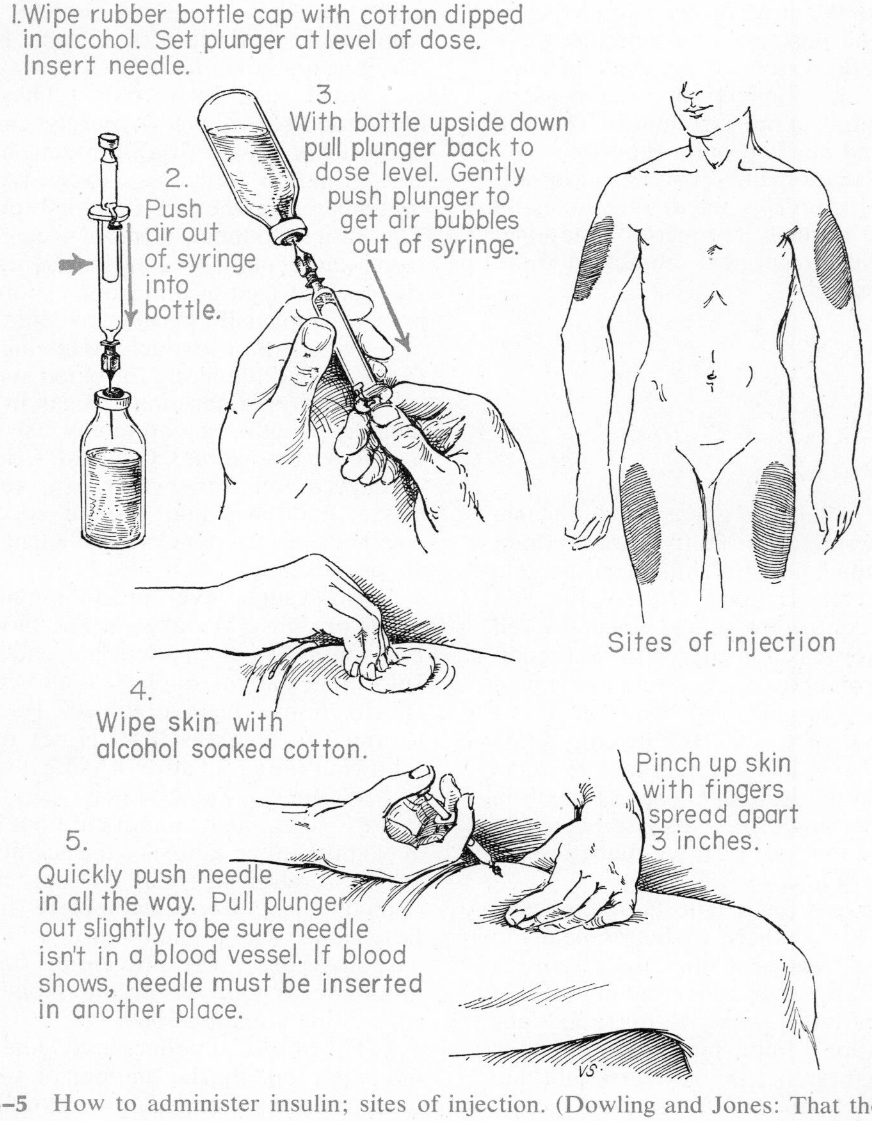

1. Wipe rubber bottle cap with cotton dipped in alcohol. Set plunger at level of dose. Insert needle.

2. Push air out of syringe into bottle.

3. With bottle upside down pull plunger back to dose level. Gently push plunger to get air bubbles out of syringe.

4. Wipe skin with alcohol soaked cotton.

5. Quickly push needle in all the way. Pull plunger out slightly to be sure needle isn't in a blood vessel. If blood shows, needle must be inserted in another place.

Pinch up skin with fingers spread apart 3 inches.

Sites of injection

FIGURE 45–5 How to administer insulin; sites of injection. (Dowling and Jones: That the Patient May Know.)

TABLE 45–1   SERIOUS COMPLICATIONS—DIABETES.

COMPLICATION	CAUSE	SIGNS AND SYMPTOMS	TREATMENT
Insulin shock	Too much insulin	Nervousness, dizziness, perspiration, headache, blurred vision, weakness, hunger, tremor, numbness of tongue and lips, stupor, unconsciousness.	Eat a piece of hard candy or a lump of sugar, or drink a glass of orange juice. I.V. glucose. Stomach tube for direct feeding.
Acidosis leading to diabetic coma	Neglected or undiagnosed diabetes	**Early signs:** Flushed skin, sweet odor on breath, nausea, vomiting, abdominal pain, tiredness. **Later signs:** Greater weakness, increased respirations, air hunger, severe abdominal pain, thirst, dry skin, parched tongue, soft eyeballs. Senses begin to dull. Coma.	Immediate emergency care. 1. I.V. fluids: glucose and insulin carefully prescribed. 2. Frequent urine and blood tests to determine sugar content. 3. Patient kept warm.

needs as other people so every attempt is made to provide a diet which is more like that of the average child/adult and that fits into the family dietary pattern. There is less emphasis on low carbohydrate intake; it may be a *measured diet* or a *free diet* which limits sweets and excessive high carbohydrate foods (holding sugar intake to a minimum).

Diet regulation for the child poses a problem unless family and child understand the restrictions, know how to provide them, and why they are needed. Young or old, the patient should stick to a standard day to day eating pattern which generally includes three regular meals plus midmorning, midafternoon and bedtime snacks. When taking insulin, this pattern of distributing calories and carbohydrates may be critical.

The measured diet starts in the hospital along with the administration of insulin. After several days, and following tests, the diet is discussed with the patient and his cooperation sought in planning a beneficial yet varied home diet. By giving the patient or parent (in case of the child) an "exchange list" of foods and pointing out that household measures are adequate for determining quantities, the attitude toward proper eating seems to improve. Especially is this true if the patient knows that

it is not entirely rigid, with no substitutions. Regardless of the patient's age, a proper attitude toward diabetes has a great deal to do with the individual's ability to live a purposeful life and abide by the "rules of the game."

Complications. Serious complications may occur; many of them can be prevented. A person with diabetes should carry an identification tag giving name, address, and telephone number of physician; this prevents mistakes in diagnosis and hastens treatment. Two complications—*insulin shock* and *acidosis*—are discussed in Table 45–1.

Tissue healing is slow in diabetic conditions. This makes good skin care and safety precaution important because any breaks in the skin may produce slow or non-healing lesions. When vision is impaired (commonly, among older persons) the patient may bruise himself by bumping into chair rockers or other objects. Keep the environment as free as possible of hazardous objects.

Special attention is paid to over-all cleanliness to prevent infections. Care of the mouth, feet, and nails should be meticulous. Ingrown nails need the special attention of the physician; careful cutting of all nails avoids small breaks and possible infection. Proper foot care for the diabetic is: 1. Keep feet clean; dry thoroughly after washing. 2. Cut toenails straight across. 3. Wear properly fitting shoes to avoid pressure (corns, constricting circulation). 4. Avoid burning, freezing, and otherwise injuring the feet. 5. See a physician when a foot sore is present.

Community health efforts are directed toward medical observation, detection programs, and education of the public.

Pancreatitis

Pancreatitis is inflammation of the tissues of the pancreas; a faulty chemical process permits the escape of activated enzymes into the interstitial tissues causing edema and excessive fullness of the pancreas. This fullness in turn can obstruct the pancreatic and the common duct, as well as deny an adequate blood supply to the gland. The "free" enzymes may erode the blood vessels causing hemorrhage into the pancreas and surrounding areas.

SIGNS AND SYMPTOMS. Pancreatitis may be painless; with acute attacks, however, hemorrhage, pain, and shock are found. With edema, pain and metabolic disturbances are pronounced. The pain is severe and widespread. Cyanosis, cold and clammy skin, a rapid, feeble pulse and subnormal temperature are present in severe attacks. The abdomen is tender and distended.

Jaundice is sometimes present because edema can obstruct that part of the common duct next to the pancreas and prevent the bile from moving along.

MEDICAL TREATMENT AND NURSING CARE. Acute pancreatitis ranges from mild to very severe and treatment includes: something to control pain (e.g., Demerol), treatment of shock, suppressing the secretion ability of the pancreas, preventing infections, replacing body fluids (not by mouth) and electrolytes.

Under severe circumstances, a carefully calculated solution is introduced into the peritoneal cavity through a special catheter and drained off after a certain length of time; this procedure is called *peritoneal dialysis.*

This patient is apt to have continuous gastric suction and nothing by mouth until the attack subsides. As he improves, small, frequent, low-fat meals are generally allowed. Three precipitating factors are: obesity, overeating, and alcoholic abuse.

Hypoglycemia

When the amount of blood glucose drops below a normal level the condition is called *hypoglycemia.* This condition is a symptom, rather than a disease, caused by any number of faulty ways the body deals with glucose.

The patient experiences such things as tachycardia, hunger, nausea, anxiety, rise of blood pressure, sweating and pallor; he finds that eating carbohydrates may relieve some or all of the symptoms. Untreated in severe form, hypoglycemia may lead to convulsions or coma.

The physician must find out what is at fault—why the blood glucose concentration falls below normal (50 mg. per 100 ml.). Immediate treatment may include a determination of the present blood glucose level and administration of IV glucose. Emergency treatment may include a sweetened drink if the patient can swallow (not if comatose).

LIVER AND GALLBLADDER DISORDERS

Metabolic Functions of the Liver

The liver provides several essential services. Review the seven main functions in Chapter 11 and notice how many of them relate to using, changing, and storing food nutrients. Much of the liver's work is related to metabolism of carbohydrates, fats, and proteins.

Its role in carbohydrate metabolism is chiefly one of maintaining a normal blood sugar level, taking out and returning glucose to the blood upon demand; it also readies some types of sugar for cells to use.

While fat metabolism takes place in almost all body cells, the liver takes care of some parts of fat metabolism faster; it converts a great amount of fat for cells to use.

As far as protein metabolism is concerned, the ability of the liver to convert proteins for cell use is its most important function. If this ability were somehow destroyed for a few days, a person could not live.

The liver continuously secretes bile and stores it in the gallbladder; the work of bile is to help the intestines digest fats and to ready the fats for absorption through the villi. Bile contains bile salts (they are responsible for readying the fats for digestion) which are reused several times before being discarded through the feces.

Disease can destroy liver cells, but the liver can replace these cells. It is said that about one-third of the liver has the capacity to carry on normal liver functions.

Jaundice

Jaundice is a yellow appearance of the skin (deeper tissues are also yellowish), which indicates faulty liver and gallbladder function. The yellow color is from excessive bile pigments in extracellular body fluids (i.e., blood plasma). The faulty liver destroys red blood cells at a faster rate than normal, releasing the pigments into the blood (hemolytic jaundice). Another type of jaundice comes from an obstruction of the bile ducts or from damaged liver cells (obstructive jaundice).

In diagnosing the jaundiced patient's condition, the physician finds out through laboratory tests which type of jaundice the patient has, because the type will influence the treatment. He also examines urine and observes the color of the feces. For instance, a clay-colored stool has meaning in making the diagnosis. (This is an example of why any abnormal color of a stool should be reported.)

Patients are often quite sensitive about this discoloration, and most of them prefer to be by themselves. Provide privacy when and however possible; they appreciate it.

Hemorrhage occurs more readily when a patient has a liver disorder that upsets the bile function. Blood fails to clot normally, and this makes the patient a poor surgical risk. Excessive bleeding occurs from such simple medical procedures as puncturing a vein to withdraw blood.

Pruritus is an intense itching. It has many causes, one of which is thought to be deposits of bile pigment in the skin. Skin care includes the use of soothing lotions to allay the itching and prevent drying.

Hepatitis

Hepatitis is an inflammatory and infectious condition in the liver which causes death of liver cells. The organism causing the infection usually reaches the liver by traveling from the intestine through the bile duct or is brought by the blood.

Acute viral hepatitis (infectious) is a common acute inflammatory disease of the liver caused by a virus or viruses. It is spread by oral and fecal contamination (e.g., poor sanitation, fecal contamination of milk, water, shellfish from polluted sea water), by carriers—people who carry the virus without being aware of it, by contaminated transfusion fluids (e.g., blood, plasma, even vaccines) and by contaminated or inadequately sterilized syringes, needles, dental and surgical instruments, tattoo needles and razors. All of these factors make infectious hepatitis a widespread, serious disease (often producing "explosive" epidemics). It attacks all age groups. *The virus is resistant.*

It is difficult to control the spread of infectious hepatitis because some of the viruses causing it are not easily destroyed. They resist heat, cold, and chemicals.

Proper sterilization means autoclaving or boiling, not simply using chemicals (antiseptic solutions). Disposable equipment is the best thing to use if it is available. Avoid self-infection by promptly and carefully disposing of used equipment. A break in the skin (e.g., hands of the nurse) becomes a port of entry for the virus. One type of virus (causing hemolytic hepatitis) is carried only in the blood; the other types are carried in the gastrointestinal tract.

There is no sure way to immunize against viral hepatitis, nor is there a specific treatment. It is a serious long-term disease; while most people recover (children sooner than adults) after a long convalescence, some patients become so dehydrated that they become comatose.

SIGNS AND SYMPTOMS.   These include poor appetite, fatigue and malaise, nausea and vomiting, fever, jaundice and dehydration.

MEDICAL TREATMENT AND NURSING CARE.   There is no specific treatment for infectious hepatitis. The patient's signs and symptoms dictate much of the medical treatment and nursing care. The fact that the virus spreads so easily and rapidly dictates the necessity for isolation techniques and strict aseptic practices. This patient must be protected from getting any other infections; his body needs all possible assistance to fight off the viral infection it already has. In addition, his virus should be confined to his unit and not spread to others.

Bed rest is essential; the lack of it aggravates the symptoms. There is little or no ambulation permitted during the early stages. This order translated into nursing action means that it is necessary to provide much assistance to this patient so that he can conserve his energy. Likewise, he needs appropriate diversional activities. Keep his bed as comfortable as possible. Arrange his bedside table for his convenience so that he has access to the things he needs.

The patient's poor appetite may cause him to be fretful about food. Small and frequent portions are more appealing than large ones. In isolation, disposable dishes are used. See that the tray is attractive. Serve the food while it is hot or cold, whichever it is supposed to be. The idea behind any nourishment is to get this patient to eat. Vitamin supplements usually accompany the diet.

Dehydration is a problem to be avoided; fluids are usually pushed (ordered) and parenteral feedings (glucose or normal saline) are given.

Sedation is sometimes required (especially in children) to quiet epigastric distress. Cleansing enemas may be ordered.

The age of the patient influences his need for assistance. The young child confined to his bed for long periods of time does not understand the need to rest. It is a challenge to divert his attention so that he gets the best possible results from staying in bed. Nourishment problems are a challenge too.

Cirrhosis

Cirrhosis of the liver is a progressive degenerative process; this means that liver cells die. If new cells are formed, they are not organized to work together as the original cells did; this upsets the way the liver functions. In addition, fibrous connective tissue takes the place of liver cells, giving this disorder the common name of "hardening of the liver." The disorganized liver cells and fibrous tissue interfere with portal circulation and may cause ascites and bleeding varicose veins in various parts of the body. Fibrous tissue can cause obstruction to the bile duct. Cirrhosis of the liver can occur in any age group.

Cirrhosis can follow a number of other liver disorders that destroy liver cells. The exact cause is often difficult to pinpoint. Even after the initial infection or disorder subsides, cirrhosis may continue. Some infections which can lead to cirrhosis include infectious

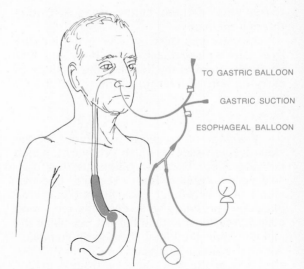

FIGURE 45–6   A Blakemore-Sengstaken tube in place.

hepatitis, bacterial infection of the umbilical cord in the newborn, syphilis, and malaria. Chronic alcoholism is another condition that leads to liver degeneration and cirrhosis.

SIGNS AND SYMPTOMS.   These include loss of appetite leading to malnutrition, edema, ascites, and internal bleeding from varicose veins.

MEDICAL TREATMENT AND NURSING CARE.   A high caloric diet (as tolerated) is ordered; vitamin B supplements and intravenous feedings of glucose are used, but salt is rigidly restricted when ascites and edema are present. Diuretics may be used to reduce body fluid; paracentesis is sometimes used when ascites is severe. Antibiotics are also used.

If the patient has internal bleeding, the physician may order sedation and transfusions of whole blood; food by mouth must be stopped and a nasogastric tube that is inflatable and can press against the bleeding area inserted. Notice the three-way tube in Figure 45–6 and the inflated balloons pressing against the esophagus and the stomach opening. The gastric suction part of the tube permits clearance of blood and fluids and irrigation. Internal bleeding is a very serious complication and often causes death.

The practical nurse would be a task performer (Role II) in a patient situation requiring this type of complex therapy. Your responsibilities usually would be specified. An important observation would be to note and record the character of the stool. Vital signs and blood pressure are closely observed.

Skin care is essential in avoiding decubitus ulcers and infection. Turning the patient frequently (if permitted) and keeping the bed dry and smooth help his comfort as well as his skin condition. This patient needs to rest and avoid any activity that will aggravate his symptoms. His environment should be quiet.

Today the physician uses many tests to determine liver function and to account for symptoms of malfunction. Observe orders for any special precautions, requirements (e.g., withholding food, collecting urine specimens, weighing the patient). Be certain that you understand your responsibilities beforehand. Do not hestitate to ask if orders are unclear or a new test is to be used.

Gallbladder Disorders

The liver produces bile, but the gallbladder is the storehouse for supply until it is needed in the small intestines to aid digestion. Review Figure 11–7 and note the dotted lines showing the cystic duct joining the hepatic duct. They form a "Y" and together become the left-hand branch of the common bile duct—a larger "Y" joining the duodenum. This is the route bile takes from the gallbladder to the small intestines.

The gallbladder is subject to the same types of disorders found elsewhere in the body. For instance, it can become inflamed and infected, it can rupture, and there can be an obstruction that blocks the release of bile (Fig. 45–7).

Stones can traumatize the bladder, causing inflammation and ulceration; this may lead to a rupture. Cancer attacks the gallbladder, the same as other body parts.

Terms associated with gallbladder disorders include:

1. Cholelithiasis—stones in the bladder or tract (gallstones).

2. Cholecystitis—inflammation of the gallbladder.

3. Cholecystectomy—surgical removal of the gallbladder.

4. Cholecystostomy—surgical opening into the gallbladder to permit drainage.

GALLSTONES (Cholelithiasis). The pres-

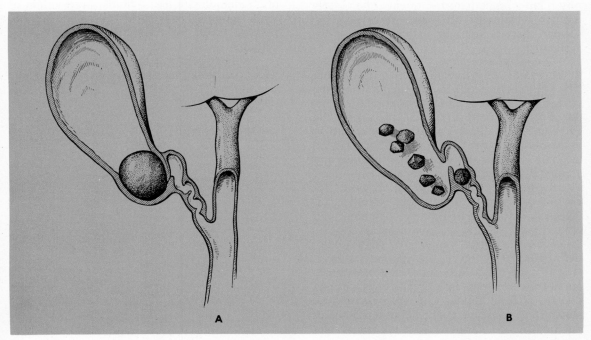

FIGURE 45–7   Causes of acute cholecystitis. A, Obstruction by a large gallstone in the bladder exit. B, Obstruction in the cystic duct by a gallstone that cannot move through the duct. (Cecil and Conn: The Specialties in General Practice, 3rd Ed.)

ence of gallstones in the gall bladder is common; it is estimated that one person in 10 has them. Many people never know they have gallstones because there is no indication that they are there.

Difficulty arises when the stones block the gallbladder exit to the cystic duct and bile cannot be released, when they get wedged in the duct, or when they traumatize the bladder by pressure or position.

A gallbladder attack comes when a stone has difficulty moving through the cystic duct. The patient experiences repeated severe colicky pain, nausea, vomiting, and chills. When the stone passes into the duodenum, the attack subsides.

When the normal flow of bile is interrupted (as with stones obstructing the passageway or from scar tissue), the patient may be jaundiced.

INFLAMMATION AND INFECTION (Cholecystitis). As stated previously, stones may traumatize the gallbladder causing inflammation, ulceration, and rupture. A ruptured gallbladder produces bile peritonitis which is often fatal in elderly patients. Bacteria may also cause these same conditions. The age of the patient with cholecystitis influences the physician's immediate treatment. The elderly patient has surgery (often emergency surgery) sooner than a younger patient because his resistance is lower.

One diagnostic test sometimes used is an x-ray examination called a cholecystogram. The x-ray picture tells the physician where the stones are located. Diet restrictions are ordered prior to the test (i.e., fat-free supper the evening before). A dye is given (by mouth or vein) and the patient eats no food for a period of hours; the dye outlines the gallbladder and stones, if any, in the x-ray picture.

Signs and symptoms of cholecystitis include fever (may be low-grade), jaundice, indigestion, a feeling of fullness, belching, and colicky pain (severe, sharp, excruciating).

Prior to surgical removal of the gallbladder (cholecystectomy), the patient's diet is strictly controlled; fatty foods and seasonings are not allowed (e.g., fats, cream, eggs, cheese, greasy or fried foods, rich spicy dressings, alcohol). An enema might be ordered to reduce flatulence. Stools are usually light colored, and urine is dark.

The pain may be so intense that a narcotic (e.g., morphine, Demerol) is needed to relieve

it. Bile salts are sometimes ordered to aid bile functions, and antibiotics are used to treat the inflammation or infection.

These treatments may cause the cholelithiasis to subside entirely. However, owing to the possibility of more serious complications, it is common medical practice to remove the gallbladder.

The preoperative orders are the usual ones. The patient usually returns from the operation with a tube inserted to drain off bile which might otherwise accumulate in the common duct (Fig. 45–8). This tube is connected to some type of container or device to allow the bile and exudates to drain. Since the patient's position can help promote drainage, the backrest may be slightly elevated after he is fully awake from the anesthetic. Observe the tube to see that there is no pull on it. The "T" portion can be pulled out of the common duct if care is not used to anchor the tube leading to the container; caution must also be used in turning the patient. Check the tube to see that it permits a free flow of drainage; tell the patient about the need for this, too, so that he will not mistakenly cut off the flow in moving about in bed.

In addition, immediate patient needs often include parenteral fluids, observation of vital signs, a nasogastric tube and suction, nothing taken by mouth, and an indwelling catheter.

This patient presents a complex nursing situation. Note that not only do bile drainage,

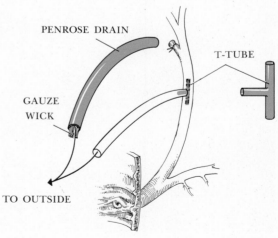

FIGURE 45–8 After cholecystectomy the Penrose drain helps to remove drainage from the area. The T-tube drains bile to the outside.

intravenous fluids, gastric suction, and an indwelling catheter all require care, the other postoperative needs of patients do too.

Sterile dressings are placed over the incision when the tube is removed, to catch any drainage. These dressings are changed frequently to protect the skin area and prevent infection. The surrounding skin area may be protected by vaseline gauze or some other type of protective paste ordered by the physician.

Important observations include drainage, condition of the skin around the drainage site, urine, stools, the presence of jaundice, and appetite.

Other Endocrine Disorders

Pituitary insufficiency results from destruction of the anterior pituitary gland; this in turn adversely affects the other endocrine glands (gonads, thyroid, adrenal). Destruction may be caused by a cyst, tumor, or postpartum necrosis of the gland.

Treatment may include radiation therapy, surgery, cortisone and other drugs to promote more normal endocrine functions.

Addison's Disease (primary adrenal cortical insufficiency) is caused by destruction or atrophy of the adrenal cortex. The cortex can be destroyed by tuberculosis, fungal infections, and similar conditions. The patient gradually becomes weak, disinterested in any exertion, loses his appetite and the body seems to waste away. The pulse is feeble; mental confusion may come and go; and the general decline leads to death unless treated.

Substitute therapy includes supplying the body with the needed adrenal hormones and sodium chloride to replenish extracellular fluids. Close attention is paid to drug dosages when infection is present to help maintain body defenses.

The use of synthetic corticosteroids has made it possible for a person with Addison's disease to live a productive life; each patient is advised to wear some type of identification on his person stating that he has adrenal insufficiency with directions of what to do if an emergency occurs (e.g., injury, vomiting, loss of consciousness).

SUMMARY

Dysfunction along the gastrointestinal tract creates local and general signs/symptoms of illness—from local discomfort to "feeling sick all over." The process of digestion and metabolism are related; the work of the liver and help from the bile and the pancreatic juice assist the digestive tract in preparing food elements for cell use. Anything that upsets the normal production and flow of digestive juices necessarily upsets the chemical digestion of food. When physical barriers (e.g., obstruction) are present, the process of physical digestion is upset. Sometimes both interfere.

Many signs/symptoms of illness associated with gastrointestinal disorders are common to other systemic diseases (e.g., pain, fever, fatigue, anorexia) and so are many of the nursing measures used to relieve them. A patient's ability to consume food may be directly related to some disorder of the gastrointestinal tract and present its own unique problem(s), however, a disorder elsewhere may rob him of his appetite and interest in food, making it equally difficult to consume it.

A great variety of tests and treatments are used for patients with gastrointestinal diseases and metabolic disorders; they include intubation, drainage, irrigation, the use of scopes (gastro, procto, sigmoid), x-ray and fluoroscope picutres with barium sulfate and many laboratory examinations of specimens.

Surgical treatment includes (among many others) gastric resection, exploratory abdominal surgery to find the cause(s), emergency abdominal surgery (e.g., obstruction, perforation), appendectomy, colostomy, hemorrhoidectomy, cholecystectomy, and thyroidectomy.

New synthetic drugs have made it possible to medically manage diseases that previously were fatal such as Addison's disease.

GUIDES FOR STUDY AND DISCUSSION

1. What are some disease conditions of the mouth? Which ones usually present nourishment problems?

2. What is an obstruction? Where can they occur in the digestive system?

3. What is the purpose(s) of gastric intubation? How might you be involved?

4. How are accumulations removed from body cavities?

5. What means are used by the physician to "see" the condition of the gastrointestinal tract? In each instance, what might your responsibilities be?

6. What are the purposes of irrigations? What are your responsibilities?

7. Some gastric disorders are functional; some are physical. What is the difference?

8. From your reading, make a list of diagnostic tests and instruments a physician might use when examining/treating a patient with a gastrointestinal disorder.

9. Use this chart in your notebook to organize your thoughts about the various diseases discussed in this chapter. Notice what (if anything) is similar among the signs/symptoms and nursing care.

Disease/ Disorder	Definition	Signs/ Symptoms	Treatments Including Surgical	Nursing Care

10. Prepare a list of questions you would like to have discussed in class. Use this opportunity to help confirm your understanding or clear up any confusion you may have regarding your nursing responsibilities.

SUGGESTED SITUATIONS AND ACTIVITIES

1. This chapter includes much about diagnostic/therapeutic tests and equipment. Displays will acquaint you with them. Use the classroom to assemble equipment; label each part and provide summarized information about each, pointing out any specific nursing responsibilities involved. You may wish to group equipment according to purpose, such as: gastric analysis, gastrointestinal siphonage, drainage, examination by "looking," irrigation, etc.

CHAPTER 46

PATIENTS WITH RESPIRATORY DISORDERS

TOPICAL HEADINGS

Introduction
Noninfectious
  Disorders
Allergies
Infectious Disorders

Special Treatments
  for Respiratory
  Disorders
Surgical Treatments
  for Respiratory
  Disorders

Summary
Guides for Study
  and Discussion
Suggested Situations
  and Activities

OBJECTIVES FOR THE STUDENT: Be able to:

1. Trace the journey of inhaled air.
2. Describe five conditions which may cause interference with breathing.
3. Explain why anxiety often accompanies difficult breathing.
4. Compare postural drainage with open chest drainage as to purpose and procedure.
5. Explain the need for medical asepsis in two instances of respiratory diseases.
6. Name four common signs/symptoms of respiratory disorder.
7. Describe three nursing care concerns you will have with patients with treatments of thoracentesis, closed chest drainage, and bronchoscopy.
8. Given a list of common respiratory conditions, describe each and list the special nursing considerations for each.

SUGGESTED STUDY VOCABULARY*

anoxia
dyspnea
cyanosis
orthopnea
cough
rales
hemoptysis
exudate
purulent
malaise
pallor

suffocation
pulmonary edema
emphysema
prognosis
atelectasis
tenacious secretions
hypersensitive
bronchial asthma
rhinitis
pharyngitis

tonsillitis
sinusitis
laryngitis
influenza
epidemic
pneumonia
irrational
tuberculosis
bronchoscopy
laryngectomy

---

*Look for any terms you already know.

INTRODUCTION

A review of Chapter 9 points out the process of respiration and how this system is responsible for delivering oxygen to the blood. You will recall that an exchange of gases takes place in the lungs; fresh oxygen is traded for carbon dioxide. The blood takes on the fresh oxygen and gives up the carbon dioxide to the lungs. The blood then transports the new oxygen to every living body cell and trades it for the carbon dioxide the cell throws off as waste.

Anything that hinders the lungs from carrying on their vital work also hinders the work of each living cell, because each cell must have a constant supply of oxygen to live and function. Likewise each cell must get rid of its carbon dioxide.

Trace the air route in Fig. 9–1 starting with the nostril to the bronchi. Then examine Fig. 9–3 and continue tracing the route from the bronchi to the alveolar sac. Anywhere along this route there can be an inflammation, infection, growth, wound, swelling with edema, anomaly, or foreign object.

The lungs produce distress signals when they are not functioning properly. Chapter 41 describes four signals: dyspnea, cyanosis, orthopnea, and cough. No difficulty is more frightening to a person than the inability to "get air"; the body cannot exist without a constant supply.

In this chapter respiratory disorders are arranged into three groups: noninfectious, allergic, and infectious. In addition, special treatments, measures, and selected surgical procedures related to the respiratory tract are included.

NONINFECTIOUS DISORDERS

Epistaxis (Nosebleed)

Common causes of nosebleed include external violence, picking nasal membranes with a fingernail, rubbing the nose hard, acute inflammation of nasal membranes (e.g., colds, sinusitis) and high fever. Bleeding also occurs with such disorders as hepatitis, hypertension, leukemia, and nasal tumors.

Any part of the nose may bleed. Usually the bleeding is easily controlled simply by firmly squeezing the soft part of the nose between the thumb and forefinger while the patient sits with his head held slightly forward. This position prevents the blood from going down his throat. Have the patient breathe through his mouth. If the bleeding persists, the physician may pack the nostrils with cotton plugs moistened with epinephrine (1:1000 solution). Further treatment includes cauterizing (searing) the tissue with electricity or chemical caustics (e.g., silver nitrate).

Acute Pulmonary Edema

Pulmonary edema means there is fluid in the lungs. It is a complication (not a disease) that comes from abnormal movement of fluid through capillary walls into the surrounding tissue spaces. As the amount of fluid increases it moves into the alveoli and if its formation continues the patient drowns in his own fluid. Pulmonary edema is often associated with hypertension and some cardiac disorders, but it may occur as a result of injury to lung tissue, inhalation of toxic fumes, self-administered large doses of heroin, some other drugs, tuberculosis, hypersensitivity to a single blood transfusion, or sometimes to prolonged use of a high concentration of oxygen.

Acute pulmonary edema is a condition in which the lungs are flooded with fluid. Sometimes this occurs suddenly, as when a cardiac patient happens to lie flat in bed permitting the fluid to settle there.

SIGNS AND SYMPTOMS. They include an acute onset of chest pressure and breathlessness, dyspnea, apprehension and fear, cyanosis, and a cough producing large amounts of frothy pink fluid. Noisy rales can be heard without stethoscope.

MEDICAL TREATMENT AND NURSING CARE. Treatment includes general and specific measures. Drugs may include digitalis, antihypertensive drugs, morphine (often producing dramatic relief), and diuretics. Oxygen (sometimes with intermittent positive pressure breathing) may be administered. A sitting position (legs dependent) should permit easier breathing and pool blood in the legs to relieve the lungs. In a severe case a venesection (open a vein for blood letting) may provide relief.

This patient is fearful of suffocation; if possible stay with him and explain anything being done in his behalf, if it appears appropriate. For example, tell him about the oxygen mask before it is applied.

Emphysema

This condition is usually associated with chronic bronchitis, asthma, and bronchiectasis. Emphysema is a lung condition in which the air sacs (alveoli) are permanently dilated and have lost their elasticity. They do not empty as they should, and air is trapped in the sacs producing abnormal air spaces.

It is a discouraging illness because the patient will not experience pronounced improvement. Unless he learns to live with his limitations and follow the physician's orders carefully, he may be in constant distress, especially as the condition worsens. The prognosis is not encouraging to date. Some work is being done to rehabilitate patients by teaching them to use abdominal muscles for breathing rather than chest muscles.

SIGNS AND SYMPTOMS. Dyspnea, even at rest, may be severe. The patient shows signs of wheezing and coughing, and may have orthopnea accompanied by anxiousness.

MEDICAL TREATMENT AND NURSING CARE. The physician orders drugs to increase the efficiency of the lungs. Lung secretions must be removed if possible; this condition is helped by drugs which dilate the bronchi (e.g., Adrenalin, aminophylline) and expectorants; postural drainage also helps (Fig. 46–1). Sometimes the physician uses intermittent positive pressure mask treatment (compressed air or oxygen) for lung aeration. One type of equipment for this is the Bird respirator.

This patient should avoid any type of respiratory infection due to his limited lung power and low resistance.

Atelectasis

Atelectasis is a condition in which the lung collapses because one or more bronchi are blocked off by "mucus plugs," tenacious secretions which prevent air movement in the lungs. It is a complication following chest and abdominal surgery. The lung secretions can accumulate if the patient does not cough enough to expectorate them. Restricted movement and sedation also contribute to this condition.

SIGNS AND SYMPTOMS. Often atelectasis is characterized by an abrupt onset of elevated temperature, elevated pulse, elevated respirations, and pain in the chest.

MEDICAL TREATMENT AND NURSING CARE. The "mucus plugs" or tenacious secretion mass is removed by the physician (bronchoscopic aspiration). If the patient is weak, a tracheostomy may be needed so that aspirations can be repeated as necessary. Other treatments and care include early ambulation, frequent turning, deep breathing, and coughing.

Foreign Bodies

Any object that gets lodged in the air route (any location) is called a foreign body. The list of such objects is limitless and it can occur to anyone at any age. Small children push such objects as buttons, beans, and parts of toys into the nose; they swallow coins, pins, and tacks which may as easily slip into the trachea as the esophagus. Food in the trachea (e.g., a piece of meat) can cause death by suffocation; this can happen to anyone.

The most important symptom of a foreign object in the bronchial tree is wheezing; others include dyspnea, cough, hemoptysis, gagging, and choking.

The physician determines the location and the position of the object usually by fluoroscope and x-ray examination; it is then removed by bronchoscopic means.

ALLERGIES AND AIR POLLUTION DISORDERS

An allergy is a condition in which the patient is hypersensitive to something (e.g., dust,

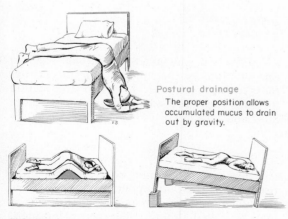

Postural drainage
The proper position allows accumulated mucus to drain out by gravity.

FIGURE 46–1 Postural drainage using the patient's bed. (Dowling and Jones: That the Patient May Know.)

certain food, pollen, cosmetics). The body reacts (locally and generally) with sneezing, watering of the eyes and nose, edema, skin eruptions, itching, nausea, vomiting, diarrhea, dyspnea, and abdominal pain.

Two allergic conditions of the respiratory tract are hay fever and bronchial asthma.

Hay Fever

Another name for hay fever is *allergic rhinitis*. Rhinitis is an inflammatory condition of the mucous membranes of the nose. The membranes swell and make breathing difficult. There is an increased production of watery nasal secretion accompanied by intermittent dryness; some pain and soreness are present. The eyes water, burn, and are red and swollen.

Hay fever is a seasonal type of allergy. The patient is allergic to certain pollens. Some change their place of residence at "pollen time" or permanently to avoid hay fever attacks.

Treatment consists of antihistamines to relieve sneezing and itching, and to dry up secretions. Many of these preparations produce such side effects as nausea, dryness of the mouth, drowsiness, and blurred vision. Therefore, any such drugs should be taken under medical supervision. Additional treatment includes desensitizing the patient by giving him a series of injections (usually weekly) of specific allergens; a series of skin tests determines the proper allergens to use.

Bronchial Asthma

Bronchial asthma is a condition in which the bronchioles swell and produce excessive secretions. There is spasm of the bronchial muscles and thick secretions block air passages; this causes the patient to work very hard to draw in fresh air to replace the trapped air. Such respirations are accompanied by loud wheezing.

Factors which are thought to cause bronchial asthma are allergies, emotional stress, infection, and marked temperature changes. Asthma may occur in any age group; it can also lead to emphysema, a condition which might especially occur in older patients.

SIGNS AND SYMPTOMS. The onset of difficult breathing comes with sudden cough; the cough becomes productive. The patient experiences chest tightness, dyspnea, wheezing, and cyanosis if the attack is acute. His pulse may be weak, perspiration may be profuse, and feelings of apprehension and anxiety may be present.

MEDICAL TREATMENT AND NURSING CARE. Every effort is made to conserve the patient's strength and to reassure him. A sitting position or Fowler's position is usually the most comfortable. During the attack (which may last from minutes to hours), sedatives are administered to quiet the patient; expectorants are given, as well as drugs to relieve the spasm of the bronchial muscles (e.g., epinephrine). Oxygen may be required; inhalation (steam, with or without medication) is also used successfully with some patients.

Prevention of attacks is the best treatment. If the patient can learn how to reduce or eliminate stressful situations, maintain good body nourishment and get sufficient rest and relaxation, it is felt that some attacks can be prevented.

Air Pollution

As mentioned in Chapter 24, air pollution is becoming a major health problem. Large air polluting industrial plants in entire cities have been shut down during critical atmospheric times to avoid large scale respiratory disorders and death. Highly populated areas face serious problems because of air pollution from automobile fumes.

INFECTIOUS DISORDERS

INFECTIONS OF THE UPPER RESPIRATORY TRACT

Infection and inflammation can occur in one or more of the upper respiratory structures at the same time. The following section includes the more common disorders of the nose and throat.

Common Cold (Rhinitis)

The term "common cold" is most often used to refer to any upper respiratory infection; when referring to its specific location, it may be called rhinitis, pharyngitis, laryngitis and "chest cold."

The cold is caused by viral infection of the upper respiratory passages. In its true sense, the common cold is not accompanied by fever and its signs/symptoms are milder than other respiratory infections where fever is present.

Many viruses can cause the common cold; there is no specific cure. Treatment includes taking plenty of fluids, bedrest, avoiding chills, antipyretics, steam inhalation, decongestants, and expectorants. Any indication of a cold before surgery should be reported immediately.

There is no vaccine for protection against the common cold; too many different viruses are involved. Progress is being made with vaccines for some specific groups of viruses.

Acute Pharyngitis

This is an inflammation of the membranes of the pharynx. It is usually caused by an organism, but other causes may include chemicals, smoking, dust, and fumes. It may produce a septic sore throat. Complications of pharyngitis may include a middle ear infection, sinusitis, bronchitis, and pneumonia.

Signs and symptoms include a dry scratchy throat, difficulty in swallowing, and a dry, tickling cough. The patient may have a slight fever, accompanied by chills, headache, and muscle ache; his throat membranes may be red and inflamed.

Treatment includes bed rest, fluids, and a nutritious diet. Moist air (e.g., steam inhalation) and throat irrigations are sometimes ordered. Aspirin or a similar drug is usually ordered; in severe cases, antibiotics or sulfonamides may be prescribed.

Acute Tonsillitis

Acute tonsillitis is an inflammation and infection of the tonsils, accompanied by the presence of a yellowish white, purulent exudate. Complications may result if infection spreads to the sinuses, middle ear, larynx, and bronchi.

Signs and symptoms include a sudden onset of chilliness, discomfort, and fatigue. Fever (usually higher in young children) and sore throat are present. The patient experiences difficulty swallowing; his tongue is coated and his breath foul.

Treatment includes bed rest with little exertion, fluids, and an easily swallowed diet.

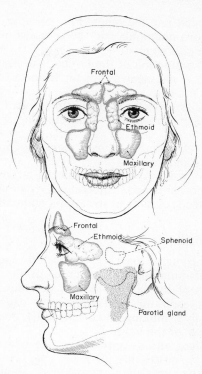

FIGURE 46–2 The paranasal sinuses. (Dowling and Jones: That the Patient May Know.)

Gargles and an ice collar may be used. Drugs usually include something for pain, sedation, lozenges, and antibiotics.

Sinusitis

Sinusitis is an infection of the membranes in from one to all of the anterior or posterior sinuses (Fig. 46–2). The maxillary and ethmoid sinuses are the chief sites of infection in children.

Signs and symptoms include fatigue, headache, fever, pain, tenderness (maxillary), and an irritating cough. Pain may be more severe with ethmoid sinusitis. Poor appetite may be present.

With maxillary sinusitis an upright position is less comfortable. Treatment includes bed rest, pain medication, local heat, nose drops or spray, and antibiotics.

INFECTIONS OF THE LOWER RESPIRATORY TRACT

An infection in the upper respiratory tract can spread to the lower respiratory tract—to the larynx and the lungs. For example, bronchitis or pneumonia may be complications of severe pharyngitis.

The function of the larynx is to serve as:

1. A passageway for air from the throat to the trachea.

2. A protective means to prevent fluids or foreign substances from entering the trachea.

3. A phonatory instrument—to produce sounds and voice.

As with any other organ, the larynx may become inflamed, ulcerated, traumatized, paralyzed, or subject to tumors and cancer.

Laryngitis

Laryngitis may be acute or chronic. It is an inflammation and infection of the membranes of the larynx. It may accompany an upper respiratory infection or be caused by excessive smoking, chemicals, dust, or excessive use of the voice.

Signs and symptoms include hoarseness and a fever (usually low).

Any persistent hoarseness should be diagnosed since the cause may be more serious than an infection from the nose or throat (i.e., cancer, tuberculosis). Treatment includes resting the voice, breathing humid air (e.g., steam inhalations), and avoiding smoking, dust, and fumes.

The amount or degree of fever and the presence of other infections help the physician determine what, if any, antibiotics and other drugs to order. This patient needs to rest his voice; he may or may not be ambulatory. Arrange his environment so that he can participate in self-care activities (if allowable) with the least amount of verbal communication. If steam inhalations are ordered, observe all safety precautions and take into account the patient's age and ability to cooperate in following directions.

Influenza

This infectious disease attacks both the upper and lower respiratory tracts. Influenza is caused by a virus and spreads rapidly. Epidemics (rapid, widespread, and involving many victims) occur in cycles; the death rate is not as high as it was before influenza vaccines were used. However, if the attack is mild or severe, precautions should be taken to prevent such complications as middle ear infection, sinusitis, and pulmonary complications (e.g., primary influenza virus pneumonia).

The adult is apt to be more seriously ill longer than the child; therefore it is most important that adults as well as children be immunized. A patient of any age suffering from chronic kidney, heart, metabolic, or pulmonary diseases should be immunized.

Signs and symptoms include cough, dryness/soreness of the throat, nasal discharge, headache, fever, muscle ache, poor appetite, and nausea.

The patient should be isolated and medical aseptic precautions used to prevent the spread of the disease. Nasal discharges should be carefully disposed of.

Although there is no specific treatment for the flu, bed rest, a warm room, plenty of fluids (including citrus fruit juices), and aspirin may be ordered. The patient needs to rest; good mouth care and daily hygiene will make him more comfortable.

Influenza may be prevented, or less serious symptoms presented, by injections of vaccines. The protection lasts about a year. It is especially advisable for people who have chronic cardiac and pulmonary diseases, for groups essential to community life (policemen, doctors, nurses, military) and groups in institutions such as students, soldiers, etc.

Pneumonia

Pneumonia is often named for the area of the lungs affected. If the infected area is the lobes, it is called lobar pneumonia; if it is in the bronchi, it is called bronchopneumonia. Notice the areas involved in Figure 46–3.

Pneumonia is an infectious, inflammatory condition of the lungs commonly caused by pneumococci organisms; however, many other organisms can and do cause it. The early use of antibiotic medications has greatly reduced the death rate so that better than nine patients out of 10 who have been properly treated recover.

Pneumonia remains a serious disease. Although its incidence is low, it is constantly present. Today deaths occur more frequently in the very young or the elderly. Because of the increase in the aging population, this disease may once again increase in incidence. Predisposing factors include chilling,

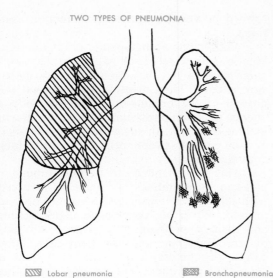

TWO TYPES OF PNEUMONIA

▨ Lobar pneumonia   ▦ Bronchopneumonia

FIGURE 46–3 The two main types of pneumonia. Lobar (on the left) involves the entire lobe or more of a lung. Bronchopneumonia (on the right) includes all pneumonias that produce massing together of lung tissue less in extent than a lobe. (Barbata et al.: A Textbook of Medical-Surgical Nursing. G. P. Putnam's Sons.)

dampness, cold, changing temperature, and lowered resistance.

This disease is spread by direct contact with patients having the disease or convalescing; people are known to carry the organisms after being in contact with the patient. When body resistance is lowered, the organisms gain a foothold in the lung tissues.

As the organisms multiply in the air sacs of the lungs, the pneumonic exudate begins to fill the air sacs and replace the air. This fluid is mixed with white and red corpuscles. The greater the amount of exudate, the more difficult it is to breathe; this causes coughing and may produce blood-tinged sputum. Body defenses attempt to destroy the organism faster than it can multiply.

SIGNS AND SYMPTOMS. Pneumonia usually has a sudden onset, and is accompanied by severe chill, high fever, stabbing chest pain, flushed face, productive cough (rust-colored expectoration), nausea, and malaise. Breathing is difficult and the nostrils spread as respirations become shallow and rapid. Fatigue is due to difficult breathing, and the patient may have a poor appetite.

MEDICAL TREATMENT AND NURSING CARE. Antibiotic therapy (especially penicil-lin) is used for the most common types of pneumonia and within a matter of hours assists the body in eliminating the organism. The lungs, with an abundance of capillaries, are soon able to reabsorb some parts of the exudate and expectoration takes care of the rest; the lungs become clear. This rapid response to medication makes it possible, in many instances, to treat the sick child at home. Less chance is taken with older patients who have lower resistance and slower recovery power.

Supportive treatment includes bed rest, few, if any, visitors, pain medication— depending upon severity (e.g., codeine, morphine), sometimes a tight chest binder to "cough against," medication for restlessness and insomnia, oxygen for dyspnea and cyanosis, fluids and electrolytes.

Nursing care is focused on conserving the patient's energy; thus, all nursing measures are carried out with the least possible patient exertion. The patient will be kept in bed until his temperature is normal; provide a comfortable bed and position the patient for the easiest possible breathing with rest (support with pillows). Use light weight warm bedding and siderails if the patient is irrational or otherwise not responsible.

The mouth and nose require careful attention because blisters and crusts form and are painful. The tongue becomes coated and sores develop. The areas are cleansed and then treated with something that will soothe and soften them.

In addition to making the usual observations, pay particular attention to the type and rate of respirations and the patient's reaction to any difficult breathing. Observe type and frequency of stools, intake and output (as ordered), and encourage fluid and nourishment intake.

Complications do not occur as frequently as they did in past times because of the use of antibiotics. Possible complications may include heart failure, pus in the pleural spaces (empyema), septicemia, middle ear infection, and sinusitis.

Tuberculosis

This disease may invade any part of the body but most commonly affects the lungs. It is a communicable disease caused by the tubercle bacillus that may be passed from one person to another through a drinking glass, a cough, a sneeze, a kiss, or from something which has been in contact with the patient. *Sputum of the patient is a most important source of infection.* This fact means protective action not only by the nurse and family but also on the part of the patient himself when coughing, sneezing, or expectorating. It also means that medical aseptic practices are observed.

Following are some general facts about tuberculosis:

1. Tuberculosis is not inherited; the organisms come from patients suffering from the disease.

2. It can be prevented.

3. It can be cured.

4. New drugs give invaluable assistance to cure, especially if infection is discovered early.

5. Bed rest is still important.

6. Chest surgery removes damaged, unhealed lung tissue.

7. Rehabilitation helps to return the patient to his place in the community.

8. Immunization is questioned by some.

9. It usually affects the lung in the early years of life but anyone who is in poor general health, undernourished and overtired, seems to be more vulnerable. It is increasing among the older segment of the population.

10. The public needs to be educated in the ways to prevent and detect tuberculosis.

SIGNS AND SYMPTOMS. The onset is slow with a severe cough in the morning which is usually productive and may be blood-tinged. Sweats occur during sleep (night sweats) and weight loss is pronounced in the late stage. Chest pain and hoarseness may or may not be present. Indigestion sometimes occurs, along with fever (usually in the evening) and dyspnea (late stages of illness).

MEDICAL TREATMENT AND NURSING CARE. Treatment is lengthy and may take from a few months to a year or two. The government provides care for patients who cannot afford such expense. It is a natural thing for a person to be discouraged and feel depressed at times about how long it takes him to get well. A happy, relaxed frame of mind is helpful to the patient and he will be more content and consequently less restless in bed or out.

Not every case of tuberculosis is cured; if it is far advanced when discovered, cure may be impossible. Despite the decline in the number of cases of tuberculosis during the past 10 years, it remains a problem and efforts toward prevention and early detection continue.

Certain chemotherapeutic drugs (in combination) are widely used to combat the tubercular bacillus, but they do not necessarily assure a cure. They arrest or slow down the growth of the organism, giving the body a chance to build up resistance. Other treatment includes bed rest, an adequate nourishing diet, and the patient's proper attitude toward a long convalescence.

This patient needs to be with others in pleasant surroundings; he can be involved with self-care activities and be taught how to properly cover his cough with paper tissues and dispose of them. Diversional activities play an important role in patient care. They can be very helpful in assisting the patient to accept his treatment and develop a positive outlook toward his future.

In instances when a patient does not respond to chemotherapy, chest surgery may be necessary. The surgical removal of a lung is called pneumonectomy; the removal of a lobe is called a lobectomy. Sometimes a lung is purposely collapsed to allow it to rest and heal.

Under desirable and appropriate conditions, the patient may receive home care rather than hospital care. Many factors have to be taken into consideration in making this medical decision, including the patient's attitude toward his illness, the severity of the illness, drug therapy required, and any possibility of infecting others in the household.

Rehabilitation is a vital part of medical treatment from the start. The patient is taught self-care and encouraged to be as independent as possible in all respects. Vocational rehabilitation is very necessary for this patient; it is essential that he gradually return to earning a living.

SPECIAL TREATMENTS FOR RESPIRATORY DISORDERS

Some types of respiratory conditions require that *medical asepsis* and *isolation* techniques be used. The purposes of asepsis are discussed in Chapter 42.

Postural drainage means positioning the patient so that gravity may aid in draining lung secretions. Special types of beds are made for this purpose. The patient may be positioned using his own bed (Fig. 46–1). The part of the tract to be drained determines the position;

the head must be lower than the rest of the tract.

The age and the condition of the patient must be considered in placing and keeping him in position. Some cannot tolerate an extreme position for very long periods of time (at least at first) because they become faint and dizzy. Ask the patient to breathe deeply and cough while he is in position. Avoid this treatment right after meals to prevent nausea. Assist any patient throughout the treatment, unless he is able with practice and ability to assist himself safely.

Suction is a safety measure used to suck or aspirate mucus and secretions from body cavities. Chapter 42 describes the purposes and precautions to use when suctioning the mouth and nasal passages.

Inhalation therapy (including the use of oxygen) means that treatment is given by way of the lungs. The source of the patient's difficulty may be in the lungs themselves or it may be a combination of lung-blood circulation disorders. Chapter 42 describes types of inhalation therapy with special emphasis on oxygen therapy.

Sputum specimens are frequently needed for diagnostic and treatment purposes.

Chest Drainage

When conditions require it, it is necessary to remove fluids, thick exudates, and air from the pleural cavity. Three means for doing this are: 1. thoracentesis; 2. closed chest drainage; and 3. open chest drainage.

Thoracocentesis is a procedure for removing fluid in the pleural cavity to relieve the patient and furnish a specimen for diagnostic purposes. This is a surgical aseptic procedure; the packaged sterile equipment is usually set up as a tray available from Central Supply.

The patient is placed in a sitting position, leaning forward and supported by laying his arms and head on an overbed table. The physician uses a local anesthetic at the site of the needle injection. In some instances a plastic tube may be inserted into the pleural space to remove the fluid. The method for creating the pull or vacuum is selected by the physician.

The practical nurse acts in Role II if she assists with this procedure. Respect the patient's need for privacy and a comfortable position throughout. Observations include color, respirations, pulse, and cough (whether or not productive). Determine beforehand if a specimen is needed; if so, have an appropriate

container ready. Note the amount and character of the drainage. Keep in mind that the physician will use a surgically aseptic technique; this means that any assistance you might render with equipment and use of the sterile field should likewise be aseptic.

Closed chest drainage (water-seal drainage) of the pleural cavity is used to remove a quantity of fluid, blood or air. The word "closed" means that outside air is not allowed to enter the pleural area. This type of drainage is often used following major chest surgery. The tube(s) is secured in place in the operating room with the end(s) clamped off until it is securely fastened to whatever type of drainage equipment is to be used—either with or without suction.

In *"no suction" water-seal chest drainage* the clamped outer end of the chest tube is connected to a glass tube inserted through a stopper into a glass jar (i.e., gallon size or larger) containing a measured amount of water; the tip of the glass tube is placed well below the water surface. When the patient inhales, a small amount of water rises in the glass tube; when he exhales, the water is driven back down the tube and air bubbles are present in the water. To measure the amount of drainage, subtract the measured amount of water from the total volume. Replace the same amount of water in the jar.

Closed chest drainage with suction uses a more complicated system of bottles. Sometimes two connected water-seal bottles are used and at other times three connected bottles. The choice is made by the physician. The chest tube is connected to one bottle and the suction tube to the other. In case of two chest tubes three bottles must be used because each chest tube must have its own water-seal drainage bottle.

The nurse is responsible for observing the working order after the drainage system has been set up. In a properly working suction bottle (the one with the open end glass tube reaching down into the water) the water in the open end glass tube goes up and then empties, pulling in air and creating bubbles in the water. Observe to see that this happens regularly; if not, report the malfunction immediately. It could be caused by air leakage in the set-up, leakage into the pleural cavity or the pump may need attention.

Open chest drainage means that outside air can enter the chest through the drainage tube. This is used to drain heavy exudates from the pleural space (i.e., emphysema). The tube(s) is placed in the cavity (a surgical procedure) and the outer end is securely fastened (taped or sutured) to the outside of the chest wall where it is attached to some type of suction or covered by dressings. To handle the thick drainage, the tube(s) must be large and flexible; it also serves as a means to irrigate the cavity and instill solutions.

Bronchoscopy is an examination of the bronchus for viewing the condition of the tissues, observing for possible growths, locating and removing a foreign body, and securing tissue for a biopsy or a specimen of secretions for a laboratory examination. The instrument used for this purpose is a hollow tube called a bronchoscope. It is disagreeable for the patient to have this tube passed through the trachea. However, regardless of his age, the procedure is usually performed with premedication and local anesthesia unless there is reason for a general anesthetic.

Preparation of the patient includes any preexamination medications, mouth care, and removal of dentures and bridgework. Food and drink are usually withheld for several hours (eight to 12) prior to the examination to prevent vomiting. The patient may ask many questions about the examination and express concern about how he will breathe while the bronchoscope is in place. Secure the assistance of the charge nurse or physician to explain this procedure to him.

Following the examination, the patient will experience throat irritation for a day or two. Usually the orders call for nothing by mouth until he can swallow and the gag reflex has returned.

Sputum may be blood-streaked; if it is bright red, report this immediately. Observe his respirations to see that air is passing through the trachea freely. Sometimes there is swelling, and breathing becomes difficult.

SURGICAL TREATMENTS FOR RESPIRATORY DISORDERS

Tonsillectomy-Adenoidectomy

Tonsillectomy-adenoidectomy is the surgical removal of the tonsils and adenoids (in children). In adults only the tonsils are removed.

Nursing care for a tonsillectomy-adenoidectomy (T and A) patient means making the same observations necessary for all general anesthesia patients—the vital signs, bleeding, free airway, warmth, rest, safety, and a return to consciousness.

This patient must lie on his abdomen, with his head turned to one side (resting on his arm) to permit drainage from the mouth until he is conscious and can control swallowing. Observe for bleeding. Some mucus and bright red bloody discharge are normally present, but increased pulse rate, restlessness, pallor, and attempts to swallow are signs that there might be hemorrhage; these signs need prompt attention.

Orders for treatment after the patient awakens usually include small amounts of chilled water that are gradually increased, followed by juices (no citrus juices because they sting). Soft bland foods—custards, ice cream, soups—are usually ordered for several days. Medications are ordered for pain and restlessness. Ice collars and warm mouth washes and gargles are soothing to the throat.

The patient usually leaves the hospital after 24 hours and is in bed at home for a couple of days. Activity is limited for a couple of weeks. Adults generally need more time for convalescence than children.

If the tonsils are removed under local anesthesia, the patient's postoperative position should be slightly elevated with a backrest. Other observations and treatments are the same.

Tracheostomy

A *tracheostomy* is a surgical opening through the neck into the trachea for the purpose of inserting a tracheostomy tube to permit breathing. Such a measure is necessary when something (trauma, burns, foreign object, laryngectomy) has made it impossible for the patient to breathe normally. The tube also provides a means for suctioning secretions from the trachea. See Figure 46–4 for the three parts of the tracheostomy tube. A tracheostomy may be an emergency measure to prevent asphyxiation when there is a sudden obstruction of the larynx.

The most important thing to remember about caring for this patient is to *keep the tube open at all times*. Mucus accumulates and must be cleaned out. The inner tube can be removed for cleaning, but the outer tube is

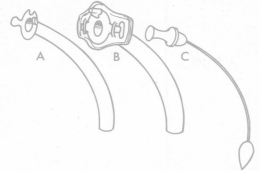

FIGURE 46–4   Three parts to the tracheostomy tube. (A, Inner tube. B, Outer tube. C, Obturator.)

never removed by the practical nurse. In fact, a physician is generally the one to replace the outer tube when this is necessary.

Cleaning the inner tube (after removal) requires soap and cold water plus brushing or rubbing; the mucus is difficult to remove and the tube should be inspected to see that the lumen is clear and clean before it is replaced. Be certain that the inner tube is securely locked in place.

The outer tube is tied in place with tapes around the neck. Gauze squares surround the outside portion to absorb secretions. An extra tracheostomy set of the same size that the patient is using is kept in the patient's unit for emergency purposes.

Communicating with this patient may take more time since he is unable to talk; he should write if he can. Patients with permanent tracheostomy tubes learn how to clean them and take all necessary precautions and with special training, they learn to talk. See Appendix III, Tracheostomy Care.

Submucous Resection

Submucous resection is a surgical procedure to correct a deformity of the nasal septum. It is not usually performed on children but rather after the nose and face have attained full growth.

The deformity may be in the cartilage or the bony part of the septum, or both; it may be due to faulty bone development, trauma, or adenoids which cause abnormal breathing space and bone placement. Some types of deformities hamper the patient's ability to breathe more than others.

The surgical procedure corrects the deformity so that the patient can breathe through both nostrils normally and the sinuses can drain. It is done under local anesthetic. The patient returns with mask or mustache dressing; the gauze under the nose absorbs drainage and must be changed as needed. An upright head position helps to relieve discomfort and swelling.

Laryngectomy

Laryngectomy is surgical removal of the larynx; this means that the voice box is gone and the passageway between the trachea and nose is closed. This patient has a permanent tracheostomy; he must breathe through it and learn to speak by developing an esophageal voice or using an artificial larynx. Communication is a problem for this patient, but if he is determined, he can be instructed by a speech therapist to develop an esophageal voice.

The physician explains to the patient what the surgery means. The prospect of losing the voice can be very frightening to the patient. Sometimes a former patient who has adjusted well to his permanent tracheostomy can be helpful; the patient has opportunity to see first-hand that people can live active, independent lives with a permanent tracheostomy. Every effort in planning and providing nursing care should be directed toward helping this patient return to self care and independence.

Preoperative care includes the usual preparations—withholding of foods and fluids, preparing the site, administering medications, and so forth. Postoperative care preparations include having at hand suction and oxygen equipment, materials to clean the inner tracheostomy tube, and an extra tube. Equipment for taking vital signs, recording intake and output, giving parenteral fluids, and the like should also be at hand when the patient returns so that the nurse can stay with the patient. His tracheostomy tube will need frequent suctioning (every five to 10 minutes), and the inner tube should be removed and cleaned often. This type of assistance is reassuring to the patient. Provide him with some means for writing his messages.

Very early in his recovery (either the second or third day), the patient is instructed how to suction and clean the inner tube (see Fig. 39–2).

SUMMARY

Any factor which hinders breathing can be distressful to a patient. The more severe the hindrance, the greater is his anxiety because oxygen is essential to living body tissues and life cannot survive long without it. In some instances, emergency measures are used (e.g., tracheostomy) to restore breathing.

Four main respiratory distress signals are dyspnea, cyanosis, orthopnea, and coughing. Positioning the patient with respiratory distress can be very important to his comfort; every effort is made to make breathing as easy as possible so that he uses the least amount of energy.

Some respiratory disorders such as emphysema are long-term and chronic and often show little, if any, improvement. The patient may or may not be willing to live within his restrictions and may become discouraged with his progress.

Rehabilitation is a vital part of patient (and family) acceptance and education in such long-term diseases as tuberculosis. Government and private agencies contribute to rehabilitative efforts.

Infection can move from the upper respiratory tract to the lower tract or in the other direction, producing serious complications in either case.

Special treatments and measures for respiratory patients include medical asepsis, isolation techniques, postural drainage, closed and open chest drainage, tracheostomy (temporary or permanent), inhalation therapy, and sputum collection and specimens.

Some procedures, surgical or otherwise, for these patients are very complex; they involve complicated equipment and background knowledge possessed by the physician.

GUIDES FOR STUDY AND DISCUSSION

1. In your opinion, why is it important to conserve the energy of the patient with respiratory distress?

2. Why are these patients so often placed on an elevated back rest?

3. How is the sign of cyanosis related to respiratory difficulty?

4. Why does a patient become anxious when experiencing orthopnea?

5. What can happen to the respiratory tract to cause difficulties?

6. Drainage is used to treat lung conditions. What is postural drainage? open chest drainage? closed chest drainage?

7. Some respiratory conditions require strict medical aseptic practices. Which conditions require this?

8. What is a thoracentesis? a bronchoscopy? a tracheostomy?

9. Use this chart in your notebook to organize your thoughts about the various diseases discussed in this chapter. Notice what (if anything) is similar among the signs/symptoms and nursing care.

Disease/ Disorder	Definition	Signs/ Symptoms	Treatment Including Surgical	Nursing Care

10. Prepare a list of questions you would like to hear discussed in class. Use this opportunity to confirm your understanding or to clear up any confusion you may have regarding your nursing responsibilities.

SUGGESTED SITUATIONS AND ACTIVITIES

1. Using the 10 basic needs, determine how any or all would be adjusted for an adolescent boy who has been admitted with lobar pneumonia.

2. Visit community agencies that share in patient rehabilitation, public education, and other services related to respiratory disorders. Prepare an exhibit of printed materials provided by the agencies to help the public understand the problems and needs of people with respiratory disorders.

3. Prepare a bulletin board display of news articles about air pollution problems facing this country.

CHAPTER 47

PATIENTS WITH HEART AND CIRCULATORY DISORDERS

TOPICAL HEADINGS

Introduction

General Information: treatment and nursing care

Diseases and Disorders of the Heart

Diseases and Disorders of the Blood Vessels

Diseases and Disorders of the Blood

Summary

Guides for Study and Discussion

Suggested Situations and Activities

OBJECTIVES FOR THE STUDENT: Be able to:

1. Explain the work of hemoglobin and the leukocytes.
2. Trace the normal route of pulmonary circulation.
3. Describe three things which can cause the heart to malfunction.
4. Name ten general signs/symptoms of cardiac distress.
5. Describe a situation which shows how nurse observation(s) assists the physician with the care of a patient.
6. Given a list of seven types of drugs used to treat cardiac patients, explain the purpose of each type.
7. Tell how to conserve the energy of a patient who is on complete bedrest by giving three examples.
8. Identify three nursing actions which could be common among cardiovascular patients.

SUGGESTED STUDY VOCABULARY*

pericardium
epicardium
myocardium
atria
ventricles
pallor
edema

dyspnea
Cheyne-Stokes respiration
diuretic
necrotic
lumen
coronary occlusion
sternal region
epigastric region

anti-coagulant drugs
cathartics
lesions
embolism
congenital
malfunction
phlebitis
thrombus

*Look for any terms you already know.

INTRODUCTION

Cardiovascular diseases account for more deaths in this country than any other disease; they strike all ages and both sexes. Some types occur most often in children, others in the middle-aged and still others in the elderly.

The heart and circulatory system are subject to a great variety of disorders. The list ranges from failure of the heart, shock and circulatory collapse, disease due to congenital anomalies, chronic valve disorders, deficiency of blood in the heart muscle, vein blockage, conditions of the aorta, irregular beating of the heart, inflammatory conditions of the heart tissues and others. With the possibility of so many cardiovascular disorders (or combinations of them), the physician is faced with trying to make a specific diagnosis. He has a great many means to assist him; likewise there is an array of drugs and equipment for treatment.

There is fear and uncertainty in the minds of people about heart disease and circulatory disorders. Many people believe that the presence of heart disease means certain death, or that the patient must live a sheltered, restricted life. Neither is true in all instances. Heart disease can and does cause sudden death; it can and does force some patients to restrict their activities, watch their diet, and alter their way of life. But many patients are able to carry on unrestricted, reasonable living and working activities.

Cardiovascular diseases/disorders may be grouped in a number of ways. In this chapter, notice that they are grouped as follows: *Diseases and Disorders of the Heart, Diseases and Disorders of the Blood Vessels,* and *Diseases and Disorders of the Blood.* Some fifteen different conditions are included and this is but a partial listing. What is stressed, however, are the signs/symptoms which influence medical management and nursing care. You will find many common signs/symptoms and many common nursing measures among the various conditions. It is more profitable for you to know what is involved, for example, when the order "complete bedrest" is written, than it is to know the details of the pathology which prompts the physician to write that order. The emphasis is on nursing care and much of that care is directly related to the patient's signs/symptoms rather than to the name of his disease.

GENERAL INFORMATION: TREATMENT AND NURSING CARE

The heart is a rhythmical, pulsating muscle that possesses the built-in ability to excite the muscle itself and keep it pulsating (or pumping blood). It is contained in a loose-fitting sac (pericardium) that has an inside surface called the epicardium. The slight space between the heart and the epicardium is moistened by a few drops of fluid to prevent friction as one surface might rub on the other.

The heart wall is the muscle called the myocardium. Inside there are four chambers: right and left atria and right and left ventricles. The wall that divides the right side from the left side has no openings in it under normal conditions. Valves control the flow of blood from the upper chambers to the lower chambers, and under normal conditions the valves serve as trap doors that prevent the blood from backing up.

Chapter 10 explains the various systems within the circulatory system: systemic, coronary, pulmonary, hepatic portal, and cerebral.

General Cardiac Distress Signals

Following is a list of general cardiac distress signs and symptoms that may occur in varying degrees with any heart disease.

1. Respirations, mildly to severely labored.
2. Pulse, irregular, ranging from very fast to very slow.
3. Cyanosis.
4. Edema.
5. Nausea.
6. Vomiting.
7. Pain, ranging from mild to sharp and crushing, in chest, shoulder, arm, abdomen, and epigastrium.
8. Weakness and fatigue.
9. Excessive perspiration.
10. Pallor.

General Medical Management of the Cardiac Patient

Many different *examinations* and *tests* are used for more accurate treatment and diagnosis. Some may be carried out by the physician and others by laboratory personnel, either at the bedside of the patient or in the laboratory. The more common tests and examinations include:

1. electrocardiogram (EKG)—to picture the rhythmic patterns of the heart (cardiac cycle) using a series of waves, P Q R S T.

2. phonocardiogram—to measure heart sounds and murmurs.

3. fluoroscopy—a type of x-ray showing the heart in action; barium is swallowed during the process.

4. chest x-ray—a still shadow picture showing heart size, location, and position.

5. intravenous angiocardiography—a set of x-ray pictures of the heart taken as an opaque liquid is injected by vein to instantly reveal the condition of the heart chambers and blood pathways.

6. cardiac catheterization—observing the heart by fluoroscope as a special catheter is moved through the heart; it includes a camera taking pictures, a means for measuring heart blood pressure, and withdrawing blood samples from the heart location. The patient usually has nothing by mouth several hours before hand, a pretest medication (e.g., nembutal) and an antibiotic. The test may last an hour or more. Following the test the patient is kept flat in bed (as ordered) and the pulse counted frequently.

7. blood pressure—this measurement may be taken at other than the usual sites (as ordered).

8. cardiac pacemaker—an electronic means to drive the heart (various types).

9. a wide range of blood tests.

Taking the patient's condition into consideration, the physician's treatments usually pertain to the following:

Medications will depend upon the results desired. *Stimulants*, such as adrenaline, are given to increase the heart action. *Narcotics*, as morphine or Demerol, are given to relieve severe pain. *Diuretics*, as Mercuhydrin, are given to relieve edema or remove excessive fluids from the tissues. *Anticoagulants* as Dicumarol or heparin, are given to prevent or reduce the formation of blood clots. *Vasodilators*, as nitroglycerin or amyl nitrite, are given to dilate blood vessels for easier flow of blood. *Salicylates*, as aspirin, are given to relieve pain and to reduce fever. *Hypotensives* or *antihypertensives*, as Serpasil, are given to reduce or lower high blood pressure.

Oxygen therapy is frequently ordered to assist the heart in its task of furnishing needed oxygen to tissues in all parts of the body.

Rest, sleep, and activity are usually regulated and directed. The physician's orders determine whether the patient may be ambulatory, may work, or must remain in bed.

Diet is usually regulated. One of the following is frequently used:

Reduction diet—to reduce overweight, which adds strain to the heart and blood vessels.

Low sodium diet—to prevent or relieve edema.

Restricted fluids—to prevent or relieve edema.

Surgery may be performed to correct certain deformities of the heart which are present at birth (congenital) or to correct certain conditions of the heart valves and blood vessels in the adult.

General Nursing Care for the Cardiac Patient

Depending upon the specific heart disease, its severity, and the medical management of the individual patient, the nursing care of all cardiac patients usually includes special considerations of the following:

Observations
Rest
Diets and fluids
Elimination
Personal hygiene
Weighing
Getting out of bed
  and ambulation
Pre- and postopera-
  tive care.

OBSERVATIONS. The presence of, or a change in, certain symptoms is meaningful to the physician and must be accurately observed and recorded. The physician's orders often specify certain regular observations such as taking the blood pressure every hour, two hours, or whatever, intake and output and so on.

1. Pulse. The type and character of the pulse can be of more importance than the rate.

It may be very irregular or have a certain pattern of irregularity. It may be very slow or very fast. If radial pulse is difficult to determine, another location should be used. An apex-radial count requires two nurses, one to take the heart count with a stethoscope at exactly the same time the other nurse takes the radial count. Each reading is so recorded.

Some medications given to the cardiac patient are intended to increase or slow heart action. Taking the pulse helps to indicate whether the medication is effective in bringing about the desired change. Some medications are stopped when a certain rate in pulse has been brought about.

2. Respiration. Many cardiac patients suffer some degree of difficulty in breathing.

Certain positions and activities may bring about shortness of breath or labored or difficult breathing (dyspnea). Mouth breathing is common.

Observations include any change in the type of respiration when the patient is sleeping or eating or when any nursing care is being given. Difficult breathing causes fear, discomfort, and fatigue.

3. Color. Pallor or a bluish color (cyanosis) is noted in the lips, nose tip, ear lobes, finger tips, and toes. This indicates that the circulating blood is not getting oxygen to the tissues properly. Any change in color as the patient is in a certain position or moves about and changes position should be noted.

4. Pain. Pain generally occurs in the arm, neck, shoulder, chest, or epigastric region, though it may be present elsewhere. Observe the location, type, and duration of the pain, as well as any possible contributory activity of the patient at the time. Note the color of the skin and whether there is excessive perspiration (diaphoresis). Other signs and symptoms which can accompany the pain are nausea, vomiting, and headache.

5. Edema. An abnormal or excessive amount of fluid in the tissues is noticeable in such parts of the body as the feet, legs, hands, face, and abdomen. If the patient has remained in an upright position during the day or night, the feet and legs will be more edematous. Slight finger tip pressure on the edematous part may leave indentations (pitting edema) and change the color or appearance of the area. (Fig. 47–1.)

6. Other complaints and symptoms include headache, palpitation, decreased urine, restlessness and anxiousness.

The above observations are significant in helping to plan and provide the best possible nursing care for the comfort and well-being of the cardiac patient.

Rest is needed. In response to the physician's specific orders for rest, provision for this is usually dependent upon the nurse and the care she gives. Every activity may be limited or restricted to help provide needed rest. Some patients may be permitted some

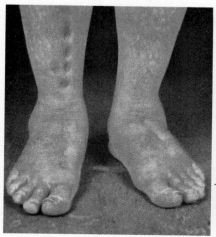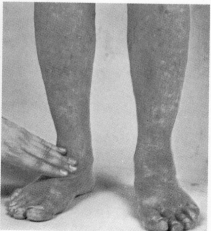

FIGURE 47–1   Left, Pitting edema of feet and lower legs. Right, the same patient after treatment relieved the edema.

self-care, others none. All nursing care is adjusted to prevent fatigue and to provide the most complete rest possible. Ways to meet these limitations are discussed in relation to the mildly and the seriously ill patients. In addition, the following considerations help this patient:

1. Avoid disturbing the patient. Anticipate and provide for his needs without his having to wait or ask for something. Do not expect or ask the patient to talk, as this requires effort. Plan nursing care to avoid disturbing the patient or causing extra effort; for instance, wearing a hospital gown and leaving it untied at the neck will require less effort for the patient when it has to be changed.

2. Avoid hurrying the patient. If it is permissible for the patient to do some things for himself, such as washing his face or feeding himself, avoid hurry or impatience. Being permitted to do something for himself may be excellent medicine for the patient. However, unnecessary or prolonged time may be very tiring to some patients.

3. Provide a comfortable position. The patient experiencing difficulty in breathing will be more comfortable and will rest better in an upright position. Pillows, over-bed tables, and other devices should be used to support the arms, shoulders, and feet. This position is used during the day and night. Necessary precautions are taken to avoid falls from the bed.

4. Control environmental conditions. Provide quiet, comfortable surroundings for the patient so that he can get constant rest and not be aggravated by some irritating condition in his close environment.

5. Provide for adequate sleep. Although the patient may sleep a little during the day he should sleep during the night, if possible. Sleeplessness often produces restlessness. Prepare the patient for sleep before giving the sleep medication; it will then be more effective. Frequent visits during the night provide opportunity to observe the patient.

6. Control pain. Pain is frightening to the cardiac patient. Medications are usually ordered to help keep him relaxed and to help relieve any pain. He will be able to breathe more easily and get needed rest.

7. Visitors are usually restricted. The physician frequently permits a close relative or friend to remain. Many patients are more relaxed knowing that someone is close at hand. They help the patient (eating, reading, using the bedpan). The presence of the mother is particularly important to the sick child.

8. Reduce activity of patient. The physician may limit or restrict the activities of the patient. Be certain that you understand what the patient may or may not do and to what extent. Such orders will determine, for example, if the patient is to be fed, to be turned, and even how often he may be given a bath. The patient should be told about his restrictions if he is capable of understanding.

DIET AND FLUIDS. Generally a special diet is ordered. If the patient is overweight a reduction diet is ordered. Soft foods, or even several smaller feedings a day, are often used to aid in ease of digestion. A salt-free diet helps reduce fluid in the tissues. The amount and type of fluids may or may not be restricted. However, the fluid intake and output are usually measured and recorded. The patient may or may not be able to feed himself.

ELIMINATION. Certain medications (diuretics) may be given to help remove fluids from the body tissues, and this means measuring the output of urine. Observe bowel elimination for frequency and type of stool. Straining to have a stool causes fatigue and adds to the difficulty of heart action and respiration. Such should be noted. A laxative or oil enema may be ordered to help soften the feces for ease of defecation. The patient should not be hurried with elimination. Assist the patient in getting on and off the bedpan or the commode and remain with him to give support and to prevent his falling.

PERSONAL HYGIENE. Care and attention must be given to the lips and mouth if the patient has dyspnea and breathes with his mouth open. Fluids may accumulate in the throat. Keep the skin clean and dry, especially over bony prominences and pressure areas. The position of the patient must be changed and the bed linen kept smooth to help prevent reddened areas and decubitus ulcers but *do not massage any area or part of the body without an order from the physician.* The cardiac patient may perspire excessively; therefore, his skin should be kept clean and dry to prevent odor and to provide comfort. His gown and bed linen should be changed as often as necessary.

WEIGHING. Very often the cardiac patient is weighed daily or several times a week. Determine how often and at what time of day he is to be weighed, as well as other directions or orders for weighing. Frequent checking of the weight helps the physician to determine whether the diet or the drugs are effective.

GETTING OUT OF BED AND AMBULATION. The physician will specify when and how the patient is to get up. You should be with the cardiac patient to give support and make observations such as change in his color, pulse rate, and respiration. Any complaint or evidence of fatigue or pain means that the patient must be returned to his bed and his condition immediately reported. Getting the patient up and out of bed should be a slow process to prevent fatigue, undue fear, or complications.

Convalescence may take many months. This takes place in the hospital, in a nursing home, or in his own home with his family. The patient and his family will be instructed by the physician (or professional nurse) regarding activity, diet, rest, and return to work or school.

PRE- AND POSTOPERATIVE NURSING CARE. Cardiac surgery is common but it requires specially trained medical and nursing personnel both during and following the operations. Preoperatively, emphasis is placed upon the careful mental and emotional preparation of the patient and his family. The postoperative patient is usually detained in an intensive care area until his condition is stable enough to be moved to a regular patient unit.

DISEASES AND DISORDERS OF THE HEART

HEART FAILURE

The heart could fail to fulfill its function for any one of several reasons related to the heart itself and to the circulation of the blood. Specifically, the disorder called *heart failure* (or congestive heart failure) means the heart muscle (myocardium) is failing to carry out its work properly. Other names for it are myocardial failure and cardiac insufficiency. The failure of function is in the ventricle (either one); this leads to signs/symptoms in other parts of the body depending upon which ventricle is involved. The heart becomes enlarged.

Signs and Symptoms

1. The pulse alternates a strong beat with a weak beat and the rhythm is irregular.

2. Pain is unusual unless there are complications.

3. Congestion in the lungs leads to edema and dyspnea; in a reclining position it becomes orthopnea. Slight exertion causes breathlessness and fatigue.

4. Cough and expectoration may interfere with sleep. Hemoptysis, rusty sputum; pink frothy fluid.

5. Breathing is irregular alternating between periods of hyperventilation and apnea.

6. Anxiety is part of the patient's response to what is happening to him whether he can be specific about it or not.

7. Others include cyanosis, nausea, vomiting, anorexia, ascites and edema of the feet and ankles. (Fig. 47–1.)

Medical Treatment and Nursing Care

Treatment is aimed at assisting the heart muscle to function more effectively to increase the cardiac output; this in turn relieves the signs/symptoms. At first the results may be pronounced, but as the myocardium deteriorates and the therapeutic agents become less effective, the patient's condition worsens.

Rest (both physical and mental) is required to relieve the heart. This patient needs reassurance and sedatives/tranquilizers are usually ordered for relaxation and sleep.

Position helps relieve dyspnea; the sitting or the semisitting position (bed or chair) makes breathing less work. Watch the patient's sleeping position; support him so he does not slip down during sleep and awaken gasping and frightened that he is suffocating.

Oxygen by nasal catheter seems to relieve dyspnea.

Improving the work of the heart muscle is most often done by using the drug digitalis; its dosage and administration are carefully determined depending on what is to be accomplished.

Edema must be dealt with. Sodium intake is controlled from the start and diuretics help reduce excess fluid. Daily weighing is a gauge to fluid weight loss/gain. Intake and output records help too.

Rest is the key word in providing nursing care. In addition to sedation and tranquilizers, you can promote rest and reassurance by what you do and say.

Carry out measures for personal hygiene in a manner which conserves the patient's energy. Listen to him if he says he feels too tired to have a bath; gauge the extent of what you do accordingly—maybe it should be just enough to refresh him and make his bed comfortable.

Rest has mental as well as physical aspects. Sometimes anxiousness and even irritability are present. Find out why if possible. Two things which often concern this patient are constipation and urinary retention. He can be restless because of breathing difficulties or be worrying about their return.

As mentioned earlier, position is important to easier breathing. Firmly support the patient in a semi-sitting or sitting position; oxygen at hand is reassuring even when it is not being used.

Measures taken to control edema (salt restrictions, diuretics, daily weight, intake/output) may need explanation especially with respect to complaints about the diet. Be observant about "no salt shaker on the tray" if ordered; this oversight may worry some patients who consider it carelessness and develop doubts about other things you are doing for him.

If this patient can assist in self-care activities, find out to what extent he can be involved before you start.

CORONARY ARTERY DISEASE

The coronary arteries furnish the heart muscle with its blood supply. When something occurs in one of these vessels to prevent sufficient blood from reaching a part of the heart muscle, that portion of the heart becomes necrotic due to lack of oxygen and nourishment. One of the main causes of coronary artery disease is the gradual accumulation of substances on the lining of the vessel; these deposits make the lumen smaller. When a blood clot forms and plugs the artery, this is called a *coronary occlusion*. Why this occurs is still an unanswered question, but some of the substance in the artery lining is fatty and is thought to be related to metabolism and diet. Cholesterol is one fatty substance under question. The "fat controversy" is mentioned in Chapter 26 under Dietary Needs of Patients.

Coronary artery disease can occur at a young age, but is most commonly seen during the middle and later years of life. Medical science is studying this health problem, looking at such factors as weight, diet, smoking, exercise, and stress. Two coronary artery diseases are *angina pectoris* and acute *myocardial infarction*.

Angina pectoris (angina) is characterized by pain that may range from mild to very intense. It may be a vague ache or develop into pain that forces a person to seek immediate help. Angina is often described as a pressing or boring sensation where the chest feels tight and breathing seems difficult. It may be associated with abdominal distress and belching, causing the person experiencing it to say, "it is indigestion."

The intensity of the pain is not crushing and searing as is the pain with myocardial infarction. It radiates typically to the left shoulder and arm and occasionally to the right arm too; likewise the deep aching sensation may radiate to the back and neck.

Angina is periodic and brought on by physical exertion (climbing stairs, hill), a heavy meal, cold weather, emotional experiences and sometimes without any apparent cause.

Postmortem studies show that most patients with angina had occlusion of one or more major coronary arteries and hardening of the walls of the arteries.

Medical Treatment and Nursing Care

What is prescribed for the angina victim is based upon the severity of the episodes and the factors which bring on the attacks. Modified physical activity and drug therapy (e.g., nitroglycerin) are common for immediate relief. Depression is sometimes present as patients think of less activity as meaning they are less able or getting old. Both the nurse and the physician have to help the patient deal with this in a realistic way when hospitalized. The outpatient likewise is helped to understand how he can carry on his daily living activities to work and enjoy his family relationships.

Treatment also includes concern about overweight, diet and smoking. Other drugs include sedatives and blocking agents (e.g., propranolol) which reduce the frequency and severity of the pain.

Surgery is used to provide additional coronary supply or to relieve obstructed blood vessels.

Angina may be tolerated and lived with (even disappear) for many years. However, if the patient is hospitalized, treatment generally includes sedation, treatment for increased blood pressure (if present), anticoagulants and bed rest. Determine what, if any, self-care activities are permitted.

Myocardial infarction is characterized by pain that is more severe and prolonged than angina. An area of the myocardium is denied oxygen due to an obstruction which in turn produces necrosis of tissue. The pain is crushing inside the chest and may last a few minutes to several hours; it may radiate the same as angina. The sudden onset of the severe pain creates intense fear. The patient's face is ashen, nailbeds cyanotic, skin cool and sweating and he is restless and apprehensive. Sudden death occurs in about 30 per cent of acute myocardial infarctions even when preceded by apparent good health. Post mortem findings usually show advanced coronary artery disease.

Medical Treatment and Nursing Care

The patient is generally admitted to the coronary care unit where there is constant monitoring of heart rate and rhythm.

Rest and relaxation are essential; therefore, the environment should be quiet and calm. Visitors are limited and so are outside world contacts such as television, radio, and news publications.

Drug therapy generally includes something for pain and apprehension, hypotension and bradycardia. To avoid straining at stools and maintain normal bowel function, a cathartic such as milk of magnesia is ordered.

Strict bed rest is usually maintained for a considerable time; be sure you know the physician's plan for gradual ambulation.

Other nursing care may include attention to an indwelling urinary catheter and any dietary restrictions (i.e., salt limitation). With restrictions and apprehension, this patient may have mood changes which you will need to accept.

CHRONIC VALVULAR HEART DISEASE

Return to Figure 10–1 and locate the following heart valves: tricuspid, pulmonary, mi-

tral, and aortic. Heart valves, when defective, may upset the normal flow of blood through the heart, into and out of the lungs and out of the heart into the systemic circulation.

Previous disease can be responsible for scarring and otherwise changing valvular tissue such as may occur in the mitral valve or the aortic valve following rheumatic fever. The valve retracts, becomes rigid and the opening narrows (stenosis). Depending upon the particular valve involved and the presence of or the lack of symptoms, treatment includes some limits on the amount of activity and the type of work a person might do. As the stenosis increases so does the tendency toward dyspnea, finally making it necessary for the patient to carry on very limited activity.

Heart catheterization (right or left) is often used to determine the nature of the problem so that treatment (surgical or otherwise) may be more specific.

Treatment (when symptoms are present) usually includes salt restrictions, diuretics, digitalis, and detecting/treating infections and anemia. Surgical treatment may/may not be indicated. With a severely damaged valve, replacement of it may be carried out if the valve itself cannot be repaired to provide patient relief.

RHEUMATIC FEVER

Rheumatic fever is a condition in which lesions are found in the connective tissue of the heart and elsewhere. These lesions may follow such diseases as acute tonsillitis, scarlet fever, and upper respiratory diseases where a certain type of streptococci is present. Attacks may recur if means are not used to prevent the causative infection. Rheumatic fever may occur at any age, but it usually begins in childhood, and it is one of the leading causes of chronic illness and death among children.

Signs and Symptoms

The symptoms usually include a high temperature, rapid pulse and respiration, swollen, painful joints. Muscles and joints ache and become tender and warm. Some of these symptoms may appear before others; some may be mild, others more severe. Fatigue, loss of appetite, abdominal pain, excessive sweating, loss of weight, unusual irritability, and twitching or jerky motions may be present.

Medical Treatment and Nursing Care

Early, complete bed rest is important to prevent or limit heart damage. Medications are ordered to control the infection, to relieve the symptoms, and to help make the patient comfortable.

All nursing care must be planned to save the energy and activity of the patient. This patient has painful joints. Care must be taken not to jar the bed, and devices (bed cradle) are used to keep the top bedding off the affected joints. Pillows are used for support. Usually some form of heat is ordered to help keep the patient warm and to relieve pain. Because of the excessive sweating, care should be taken to prevent chilling. Cotton flannel or some lightweight absorbent material may be used in place of sheets, and to clothe the patient. Frequent bathing and linen changes are necessary; these are done quickly but carefully to avoid chilling and any discomfort. Observations of the temperature, pulse, and respirations are frequent.

Fluid intake is observed. Usually the physician orders the fluid intake increased to a certain amount each day. A diet high in vitamins and other requirements is given. The patient is fed by the nurse, if necessary.

Convalescence is long; help the patient to understand why his activities are restricted. As he begins to feel better—especially if he is a child—it may be difficult to keep him sufficiently quiet. Meeting his diversional needs is essential if his bed rest is to be effective. Very often the family can be of assistance; they too must understand what is required during the long recovery.

CONGENITAL HEART DISEASE

The term *congenital heart disease* might be called a broad term because it is used to cover any one of a great number of defects present in the heart or the great vessels leading to and from it.

Why heart defects occur during fetal life is not understood. It is known that the health of the mother during pregnancy is important. For example, German measles during the early weeks of pregnancy may influence the development of the fetus and create defects in the heart, eyes, ears, and other body parts. The role of drugs, malnutrition and infections during pregnancy are being studied for their relationship to congenital deformities. The role of heredity in congenital heart defects is not understood.

Some of the more common types of congenital heart defects occur in the large blood vessels leading to and from the heart, in the heart valves, and in the dividing wall between the right and left sides of the heart.

Signs and Symptoms

Cyanosis may or may not be present at birth, and may increase during early months of life, making its appearance around mouth and lips. The skin is a dusky blue. The gums bleed easily. The patient has dyspnea upon exertion and sometimes following eating or crying. There may be clubbing of the fingers and toes. The patient is weak and irritable and his growth and development are delayed.

The treatment is surgical; the defect is repaired and the child can lead a normal or a nearly normal life.

One of the most serious nursing problems is to understand the needs of the child and the parents. Because the child has had difficulty in breathing and has been unable to participate in regular childish activity, his parents have protected him. Knowing this, and knowing that such anxiety is natural for the parents, you may have to work with a fearful mother and a spoiled child. Talking with the mother and finding out how she has provided for her child's well-being may help her to appreciate your interest in the patient.

When surgery has been done, the physician discusses with the parents the activities the child will ultimately be permitted to carry on. In some instances the child will need additional guidance to help him adjust to a new life.

Congenital heart defects may show up later in life and may possibly require corrective surgery. Adults are often fearful unless special precautions are taken to help them and the members of their families to understand the possible value of such surgery.

DISEASES AND DISORDERS OF BLOOD VESSELS

Blood vessel tissue is influenced by the aging process in the same way as other body tissues. The aging process is still a mystery; the results are better known. For example, it is known that blood vessels become less elastic with age, that they can feel more firm to the fingertips. As mentioned under coronary artery disease, substances can accumulate on the lining of arteries and narrow the lumen. Anything that prevents the blood vessels from moving blood freely around the body creates problems. Some are local; others are generalized.

PERIPHERAL VASCULAR DISEASES

Peripheral vascular diseases are primarily related to disorders of the blood vessels of the extremities. They can occur in any age group, but older people are more often affected. In general, these disease conditions develop over a period of time and are difficult to prevent. They are often chronic, and treatment must extend over a long period of time.

As with diseases of the heart, most of the peripheral vascular diseases share common symptoms and call for similar treatment and nursing care. These general factors will be discussed before specific disease conditions are described.

Signs and Symptoms

The symptoms of peripheral vascular diseases may be mild or severe, with or without complications. Some symptoms develop slowly and may be unnoticed by the patient. It is the lack of proper circulation in a part of the body that brings about certain symptoms. Pain is usually present in the extremity or part and it may be mild, continuous, and throbbing, or sudden and severe. The patient may complain of tingling and numbness in the toes and fingers and of his hands and feet being cold. Discoloration of the skin may develop; it may be blue, then mottled and darker with the area hardened. The skin may become irritated or broken.

Medical Treatment and Nursing Care

Treatment usually includes means to help improve the circulation of the blood to the extremity and to protect against trauma, infections, blood clots, and other complications. Posture, position, and exercise are usually specified for the bed patient, as well as for the patient who is up and around or who may be at home.

Orders and instructions are given (usually by the physician) to the patient concerning any restrictions regarding diet, smoking, shoes, and clothing and the use of heat. However, because peripheral vascular diseases are usually chronic and occur frequently in the elderly, you may be asked or expected to give some instructions to the patient about his care or the prevention of complications.

In many respects the important considerations in nursing care are similar among the more common peripheral vascular diseases. These include such things as:

1. Personal cleanliness.
2. Preventing infections and complications.
3. Providing for warmth.
4. Medications.
5. Diet and fluids.
6. Body alignment and exercise.
7. Emotional needs and problems.
8. Pre- and postoperative care.

Personal cleanliness emphasizes the prevention of infections. Because the circulation is poor, the skin is easily broken or burned. These precautions should be taken:

1. Bath water lukewarm to prevent burns.
2. Mild soap to avoid skin irritation.
3. Washing and drying with gentle strokes to avoid breaking skin.
4. Dry carefully between toes and where skin surfaces touch.
5. Lanolin cream or lotion used on the skin rather than alcohol.
6. Hose changed daily or more often.
7. Observations of the skin and nails to include any rough, dry, or cracked areas; any red, blue, or discolored areas; swollen, soft, or hard areas; painful areas.

Preventing infections and complications requires attention. Any break, scratch, blister, or crack in the skin predisposes him to an infection with the possible development of an ulcer. The physician will indicate the treatment in order to prevent further complications.

Nails should be trimmed carefully and only as necessary. Toenails should be cut straight across and not too short or close. Avoid injury to the skin and tissue close to the nail. Ingrown toenails, corns, and calluses should receive special handling.

Providing for warmth helps to improve circulation to the part. General body warmth rather than locally direct heat is more desirable. The room should be warm with no drafts. Clothing should be sufficient (and loose to allow for circulation) for warmth without causing the patient to perspire. Avoid chilling because of the poor circulation to the extremity.

Local or direct applications of heat or warmth to the extremity (e.g., hot water bottles, hot sodas, and heating pads) are not to be applied without a written order.

Medications ordered include those to relieve pain, to dilate the blood vessels, and to decrease the clotting time of the blood. Some of these drugs may produce toxic reactions; observe for signs of toxic reactions (e.g., nausea, vomiting, skin irritations).

Diet and fluids are usually specifically ordered. Certain amounts and types of food and fluid help to regulate circulation and to prevent infection of tissue. Calories, fats, proteins, and vitamins are regulated according to the weight and age of the patient and his nutritional and other illness needs.

BODY ALIGNMENT AND EXERCISE. It is essential to understand the physician's orders regarding position, change of position, exercise, and rest, because the type, rate, and duration of exercise to help improve circulation are specifically regulated. Frequent change of position is usually ordered, but be very certain which positions should be avoided and whether or not the extremity should be elevated and, if so, for how long.

The rocking or oscillating bed may be used to improve circulation (Fig. 47–2). An electric motor on the bed lowers first the head and then the foot of the bed slowly. The rate and degree of tilt are regulated. The bed may be kept in operation for specific periods or during the day and night as the patient becomes accustomed to it. It is stopped for meals, nursing care, and other treatments.

Emotional needs and problems should be recognized. Many of the peripheral vascular diseases occur in the older age group and are of long-term duration. These patients become discouraged for many reasons.

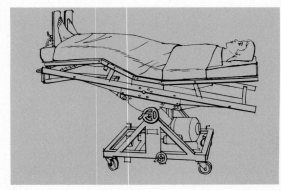

FIGURE 47–2   A patient on a rocking bed. (Sutton: Bedside Nursing Techniques, 2nd Ed.)

Treatment is slow and may necessarily be expensive, involving surgery, ranging from a simple procedure to amputation of an extremity.

PRE- AND POSTOPERATIVE NURSING CARE. In the event of surgical treatment for these conditions, the patient has the same nursing needs before and after surgery as discussed in Chapter 42. The orders will include precautions regarding position, elevation of part, movement, and important observations.

VASCULAR ULCER

The ulcer is an open area on the skin with destruction and sloughing of the underlying tissue. The local area may be quite small or it may be large. Ulcers are difficult to heal due to poor tissue nourishment, and there is always the possibility of infection.

Usually bed rest will be ordered, but the extremity or part may or may not be elevated. Bed cradles, foot boards, or pillows may be used to keep the weight of the bedding off the part.

Heat may or may not be ordered. If heat is ordered, be *sure* of the method, whether it is to be moist or dry, how long it is to be applied, and the temperature to be used. Overheating or burning can take place easily and quickly because of poor blood supply to the area.

If medicated preparations are ordered for application to the ulcer or the area around it, *sterile equipment and materials as well as sterile technique should be used.*

HYPERTENSION (HIGH BLOOD PRESSURE)

Hypertension is a sign that some parts of the body (e.g., circulatory system) are not functioning properly. It is not a disease as such, but it is often associated with vascular diseases. Blood is under pressure in the blood vessels under normal circumstances; it has to be to carry on its functions. Body mechanisms adjust the vessels during health to maintain a normal range of pressure according to age and activity. When the body fails to make these necessary adjustments, the blood pressure may drop below normal range (hypotension) or rise above normal range.

Abnormally high blood pressure most often occurs in persons over 40 years of age, but occasionally it occurs in younger adults and even children. There is no known cause for this condition except when it can be directly traced to some other disease; this is called *secondary hypertension*. When it cannot be traced to another disease, it is known as *essential hypertension*.

Certain changes occur in the circulatory system. The lumina of the arterioles are narrowed, causing poor circulation and nourishment of surrounding tissues. Because the lumen is smaller, greater pressure is needed to force the necessary amount of blood through the blood vessels. This makes the heart work harder; rate may not increase, but each beat is stronger to provide the necessary extra force. This rise in blood pressure may be present for some years before there are symptoms.

Signs and Symptoms

Fatigue, headache, dizziness, irritability, and insomnia are the usual symptoms. Changes may occur in such organs as heart, brain and kidneys as the condition worsens. For example, hypertensive heart disease results if the heart is not able to perform the extra work required, or a cerebral hemorrhage may occur.

Medical Treatment and Nursing Care

Factors that are considered either in prevention or treatment include body weight (overweight is avoided), eating habits (avoid overuse of salt), habits of rest, sleep, and relaxation, and emotional stress, and heredity.

There is no specific treatment for high blood pressure. It will vary with the patient. The physician may order a reduction diet if the patient is overweight or a low salt diet to help prevent edema. Medications are used to help produce rest and to help control the high blood pressure. The patient under treatment may remain at home or continue to work. Rest periods during the day may be part of the treatment.

If the high blood pressure progresses or becomes severe, the patient may be hospitalized. Important observations to make include headache, dizziness (vertigo), and any difficulty in, or complaints about, seeing or breathing.

ARTERIOSCLEROSIS

Often called "hardening of the arteries," this condition occurs when the wall of the artery becomes thickened and hardened and the lumen is narrowed by a filling or deposit. It occurs in all age groups but more frequently after 50 years of age and more often in men than women. Many factors are thought to influence the condition, including nutrition, fat metabolism, heredity, emotions, and certain habits such as the use of tobacco. There is no exact treatment for the generalized condition of arteriosclerosis, which takes place over a long time, often years.

The circulation and pressure within the arteries determine the symptoms. The symptoms appear when the changed condition of the artery will no longer permit enough blood to circulate to furnish oxygen and nutrients to tissues or remove the waste products from the tissues. As a result, scar tissue forms and the functions of the different organs (e.g., heart, kidneys) are disturbed.

All of the arteries are affected by arteriosclerosis, some more frequently than others. The coronary arteries (arteries supplying the heart) and the large vessels in the trunk, thighs, and legs are commonly affected. As the artery becomes hardened and filled, a thrombus may easily form and entirely shut off the flow of blood to the organ or part (e.g., coronary thrombosis, cerebral thrombosis).

ARTERY OBSTRUCTION OR OCCLUSION

An artery may become obstructed rapidly due to embolism or gradually due to arteriosclerosis, which more frequently affects the lower extremities.

Signs and Symptoms

It begins with cramplike pain in the lower leg, tingling and numbness in the toes, cold feet and toes, and a dusky blue discoloration of skin. As the condition progresses there are tissue changes, with ulceration, infection, and gangrene.

Medical Treatment and Nursing Care

Treatment is focused on keeping the extremities warm, maintaining good skin care, preventing infections, bruises, and scratches, and exercising and positioning the patient to permit the best possible blood circulation. The application of local heat, rubbing, or massage must have a physician's order.

Surgical treatment may involve the removal of the substance obstructing the vessel, replacement of the diseased vessel with a man-made material (i.e., nylon), or amputation if there are gangrene and infection.

Buerger's and Raynaud's diseases are two diseases in which there is interference in the circulation in the arteries, especially of the extremities. The causes of the two diseases are not known. The signs and symptoms are similar to those described above for artery obstruction or occlusion.

THROMBOPHLEBITIS

This is a condition in which the vein may become partially or completely obstructed with a thrombus, resulting in inflammation. The blood clot may be a result of *phlebitis* (inflammation of the walls of the veins) caused by injury, pressure, or infection. In thrombophlebitis there is the possibility that the clot, or a part of it, may be loosened and carried into the pulmonary circulation, producing an embolism.

Thrombophlebitis may develop from any condition that interferes with the venous circulation. It may be a complication of pregnancy or due to inactivity after surgery. For this reason attention has been given to early ambulation in preventing its occurrence. Pel-vic and leg veins are the most common sites of occurrence.

Signs and Symptoms

Swelling, redness, warmth in the local area, fever, and pain, especially if deeper veins are affected, are all common symptoms. The local area appears blue and mottled. The patient suffers from fatigue and has poor appetite.

Medical Treatment and Nursing Care

The treatment usually includes rest, continuous moist heat to the extremity, and drugs to control clotting and circulation. The physician may ligate one or both of the femoral veins. The written orders should indicate whether or not the extremity is to be elevated.

Complete bed rest and immobilization are usually emphasized to help prevent the thrombus from breaking away and producing pulmonary embolism. However, not all physicians are in agreement on this point. Be sure you understand what, if any, exercise or leg elevation the physician wants the patient to have. Sudden, difficult breathing, coughing, spitting of blood, and any signs of shock must be reported at once. These changes may indicate a pulmonary embolism.

Some physicians may order the patient to wear an elastic stocking or bandage following treatment and recovery, especially if there is a tendency for the condition to occur again. If so, the patient is measured for the elastic stocking and instructed how and when to put it on and wear it. Some patients need to wear one constantly; others only during the day.

VARICOSE VEINS

A varicose vein is one in which the valves in the veins do not function correctly. Instead of forcing the blood to move in one direction, they permit it to flow both ways. The vein becomes dilated and tortuous. As a result, the venous circulation is greatly impaired. There are a number of factors which may cause a varicosity:

1. Obstruction in the vein interfering with venous flow.
2. Pregnancy.

3. Wearing clothing that is too tight around the waist, trunk, or legs.

4. Work requiring continuous heavy lifting.

5. Long, continuous periods of standing. The veins of the leg are the most frequently affected. Other commonly varicosed veins are those of the lower rectum (hemorrhoids or "piles") and those of the testicles (varicocele).

Signs and Symptoms

Symptoms include an aching, tired, heavy feeling in the part, cramplike pains in legs at night, and "knots" in the veins. Later symptoms include edema of the feet, skin discoloration, and sometimes an open ulcer.

Medical Treatment and Nursing Care

An elastic bandage or stocking may be used on the affected leg. Orders are usually given regarding bed rest and elevation of the leg. Other treatments may include injections of drugs; surgery to ligate (tie) the affected vein and the removal of the varicosed or ulcerated part; and the application of a paste bandage or boot.

Special emphasis in nursing care includes: the prevention of burning, the prevention of infection and the prevention of a possible breaking away of a blood clot, and care not to scratch or bruise the skin. When an ulcer has developed, aseptic technique must be used in changing the dressings to avoid infection. Healing is difficult and slow. The patient is uncomfortable and easily becomes discouraged. Diversion is one of his basic needs; permit him to participate in self-care activities to the extent of his abilities.

DISEASES AND DISORDERS OF THE BLOOD

Review Table 10–2, Blood: Formed Elements and Plasma. The diseases and disorders of the blood and its formed parts are many and varied. There are conditions in which there are too many white blood cells, too few red blood cells, misshapen blood cells, too little blood volume, or an inability of the blood to clot in a normal manner.

THE ANEMIAS

Anemia is a condition in which the number of red blood cells is decreased and there is less hemoglobin. Less hemoglobin means less ability of the blood to transport oxygen and carbon dioxide. Among children, anemia is the most common blood disorder. Elderly people have the least bone marrow; therefore, they have less built in power to manufacture red blood cells. Anemia may result from hemorrhage (acute or chronic), destruction of red cells, or faulty formation of red cells.

Anemias are typed or classified according to the cause, which may be iron deficiency, nutritional deficiency (pernicious anemia) blood loss, heredity (sickle cell anemia), or faulty bone marrow function (aplastic anemia).

General Signs and Symptoms

The general signs/symptoms are much the same regardless of what causes the anemia.

1. skin color ranges from mild pallor to gray, white or a faint yellow.
2. weakness and fatigue.
3. headache and ringing in the ears.
4. dyspnea.
5. elevated temperature.
6. digestive disturbances.

Iron Deficiency Anemia

This disorder is due to iron deficiency or lack. The body does not get enough iron to meet its needs. This leads to a lack of hemoglobin because iron is used in making hemoglobin. Too little hemoglobin means that the blood lacks the capacity to transport enough oxygen to the body cells. The patient feels tired and weak, has little interest in food, and is pale.

Rapid growth and a poor diet or poor eating habits can contribute to iron deficiency. Between the ages of 11 and 15, the body produces more hemoglobin to meet the ordinary demands for growth. However, if growth is unusually fast and the diet is lacking in iron, it is not uncommon for children to show signs of anemia. The treatment consists of additional iron and a diet high in iron, proteins and vitamins.

Iron therapy is usually by mouth (ferrous sulphate) before or after meals, depending on the physician's preference. Iron is known to be irritating to the stomach and intestines. If an intestinal disease such as colitis is present, the iron may be given by intramuscular injection (liver extract). Special care must be given to the teeth and mouth after liquid iron is given because it stains the teeth and has a disagreeable taste, and the mouth may be sore and the gums tender. The stools are apt to be dark and tarry; this should be explained to the patient so that he will not be alarmed. If the patient is a child, the parents should understand the change in the stool. Constipation may be a problem.

Personal hygiene includes special care to the skin to prevent irritation and infection. The patient often complains of being cold, and sufficient clothing and bedding should be provided. Attention should be given to the temperature of the room so that the patient is comfortable.

Due to his poor appetite the patient may need encouragement to eat and to feed himself. Children and elderly patients often require closer assistance to meet their nutritional needs. Involve a family member if appropriate.

Pernicious Anemia

This type of anemia is a nutritional condition too, but it is due to the inability of the body to absorb vitamin B_{12} properly. This affects the production of normal, mature red blood cells. The body needs assistance to use vitamin B_{12}; proper diet alone is not enough. Treatment includes giving the patient vitamin B_{12} intramuscularly or by mouth.

In addition to some of the general signs and symptoms of anemia listed above, the patient with pernicious anemia usually has a sore mouth and tongue along with gastric distress and diarrhea. He may be discouraged and irritable at times. Early treatment of this disorder is beneficial in reducing the signs and symptoms. Delayed treatment often permits permanent damage to occur in the nervous system.

THE LEUKEMIAS (see Chapter 43, Patients with Cancer)

INFECTIOUS MONONUCLEOSIS (GLANDULAR FEVER)

This disease is a generalized infection that may have a sudden or slow onset. It is communicable, generally appearing in the spring and fall, and at times there may be an outbreak involving many people. Infectious mononucleosis is most commonly seen among adolescents and young adults; however, it may occur among others. The exact cause of this disease is not known, but it is thought to be a virus. The prognosis is usually good, even though the patient is confined to bed for two or three weeks (children for less time than adults as a rule). One serious (even fatal) complication is a ruptured spleen thus the need for quiet and bed rest.

Signs and Symptoms

To begin with, the patient has irregular fever, which may last for several weeks, and

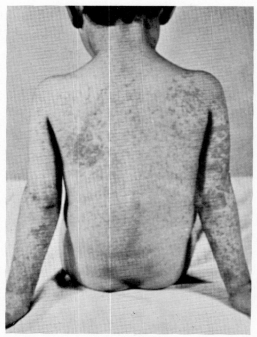

FIGURE 47–3 Skin rash in mononucleosis. (Nelson: Textbook of Pediatrics. 9th Ed.)

fatigue and weakness that last a long time; a sore throat and enlarged lymph nodes may or may not appear early in the disease. Later he develops skin rash, jaundice, headache, stiff neck, blurred vision, and mental confusion. See Figure 47–3.

Medical Treatment and Nursing Care

There is no known specific treatment. Bed rest is required and following that activities are gradually increased as the patient's fatigue and fever diminish.

Medications may include something for fever and pain, vitamins and antibiotics if a secondary infection occurs. A high protein diet is usually ordered. Nursing care focuses on providing this patient with as much rest and quiet as possible. Plan his care with his state of dependency in mind. At first, he may be allowed to do little for himself, gradually becoming involved in self-care activities.

Because of a long convalescence, quiet diversion becomes a prominent daily need. Children and adolescents may find their confinement difficult.

SUMMARY

Heart and circulatory diseases and disorders account for the greatest number of deaths in this country. No age group escapes them, but during certain periods of life some types of disorders are more common than others. The natural aging and maturing process in body tissues accounts for many of the diseases of the heart and blood vessels among the middleaged and elderly. Malformations and infections are more commonly responsible for heart and circulatory disorders in children and young adults.

There are many common signs and symptoms that show up in patients with heart and circulatory disorders, whatever the particular disease that causes them. Nursing care is geared to assisting the patient according to his particular signs and symptoms. It is more essential that the practical nurse know *how* to conserve the patient's energy while giving daily care than it is to know the pathology that makes it necessary for the physician to order "complete bed rest."

GUIDES FOR STUDY AND DISCUSSION

1. Review the formed elements of the blood and their functions, pulmonary circulation, systemic circulation, and coronary circulation.

2. What means does the physician have for getting information about the condition of the patient?

3. What are the main signs/symptoms of heart disease?

4. It is common to read "he suffered a heart attack." As you understand it, what is a heart attack?

5. Why are the nurse's observations so essential? What should they include?

6. Why must the patient with heart disease conserve his energy? How does the nurse help him do this?

7. What *types* of drugs are commonly used for cardiac patients? What is the purpose of each type?

8. Among the diseases/disorders discussed in this chapter, the need for bed rest is often mentioned. See how many types of these patients require bed rest. What nursing problems may be encountered because of this?

9. Use this chart in your notebook to organize your thoughts about the various

diseases discussed in this chapter. Notice what (if anything) is similar among the signs/symptoms and the nursing care.

Disease/ Disorder	Definition	Signs/ Symptoms	Treatment in- cluding surgical	Nursing Care

SUGGESTED SITUATIONS AND ACTIVITIES

1. Plan a role playing situation for one of the following patients which shows your ability to provide effective nursing care:
   a. A 45 year old male patient on complete bed rest with a myocardial infarction.
   b. A 17 year old female patient with iron deficiency anemia and no appetite.
   c. An elderly woman with peripheral vascular disease who is discouraged with her slow progress.
2. Visit an intensive care unit and observe as many lifesaving and life preserving pieces of equipment as you can. Why does this specialized hospital area require highly trained personnel?

CHAPTER 48

PATIENTS WITH GENITOURINARY DISORDERS

TOPICAL HEADINGS

Introduction
Diseases and
 Disorders of the
 Kidneys, Bladder,
 and Related Parts

Diseases and Disorders of the Reproductive Organs
Summary

Guides for Study and
 Discussion
Suggested Situations
 and Activities

OBJECTIVES FOR THE STUDENT: Be able to:

1. Describe the main function(s) of the parts of the male reproductive system; the female reproductive system.
2. Identify two similarities and two differences between the male and the female urinary systems.
3. Name three pertinent observations in caring for a patient with kidney/bladder disorders.
4. Explain the need for strict aseptic practices when caring for a patient with a genitourinary infection.
5. Describe two precautions taken concerning the use of the indwelling catheter.
6. Given a list of terms describing abnormal urination, define each.
7. Give an example of a careless nursing practice which could lead to a genitourinary infection.
8. Tell why venereal disease can be called "the silent epidemic."
9. Describe three nursing measures generally carried out for a post-operative vaginal hysterectomy patient.

SUGGESTED STUDY VOCABULARY*

inflammation	pyelitis	syphilis
infection	pyelonephritis	amenorrhea
dysuria	septicemia	dysmenorrhea
oliguria	toxic	leukorrhea
polyuria	leukocytosis	cervicitis
hematuria	acute	vulvitis
anuria	chronic	vaginitis
nocturia	nephritis	sterility
sepsis	disoriented	prostatitis
abscess	sedation	orchitis
obstruction	nephrosis	epididymitis
residual urine	renal calculi	vaginal repair
aseptic technique	uremia	perineorrhaphy
urethritis	hemodialysis	hysterectomy
cystitis	gonorrhea	

*Look for any terms you already know.

INTRODUCTION

One reason for including the urinary and the reproductive systems in one chapter is that they are anatomically close to each other and, in the male, some of the structures serve both systems. However, strictly speaking, each system has its own work to perform.

Like any other system, these two systems produce distress signals when they are not functioning properly: pain, fever, chills, hemorrhage, inflammation, sweating, weakness, and dehydration. The urinary system has its own ways of showing that it is not working properly, such as urinary retention and incontinence.

Both systems are subject to the same general disorders as other systems — they can suffer from inflammation, infection, obstruction, cancer, congenital malformation, injury, and malfunction.

Review Chapters 13 and 41.

DISEASES AND DISORDERS OF THE KIDNEYS, BLADDER, AND RELATED PARTS

The work of the kidneys is closely related to the circulatory system. The kidneys are body regulators; they: 1. Filter liquid metabolic wastes from the circulating blood. 2. Regulate body fluid balance. 3. Regulate the acid-base balance in the blood. Sometimes the list of the leading causes of death includes a grouping called "cardiovascular-renal diseases" because one system is so tied in with the workings of the other. Consequently, some signs and symptoms are common to both the circulatory and the urinary systems (e.g., edema, weight increase, and irritability), and patient care involves many of the same nursing measures.

The disorders included here represent some of the more common types of conditions involving the urinary system. Notice the common signs and symptoms among them.

Pain and Urine Irregularities

Three types of observations are particularly helpful to the physician in diagnosing and treating patients with kidney and bladder disorders; they are observations about the nature, extent and location of any pain, what, if anything, is abnormal about urination, and what, if anything, is abnormal about the urine.

PAIN. Chapter 41 points out how you can secure information (subjective and objective) from the patient who is experiencing pain. The personal nature of pain makes it difficult to determine what it is like and, sometimes, to determine where it is located.

Pain associated with the urinary system may be local or it may spread out to other parts of the body; it can range from a constant, dull ache to severe stabbing attacks. Any observations (subjective or objective) of pain experienced by patients with urinary disorders should include:

1. location and type.
2. relief (if any) provided by medication.
3. accompanying symptoms (e.g., nausea, vomiting, abdominal distress).

ABNORMAL URINATION. The main causes of abnormal urination (abnormal in amount, in sensation during or following, or in frequency) include obstruction of some type, paralysis, infection, and irritation. Terms describing abnormal urination include dysuria, oliguria, polyuria, hematuria, anurea, and nocturia (See Chapter 41, Urinary Distress).

ABNORMALITIES OF URINE. Observe for *any* abnormal color, odor, appearance, or presence of foreign matter in urine specimens, whether the patient has a known urinary disorder or not. Watch for such things as blood, pieces of tissue, shaped or formed masses of blood clots, gravel, stones, and pus.

Sepsis Due to Infection

Sepsis means poisoning from the presence of harmful bacteria and their by-products. The normal urinary tract is free from bacteria except near the external meatus. The normal state of urine is unfavorable to bacteria and its outward flow through the urinary meatus has a washing-out effect; both of which serve as barriers to urinary tract infection (bacteriuria).

Bacteriuria may cause the body to react to the sepsis in an overall way producing such signs/symptoms as fever, chills, dehydration, constipation, headache, pain, fatigue, poor appetite and malnutrition.

The invading organism must have a source; finding that source and identifying the organism(s) are two steps in treatment. Sources of infection include: 1. an abcess in the tract. 2. an obstruction (e.g., stone, tumor, stricture) somewhere along the tract that causes urine to collect and serve as a breeding place for organisms. 3. organisms brought to the site by the circulating blood. 4. an ascending infection that starts in the urethra and moves up the tract (particularly hazardous in the male due to the relationship of secondary sex organs to the urethra). Studies show that the large bowel furnishes most of the bacteria which invade the urinary tract. This fact should caution you about the need to observe strict aseptic technique when irrigating the urinary bladder and inserting a catheter; likewise it is reason enough to use proper cleansing and bathing techniques with respect to the genitalia. Bowel incontinence requires continuous precaution against urinary tract infection.

Treatment is focused on removing the cause of infection. Sometimes this is a difficult and slow process. If there is a specific antibiotic for the causative organism, the infection may be brought under control. However, when the bacteriuria persists, drugs called antiseptics (e.g., mandelic acid, mandelamine) are sometimes used to maintain the urine in a state that is unfavorable to bacterial growth. This may need to be an on-going treatment. Treatment also involves frequent urine specimens collected as ordered (e.g., "sterile voided," "sterile"), bladder irrigations, drugs instilled in the bladder, indwelling catheters changed periodically and not left in place over an extended period of time, and keeping a record of intake/output.

Infectious Disorders

URETHRITIS. Urethritis is inflammation of the urethra caused by organisms that have invaded the lining. If the urethral lining is damaged it is an open invitation to invasion by organisms. It has been proven that careless techniques in irrigating the bladder, in catheterizing, and in examining the bladder with instruments (cystoscopy) may lead to urethritis; an indwelling catheter is another cause of irritation and trauma.

Signs and Symptoms. The symptoms are a burning sensation on urination, frequency and urgency of urination, and drainage of pus.

Medical Treatment and Nursing Care. Treatment is divided into two main categories: 1. Local treatment, such as sitz baths and thorough washing and cleansing of the urethral area. You may need to wash the area for the patient, paying strict attention not to use strokes that might bring contamination from the anal region. 2. Systemic treatment, which includes drug therapy (chemotherapy, antibiotics), adequate diet, increased fluid intake, and sufficient rest to help the body ward off the infection.

Every means should be used to prevent reintroduction of organisms. Handwashing should be very much a part of the nurse's (and the patient's) procedure. Urinals and bedpans should have thorough daily cleaning (sterilizing or boiling).

CYSTITIS. Cystitis is inflammation of the lining of the urinary bladder. This condition is more common among women than men. It can be acute or chronic.

The urinary bladder (normally) has good resistive power; it stores and discharges urinary wastes under "sterile" conditions. In other words, a normal bladder is able to resist inflammation under ordinary circumstances. Cystitis usually comes from some source outside the bladder (a secondary infection), such as a kidney infection, renal tuberculosis, an obstruction, or an ascending infection from the urethra.

Signs and Symptoms. Symptoms are frequency and urgency of urination (day and night), burning sensation on urination, pain (before, during, and following urination), uncontrolled urination, fever and chills (may not be present), and hematuria.

Medical Treatment and Nursing Care. The cause of the infection must be determined and removed (if possible). The physician will usually order urinalysis (various types), chemotherapy, forced fluids, and bed rest if the patient has a fever. If recovery is slow, the patient may become discouraged. Children need diversional activities if they are confined to bed rest for a long period of time.

PYELITIS AND PYELONEPHRITIS. These infections are discussed together because pyelitis (simple inflammation of the kidney pelvis) easily becomes pyelonephritis (inflammation of the kidney tissue), which involves much more kidney tissue. Pyelonephritis may become a serious kidney disease that destroys kidney tissue and limits its filtering ability. Abscesses may form and septicemia may occur as a result.

Signs and Symptoms of Acute Pyelonephritis. Patient may have fever and chills and loss of appetite. Sweating, leukocytosis, and vomiting may occur. Pain and tenderness may or may not be present, and there are pus and bacteria in the urine.

Medical Treatment and Nursing Care. The patient is confined to bedrest and may require considerable assistance in meeting his personal care needs, especially if he has a high fever and is toxic. Fluids are pushed (3 to 4 quarts per day), bowels are regulated, and antibiotic drugs are ordered. Blood and urine specimens are frequently examined. In severe cases surgery may be required to drain the kidney or, if necessary, to remove it. The patient with acute pyelonephritis is not interested in food and eating; this poses a nursing challenge, especially with young children.

When the disease is chronic, the physician tries to find and remove the source of the infection (e.g., infected tonsils, appendicitis, infected teeth, or colitis). The patient's symptoms are not as pronounced and severe, but chronic pyelonephritis can permanently destroy kidney tissue. Treatment (chemotherapy or removing infection elsewhere) is directed toward holding kidney damage to a minimum; this often is a long, slow treatment process and patients can easily become discouraged.

Nursing care includes the special concerns one has with long-term patients who are not ambulatory.

Noninfectious Disorders

NEPHRITIS. Nephritis is inflammation of kidney tissue. You might think of it as a family name, because there are many types of nephritis (e.g., gomerulonephritis, arteriosclerotic nephritis, and congenital nephritis). This progressive disease attacks kidney tissue and permanently damages it. The patient gradually loses kidney power to regulate body fluids.

Nephritis is not caused by bacteria that directly invade kidney tissue; it follows an infection that has occurred elsewhere, such as tonsillitis, upper respiratory, scarlet fever, sinusitis, or rheumatic fever. What happens in the kidney is thought to be a delayed response to the earlier infection; the delay may be two or three weeks.

Nephritis may be acute or chronic. The acute stage may pass; the patient recovers. However, there is no assurance that the recovery is either complete or final. Chronic nephritis is another matter. It continues and seriously disrupts the cardiovascular system, the urinary system, and body fluid balance. Anemia is usually present (mild to severe) and the blood is otherwise affected (white cells and lymph).

Children and young adults are more frequently victims of acute glomerulonephritis than older persons.

Signs and Symptoms. The symptoms include edema, beginning with the hands and face and becoming more generalized, headache, hypertension, oliguria, hematuria, and dyspnea. The patient may have loss of appetite, nausea and vomiting, fever, and disturbed vision. He may show signs of restlessness and irritability. In severe cases, he may be delirious or in a coma.

Not all of these signs and symptoms are present in all cases. At times one or more might appear for a short time and then disappear. This makes it essential that close observation be an on-going part of nursing care.

Medical Treatment and Nursing Care. The stage of development and severity of the patient's condition influence his nursing needs and medical management. The physician continues to watch the urine and blood laboratory reports. Kidney function tests are used to observe renal function. Observations include any changes in vital signs, disorientation as to time and place, appetite, skin condition, and intake and output. The patient's condition may change very rapidly.

One can see from the signs and symptoms that the special nursing needs of nephritic patients might include positioning to aid breathing, encouragement to eat (usually a modified diet), bed rest, and considerable assistance with personal care and hygiene (good skin and mouth care). Restlessness and irritability create problems for the patient; the nurse must accept these problems as part of this patient's disorder. Sedations may be ordered, but this does not relieve the nurse of responsibility for providing every comfort measure appropriate to the patient's needs. The age of the patient often influences his needs in this respect; children are especially apt to be fretful and restless.

NEPHROSIS. Nephrosis is a term used to denote kidney disease where kidney tissue degenerates and is destroyed. The body distress signals are much the same as for nephritis. Nephrosis, like nephritis, is a family name including a variety of types, and it too may be acute or chronic. It is primarily a children's disorder, but it can be very severe in adults.

Treatment and nursing care are centered around measures (medicine, diet, sometimes bed rest, fluid restrictions) that attempt to aid the kidneys while they repair themselves (if this is possible). Every effort is made to avoid any type of patient infection. Here again, strict observance of aseptic techniques should guide all nursing action.

RENAL CALCULI. Renal calculi is another name for kidney stones. The reason stones form is not completely understood. The stones may be too large to leave the kidney or bladder or they may work their way out of the kidney, down the ureter, and into the bladder, and be expelled on urination.

Signs and Symptoms. The symptoms include pain, ranging from a dull ache to a most severe knifing pain that radiates to the groin, legs, and lower abdomen (renal colic), nausea and vomiting, fever and chills, and hematuria.

Medical Treatment and Nursing Care. The physician generally uses x-rays to make the diagnosis, if possible, or does such examinations as cystoscopy and ureteral catheterization to locate the presence of stones.

Morphine is usually given (especially to adults) for the severe pain. External heat may be ordered and fluids forced. Parenteral fluids may be administered, especially if the patient vomits. The physician wants the patient to increase his urinary output.

If the symptoms do not clear up in a few days, it may be necessary to remove the stones by manipulation or by surgery.

In addition to the usual nursing measures against pain, nausea, vomiting, and fever and chills, the nurse should watch the urine closely for presence of any foreign matter. Sometimes the stone passes; sometimes it does not. Blood in the urine should be noted and described.

The patient with renal colic suffers and is subject to exhaustion and fatigue. He is apt to have little interest in his personal hygiene or eating. Sleep and rest are needed, and a quiet environment with as few interruptions as possible should be provided.

UREMIA. Uremia is a condition in which urine products get into the bloodstream and body cells and produce general toxic symptoms. The kidneys lose their ability to excrete and this quickly becomes a critical problem for the body. Uremia can arise from any renal diseases that destroy kidney tissue and cause the filtering action to break down. For example, a patient with glomerulonephritis may have uremia too. It can also occur when there is an obstruction (e.g., tumor, stones, stricture) somewhere in the urinary tract.

Signs and Symptoms. The uremia patient exhibits poor appetite, nausea and vomiting, irritability, disorientation, and drowsiness and stupor. He may have headaches and suffer from anemia, dehydration, and disturbance in the balance of body fluids and electrolytes. Delirium, convulsions, and coma may also occur.

Medical Treatment and Nursing Care. Patients with uremia may be very sick and the condition may worsen rapidly. The physician finds the cause (if possible) and treats the patient according to his symptoms. He is concerned that the patient eat a proper diet and take enough fluids. The anemia may require blood transfusions; restoration of the electrolyte balance is of great importance. If treatment does not bring the body cells into proper electrolyte balance and return the blood to a normal state, the disease becomes fatal.

Skin care (as with other kidney diseases) should be careful and thorough to avoid any infections. Medications are ordered for the patient's restlessness, to prevent convulsions and to aid the acid-base balance in the body.

To protect the patient from injury due to his confused state of mind and possible convulsion, side rails should be padded and a padded tongue blade should be at hand at all times to prevent him from chewing his tongue or strangling during a seizure.

Artificial Kidney Machine

Machines are available to do the work of the kidney. A portable machine can be used in the patient's home after family members have been thoroughly instructed in how to use, maintain, and clean it. The machine filters the blood with chemical solutions, removing materials ordinarily filtered out by the kidneys. This process, called *hemodialysis*, takes about four hours. The patient's blood is pumped through a permanent tube in the patient's arm into the machine where the filtering action takes place. The treatment must be performed twice a week.

DISEASES AND DISORDERS OF THE REPRODUCTIVE ORGANS

Venereal disease could be discussed elsewhere under another system or category as well as here, but because they are spread through sexual contact they are included in this chapter.

Male reproductive organ disorders have a direct relationship to the urinary tract; thus, reference is made to resulting urinary symptoms in this content.

Infection, tumors, and cancer are responsible for many male and female reproductive disorders. See Chapter 43, Patients with Cancer.

Venereal Disease

Venereal diseases are spread by sexual contact; one sexual contact with an infected person is all it may take. They are on the increase and have become the leading reportable communicable disease in many areas. It is called the "silent epidemic" by some, perhaps because so many cases are not reported due to the intimate nature of the way it is spread or because many times the symptoms are not apparent or are not recognized, so medical help is not sought.

There are two major venereal diseases: *gonorrhea* and *syphilis*. Both are infectious.

GONORRHEA. Gonorrhea is caused by the gonococcus organism invading (infecting) the lining membranes of the reproductive tract and adjoining tissues.

The disease usually makes itself known in the male by: 1. a sudden onset of frequent, painful (and burning sensation) urination. 2. a discharge (pus) from the urethral meatus. If the male goes untreated, the infection can spread and finally produce so much scar tissue in the urethra that urination is difficult and even prevented. This in turn can produce urinary retention with a secondary infection which may spread to surrounding gland tissue and to the kidneys.

The female may be unaware of the infection because there are no apparent signs/symptoms. If urination is somewhat painful and/or there is a vaginal discharge, they may be ignored. If the female goes untreated, the infection can spread into the cervical glands, to the Fallopian tubes and ovaries producing abscesses and pelvic infection (peritonitis). All of this may produce permanent sterility.

The gonococcus can be carried by the blood stream to other parts of the body causing arthritis and damage to the heart valves in both the male and the female. The infected mother can cause eye infection in her newborn which, if not treated (e.g., by silver nitrate drops at birth), will produce permanent blindness.

Early medical care usually consists of brief treatment with an antibiotic drug (e.g., penicillin); the dosage has increased over the years because the gonococcus has become resistant to penicillin. Females may require larger dosages than males.

SYPHILIS. Syphilis is called "the great imitator" because during its advanced stages signs/symptoms of other types of diseases begin to appear. It is caused by a spiral-shaped organism (spirochete) that can invade any body tissue. Like gonorrhea, syphilis is spread through sexual contact with an infected person. The spirochete is fragile and does not long survive outside the body; therefore spreading of the disease by dishes or a toilet seat is not likely. Transmission by kissing is rare.

The fetus can acquire syphilis from the infected mother through the placenta; this is called *congenital syphilis* and can cause such things as deformed bones (e.g., skull, long bones) and teeth, blindness, deafness, and mental retardation.

Signs and Symptoms. Syphilis progresses in definite stages. From the time of transmission (direct contact with infected lesion), the incubation period averages three weeks (ranges from 10 to 90 days). The *primary* stage (1-5 weeks), a highly communicable stage, follows when a lesion (chancre) appears; the blood test is then positive and a body rash may be present. In the *secondary* stage, which may last for a few months to a year or more, the chancre has disappeared (after 3 to 6 weeks). The organisms have invaded the body and are in the bloodstream. The blood test is positive. The female is infectious and can pass the disease to the fetus. The *third (tertiary) stage* follows a long, quiet period of several years, when no symptoms are present, showing itself by blindness, crippling and paralysis, mental illness and death. The nervous system, heart, blood vessels, skeletal system, and skin are affected. The damage is permanent. The mother can infect the fetus.

Medical Treatment: The diagnosis of primary syphilis is best confirmed by a laboratory procedure called a "darkfield examination," a microscopic examination of live, moving spirochetes against a dark background.

Since 1946 the best treatment for syphilis has been penicillin; the recovery rate is very high. However, the knowledge that there is a "quick cure" and the relaxed attitudes about sexual haphazardness have moved syphilis from a controllable disease to one of epidemic proportions. Follow-up examinations (blood, chest x-rays, spinal fluid) should be made to determine whether or not the initial treatment was effective. Failure to do this may be another reason why syphilis is on the increase; patients may assume they are fully cured when they are not.

Infertility and Sterility

These terms mean the inability to conceive or to produce young. For one or more reasons the husband or the wife is incapable of reproduction.

Factors that the physician considers in examining the husband include his present state of health, age, past medical history (e.g., mumps, genital infections, injuries and trauma to the genitalia, venereal disease, prostatic difficulties, and urethral discharges), occupation, and mode of life. If the medical history indicates reasons for a complete physical examination, this is done.

Gathering evidence about the wife may involve more tests and time than it does for the husband. The physician does a pelvic examination and takes a complete past history as to pelvic surgery, endocrine disorders, inflammatory pelvic conditions, marital history, and menstrual history (e.g., pain, absence of menses, irregularity of cycles).

Follow-up visits may include extensive laboratory tests and further examination of the body structures involved.

Male Disorders

INFECTIONS. Review Figure 13–5. Locate the prostate gland, seminal vesicle, epididymis, and testes, noticing what easy access organisms have from one part of the male sex organs to another. The urethra serves as a common pathway for urine and semen, making it possible for inflammation of the urethra to invade both the urinary tract and the adjoining reproductive structures.

PROSTATITIS AND SEMINAL VESICULITIS. Organisms can reach the prostate gland as an infection ascending by way of the urethra or descending from the kidneys, the bladder, or the epididymis. Organisms from an infection elsewhere in the body (e.g., tonsils, sinuses) may be transported to the gland via the bloodstream.

PROSTATITIS. Prostatitis is inflammation of the prostate gland due to infection. Seminal vesiculitis is inflammation of the seminal vesicle due to infection. Due to the close anatomical relationship between the two, an infection in one can easily reach the other. Infection of these structures may be acute or chronic.

Acute prostatitis produces such signs and symptoms as fever, soreness of the vesicle, pain and feeling of fullness in the rectum and perineum, and possibly obstruction to unination. The gland itself is enlarged and tender.

Treatment usually includes penicillin and sulfa drugs or other antibiotics. Rectal suppositories (e.g., opium and belladonna) may be ordered to relieve symptoms. When the patient has difficulty voiding, an indwelling catheter may be used for several days.

If an abscess is present, fever and chills are pronounced and may lead to toxemia. Chronic prostatitis may produce few if any symptoms; this condition is quite common. The more usual complaints include some difficulty on urination, urethral discharge (scant to profuse), and pain in the testes, rectum, perineum, groin, lower back, and vesicles. This discomfort may influence sexual functions.

Treatment centers around finding and removing the cause and origin of the infection (if possible), establishing good drainage, and preventing reinfection. This means that the urine must be kept sterile. Surgery may be necessary. Partial or total removal of the prostate gland is called a prostatectomy.

ORCHITIS AND EPIDIDYMITIS. Orchitis is inflammation of a testis; it is most often associated with inflammation of the epididymis, called epididymitis. About the only time this is not true is when orchitis is a complication of mumps.

During acute orchitis, the patient experiences pain in the testis. The testis is swollen, tender, firm, and heavy. Nausea and vomiting may or may not be present.

The patient is usually kept on complete bed rest with the scrotum elevated to relieve pain. Hot or cold applications may be ordered.

The organisms responsible for epididymitis may come from the surrounding organs and parts (e.g., urinary tract, prostate) or may be brought to the area via the bloodstream.

During an acute attack of epididymitis, the patient usually experiences severe local pain. The scrotum is reddened, swollen, and very tender, and fever is present (sometimes with chills).

To provide comfort, the patient is on bed rest with the scrotum elevated; hot or cold compresses or ice packs may be ordered. Penicillin and other antibiotics are generally ordered. When the patient becomes ambulatory, a scrotal support is worn to aid comfort. A chronic infection may require surgery (epididymectomy).

Female Disorders

MENSTRUAL DISORDERS. *Amenorrhea* is the absence of menstral flow. Besides pregnancy and menopause causes of amenorrhea may be some lack on the part of the ovary (e.g., failure to supply estrogen and progesterone), or some other endocrine disorder, such as a faulty pituitary gland. Amenorrhea may also be due to an anatomical reason, such as the lack of a genital canal to permit the escape of the flow.

Other factors which may directly or indirectly contribute to dysfunction of the ovaries or the pituitary glands are longterm, chronic disorders (e.g., heart disease, diabetes, nephritis, tuberculosis), anemias, thyroid disorders, malnutrition, psychic reasons (e.g., fear, shock, emotional distress), tumors, and environmental changes.

To treat the patient, the physician determines the cause, if possible. One can see from the rather long list of reasons above (and there are others) that treatment necessarily will differ from one patient to another.

Review Figure 13-2. Locate the cervix, vagina, uterus, uterine tubes, and ovaries.

Dysmenorrhea means painful menstruation. Normally there is no pain or disability due to menstruation. It is a bodily function common to all females from puberty to menopause and should be as natural a process as breathing or digestion. It is not a period of being "unwell" or of inability. When there is pain, the cause should be determined by a physician, and not treated with home remedies, by taking self-prescribed medications, or by staying in bed with the heating pad.

Surgical treatment may be necessary to correct the disorder or it may be corrected with medication prescribed by the physician. Improved posture, regular nourishing meals, activity to produce better circulation, including trunk and hip exercises, and loose clothing to avoid abdominal pressure may be simple ways of preventing discomfort; a right attitude toward menstruation is also beneficial.

Daily hygiene is carried on as usual. Strenuous exercise, such as horseback riding, running and jumping, should be avoided to prevent undue movement of the congested uterus or stretching of the ligaments which support it.

INFECTIONS. *Leukorrhea* is an abnormal genital discharge (blood-free); it is not a disease but a symptom of some type of dis-order. The discharge may be due to gonorrhea, syphilis, infections of the ducts and glands, tumors that create dysfunction, or by organisms that attack the lining of the vagina and the cervix. Here too treatment is based upon the factors causing the discharge; the physician seeks the reason for the abnormal discharge and prescribes treatment accordingly.

Pathogenic organisms may invade and infect any part of the female reproductive system. Infections in the various anatomical parts have specific names. Brief descriptions of the more common conditions are given in Table 48–1.

Surgery

Surgical treatment is used to repair damaged tissues and to remove tumors, cysts, and malfunctioning organs partially or totally. Table 48–2 describes some of the common types of treatment.

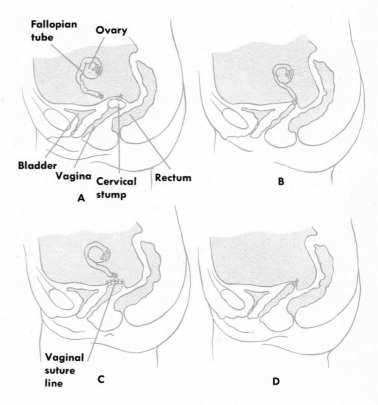

FIGURE 48–1 A, Cross section of a subtotal hysterectomy. Note that the cervical stump, fallopian tubes, and ovaries remain. B, Cross section of a total hysterectomy. Note that the fallopian tubes and ovaries remain. C, Cross section of a vaginal hysterectomy. Note that the fallopian tubes and ovaries remain. D, Cross section of a panhysterectomy. Note that the uterus, fallopian tubes and ovaries are completely removed. (From Shafer, Kathleen Newton, Sawyer, Janet R., McCluskey, Audrey M., Beck, Edna Lifgren, and Phipps, Wilma J.: Medical Surgical Nursing, 5th Ed. St. Louis, The C. V. Mosby Co., 1971.)

TABLE 48-1.   COMMON INFECTIONS OF THE FEMALE REPRODUCTIVE SYSTEM

Infections	Signs and Symptoms	Remarks
Cervicitis: inflammation of the cervix, surrounding mucosa, and cervical glands	Enlarged, edematous cervix; vaginal surface red and inflamed; purulent discharge (leukorrhea); pain (may not be present)	Common cause is gonorrhea. This condition may be related to a urinary tract infection Treatment may include smears and cultures, cervical and vaginal antibiotics, if patient can tolerate them, and topical drugs as warranted
Vulvitis and vaginitis: inflammation of one often leads to inflammation of the other — sometimes called vulvovaginitis	Redness and swelling; itching, pain (may not be present); and discharge (may not be present)	The vulva encounters many things to cause inflammation: urine, feces, menstrual flow, vaginal discharge, tight clothing, infected hair follicles, sebaceous cysts, ulcerated areas, fungus, ringworm, gonorrhea, and syphilis. The anal-rectal areas easily become involved as well Treatment is often given in the physician's office; the cause must be determined (if possible) so that specific drugs can be used effectively
Pelvic inflammatory disease, inflammation of pelvic organs, not including the uterus Oophoritis: inflammation of the ovaries Salpingitis: inflammation of the fallopian tubes (may result in sterility). Infection in the tubes may lead to generalized peritonitis or to an abdominal abscess.	Infectious discharge; pelvic and abdominal pain; backache; nausea and vomiting; fever; urinary symptoms, such as burning on urination (may not be present)	Organisms may enter the pelvic organs from the vagina or by way of the bloodstream or the lymphatics Treatment includes bed rest and positioning to promote drainage. Antibiotics usually are ordered. Local heat (e.g., sitz bath) may be ordered. Drainage and discharge may require perineal care and perineal pads. Isolation technique may be ordered. Strict medical aseptic technique should be practiced
Endometritis: inflammation of the lining of the uterus; the uterine muscles can easily become involved	Fever, low to moderate; elevated white blood count; uterine area firm and tender; and purulent or bloody discharge	A variety of organisms can cause this condition. Infection can follow abortion or use of instruments within it, or come as ascending infection or via the bloodstream or the lymphatics Treatment is directed toward preventing the spread of infection to surrounding areas. The uterus is drained through the cervix. Antibiotics may be used. If a foreign body is causing the inflammation it may require surgical removal

TABLE 48-2 TYPES OF SURGICAL TREATMENT

NAME	USE	REMARKS
Vaginal repair	To firm up vaginal wall.	Preoperative preparation: in addition to regular preparation, may include cleansing douche.
Anterior colorrhaphy	Repair a cystocele-bladder herniated into vagina.	
Posterior colorrhaphy	Repair a rectocele-rectal wall herniated into vagina.	Cathartic and cleansing enema to rid the bowel of feces.
Perineorrhaphy	Repair of damage to the pelvic floor.	Postoperative: emphasis on prevention of infection and of pressure on sutures, perineal care (cleansing strokes from vagina toward anus); other orders may include: heat lamp, local application of cold, sitz bath, douche, special orders re: bowel movements and urination.
Hysterectomy subtotal vaginal panhysterectomy	Removal of the uterus for therapeutic and preventive measures. See Figure 48-1 for types.	Preoperative preparation: regular for abdominal surgery plus perineal shave; vaginal douche may be ordered. Postoperative care: may have abdominal dressing and perineal pad. Or, if vaginal, only sterile perineal pads held in place by T binder. Observe for bleeding frequently over first eight hours. Foley catheter or catheterize after voiding. Food and fluids restricted for a time. Watch for abdominal distention. Exercise feet and legs—move about, change position and support with pillows. Observe for complaints of pain and voiding difficulties.

SUMMARY

The nurse caring for patients with genitourinary disorders should keep in mind how closely related the reproductive and urinary systems are to each other. Careless handling of equipment and less than strict aseptic techniques can cause infection, with serious results for the patient.

Both systems are subject to the same general disorders as other parts of the body: injury, tumors, cancer, tuberculosis, infection, inflammation, obstruction, congenital deformity, and malfunction.

The kidneys, in their role as body regulators and waste removers, are directly related to the circulatory system and to the acid-base balance in the body. These relationships make kidney diseases serious medical-nursing responsibilities that often require close observation (for pain, urine, urination, intake and output, and electrolyte balance), continuing laboratory examination of specimens, supervision of diet, control of pain, skin care, positioning, and general comfort measures.

Infection in the urinary tract may easily spread to the reproductive tract, and vice-versa. Nursing action should be guided by the use of aseptic technique for protection of the patient and the nurse.

GUIDES FOR STUDY AND DISCUSSION

1. In the male, what structure is common to both the urinary and the reproductive systems?

2. In the female, the urethra is shorter than in the male. How might this account for the fact that cystitis is more common in the female?

3. The work of the kidneys is closely related to the circulatory system. What do the kidneys have to do with the blood? Why is kidney malfunction such a serious condition?

4. Why should you always observe the condition of urine? What do you look for?

5. What is the reasoning behind the frequent changing of indwelling catheters or not leaving one in place over a period of time?

6. How should the following fact influence your nursing actions? Most bacteria found in urinary tract infection come from the bowel.

7. What nursing observations are particularily helpful to the physician treating a patient with some type of bladder or kidney disorder?

8. What nursing measures might be required for a child with pyelonephritis who has fever, chills, sweating, loss of appetite, nausea, vomiting, pain, fatigue and constipation?

9. What nursing measures might be required for a child with nephritis who has generalized edema, headache, oliguria, dyspnea, loss of appetite, nausea, vomiting, fever, disturbed vision, restlessness, irritability and disorientation? What measures are common between the patients in questions eight and nine?

10. In your opinion, what are two of the most essential nursing actions in caring for a patient with pelvic inflammatory disease? Be ready to defend your answer.

11. Why would the chance for infection run high for a patient with a vaginal repair or a vaginal hysterectomy? Why should the cleansing strokes (perineal care) be from the vagina toward the anus?

12. Venereal disease is on the increase. Why is this happening when there is an available cure?

13. Use the same type of chart form as suggested in the previous chapter to organize your thoughts about the various diseases and conditions discussed in this chapter.

SUGGESTED SITUATIONS AND ACTIVITIES

Strict aseptic nursing practice has been emphasized several times in this chapter. Select one such instance and prepare a one-two minute talk on how you would carry out the nursing measures. Use any equipment or visual aid you may need.

PATIENTS WITH BRAIN AND NERVE DISORDERS

OBJECTIVES FOR THE STUDENT: Be able to:

1. Name three things that can cause nervous system disorders.
2. Demonstrate how a suspected back injury patient should be moved.
3. Given three essential observations of a patient with an acute head injury, describe what you would watch for in each.
4. Arrange a bed that will help prevent foot or leg deformity of a paralytic patient.
5. Tell how to prevent pressure areas on the skin of a paralytic patient by describing three nursing measures.
6. Describe three signs/symptoms commonly seen among patients with nervous system disorders.
7. Explain how to protect the safety of a restless, semi-conscious patient.
8. Describe two ways to help rehabilitate a paralyzed patient.

SUGGESTED STUDY VOCABULARY*

cortex
hydrocephalus
cerebrospinal fluid
atrophy
meningocele
contusion
concussion
subdural hematoma

intracranial
delirious
degenerate
regenerate
multiple sclerosis
abscess
meningitis
encephalitis

lethargic
convulsion
poliomyelitis
neuritis
epidemic
amnesia
cardiovascular accident
stroke

*Look for any terms you already know.

INTRODUCTION

You will recall that the brain and the nerves make up the body's communication system and that this communication system has two main functions:

1. To alert man to what is happening around him so he can respond accordingly—"a connection between man and his external environment."

2. To be an "intercom" mechanism within the body to control and coordinate the many and continuing internal body activities.

There is an on-going exchange of information in the nervous system with the brain serving as the control station. When there is some disorder in the brain or in the pathways (the nerves) leading to or from the brain, the exchange system is interrupted. Messages (stimuli) do not get through and the patient cannot respond in a normal way. It is by trying to locate or determine these abnormalities that the physician seeks a diagnosis.

Under ordinary circumstances a person is alerted to his external environment through his normal senses of sight, hearing, touch, smell, balance, and taste; he is aware of temperature, pressure, and pain. If the message going in (stimulus or input) is interrupted for some reason, or if the brain, as the receiving center, is unable to receive or to use the incoming message properly, the person has difficulty responding in an appropriate manner. This difficulty may show up in such things as speech, reasoning ability, facial expressions, and eye expressions and movements. Muscle coordination may also be affected. For example, the patient may not be able to write very legibly, or to walk with a normal gait. The list of signs and symptoms includes many more; three are discussed in detail in Chapter 40 (unconsciousness, convulsions, and fainting). Review Chapter 15, the Nervous System, and Table 15–1, Nervous System, Levels of Function.

The content in this chapter is divided into two parts, Conditions of the Brain and Conditions of the Spinal Cord and Nerves. There is much that is related to both the brain and the spinal cord, but for convenience of study various common conditions of each are discussed separately.

CONDITIONS OF THE BRAIN

The brain is a very complex organ; it carries on many independent functions as well as many interrelated functions. Local nerve cells (e.g., in the cortex) take care of specific things in particular areas (e.g., vision and speech). In addition, there are endless numbers of interconnecting pathways that tie the functions of one brain area to another and to another. Knowing this helps you to understand why, in some cases, a patient shows more than one distress signal (e.g., difficulty in speaking, remembering, and reasoning).

A wide variety of things can happen to brain tissue to cause it to malfunction. Some of the better known conditions are included here.

Congenital Deformities

The causes of malformations during uterine growth still puzzle medical scientists. Sometimes signs of abnormal brain development are very apparent at birth, while other times it takes a while for these abnormal functions to appear.

Early diagnosis is often difficult, but to make early treatment available and helpful certain information is sought routinely. One routine test (PKU) for mental retardation in the infant is for the presence of phenylketonuria due to an inborn error in metabolism. Diet regulation seems to prevent mental retardation when this condition is discovered early.

Much research is being carried on to determine what causes mental retardation and congenital deformities.

Hydrocephalus is a condition that produces a larger than normal head. For some reason the passageway for circulation of cerebrospinal fluid is restricted. This causes the fluid to accumulate in the ventricles of the brain. Pressure results and causes the brain to atrophy or prevents it from being its normal size. At the same time, the accumulated fluid causes the head to enlarge. If the condition is not corrected the patient becomes progressively worse.

An adult may develop hydrocephalus when inflammation of the brain covering produces scar tissue and prevents normal circulation of cerebrospinal fluid.

A *meningocele* is a condition in which the cranial cavity is not completely closed and brain tissue is forced through the opening.

Trauma

Brain injury is a common type of trauma resulting from motor vehicle accidents, falls, and being struck by fast and piercing objects. Sometimes the skull is fractured and pieces of bone, glass, dirt, or other foreign objects are driven directly into brain tissue. At other times, little or no outward sign of damage is visible, but the brain is damaged. Brain trauma claims over 100,000 lives each year.

The brain and the skull do not move at the same rate when there is a blow to the head; the brain moves as a mass striking the inside of the skull. If it is thrown against a sharp, irregular surface brain tissue is torn and bruised. The blow can cause the brain to rotate breaking fragile blood vessels and draining blood into subdural spaces. A head injury causes additional cerebral blood to flow immediately (due to dilation and loss of normal automatic regulation) and this in turn creates increased pressure within the cranium.

In nine out of ten cases of severe non-penetrating injuries to the head, cerebral contusions and lacerations occur. A *brain contusion* is injury to underlying tissue due to a blunt blow; a blow that does not break the skull but throws the brain mass against the inside of the skull sometimes turning it as well.

A *concussion* is a loss of consciousness following a head injury without the presence of brain lacerations and contusions. Recovery may be prompt in less severe injuries or may lead to long periods of unconsciousness or death. Amnesia may follow recovery of consciousness as well as forgetfulness, fatigue, irritability, and unsteadiness.

Sometimes trauma before, during, or after birth causes a sizable blood clot to form beneath the dura mater and create pressure on the brain. This is known as a *subdural hematoma*. The clot plus the fluid that accumulates at the site can cause damage to the fast-growing brain of the baby; early detection and removal are essential if brain damage is to be prevented or held to a minimum. Some early signs of a subdural hematoma are convulsions, vomiting, lethargy, fretfulness, and failure to suck or nurse in the usual way. In time the head may start to enlarge.

Adults may have subdural hematomas too, but because the brain has attained full growth by that time, the condition is not as critical as it is in the infant. The clot and fluid can be removed with less danger to the patient.

Signs and Symptoms. The most serious result in brain injury is hemorrhage. Sometimes the bleeding is slow and the results do not show up for hours after the accident. Intracranial bleeding and edema increase the pressure within the skull and push against the brain tissue. The results include headache, dizziness, vomiting, drowsiness, restlessness, disorientation, delirium, convulsions, labored breathing, and bladder and bowel incontinence. The patient may be unconscious or in a coma. He exhibits increased blood pressure and decreased rate of pulse and respirations.

Medical Treatment and Nursing Care. During the initial examination of a patient with an acute head injury, the physician will be looking for evidence of an intracranial clot. The duration of the unconsciousness (even if brief) is essential to know as well as any change of consciousness, breathing, change in eye pupils, speech, vision, or muscle strength.

The vital signs are taken frequently and observed for any instabilities. Likewise, the patient is watched for onset of stupor and coma, or stupor that progressively deepens. For example, does the alert patient become drowsy or difficult to arouse?

Keep the environment quiet and restful. Determine what, if any, activity is permitted. Be sure to plan such things as personal care in keeping with any orders related to rest/activity. Restraints may be ordered for restlessness or deliriousness.

The patient needs an adequate airway; if he is unable to clear his throat, a tracheostomy is usually done and respirations closely observed. Sedation is avoided to prevent further depression of the damaged brain and the respiratory process. To prevent further brain edema, the management of fluids and blood replacement is carefully controlled and usually mildly restricted.

Degeneration

When tissue degenerates it becomes less healthy and less useful to the body. Degeneration is the process of this decline in usefulness. This decline may come on slowly, going on for months and even years, and cause a chronic state of disorder; or it may show up in weeks; or it may come on suddenly, causing an acute state of disorder.

The reasons for brain tissue degeneration are many, and very often the physician must gather information from several sources (e.g., talking with patient and his family, tests, examinations, nurse's observations) before he can make a diagnosis, if he can at all.

A degenerative process that shows symptoms in weeks/months may be caused by a hematoma (blood clot and fluid) in the brain or a brain abscess (localized infection). Abrupt brain tissue changes can result from trauma and hemorrhage; brain tissue reacts to toxic factors in the bloodstream such as poisons, alcohol, and poisonous gases. Anoxia quickly causes brain damage and deterioration. Senility and mental illness are associated with brain tissue changes.

Slow, progressive brain tissue changes may be due to a slow-growing brain tumor or to actual change within brain cells themselves.

MULTIPLE SCLEROSIS. An example of a slow degenerative nerve tissue disease is multiple sclerosis. The nerve coverings in the brain and elsewhere develop patches of deteriorated tissue that interrupt the normal input and output flow of stimuli. Multiple sclerosis occurs most frequently among adults from ages 20 to 40.

Signs and Symptoms. The symptoms include visual disturbances (e.g., double or blurry vision or blindness), poor motor coordination (clumsiness, atonia), tingling and numbness in extremities, even paralysis, tremor of the hands, personality changes, and slurring of speech. These symptoms may disappear entirely for periods of time, only to recur later.

Medical Treatment and Nursing Care. There is no known cure for multiple sclerosis. This means that the physician may try many different therapies (e.g., drugs, diet) in his search for something to relieve the symptoms and hopefully to check the progress of the degenerative process.

Because this disease may progress for a period of years, one of the patient's greatest needs is for diversion and outside interests. The amount and the type of diversion depends upon the patient's ability to tolerate activity, people, and events.

The patient tires easily and needs extra rest. His general state of health is protected as much as possible to prevent his contracting such infectious diseases as colds or influenza. This patient is not confined to bed rest, as a rule, unless it is absolutely necessary. When he is, one special concern is to see that pressure areas do not develop; this means good skin care. Sometimes constipation is a problem. Diet is usually watched closely and often is low in fat.

Vascular Lesions

Stroke is the common name for *cerebrovascular accident (CVA)*; it is third in the list of the causes of death and occurs most frequently in older persons. The "accident" refers to an interference with the blood and oxygen supply to the brain. Three circulatory disorders commonly associated with the stroke are: 1. *cerebral thrombosis*—the presence of a forming clot in an artery of the brain. 2. *cerebral embolism*—the blocking of a blood vessel in the brain by a clot moved in by the blood stream. 3. *cerebral hemorrhage*—bleeding in the brain from a ruptured blood vessel; the bleeding may be slow and a small amount or massive, causing a severe stroke.

The stroke patient may suffer temporary or permanent brain damage—depending upon the extent of bleeding and/or the area involved.

Immediate signs/symptoms of the "accident" depend upon the extent of the cause. With cerebral hemorrhage, the rupture of a large vessel with massive bleeding may cause immediate loss of consciousness and convulsions. Or with less severe hemorrhage, unconsciousness may come on slowly and last a short time or a long time showing gradual improvement. On the other hand, the unconsciousness may deepen and result in death. Other signs/symptoms include: a rapid, bounding pulse, stertorous breathing, and elevated blood pressure. The patient may be unable to speak; one side of the body may be weak or limp and vomiting may occur.

Emergency care includes turning the patient on the affected side (this cheek is usually puffy) to permit mouth drainage and prevent aspiration; slightly elevate the head. Loosen clothing about the neck and keep the patient quiet. Prevent chilling.

The first few days are critical and the prognosis guarded; if the patient survives this period, consciousness may slowly return and the paralysis gradually disappear. It should be emphasized that *rehabilitation begins the day the patient has the stroke.* As a practical nurse, you will share in this rehabilitation. When consciousness returns, the patient may begin to realize some of his limitations (e.g., drooling, speech difficulty or inability to speak, limited or no use of an arm or a leg) and be upset and discouraged. Reassure him that his progress has already started and you are going to help him help himself. Remember that the way a stroke patient acts and feels at first is no indication of how he may be as time goes on. He is the same person he was even if some of his actions and abilities seem changed. One focus of his care is directed toward self-involvement as soon as possible.

Early care may consist of eye care if the blinking reflex is affected and the eye remains open; orders could include eye irrigations followed with eye drops to prevent damage to the cornea. Eye pads or eye shields are also used.

Fluids and nourishment. The comatose patient will receive nothing by mouth; nourishment will be administered by intravenous infusion or hypodermoclysis. For the conscious patient with swallowing difficulties, giving fluids and nourishment requires time and patience. Be persistent and avoid being hurried so the patient does not give up because he is taking too much time. As he improves, tell him so even if his progress is slight. As soon as possible involve him in helping to feed himself.

Mouth care several times a day is essential; be sure that food does not remain lodged in the affected side. The patient with dentures should wear them if at all possible.

Rest is important because the stroke patient tires easily. Do not hurry him to cause undue fatigue or frustration because he cannot perform as he once did; provide for quiet and relaxation.

Make needed adjustments in helping the patient meet his daily living needs. Involve him as much as possible so he can experience some independence. Encourage him; be sympathetic but avoid pity. Treat him as the person he is; listen to him and ask his opinion.

Communication is often a frustrating experience. If the patient cannot speak, see if he can answer you by nodding "yes" or "no" or by writing. Stand where he can see you and give him your attention when he is speaking. It may be slow and halting, but try not to interrupt him. Remember, it is a difficult, often discouraging experience for him; he needs your help and your understanding.

Bowel and urinary bladder incontinence are somewhat common; either or both may show improvement as the patient progresses. Let him know this and provide the urinal/bedpan right after eating. Observe stools, watching for signs of constipation, diarrhea or possible fecal impaction (a collection of hardened feces in the rectum).

Positioning must be proper to prevent contractural deformities. Deformity of the feet (the most common) of the stroke patient is prevented by using devices shown in Figure 36–6. Reposition the patient often (sides, prone, supine) to promote drainage of secretions and because it is especially helpful in preventing deformities of the hips, knees and shoulders. Range of motion exercises are useful in eliminating unnecessary crippling.

It is easier (and takes less time) to prevent pressure sores than it is to treat and cure them; more than that, consider how the patient is spared pain and discomfort. Many items are said to help prevent pressure sores, but protection of *any* slight indication of a reddened area to prevent a skin breakdown is the first thing to do. The surest way to prevent pressure areas is to change the patient's position about every two hours; support the body properly and rotate the position from prone to right and left sides and supine.

Determine how soon the patient may sit on the edge of the bed and stand on the unaffected leg. Provide safe support and encouragement to help the stroke patient move toward ambulation as early as permitted.

The Physical Therapy department can evaluate the physical impairments and outline a program of exercises. Be sure you understand how the patient is to carry out features of this program when he is sitting in a wheelchair, sitting or lying in bed or in an upright position. Get special instructions if you need them. Many stroke patients can benefit from the joint efforts of "the team" as it tries to: 1. prevent complications; 2. reestablish function in paralyzed limbs; 3. alter function in undamaged areas of the brain to gain maximum use.

Arteriosclerosis in the brain is a common disorder of aging individuals. The lesions lead to patches of degeneration of brain tissue and account for a great many symptoms of brain damage observed in aging people. This condition ranks high in the leading causes of death for people over 65 years of age.

Inflammatory Conditions

The brain and its covering may be invaded by infection-causing organisms that produce brain damage. The organisms may enter the brain tissue by way of the blood-stream or by direct extension from a middle ear infection, sinus infection, or a skull fracture.

MENINGITIS. Meningitis is an example of an inflammatory condition of the brain; the meninges (membranes covering the brain) become inflamed and affect mental and motor activities. This is a most serious disease; often fatal.

Signs and Symptoms. The patient's temperature is quite elevated, and he complains of pain, stiffness of the neck, severe headache, and visual difficulties. He is nauseated and vomits. In acute cases, these symptoms may rapidly lead to coma and death within days, or even hours.

Medical Treatment and Nursing Care. The physician needs to know which organism is responsible; he determines this by examining a specimen of spinal fluid secured by doing a spinal tap. The type of causative organism influences his decisions about the type of treatment and the drugs he will use.

The patient with meningitis is very sick. In addition to specific drug therapy, measures to lower his temperature and protective siderails, perhaps padded, are employed. Observations are made of his level of consciousness and his reactions to light and sound. The environment is to be quiet and the amount of light controlled if this seems to bother him. Observations also include evidence of dehydration, constipation, or urinary retention.

ENCEPHALITIS. Encephalitis is inflammation of brain and spinal cord tissue. The epidemic form is commonly known as "sleeping sickness" or lethargic encephalitis. Complications include urinary tract infections and pneumonia; a chronic condition known as Parkinson's disease may be a result of brain tissue destroyed during the disease.

The main signs and symptoms include highly elevated temperature, stiff neck, visual difficulties, severe headache, nausea and vomiting, and drowsiness. Mental processes are slowed, some speech difficulties are present, and a tremor of the hands and convulsions may be present at times.

If the patient is comatose, he may receive tube feedings and parenteral fluids; he will need to have mouth and nose secretions suctioned and will require special attention to the mouth and the skin. The environment must be kept quiet and the amount of light subdued because light will hurt his eyes. Additional treatments may include oxygen and an indwelling catheter.

CONDITIONS OF THE SPINAL CORD AND NERVES

Nerve tissue, wherever located, is very sensitive to environmental changes and toxic influences. It does not have the power to regenerate that so many other body tissues do. Most organs have built-in reserve tissue they can use. When disease destroys some of it they still continue to function. This is not true of nerve tissue for the most part, although nerve fibers in some parts of the body can regenerate under certain conditions. When they cannot regenerate, any destruction means loss of that much nerve function.

As with brain cells, the nerve fibers in the spinal cord have special functions, and once the cells or fibers are damaged they cannot be repaired. The functions previously performed by those damaged nerves are lost. For example, damage at a certain place in the spinal cord can cause paralysis of the lower extremities and loss of bladder and bowel control. At another level, the use of muscles for breathing can be lost, making it essential for the patient to use a respirator to promote his breathing. If damage occurs to the cardiac and respiratory nerve centers in the medulla, the condition is fatal. Therefore, every effort is made to prevent damage to nerve tracks and the spinal cord. Chapter 51, *The Accident Victim*, makes special mention of the need for care in handling accident victims to avoid trauma (or further trauma) to the spinal column and spinal cord.

Inflammatory Conditions and Degeneration

POLIOMYELITIS (infantile paralysis). This is a viral infection of spinal cord nerve tissue. If the inflamed nerve tissue suffers permanent damage the resulting paralysis is also permanent. Many paralytic poliomyelitis patients recover completely and some have a return of some degree of muscle function. Overall the mortality rate is about 5 per cent.

The incidence of poliomyelitis and resulting paralysis has been drastically reduced since the discoveries of vaccines (Salk, Sabin,

Cox, Kropowski); it is felt that the disease could be eliminated if a thorough vaccination program were used by the people.

The virus is thought to enter the body by way of the mouth. It multiplies in the throat and lower intestinal tract and escapes through throat secretions and stools. The virus attacks selected spinal cord nerve tissue causing muscle pain, spasms and possible paralysis.

One type of poliomyelitis called abortive or nonparalytic results in complete recovery. The patient is treated for his symptoms of headache, back pain and leg spasms. Sometimes orthopedic follow-up is needed to correct minor muscle weakness.

Paralytic poliomyelitis ranges from a mild attack with complete recovery to a profound attack on vital areas producing death and all stages in between. Types include: spinal, bulbar, bulbospinal and polioencephalitis.

Signs and Symptoms. The appearance of signs/symptoms follows no set pattern. They may start with a fever, stomach upset, diarrhea, headache and malaise and then disappear for a few days after which the fever returns along with the appearance of paralysis. Generalized muscle and bone discomfort may be present from the start. Children often experience upper respiratory symptoms. All patients usually have one or more of the following: neck and back stiffness (slight to extreme) and cramping pain in some muscles (slight to severe). The location of the muscle weakness/dysfunction depends upon the area of the spinal cord affected.

Medical Treatment and Nursing Care. Strict isolation technique should be used in caring for patients during the acute, infectious stage. Life saving measures (tracheostomy, respirator) are taken when vital functions (e.g., breathing) are involved. Extreme care should be used when suctioning this patient to avoid infection.

During the preparalytic stage, treatment and care (isolation technique) are centered around relief of discomfort, rest, prevention of complications with immediate treatment if they occur, prevention of deformities by maintaining weak muscles until they begin to return to function.

Relief of muscle discomfort may include hot wet packs, diathermy, warm baths, dry heat, analgesics, moving the patient around in bed and changing positions of paralyzed limb(s).

The type of respiratory problem determines what type of assistance the patient needs (e.g., respirator tank, chest-type of respirator, rocking bed).

Meeting the emotional needs of the patient will require the coordinated effort of the physician and the nurse; sometimes the psychiatrist is needed. Other team workers likewise must know how to support and encourage this patient — the social worker, physiotherapist, vocational rehabilitation worker.

The patient's needs are best met when a team approach is used from the start; in this way he receives the therapy he needs when it is the most valuable to him. This approach helps to prevent unwanted after-effects and helps relieve fears and uncertainties in the mind of the patient and the family.

Other inflammatory conditions of the spinal cord include spinal meningitis and abscesses. Syphilis causes nerve deterioration.

Spinal meningitis is infection of the meninges covering the cord in the cervical region of the column and the medulla of the brain. You will recall that the medulla contains such vital centers as the cardiac and respiratory centers, so infection in this area can easily produce fatal results.

Spinal cord damage can result from local abscesses in the vertebral column, as in the case of tuberculosis or osteomyelitis. Syphilis causes deterioration of the nerve cells in the cord and is responsible for such symptoms as a peculiar shuffling gait and lack of balance.

Trauma

The spinal cord is encased in the bony cage of the vertebral and spinal column. This column is made up of 26 bones (vertebrae) set one upon another and fastened together to permit movement. The greatest area of movement is the cervical region. When something happens to cause one or more of the vertebrae to get out of line, collapse, or otherwise interrupt the normal channel housing the spinal cord, it is possible to pinch, sever, bruise, or injure cord tissue. Hemorrhage and edema (also a tumor) can occur and create pressure against and within the spinal cord and the spinal nerves. With these possibilities in mind, can you see why extreme care and good judgment must be used in moving, turning, and lifting a patient who has suspected back injury?

The most essential thing is to have a physician determine the exact location and the extent of the injury before anything else is done. If the patient must be moved first, keep him flat and well-supported in good alignment to prevent as much body movement as possible.

The location of the injury and the extent or severity of it influence the immediate signs and symptoms, or lack of them, and the treatment to follow. It is possible for the spine to be fractured or vertebrae dislocated without injury to the spinal cord. Here again, the physician tests the patient's sensory levels and motor functions to determine the site of injury and what (if any) cord damage there is. X-ray pictures may be useful to the physician, but only as one means to help him determine the extent and location of injury.

Signs and Symptoms. Paralysis may or may not be present. There are usually pain, at times severe, nausea and vomiting, loss or change in sensations, bladder and bowel incontinence, difficulty in swallowing and breathing, and shock.

The location and extent of the injury dictate which parts of the body, if any, are paralyzed. For example, if the cord and nerve injury are in the lumbar region (mid-back) any resulting paralysis would be below this mid-

back area. If the damage is in the cervical region, much more of the body could be paralyzed.

Study Figure 49–1, and note the shaded parts that show general areas of paralysis or involvement.

Medical Treatment and Nursing Care. When the physician has determined the location and extent of damage, he will know how to proceed to relieve and try to correct the situation. Here again the location and the extent of injury dictate whether surgery is needed at once or later and whether traction, a special bed, such as the Stryker frame, or a brace or cast will be used, and whether early ambulation will be permitted.

Nursing care is influenced by the patient's state of immobility and the equipment used to provide such things as traction and body alignment. It is also influenced by the extent and location of paralysis. In relation to meeting his daily living needs, he may be entirely dependent upon others for assistance, or he might be able to engage in some self-care activities. Knowing that it is important for patients to be self-reliant when possible, keep in mind the need to plan and provide for these activities as soon as the physician says it is possible.

Proper exercises and body alignment, ad-

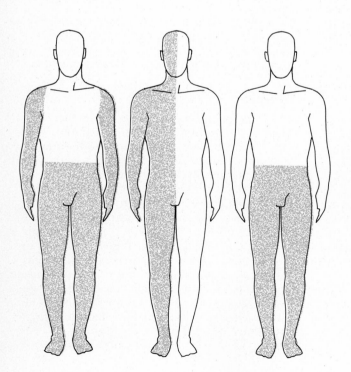

FIGURE 49–1 Areas of paralysis. A, All extremities (quadriplegia). B, One half of the body: one side from head to foot (hemiplegia). C, The lower extremities (paraplegia).

equate skin care, attention to bladder and bowel elimination, prevention of infections (e.g., ascending infection due to indwelling catheter), diet and fluid requirements, sleep and rest, diversion, and emotional support are some of the factors that must enter into the plan for this patient's nursing care.

If the patient has had surgery, his immediate pre- and postoperative needs and assistance are the same as for any surgical patient, plus any special medical orders due to the state of immobility.

The correction and repair of spinal injuries can be a long, complicated process requiring much time and complex equipment. At certain stages of patient recovery, the practical nurse may be performing selected tasks (Role II) and later move into a Role I position, where she is doing all or most of the tasks required for the patient.

Peripheral Nerve Disorders

A peripheral nerve disorder may be body-wide (systemic), regional, such as in the right foot, or local, when a particular nerve is involved (e.g., trigeminal nerve in the face).

The peripheral nerves keep the body in direct contact with the external environment. Chapter 50 deals with the chief means (special senses) the body has for keeping in touch with and reacting to the external environment. By now you know that illness or body disorders may come from microorganisms, body deformities, improper nourishment, abnormal functions, trauma, environment, climate, and heredity. Any one or more of these can contribute to peripheral nerve disorders, as they would to disorders in any other part of the body.

The factors contributing to numbness in the feet, for example, may be poor systemic circulation, a tumor blocking the free flow of input and output sensation, a chemical imbalance in the nerve cells at a particular spot that prevents the cell from carrying its local work load, or local infection in the nerve tissue. A cluster of local nerves may have been cut or severed when the foot was injured. *Neuritis* is somewhat a family name for inflammation of peripheral nerves. The nerve tissue becomes inflamed, producing swelling, pain, heat, and total or partial impairment of local function. When the inflammation continues or persists, the local nerve tissue can degenerate and lose some, most, or even all of its power to work.

Inflammation of this sort may be due to toxic substances brought to the area via the bloodstream from an infection elsewhere in the body (e.g., from infected tonsils or an abscessed tooth) or from poisonous substances inhaled, ingested, or absorbed by the skin. Examples of these include lead, alcohol, insecticides used on food that was improperly prepared for market, and air polluted with noxious gases. Constant external local pressure may produce sufficient inflammation and swelling to numb the area. A dietary lack in certain minerals may cause an imbalance in nerve tissue metabolism and create abnormal functioning. Actually, the causes of peripheral nerve disorders can be varied and many.

Trigeminal nerve disorder (tic douloureux) can be a most painful condition. Review Table 15–2, The 12 Cranial Nerves, to help you recall how the three branches of this nerve serve the body and to understand why a disorder in this nerve causes such widespread facial discomfort.

The cause of the pain is not always clear. Something triggers or causes painful cycles to occur; they last a few seconds, fade away, and return again. The patient knows the cycle and comes to dread it. He tries to hold his face or facial expression in a position that makes the pain more bearable, hence you will notice what might look like a grin on a patient's face during the painful spasm. The patient also discovers through experience some of the things that set off the pain and tries to avoid them if at all possible (e.g., rapid change in environmental temperature and vibrations, such as loud sounds, music, chewing, or shaving).

The treatment includes injecting the nerve with alcohol, which gives relief for several months, or surgically resecting part of the nerve to provide permanent relief.

If the patient loses some sensation around the mouth because of the removal of part of the nerve, he will need to pay particular attention to regular, careful mouth care after every meal to remove any remaining food particles and to avoid biting his tongue, and he must be sure to swallow correctly.

When the surgical treatment involves the branch that serves the eye, eye irrigations or washes will become as necessary as regular mouth care because the ability to blink normally will be gone and the eye will not cleanse itself as it normally does.

SUMMARY

Any factor that causes interruption in the input or output of nerve stimuli or prevents the brain from sorting out the impulses and deciding how to use them creates nervous system disorder. The disorder shows up in a wide variety of signs and symptoms, ranging from a person's mood, ability to organize words into reasonable expressions, ability to swallow, walking gait, use of his hands, the size of the pupil in the eye, or a pain in the foot, to list a few.

Conditions that cause malfunction of the nervous system include congenital deformities, trauma, degeneration of nerve tissue, toxic substances, infections, and pressure due to hemorrhage and edema.

Some of the common distress signals of nervous system disorder are dizziness, drowsiness, disorientation, delirium, coma, vomiting, fainting, convulsions, decreased pulse and respiration rates, increased blood pressure, bladder and bowel incontinence, personality changes, and slurred speech.

Nursing care problems include special attention to the condition of the skin, to avoid pressure areas and to keep the skin around the buttocks clean and dry when the patient is incontinent. Avoid infection; watch particularly for an ascending infection if the patient has an indwelling urinary catheter.

Patient position, body alignment, and muscle reeducation to prevent contractures and to reestablish use of body parts also present a need for special nursing skill and emphasis. Constipation, poor appetite, discouragement, anxiety, and disinterest in self and in optimum recovery are other nursing problems to be met.

Many patients with nervous system disorders may not need to be hospitalized; however, for those who are, the stay may be long and sometimes discouraging. Keep in mind that they will need emotional support, involvement in as many self-care activities as possible, and purposeful diversional outlets.

GUIDES FOR STUDY AND DISCUSSION

1. Why would a comatose patient receive nothing by mouth?
2. What can cause brain disease and disorder?
3. Change of consciousness, frequent taking of vital signs, and an adequate airway are three essential observations of a patient with an acute head injury. What do you look for in each instance?
4. How many devices to prevent foot and leg deformity can you describe?
5. When does rehabilitation start for the stroke patient? What can you do to promote it?
6. Why is isolation technique used with the poliomyelitis patient? When is it discontinued?
7. In your opinion, what would be two nursing care problems common to both the stroke patient and the paralytic poliomyelitis patient?
8. What can cause spinal cord disease/disorder? With respect to meeting the basic needs of a patient on a Stryker frame with a spinal cord injury, what special attention might he need?
9. A paralyzed patient needs special attention to his skin. See how many nursing measures you can suggest for his skin care. Be ready to tell why each is useful.

10. Why must an accident victim with a suspected back injury be moved in a certain way? What is the best way to do it?

11. Use the chart suggested in previous chapters to organize your thoughts about the various diseases and conditions discussed in this chapter.

SUGGESTED SITUATIONS AND ACTIVITIES

1. The physician has said that the patient must become involved in helping with his daily hygiene. The patient, a 40-year-old male recovering from a spinal fracture, is on a Stryker frame, and is resisting doing things for himself because he is afraid his back will not heal right if he moves too much.

Use your imagination and cite two of the reasons he gives you for not wanting to help with his daily hygiene. Plan how you can get him involved in a way that is acceptable to him.

2. Prepare a display of devices or means for protecting the safety of the patient with nervous system disorders. Use the common signs and symptoms of these disorders to help you decide what will be included in the display.

CHAPTER 50

PATIENTS WITH DISORDERS OF THE SKIN, EYE, AND EAR

TOPICAL HEADINGS

Introduction
Somatic Disorders
    and Burns

Disorders of the Eye
    and Ear
Summary

Guides for Study and
    Discussion
Suggested Situations
    and Activities

OBJECTIVES FOR THE STUDENT: Be able to:

1. List ways in which the skin alerts the body to the external environment.
2. Describe three sensations that a patient may experience when there is internal body disorder.
3. Identify a major concern of most patients with skin disorders of the face and hands.
4. Compare the daily hygiene care given for a patient with dermatitis with the care for a patient without it by showing how they differ.
5. Give two examples of nursing action which help prevent infection of a patient with a skin disorder.
6. Compare the immediate needs of the patient with severe burn injury with his long range needs.
7. Identify four factors to keep in mind while caring for patients with eye disorders.
8. Identify four factors to keep in mind while caring for patients with ear disorders.

SUGGESTED STUDY VOCABULARY*

stimuli
receptors
somatic disorders
pruritis
macula
papule
vesicle
pustule
allergen
urticaria

desquamation
dermatitis
acne
eczema
aseptic practices
skin graft
rehabilitation
malfunction
congenital defects
lacerations

sutures
cataract
peripheral vision
intraocular hemorrhage
glaucoma
ophthalmitis
cerumen
tympanic membrane
otitis media
otosclerosis

*Look for any terms you already know.

INTRODUCTION

The body has many receptors to receive all manner of stimuli from the external environment and to be guided by them. Some are in direct contact with the environment, such as the eye or the ear. Others are in deeper tissues and cooperate with the brain to help us keep our balance, move our bodies in an appropriate manner and keep track of the position of a body part with respect to the rest of the body.

Review Chapter 16. Under Activities you were asked to relate somatic and special sensory stimuli to patient care on an imaginary basis. Now you can relate sensory stimuli to actual patient care. In fact, many of the signs and symptoms of illness (e.g., pain, itching, nausea, dizziness, blurred vision, and impaired hearing) are clear-cut examples of body sensory mechanisms sending out distress signals. Chapter 41, *When Illness Occurs*, is a good reference to use with this chapter.

The brain and the sensory receiving receptors make up a unique communication system to keep a person in touch and in tune with the outside world and to respond in an appropriate manner. Body receptors can be disordered by many causes, both external and internal.

The content in this chapter is divided into two main parts: somatic disorders (including the skin) and disorders of the eye and ear.

SOMATIC DISORDERS

What are Somatic Disorders?

The word *somatic* means pertaining to the body. Somatic senses, or body sensations, are indexes to the body's state of well being or illness. The physician gathers information about these sensations when he treats the patient. The nurse gathers information—she observes, reports, and records what the patient says as he tries to explain how he feels and what he is experiencing. Finding words to express his sensations is not always easy and the problem takes on an entirely different dimension when the patient is too young to talk, is unable to talk, speaks another language, or is otherwise limited in his verbal communications.

Using the idea of somatic senses being indexes or indications to body disorders, think of the following terms as some the patient uses to let someone else know what he is experiencing: tingling sensation, dizziness, double vision, itching, pain (many ways to describe his personal sensation of pain), aching, stiffness, nausea, ringing in the ears, numbness, pressure, headache, and crawling sensation over the skin. You may need to use them with the patient to help him describe what he is experiencing so that you can report your observations as accurately as possible.

Somatic disorders (as used here) pertain to the various inabilities of the body's receptors to carry out their function of picking up and transmitting normal stimuli to the brain. Abnormal stimuli such as itching and pain may crowd out normal stimuli.

Disorders of the Skin

One of the most important functions of the skin is its sensory function. Receptors in the skin are scattered over the body in an uneven pattern. Consequently some parts of the body covering have greater ability to "pick up" stimuli than others. For example, finger tips are very sensitive to outside factors, as they come in contact with so many things; the skin on the back has fewer receptors.

The receptors in the skin have the ability to sense the slightest movement or pressure on its surface; they also transmit moderate, strong, sharp, or continued stimuli. The stronger the stimuli, the more receptors involved and the greater the pain, the ache, or the pressure.

Use Figure 16–5 to locate nerve receptors for warmth, pain, cold, touch, and deep pressure. Notice that the first four receptors are located closer to the body surface than the last one, which is in the fatty tissue.

Skin disorders occur in all age groups. They may be caused by internal or external factors. Some are easily cured; others resist cure and are long-term or incurable. The age of the patient has a great deal to do with the possible need for adjustments in providing specific care. A child will present problems in carrying out treatments that the adult will not. One thing is certain of almost all ages; if there is an itching sensation, there is a tendency to scratch.

Skin disorders may disfigure the body temporarily or permanently. People are sensitive about appearing unlike other people; this is especially true where the face and hands are involved. Often the patient worries about whether or not appearance may be altered. Family members need to know what to expect in cases of possible disfigurement; they can do a great deal to help the patient feel acceptable to himself and to the family group.

By nature, the skin has good healing power. Some diseases inhibit this healing power and extraordinary precautions are used in such instances to prevent the occurrence of injury and breaks in the skin. Keep in mind, when carrying out nursing measures for patients with skin disorders, that the skin will heal better and faster if you do not interfere unduly with the process. Avoid "over-nursing" the condition.

ITCHING.   Itching (pruritis) accompanies many skin disorders. It makes the patient restless and he wants to scratch; both aggravate the condition.

In giving daily care, adjustments are made to meet the specific instructions of the physician. When the skin is cleansed the action should be as gentle and nonirritating as possible. The area is patted and not rubbed. Rubbing stimulates circulation (so does scratching) and this brings additional warmth to the area, thus promoting further irritation and the urge for more scratching.

Body temperature has a great deal to do with the comfort of the patient who itches. The room should be kept at a temperature low enough to prevent perspiration and sufficiently warm to avoid chilling (usually around 70° F.). Excessive dryness of the skin can be as aggravating as perspiration. The amount of moisture in the air can soothe or aggravate the itching sensation.

Special attention should be given to the length of finger nails; sometimes the hands are covered (small children) to prevent scratching.

Sleep and rest are often interrupted by the itching sensation; sleep medications may or may not be given. When the adult patient is awakened by the itching and his scratching, suggest that he turn on his light and read or listen to the earphone radio, if available. Distracting attention from the itching sensation will help it to subside if scratching ceases. Repeating such earlier evening care measures as giving a soothing back rub or a warm drink may be sufficient to relax the patient for further sleep. Daytime activities should also be diversified and absorbing to distract his attention from his discomfort.

The physician may work long to find an exact diagnosis and cause of a skin disorder. The cause may be an external factor (e.g., allergic, chemical), an internal one such as an infection, due to a drug, an allergy or an endocrine imbalance. It may be due to some type of infectious agent as a fungus or virus.

The diagnosis guides treatment which may be *topical, systemic,* or a *combination of both.* Topical treatment (e.g., medicated baths—see Appendix III, soaks, lotions, pastes) is used to: 1. relieve itching and soothe irritated skin. 2. soften skin crusts. 3. remove odors. 4. cleanse. 5. lubricate dry skin. Heat (in some form) helps fight infection by increasing blood in the area. Systemic treatment is used to: 1. fight infection (e.g., specific antibiotics). 2. correct body chemical imbalances. 3. treat nutritional disorders. Often a combination of both is used.

Skin diseases can be unsightly. Avoid showing any distaste while treating the patient. He needs emotional support because his appearance is no doubt distasteful to him already. Dispose of all treatment materials quickly and see that his bed is kept clean of soil and debris.

SKIN LESIONS

Primary

macule—a discolored, flat spot on the skin.
papule—a small circumscribed, solid raised area.
nodule—a large circumscribed, solid raised area.
hive/wheal—whitish/pink raised area due to local edema with severe itching.
vesicle—a small circumscribed, raised area containing fluid.
pustule—a "vesicle" containing pus.

Secondary

scale—a thin layer of dead cells shed by the skin.
crust—the dried remains of the skin, exudates, and medications.
excoriation—a superficial loss of substance such as produced by scratching.
fissure—a narrow slit in the skin.
ulcer—a local skin defect produced by sloughing of necrotic tissue.
scar—the skin mark remaining after the healing of a wound or injury.
keloid—the raised skin mark after healing that is hard and shiny.

OTHER TERMINOLOGY RELATED TO SKIN CONDITIONS

Dermatology: the medical specialty concerned with the diagnosis and treatment of diseases of the skin.

Desquamation: the peeling off of the outer skin layers.

Wart: skin overgrowth.

Pigmentation: deposits of coloring matter (e.g., freckles are brown spots of pigment provoked by exposure to the sun). Complete absence of any skin pigment is called albinism. Chemicals (in industry) may cause some workers to lose skin pigments in areas or patches.

Allergen: a substance which is capable of causing a hypersensitive reaction.

Urticaria: a general term applied to red or pale, smooth, slightly raised patches that itch a great deal (certain foods may produce this condition in some people).

SKIN CHANGES. The body covering undergoes a slow but steady change from birth on. A soft, smooth, thin covering gradually becomes a thicker, firmer, drier, and then more wrinkled covering. Its power to heal and to resist infections is lessened in the elderly years as circulation is diminished. Hair follicles often become inactive, causing baldness. Disease, diet, environment, personal hygiene, habits, recreational pursuits, and employment all influence skin quality and characteristics.

GENERAL TYPES OF SKIN DISORDERS

Dermatitis. The term *dermatitis* is a broad family name covering a great variety of types of inflammatory conditions of the skin. Inflammation of the skin may be due to internal or external causes. It may be acute and short-term or chronic and last even a lifetime. In many instances, the physician has difficulty determining what causes the inflammation. He takes a detailed dermatologic history, trying to pinpoint the cause. He inquires into factors in the family history that might contribute to the disorder, the past history of the patient, and all manner of factors concerning the present disorders, such as habits of eating, sleeping, bathing, environment, emotional stresses, and the process of the disorder itself (e.g., when does or did it appear? Does it seem better at times?).

In addition, many special tests are run to examine skin tissue and exudates from skin lesions, patch tests to determine allergies, and intradermal tests. The medical examination also includes examination of the urine, blood, stool, thyroid function, and any other tests of body tissues or activity that need to be considered.

The list of specific causes of dermatitis seems almost endless when you stop to realize how many different things people can be allergic to, how peculiarly body tissues sometimes react to emotional stress, and how some tissues overact. In addition, organisms, mites, lice, and insects can attack the skin and cause their own disturbances locally or systemically. The following disorders are but a few of the most common types of dermatitis.

Acne vulgaris (pimples) is a common skin disorder among adolescents. Acne is associated with the changing body chemistry during youth. It often becomes worse during menstruation and the condition may clear up by itself. Meanwhile adolescents are concerned about their appearance and the possible after-effects such as scarring. Factors which seem to influence an eruption are worry, overwork, lack of sleep, and poor diet. Diet and constipation are often watched closely in treatment.

In addition to the raised reddish areas, pyogenic (pus-producing) organisms often invade the areas and create pustules. Squeezing these pustules aggravates this infectious condition and contributes to scarring. Scarring and pitting may occur at any stage of the disorder.

Treatment includes eating a nourishing diet (milk, meat, fish, cheese, citrus fruit, and raw and cooked vegetables) and avoiding such things as chocolate, fried foods, rich pastries, and nuts. Between-meal eating is discouraged. While skin cleanliness is important, as it is for anyone, it should not be overdone. Ointments and lotions are prescribed by the physician to aid in the skin cleansing and skin peeling process as well as to mask the blemishes. There is disagreement over the use of x-ray therapy for acne.

Dermatitis may attack the scalp, causing inflammation and severe greasy scaling; it may spread to the eyebrows and other body parts. If the areas become infected, crusts form, and there may be a loss of hair. Medicated shampoo, topical ointments and lotions, additional vitamins, usually a low fat diet, good personal hygiene habits, adequate sleep and rest, and exercise are among the things ordered for treatment.

Eczema is a term commonly used to describe inflammation of the skin with reddened lesions present in varying stages: some are vesicles with watery discharges, crusty and scaly; others are macular. Edema may or may not be present. Actually, the term eczema means the same thing as dermatitis. When contact with certain substances causes the condition, it is called *contact dermatitis*. When an infant develops a dermatitis (for any of a number of reasons) it may generally be classified as infantile eczema.

Older persons are apt to have eczema involving the legs and feet. It seems to occur more often with people who have varicose veins and who stand on their feet a great deal. Treatment includes aiding the circulation (supportive stockings, bandages) and local treatment to the area (ointments, wet compresses).

Other inflammatory conditions of the skin accompany such diseases as measles, smallpox, and chickenpox; they produce a skin rash which may cover the whole body. The pattern of inflammation varies among the diseases; some are much more serious and may cause permanent damage to the surface of the skin.

Insect bites and *contacts* can cause inflammation of the skin. Some are accompanied by severe itching. Careless personal hygiene habits and poor living conditions promote such things as body lice, bedbugs, itch mites (scabies) and fleas. Proper hygiene habits and clean clothes and environment help to control these pests. Bee stings can be dangerous and are responsible for a considerable number of deaths each year. Contact with certain vegetation (e.g., poison ivy or poison oak) can produce skin eruptions and make the victim very uncomfortable because of the severe itching.

Fungus infections attack the skin. One of the more common types is barber's itch. It is spread through carelessness. This is one reason that standards of cleanliness in barber shops are maintained through inspection by state boards of health. *Athlete's foot* is a very common type of fungus infection spread through public bathing facilities. It usually appears between the toes in the form of cracks or open lesions and may spread to other parts of the body. Good foot care and avoiding moist skin conditions of the feet (changing hose and shoes daily and using talcum powder) help to prevent the condition.

Burns

Each year several thousand persons die because of burns and conditions related to burning and fires. Burns and associated conditions are caused by chemicals, friction, and heat (flame, electricity); smoke and fume inhalation create additional problems for the burn patient. Care of the severely burned patient is an exacting and long-term matter, requiring patience and acceptance on your part.

Burns are described in many ways; one common classification is according to four degrees of damage to the skin. Damage to the skin and body may range from slight to severe.

First Degree. Local redness (erythema).

Second Degree. Local redness with blister filled with clear, serumlike fluid. Upon healing it may or may not leave a faint scar.

Third Degree. Continued exposure to heat produces death of the epidermis and exposes the capillaries in the surface beneath. This denuded surface oozes, and the body loses fluid from the blood; if it is an extensive surface, the loss of fluid creates a critical condition. There is absorption of toxic substances from the necrotic tissue into the blood; infection in the denuded areas is another danger. When more than two-thirds of the body suffers second and third degree burns, the patient's chance for survival is very slim (Fig. 50–1).

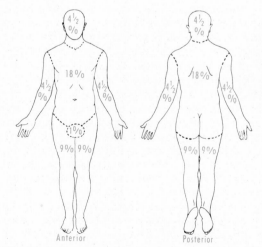

FIGURE 50–1. Rule of nines, a rapid method of estimating the percentage of body surface involved in burn injuries.

Fourth Degree. Charring and black discoloration accompany destruction of deeper tissues and organs.

SYSTEMIC SIGNS AND SYMPTOMS. The extent of damage to the epidermis and to the underlying tissues determines how severely the body will react. A large area, even though not severely burned, will cause extensive fluid loss upsetting the electrolyte balance of the body. If the lower layer of the epidermis (it produces new skin cells) is destroyed, the patient will need skin grafts. Deeper destruction (to the dermis) creates profound problems of fluid loss, edema, and creates a situation just right for bacterial growth which all but assures burn wound sepsis unless extreme care is taken such as an effective antibiotic or the wound kept free of septic material.

The cause of the burn, the length of exposure to the causing factor and whether or not the victim was in an enclosed area are important circumstances to know so that proper treatment can start promptly.

Nerve endings, raw and exposed, produce extreme pain; if the burn damage extends deeper than the sensory nerve endings shown in Figure 16–5, the patient experiences less pain.

Burns change the circulatory system. Blood leaves the area because the capillaries contract leaving the area white-looking until they dilate. Edema is present often in the form of blisters as well as in the tissues under and around the burn area and in distant parts of the body too.

The lungs can be damaged by heat, gases, and particles causing hyperventilation and set the stage for infection. Severe lung damage can occur even if burn damage is slight.

Other parts of the body reacting to burn injury may be the liver, heart, digestive system, and the kidneys.

MEDICAL TREATMENT AND NURSING CARE. Cold is being used in treating small burn areas. The early use (within the first 30 minutes or so) of cold (water or ice pack) is said to reduce pain and edema.

The first and immediate needs of the severely burned patient are to prevent shock, replace lost body fluids, control pain, and free the burned area of all foreign matter and devitalized tissue (debridement). These emergency measures are taken as safely and rapidly as possible.

Sterile instruments, gloves, gowns, and masks should be used while the exposed areas are being cleaned to hold down infection. The wounds are washed and sterile dressings applied.

Nursing a patient with severe, extensive burns requires strict observance of aseptic practices and patience; it is time consuming. The first three or four days represent a critical period for the patient. Intravenous therapy is usually continuous to replace lost fluids and to protect the electrolyte balance; whole blood and plasma are usually given. Fluids are also taken, by mouth when possible, or by a continuous drip stomach tube.

The extent and degree of skin damage determines how long it takes for healing. When skin grafts are necessary they are started as soon as possible to prevent scar tissue from forming. Scar tissue can produce a loss of function in a hand, arm, or leg, and early skin grafts cover the burned but healing area and prevent or limit formation of scar tissue. The patient's own skin is used for grafts. Tissue adhesives hold the skin in place until the grafts take.

Getting the state of body nourishment and fluid balance back to normal is a long process. Diets high in proteins and vitamins as well as calories are usually ordered. Depending upon the extent and location of the burns, it may be necessary to feed the patient for a while.

During this long, slow recovery the patient may easily become depressed and worried. His physical condition and appearance give him deep concern; he worries about the future with its possible limitations. Some patients talk more about their concern than others. At times special help is needed to assist a patient in making an acceptable adjustment to his condition. He is usually sensitive to the manner and reaction of the nurse, and this makes it most important that you react favorably to the appearance of the wounds or any disagreeable odor.

Rehabilitation is an important part of recovery. Despite the use of every possible medical and nursing measure, deformity may result. Parts of the body may need to be reconstructed (plastic surgery); this may mean repeated surgical procedures and prolonged hospitalization.

Physical therapy and occupational therapy, when available, are of direct aid in helping patients learn to use hands or to walk again. When appropriate, this patient may become involved in self-care. Returning to a state of independence is important to his well-being.

DISORDERS OF THE EYE AND EAR

THE EYE

Disorders of the eye and related structures may be due to internal or external causes. As with other body organs they may be caused by trauma, infection, malfunction, tumors, and congenital defects. The whole eye or any of its several parts may be involved. Disorder in some other part of the body may show up in the eye. Sometimes it is an eye symptom that leads the physician to the original disorders. For example, during a medical examination the eye pupil is tested with a light to see how it reacts. A single dilated pupil may be a clue to brain damage or disorder.

Trauma

The eyeball is subject to being pierced, to blunt injury, and to lacerations and abrasions. Any foreign object entering the eye may introduce contaminating material and produce infection. Hemorrhage is always a serious possibility.

Chemicals injure the eyes. You will notice the warning on many aerosol spray cans to avoid getting the spray in the eyes. Immediate flushing with plenty of water is the first step in an emergency. Industrial accidents to the eyes have lead to safety practices of wearing protective head and eye shields.

The cause and extent of the trauma dictates the treatment; however, if there is presence of or danger of rupture of an eye part, such as the iris, the patient is generally put on absolute bed rest for a period of time with both eyes covered. Lacerations require sutures. Close observation by the physician indicates whether the eye can "be saved" or must be removed.

Cataract

This is a disorder of the lens that makes it frosty or cloudy and interferes with vision.

Once the frosting or clouding process begins it usually progresses to a state of blindness. Cataracts are found most frequently among older persons, but they may occur at any age. The condition may be congenital, or it may arise as the result of an eye infection, an eye injury, or the aging process. The exact cause of the change in the lens from clear to cloudy is not known, but body metabolism is thought to play a part in it.

Treatment includes the surgical removal of the lens, and today this is a highly successful operation. With present-day techniques and careful study of the patient's specific needs prior to surgery, most operations are successful, regardless of the age of the patient.

The patient stays in the hospital for a week or more. During this time nursing care is planned and carried out to avoid putting any strain on the operative site. This precaution includes avoiding straining during bowel movements and sudden jarring or turning of the head. The eyes are covered to provide eye rest and inactivity. Knowing these facts can help you understand this patient's state of dependency and need for all manner of assistance in meeting his daily living needs. The physician's orders should indicate the position of the patient's head. Can he be turned? What if any facial movements are allowed (mouth care, chewing, face washed)? If such are not included, be sure you ask *before* you proceed to care for the patient.

One of the adjustments this patient makes after the eye is healed and is ready for his special lens is getting used to the lenses. Four main things are noticeable to the patient:

1. Colors are more colorful. He had gradually lost the ability to see colors due to the frosting effect of the lens. Now that the lens has been removed, he sees full color once again.

2. The new lens magnifies objects and this makes it difficult to judge distances.

3. If one cataract is removed at a time, the two eyes do not function in unison. The unoperated-on eye is blocked off in some way (e.g., by using a patch) to avoid seeing two different sizes of objects.

4. Vision straight ahead is good, but peripheral vision is blurred. It takes time to adjust to this by turning the head to see things.

Intraocular Hemorrhage

This means bleeding into the eyeball. The bleeding may cloud the vitreous humor entirely or it may affect the retina or choroid coat in spots. Severe hemorrhage can separate these two layers and cause blindness. However, any such hemorrhage (depending on where located) usually causes temporary loss of vision.

Intraocular bleeding may occur in patients with such conditions as hypertension (high blood pressure), diabetes, and nephritis.

Glaucoma

Increased pressure within the eyeball is called glaucoma. This pressure comes from some type of interference with the control of the amount of aqueous humor in the eye. This builds up pressure and is very painful. Blindness may result. Conditions of inflammation in the anterior chamber of the eye, injury, tumors, and cataracts may cause glaucoma, as well as primary unknown factors. Today glaucoma detection clinics are helping persons with early signs of the disease so that early treatment may be initiated.

Tumors

A variety of tumors originate in the eye and in its surrounding structures. Some grow rapidly and perforate the eyeball. They can and do occur in children as well as adults. Enucleation (removal) of the eyeball in case of certain malignant tumors does not always prevent metastasis to other parts of the body.

Ophthalmitis

This is a general term used to describe inflammation of the eye. Specific terms are used to designate the location of the inflammation (e.g., scleritis for inflammation of the sclera, iritis for inflammation of the iris).

Blood stream organisms or injuries that introduce pyogenic organisms into the eye are responsible. When the entire eye is involved it may become a complete abscess. Severe damage to some parts causes adhesions within the eyeball and damage to the lens with complete loss of vision; enucleation is then necessary.

Inflammation of the eye is very painful; some types produce a purulent exudate and strict aseptic treatment measures must be used to prevent contamination of the other eye.

Patients with eye difficulties are often fearful of the outcome; the thought of possible blindness is frightening to anyone.

Nursing Care

The practical nurse may not be responsible for carrying out some of the more complex treatments for these patients but you will assist in some parts of the nursing care.

The following points should be kept in mind:

1. The eye is very sensitive; extreme care should be used to prevent any undue pressure on it.

2. The patient needs to have confidence in his nurses. He needs to know what to expect next because his eyes are usually covered.

3. The nurse should always announce her presence in a quiet way and explain what she is going to do.

4. All parts of the patient's care should be done with careful, gentle movements. This is reassuring to him.

5. The eye can be sensitive to light (artificial or natural). The patient should not be facing a window or a light. If he is able to use his eyes, the light should come over his shoulder.

6. Treatments ordered by the physician may include: moist heat, instillation of drops, irrigation, and application of ointments.

Moist heat is applied with "wet dressings." Mineral oil applied to the eyelid before the treatment helps prevent burns. Four-inch square gauzes are placed in a basin with the ordered solution and heated to the desired temperature. The solution must remain at that temperature to be effective. The gauze squares are wrung as dry as possible with forceps and, after testing, are applied.

Each square that has been used on an eye with exudate is discarded. Separate equipment is used for each eye to prevent any cross-infection.

Instillation of drops is a common treatment. The patient needs to know how it is to be done so he can maintain the proper position (relaxed, looking upward, and gently closing eye afterwards). A small amount of medicine is put into the eye dropper which is always held so the medicine remains in the lower end of it. (Medicine should *not* enter the rubber bulb on the opposite end.) Any unused medicine is discarded and not returned to the bottle.

With the patient's head tilted slightly back and his eyes looking upward, the lower lid is gently pulled down and one drop placed inside the lower lid in the center or toward the outer corner. Care should be used to avoid touching the eye or lashes with the drop or dropper. Sudden jumping or blinking may occur if the medicine or the nurse's hands are cold. If the medication will blur or change vision for a while, tell the patient ahead of time.

Irrigation is flooding the eye to apply warmth, relieve pain, and wash out exudates and foreign bodies. The patient is turned to the same side as the affected eye. An emesis basin is placed at the outer corner of the eye to catch the solution.

A rubber bulb syringe or eye dropper is used to direct the solution toward the inner corner (Fig. 50–2). It then flows across the eyeball and into the emesis basin. (Solution should never flow from one eye across the bridge of the nose to the other eye.) Separate equipment is used for each eye to prevent cross-infection. Temperature of the solution should be tested on the wrist to be sure that it is not cold or too warm.

Ointments medicate the eye; they are known as ophthalmic drugs and usually come in small tubes. The tip of the ointment tube should not touch any part of the eye. The ointment is spread in a thin line along the inside of the lower lid, which is gently pulled forward during the application.

The patient with eye disease may be quite dependent upon the nurse regardless of his age. His activities are prescribed and limited according to his needs to prevent stress or strain. Very often complete bed rest is essential.

EAR

Ear disorders (especially those related to deafness) are more common than one might suspect. About one out of every four handicapped persons has some degree of hearing limitation. Deafness is not an affliction of the elderly alone; over one-half of persons with limited hearing are under retirement age. Deafness among the young hampers communication, learning, and the ability to adjust normally. Deafness at any age should be treated as early as possible to avoid maladjustments in living and working.

Today, three main factors account for improvement in treating ear disorders: antibiotic treatment of acute disorders, techniques to diagnose ear disorders, and techniques, anesthesia, and instruments suitable for performing ear surgery, called otologic microsurgery.

The ear is subject to trauma, congenital malformation, inflammation, infection, and degeneration, as are other body parts. Some of the more common disorders of the ear are discussed below. A common symptom among ear disorders is pain; very often it is sharp and severe.

Outer Ear Disorders

Foreign objects in this portion of the ear are common among children. The object should be removed by an ear specialist if possible; he has special instruments which may be needed to avoid further injury to the ear structure, especially the ear drum. If the object is a substance that will absorb water (e.g., a bean or peanut) he will not irrigate the outer ear to try to flush it out because the object will swell and increase in size.

Ear wax is called *cerumen*. It comes from glands in the wall of the external ear canal and may become wedged (impacted) there, producing loss of hearing in time. This is especially likely to happen if water gets in around

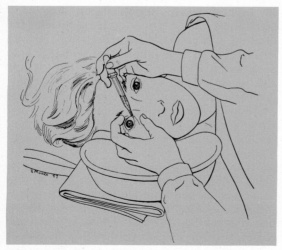

FIGURE 50–2   Eye irrigation. Note the position of the patient's head. The lids are gently separated using thumb and index finger. The tip of the syringe or dropper should touch no part of the eye.

the dried wax. The physician softens the wax with normal saline solution and cleans out the canal.

Dermatitis of the outer ear canal is another disorder. The physician determines, if possible, what causes the inflammation and treats it accordingly. Dermatitis elsewhere on the body may come to involve the external ear and even the ear drum itself. The physician treats the patient's symptoms of pain and uses topical treatment (e.g., drops and a gauze wick in the canal) and antibiotics.

The ear drum (tympanic membrane) is subject to injury from infections, which may create serous- or blood-filled blisters on its surface, from loud, explosive blasts, and from blows to the outer canal, and to burns from sparks that reach it. The ear drum may rupture or perforate because of the above causes or because of pressure from fluid or pus in the middle ear. A perforated ear drum may heal by itself or it may require surgical closure. Sometimes it is necessary to surgically perforate the ear drum to establish drainage of pus and fluid from the middle ear.

Middle Ear Disorders

OTITIS MEDIA. Otitis media is inflammation of the middle ear, otherwise known as middle ear infection. It may be an acute form, coming from a respiratory infection or communicable disease that spreads via the eustachian tube to the middle ear. Or, it may be chronic in nature and accompany inflammation of the mastoid bone (mastoiditis).

Signs and Symptoms. Symptoms in the acute form of otitis media are reddened ear drum (may or may not bulge), pain (may be severe), and elevated temperature (higher in children than adults). In the chronic form, there are a discharge from the ear, pain, slow, progressive hearing loss, and perforation of the ear drum (opening gradually gets larger).

In acute middle ear infection, if the inflammation does not clear up with bed rest and medication, surgical perforation of the ear drum may become necessary to release the fluid, pus, and blood pressing against it; otherwise the membrane may rupture. Antibiotics are used to help clear up the infection, but unreleased fluid remaining in the middle ear may result in deafness.

Chronic middle ear infection often is treated surgically; however, topical drugs are often applied to the affected area (e.g., antibiotic powders or drops).

Destruction of the middle ear structures from long-term infections require surgical reconstruction of the area. This is where modern microsurgical techniques are used to successfully restore hearing to many patients.

Deafness resulting from disorders or destruction of the mechanisms in the middle and inner ear is known as conductive deafness.

OTOSCLEROSIS. Otosclerosis is a condition of tissue and bone changes in the middle and inner ear. The chain of three small bones (malleus, incus, stapes) gradually becomes immobile. They are unable to vibrate freely to carry sound impulses across to the inner ear. Likewise, tissue changes in the inner ear cause the fluid to become less mobile. The structure becomes less sensitive to handling stimuli and less able to control body balance and motion. As the working parts of the inner ear change, the person notices ringing in the ear (tinnitus), dizziness, and nausea and vomiting, and may have an unsteady gait. At the same time, hearing ability is diminished until deafness occurs.

Ear surgery is used to reestablish the mobility of the bone chain. Sometimes this includes replacing some of the chain with plastic parts. Surgical repair also includes reestablishing the mobility of inner ear fluid.

General Nursing Considerations

Regardless of what causes the disorder or deafness, certain factors should be kept in mind when nursing the ear patient.

Communication in the usual manner may be a problem. Messages may need to be written instead of spoken. When speaking, face the patient and speak distinctly in as normal a manner as possible. If the patient reads lip movements, provide opportunity for him to do this without calling attention to it.

Treatments should be carried out with strict aseptic practices. Infection in the ear means it is close to the brain, making it doubly hazardous. Keep the skin area *clean.* Keep the patient's hair away from the affected ear.

Observe for any complaints of dizziness, pain, or facial paralysis, which sometimes occurs following ear surgery. Protect the patient's physical safety by using precautions if his equilibrium seems upset. He may need assistance getting out of bed or walking. Irrigation of the ear canal should be done with a rubber bulb syringe because the stream of solution is under less pressure, which avoids force against the ear drum. The patient is positioned to permit the solution to flow back into an emesis basin positioned under the affected ear.

Help patients and families to understand that improvement may be slow following surgery. Explain why parents should not attempt to remove a foreign object from the ear canal and explain the danger of using water in the ear to wash or soak out an object.

SUMMARY

Sensory receptors are located in all parts of the body—near the surface, below the surface, and deep within the body itself. These receptors, in cooperation with the brain, make up a unique communication system to keep a person in touch with the environment about him and his internal environment as well.

Somatic disorder is inability of the body receptors to carry on their function of picking up and transmitting stimuli in a normal manner. In fact, the disorder may create abnormal stimuli, such as itching or pain.

One important function of the skin is its sensory function. Skin receptors are capable to receiving stimuli, from the very slight to the very strong.

A person's skin is an index to such things as his age, state of health, personal hygiene habits, nutritional state, environment, work, and recreational pursuits. The patient is usually sensitive about any skin disorder that may change his facial appearance.

Skin disorders frequently are slow to improve because there are so many different factors that can cause them. The physician seeks the cause so that treatment may be specific.

Burns are usually described according to the extent of damage to skin layers; namely, first, second, third, and fourth degree burns. Every nursing action with burn patients should be guided by principles of aseptic practice to prevent or control infection.

The eye and the ear are subject to some of the same causes for disorders as other parts of the body, such as trauma, inflammation, infection, degenerative processes, congenital malformation, and hereditary factors.

Patients become very anxious about the thought of loss of sight and hearing. When they undergo surgical and medical treatment they are hopeful that positive results will show up at once. This is not always the case, and they need explanations to help them understand why. You should be alert to this need and see that it is called to the attention of the physician or charge nurse.

The delicate nature of the eyeball and the ear requires the nurse to exercise extreme care in carrying out nursing measures (e.g., irrigations) to avoid further injury. The closeness of these structures to the brain makes it essential to practice aseptic precautions to avoid spread of any infectious process to the brain tissues.

GUIDES FOR STUDY AND DISCUSSION

1. What are the purposes of topical skin treatment? systemic skin treatment?
2. The body reacts to abnormal stimuli from within, causing the person to sense that something is wrong. What are some of these common systemic sensations?

3. In your opinion, why are patients with dermatitis often discouraged?

4. Itching accompanies many types of skin disorders. Why is this true? What problems does itching cause for the patient? What can the nurse do about them?

5. Why should a person with deep burn damage be less apt to experience pain than one with more superficial burn injury?

6. Why are the chances of infection so great for the burn patient? How should this fact influence your nursing action?

7. Many conditions of the skin are unsightly and long-term in nature. How might the patient react to this? What personal resources will you need to use in great measure?

8. Complete the following chart by describing the need to prevent infection as related to each condition.

Condition	Safe Nursing Practices to Follow
1. dermatitis	
2. burn injury	
3. opthalmitis	

9. What precautions are taken while caring for a patient with eye disorders? What would you have to know about each patient?

10. What is a cataract? What precautions are taken in caring for a patient who has had a cataract operation?

11. What precautions are taken while caring for a patient who is deaf?

SUGGESTED SITUATIONS AND ACTIVITIES

1. The care of the severely burned patient includes such things as preventing infection, replacing body fluids, relieving pain, preventing contractures, bolstering the spirits of the patient, and providing adequate nourishment. Imagine yourself in Role II assisting with any one of these factors. What would you have to know and keep in mind to be an effective assistant?

2. Imagine a situation in which a blind adolescent bed patient is anxious to help with his personal hygiene. Show how he can be assisted in this self-care activity.

3. Assume that the same skin treatment (e.g., an oatmeal bath or wet soaks) was ordered for a three year old and for a 27 year old person. What different problems might arise when you administer it?

CHAPTER 51

THE ACCIDENT VICTIM: EMERGENCY AND DISASTER

TOPICAL HEADINGS

Introduction
The Problem of Accidents
Responsibilities at the Scene of an Accident
Aiding a Victim with Generalized Body Trauma
Aiding a Victim of Drowning

Aiding a Victim of Heat Stroke, Heat Exhaustion, or Frostbite
Aiding a Victim of Poisoning
Aiding a Patient with Foreign Objects in the Eye, Nose, Throat or Esophagus

The Victim with a "Hidden" Medical Problem
The LPN's Role in a Disaster
Summary
Guides for Study and Discussion
Suggested Situations and Activities

OBJECTIVES FOR THE STUDENT: Be able to:

1. Explain the difference between first aid and medical care.
2. Name two purposes of first aid.
3. Describe four types of information useful to the physician being called to the scene of an accident.
4. List the first steps to take in caring for an accident victim.
5. Demonstrate a mouth to mouth resuscitation technique.
6. Describe first aid measures for an accident victim with hemorrhage and shock.
7. Devise a step by step plan for aiding a poison victim in the home.
8. Describe first aid given to a victim of drowning.
9. Write a description of the responsibilities an LPN might be expected to carry during a community-wide disaster.

SUGGESTED STUDY VOCABULARY*

artery pressure points
tourniquet
contamination
heat stroke

heat exhaustion
artificial respiration
resuscitation
antidote

universal antidote
corrosive substance
noxious gas
catastrophe
disaster

---

*Look for any terms you already know.

INTRODUCTION

Accidents rank fourth among causes of death in the nation. Accidental deaths happen anywhere, in well-known circumstances such as highway accidents and under less well-known circumstances, such as choking on a piece of meat.

This chapter points out the "first care" that should be given to accident victims in a wide variety of circumstances. First care means first help or first aid given to a victim prior to medical care. Chapter content is divided to help you see the direct relationships of first care measures to the first care needs of the victim.

THE PROBLEM OF ACCIDENTS

The term accident, as used here, means an unforeseen happening that is injurious. Although one is apt to think of an accident as leading to the injury or death of one person, rapid travel, mass transportation, huge gatherings, large industrial plants, and other modern features create conditions in which a single accident may take so many lives at once that it is labeled a catastrophe.

Accidents claim more than 100,000 lives a year in the United States and cripple or injure many more people than that, and the problem grows. More than one half of these deaths are due to motor vehicle accidents. People of all ages are victims of a great variety of life-taking circumstances.

Sensible aid to accident victims helps to save lives and prevent further injury. As a licensed practical nurse you will have more knowledge of the workings of the body than "the man on the street" and should be expected to render more careful aid to the accident victim.

RESPONSIBILITIES AT THE SCENE OF AN ACCIDENT

Chapter 4, The Legal Aspects of Nursing Practice, includes a discussion of responsibilities in emergency situations, with special emphasis on motor vehicle accidents. Reread that section to be sure you understand that aiding someone at the scene of an accident (any type of accident) places certain responsibilities upon you. Your help (if you choose to help) is geared to the immediate needs of the victim to save his life and prevent further injury while awaiting medical help.

Some minor situations might be attended to by a lay person or a member of the family, but it is safest to have a physician see the victim or know about what has happened and direct his care. The first aid person has an obligation to call a physician to the scene of an accident and even to call the fire or the police departments if they can help with lifesaving equipment.

The physician can use certain information beforehand to direct first aid measures until he arrives and to come better prepared to meet the needs in the situation.

1. Observe patient for evidence of bleeding, difficult breathing, poisoning, burns, fractures, shock, consciousness, etc., to tell the physician what seems to be wrong.

2. Tell him how many people are involved.

3. State what (if any) first aid measures have been given. Ask for instructions.

4. Give the location of the accident.

If the victim needs your attention, ask a bystander to call the physician, instructing him what to report.

Once a person (any person) renders first aid, he should remain with the victim until the physician arrives to report necessary information.

Immediate "firsts" are:

1. Never move a patient unless absolutely necessary.

2. Stop bleeding.

3. Start artificial respiration if patient has stopped breathing.

4. Keep patient warm. No external heat.

5. Be ready to treat shock.

6. Loosen clothing. Avoid pulling any clothing from burns.

7. No liquids to a semiconscious or unconscious victim.

8. No alcoholic beverages to victim.

9. Remain calm.

10. Get medical help as soon as possible.

AIDING A VICTIM WITH GENERALIZED BODY TRAUMA

Trauma is a wound or injury. The location and the extent of trauma influence the victim's general condition, but the first steps include the following:

Moving Victim

Move victim only if absolutely necessary. The move may kill him or cripple him for life if there are internal injuries or if the spine is broken. Cover him where he lies and wait for help if it is coming. If he *must* be moved, move him lengthwise; slip something under him (e.g., a blanket) to pull him. If nothing is available, support body (full length) in a straight line to lift him.

Turn the victim's head to one side if he vomits.

Bleeding

Take immediate action if bleeding is severe. A loss of two or three pints of blood in an adult causes serious results. Have the patient lie down to prevent fainting. Press the cleanest cloth article at hand firmly against wound. Continue pressure. Do not remove saturated cloth. Add another to it. Apply pressure to nearest artery if continued direct pressure over wound fails to check bleeding. See Figure 51–1 for artery pressure points. Apply tourniquet (arm and leg wounds) *only* if necessary and if trained in its use. Prolonged use of a tourniquet is dangerous to tissues. The victim may go into shock when it is removed. Steady pressure over the wound is better, if this is possible.

Leave the bandage in place when bleeding stops; bind securely but avoid snugness that might cut off blood supply to the part. Check pulse beyond the wound to be sure that part is receiving a blood supply.

Nosebleed patients should sit upright with the head back (supported, if possible) and the nostrils pressed together firmly for about five minutes to allow clot to form. If bleeding continues, place a small roll of paper under the upper lip and press the lip firmly against the jaw. An ice bag may be applied to the back of the neck. If necessary, pack each bleeding nostril with a sterile gauze plug, allowing one end to protrude from the nostril. The patient should lie down with his head elevated. However, if bleeding persists, medical care should be sought.

Small cuts and wounds respond to local pressure.

Breathing

Take immediate action if the victim has stopped breathing. Brain tissue does not survive long without oxygen. Clear the nostrils and mouth of any foreign matter and start artificial respiration at once. The technique for the mouth-to-mouth method of respiration is described in Figure 51–2.

Shock

Shock is a state of collapse of the circulatory system. It may be due to external or internal hemorrhage or to fluid from the circulatory system passing through the capillary walls and collecting in the tissues (called a white hemorrhage). This type of shock may be brought on by extreme fright or by a distressing or acutely painful experience. Other causes are discussed in Chapter 41. Whatever the cause, blood volume must be restored as quickly as possible to prevent death.

The common signs of shock are cold, pale, and clammy skin, shallow breathing, and very weak pulse. If he is conscious, the patient is anxious and restless; he may feel chilly. Emergency care includes the following measures.

Keep the patient flat with his head lower than his feet, except in case of head or chest injuries, in which case either raise head and shoulders 10 to 12 inches higher than the feet or keep the patient entirely flat. (This is emergency care and may not be exactly the position used under medical management.) Loosen clothing. Keep air passages open; the patient needs ventilation. Keep him warm but use light covers to avoid overheating him. Use no source of additional heat. Give him only a few sips of water if he is conscious, *none if he is nauseated or has any abdominal injury.* GIVE NO STIMULANTS.

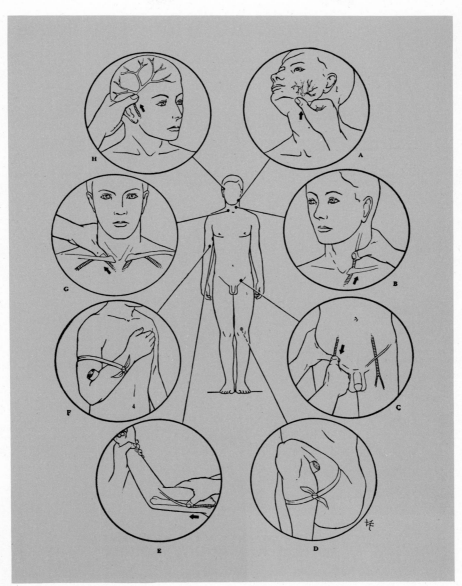

FIGURE 51–1   Pressure points on arteries. The arrows show the direction in which the blood flows through the arteries. Pressure points are located between the wound and the heart. For bleeding from: A, face. B, head and face. C, leg (inguinal ligament is shown as it passes over the artery). D, below knee. E, arm. F, below elbow. G, shoulder and entire arm. H, scalp and upper part of head. (Miller and Burt: Good Health, Personal and Community, 3rd ed.)

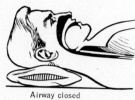

Airway closed

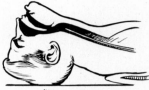

Airway open

Place one hand under the patient's chin and the other on top of his head. Lift up on the chin and push down on the top of the head to tilt the head backwards.

While holding the jaw forward pinch the nostrils closed with the other hand to prevent leakage of air through the nose.

Blowing into the lungs causes the chest to expand. When the chest has expanded adequately remove your mouth from the patient's so that he can exhale.

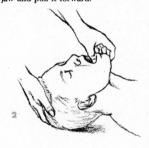

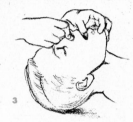

Put the thumb of the hand under the jaw into the patient's mouth; grasp the jaw and pull it forward.

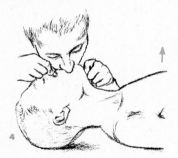

Take a deep breath; place your mouth tightly over the patient's and blow forcefully into his lungs.

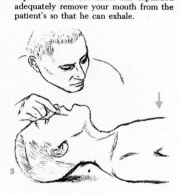

Repeat this sequence of maneuvers every 3 to 4 seconds until other means of ventilation are available.

If you cannot open his mouth blow through his nose. In infants cover both mouth and nose with your mouth. Blow gently into a child's mouth, and in infants use only small puffs from your cheeks.

TECHNIQUE OF ARTIFICIAL RESPIRATION BY MOUTH-TO-MOUTH METHOD
(Nealon)

FIGURE 51-2 Techniques of artificial respiration by mouth-to-mouth method. (From Miller and Burt: Good Health, Personal and Community, 3rd Ed.)

Fractures

First aid treatment for victims with fractures or possible fractures includes the following (Fig. 51–3).

1. Keep the patient warm.

2. Avoid moving him, if at all possible.

3. Treat him for shock while waiting for medical aid (see under Shock).

4. Stop bleeding (see under Bleeding).

5. Do not attempt to push any bone back in place.

6. Do not try to cleanse the wound over the fracture.

7. Support the part with a splint if patient *must* be moved. Use padding to protect injured part from the splint (Fig. 51–4). Avoid tying the splint too tightly.

8. Never attempt to move a victim with a fractured spine, neck, pelvis, or skull.

9. Do not assume that there are no fractures just because the victim moves. *Be sure* before you move an accident victim.

Wound Care and Bandaging

Call for medical assistance at once if the wound appears to be serious. Expose wound by quickly removing clothing. Cut them away, if necessary. Avoid further contamination: wash your hands, if possible; use sterile or at least clean pressure materials.

Cleanse area around wound with soap and water. Apply antiseptic on area around wound, not in wound itself. Let antiseptic dry before covering wound.

There are many types of bandages available today. In addition to the regular roller gauze in varying widths, there are stockinet, elasticized material, and spray-on covering. It is not likely that one would have any of these at the scene of an accident; however, it is possible to tear strips of cloth to make bandaging material. Fold the cleanest available dry cloth and place it over the wound. Bandage securely. Study Figure 51–5 to see how to use strips of bandage material (in a roll) to cover

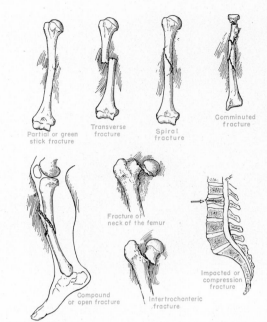

FIGURE 51–3 Eight examples of how bones can fracture. This will help you understand why the victim has pain (often severe enough to cause shock) and why moving him or trying to push a bone back in place is dangerous. (Dowling and Jones: That the Patient May Know.)

different parts of the body. Figure 51–6 shows how to fold, apply, and secure a triangular bandage (sling) to support an elbow and forearm.

Burns

Burns are wounds and caused by a number of things: heat (e.g., flame, steam, air, sun), strong acids (chemicals), friction, x-rays, and electricity. As you know, the skin encases and protects all tissues within the body; it separates the internal structures from the outside world and protects them from infection. If a large part of the skin area (one third or more) is destroyed, the results are usually fatal. Chapter 50 describes types or degrees of

FIGURE 51–4 Splinted leg. (Miller and Burt: Good Health, Personal and Community, 3rd Ed.)

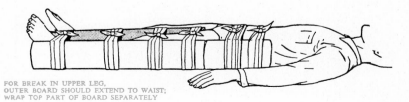

FOR BREAK IN UPPER LEG,
OUTER BOARD SHOULD EXTEND TO WAIST;
WRAP TOP PART OF BOARD SEPARATELY

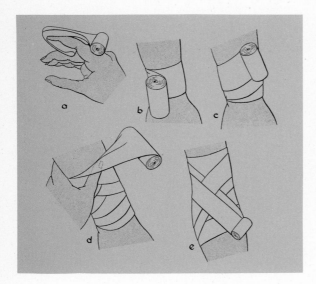

FIGURE 51–5 This type of bandage "turn" depends on the shape and location of part to be covered. A, Recurrent turn means folded back and forth over itself before securing with a circular or spiral turn. B, Circular. C, Spiral. D, Spiral reverse (note the use of thumb to bring bandage back). E, Figure-of-eight produces a criss-cross effect such as needed in an elbow bandage. (Montag and Filson: Nursing Arts, 2nd Ed.)

burns in more detail. The concern here is to know what emergency steps should be taken prior to further medical treatment.

CHEMICAL BURNS.   Flush the area with plenty of cold water to remove or dilute the chemical. Follow with the treatment that is outlined below. If the eye is involved, flush it with plenty of sterile water or normal saline if either is at hand; otherwise, use cold water. Cover with thick bandage; repeat in 10 to 15 minutes. Drop mineral oil or other mild oil into the eye.

OTHER BURNS.   Smother fire if victim is aflame: roll him on the ground or floor or wrap him in a rug, blanket, or coat. Do not let him stand or run. Place him in shock position and keep him warm, but do not apply external heat. Cut clothing away; *do not pull it*. If it sticks to the body, cut around it.

Wash your hands thoroughly, if that is at all possible. Cover the burned area with dry, sterile gauze, if that is available; if not, use clean towels or sheets. This prevents contamination, keeps air away, and helps reduce pain.

Call an ambulance or a physician at once. *Do not apply any medicine or attempt to remove or change dressing.* However, applying ice packs or cold water to small burned areas helps reduce pain and edema. Handle the patient as little as possible; pain can be intense unless the burns are so deep that nerve endings are destroyed. Give him warm, slightly salted water if he can tolerate it.

Severe sunburn needs medical attention.

AIDING A VICTIM OF DROWNING

The immediate need is to get the victim to breathe. *Start artificial respiration at once.* Valuable time is lost by shifting the patient around to try to drain water out of his lungs. Clear nostrils and mouth of anything that would obstruct air flow and start mouth-to-mouth resuscitation immediately. Lower victim's head briefly if water or stomach contents flood airway. Continue artificial respiration until help comes. Send for help as soon as possible, but don't leave.

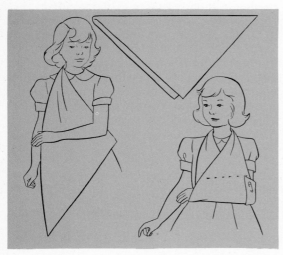

FIGURE 51–6   A triangular bandage or sling.

AIDING A VICTIM OF HEAT STROKE, HEAT EXHAUSTION, FROSTBITE

Heat Stroke

Heat stroke is serious, and can cause death. When the heat regulating system is working to full capacity and is unable to keep the blood from overheating, heat stroke results. The heat regulating center begins to falter at about 106° F. Sunstroke might be called a mild heat stroke. Unless the victim is removed to a cool place, a serious heat stroke will follow.

The symptoms of heat stroke include a rapid, bounding pulse; loud, rapid respirations; and dry, red, hot skin. The victim's temperature rises, but he does not perspire. He may complain of thirst, nausea, and drowsiness, and he may lapse into unconsciousness or coma.

Treatment is aimed at lowering the victim's temperature. Loosen or remove his clothing and place him in a cool area with his head elevated. Fanning or sponging with tepid water may help. Submerging him in a tub of ice water may be necessary if his temperature is very high.

Heat Exhaustion

Heat exhaustion is serious too. It occurs when the body has lost too much salt through excessive sweating, usually due to too much vigorous exercise in hot weather. Heat cramps are sudden muscle pains due to same cause.

The heat exhaustion victim has a subnormal temperature and a rapid but weak pulse. His skin is moist, pale, and cold; his respirations are quiet and shallow. He perspires profusely and is dizzy or faint. Heat cramps may strike the legs and abdomen.

Place the victim in a cool spot with his head lower than this trunk. Loosen his clothing and cover him lightly to ward off drafts. Have him drink fluids, preferably salt water, and make him rest. Heat may relieve cramps.

Frostbite

Frostbite is the term used to describe the condition of toes, fingers, noses, ears, or cheeks that have been exposed to low temperatures for so long that circulation has been completely shut off. The tissues receive no oxygen or foot nutrients, and ice crystals form in and around cells. This can produce death of tissue (gangrene). The victim may not have been aware that frostbite was setting in. The frostbitten part loses its normal color and takes on a gray-white dead appearance.

Take the victim to a warm area and keep him warm. Give him warm fluids and apply warmth to the frozen parts (e.g., put them in warm water). Do not rub or massage the part; the ice crystals will damage the tissues. Exercise the part gently when it has thawed.

AIDING A VICTIM OF POISONING

A poison is any substance that, by its chemical action, may cause damage to the body if swallowed, inhaled, absorbed, injected into, or developed within the body. Poisoning is the sickness it causes. Poisoning is an emergency.

Emergency care for the victim should be fast and sensible. An antidote is something given to counteract a poison. Time does not permit hunting up a specific remedy (antidote) unless that remedy is specified on the container. For one thing, you may not know the nature (chemical composition) of the poison; this makes it difficult and time-consuming to try to find a specific remedy. The universal antidote (a mixture used when the exact poison is not known) is: one part strong tea, one part milk of magnesia and two parts burnt crumbled toast.

General Action. Call an ambulance immediately. Or, call an emergency center and ask for instructions. Try to find out what was swallowed. Look for a container, smell the victim's breath. If the substance came from a container with the remedy printed on it, *follow directions.* Keep the container and take it to the hospital in the ambulance. Examine victim's mouth: remove any foreign substance and save it for the physician, and look for evidence of corrosives (something that eats away tissue), such as burns on lips, tongue, and mouth.

Dilute the poison by giving the victim, if he is conscious and able to swallow, large amounts of liquids. Milk is first choice, followed by egg, water, water mixed with mustard or baking soda, and soapy water. Give several glasses (six to seven for an adult) and then place finger well back into victim's throat to produce vomiting. Hold the victim's head down to prevent his drawing vomitus into lungs. Repeat this process in a few minutes. If you *know* an acid has been swallowed, give plenty of water and starch or water and baking soda; these are alkalines. If you *know* an alkaline has been swallowed, give plenty of vinegar and water or lemon juice and water; these are acids. Do not cause vomiting if the victim swallowed a corrosive, gasoline, kerosene, lighter fluid, iodine, or strychnine, is unconscious or is in a coma.

If the victim is unconscious, keep him in shock position. Notify the hospital or emergency center of the kind of poison (if possible) and the condition of the victim when you call, so that they will be ready when he arrives.

If a poisonous gas has been inhaled, get the victim to fresh air. Loosen his clothing, start artificial respiration, and call an ambulance. Administer oxygen continuously during the trip to the hospital.

AIDING A PATIENT WITH A FOREIGN OBJECT IN THE EYE, NOSE, THROAT, AND ESOPHAGUS

EYE.   Wash your hands thoroughly. Do not rub the eye. Close both eyes for a short time to allow the object to be washed out. If the object is still present, draw the upper lid over the lower lid to aid the washing process. If it still does not wash out, flush the eye with plain water, or roll the lid back, locate the object, and gently remove it with a moistened bit of cotton or the corner of a clean handkerchief if it is on the lid. If the object is on or against the cornea, cover the eye with cotton and seek medical aid.

NOSE.   Do not probe the nose if the object is not removable; you may injure the nostril or push the object deeper. Do not allow the patient to blow his nose violently. Seek medical aid if the object is not easily removed.

THROAT.   Encourage the victim to cough. Hold his head down and slap him forcefully between shoulders. If the patient is a child, you can pick him up by his heels and try to dislodge the object.

ESOPHAGUS.   Keep the patient quiet. Discourage swallowing or straining to remove object. Seek medical aid at once.

THE VICTIM WITH A "HIDDEN" MEDICAL PROBLEM

The American Medical Association estimates that one person in five has something different about himself that should be made known immediately when he is involved in an emergency. Quick knowledge of this "individual something"—this "hidden" medical problem—may save the person's life.

More than 200 different hidden conditions or circumstances that may be important at the time of an emergency have been identified. Some of them are blood type, diabetes, epilepsy, glaucoma, contact lenses, hemophilia (blood will not clot), multiple sclerosis, laryngectomies (neck breathers), deafness, muteness, allergy to something, certain drugs being taken, removal of an organ (e.g., lung, kidney), and amnesia. If the individual's problem is to be known immediately he must have some information on his person.

Medic-Alert Project

An organization whose main purpose is to educate the public to the need for constantly having needed information on the person is the Medic-Alert Foundation International.

Medic-Alert, a nonprofit, charitable organization (endorsed by the American Medical Association and a number of other national groups), makes it possible for a person with a hidden medical problem to carry this information on his person and to have medical information about himself on file in a central office, available to authorized persons on an around-the-clock basis.

The wearer of the Medic-Alert emblem never removes it. It states his problem, his file number in the central office, and the telephone number of that office (Fig. 51–7). He carries a membership certificate that provides further on-the-spot information. The person who joins the Medic-Alert plan pays one fee for a lifetime membership, which covers the cost of the bracelet or necklace and of maintaining the central file of information.

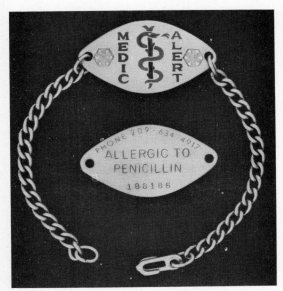

FIGURE 51–7 Medic-Alert Bracelet. Notice the identifying information on the front and back of emblem. (Courtesy of Medic-Alert Foundation International, Turlock, California.)

This method of assuring proper "first aid" is fairly new and it takes time for people to understand that it is a lifesaving effort and not something to single out the "abnormals" among us. Medical problems are common; almost every family has a "hidden" one.

THE LPN'S ROLE IN A DISASTER

The word *disaster* means a sudden and extraordinary misfortune, a destructive situation involving people and surroundings. Synonyms are calamity, catastrophe, and tragedy. Such an extraordinary misfortune brings human need with it. The sick and injured need immediate care; the dead need attention. The homeless, the frightened, the feeble, the very young, and the stunned need shelter and food and someone to care about them as well as to care for them. If the ruinous event brings widespread, lasting results with it, it takes time and much human effort to correct the situation. In the meantime, problems with shelter, the water supply, sanitation, the food supply, sickness, and people's outlooks and attitudes all must be handled.

Disasters may be due to natural causes (e.g., fires, tornadoes, floods, hurricanes, epidemics, riots, explosions, accidents involving transportation, earthquakes) or to warfare (e.g., firearms, nuclear weapons, chemicals, germ warfare). It is easy to understand from reading this list of examples that some disasters involve a small locality and others involve vast areas. The size of the disaster, the location of it, and the range of destruction (both human and otherwise) have very much to do with how and to what extent human need can be met. The loaded bus that overturns, killing eight of its 40 passengers and injuring 25 others, on the outskirts of a community with two small hospitals creates a local disaster situation that requires much from the hospital staffs as well as other community resources.

When the destructive force is widespread, community order is disrupted or broken up. Every able-bodied person is required to share in meeting human needs. The nature of the destructive force also enters into the situation. For example, the deadly effects of the force may linger in the environment, as is the case with a nuclear attack. Or, a continuing series of severe, destructive earthquakes in an area has its own psychological effect on humans as well as its continued destruction of life and property. In either example, community orderliness is broken up and the manner in which the injured, the sick, the very young, and the very old are cared for is quite different from the care given in a local situation in which the community remains intact as a functioning unit.

As a licensed practical nurse you are a valuable community member in the event of a disaster. Your education equips you to carry responsibility and to render sound judgment. That is to say, where there is medical-registered nurse management, you follow directions and function in Role I or Role II (or both) as the situations demand.

The United States Department of Health, Education, and Welfare, with the assistance of the National Federation of Licensed Practical Nurses and the American Nurses' Association, has outlined the functions of the LPN in disaster situations as follows.*

---

*The Role of the Licensed Practical Nurse in National Disaster. U. S. Department of Health, Education, and Welfare, Public Health Service, Division of Health Mobilization; Health Mobilization Series I, No. 6, 1967, pp. 6–9.

A. Participates in planning and providing nursing care for large groups of persons under extreme duress in various types of disaster situations by:
 1. Providing for the emotional and physical comfort and safety of large numbers of disaster victims with limited supplies, equipment, utilities, and personnel, through:
    a. Understanding the emotional stress caused by personal fear, problems of displacement of people and separation of families, increasing anxiety, and continuing danger.
    b. Recognizing the emotional and physical limitations of self and others during severe stress in mass care situations.
    c. Helping people with different cultural backgrounds and religious beliefs to accept and adapt to shelter and disrupted living conditions under crowded and often adverse situations.
    d. Recognizing and understanding the effect of disrupted social and economic patterns, such as personal and material loses, emotional trauma, and crowded living conditions.
    e. Encouraging patients with emotional reactions to verbalize their concerns and fears, and guiding them in performing certain tasks.
    f. Participating in the development, revision, and implementation of nursing procedures designed to insure the comfort and safety of patients and personnel under chaotic conditions.
    g. Providing for basic instruction to disaster victims in the aspects of appropriate self-care, encouraging them to further provide for their own needs and the needs of others.
    h. Helping to maintain, insofar as may be possible, a safe and healthful environment for disaster victims.
 2. Observing, recording, and reporting to appropriate persons (record and report forms may have to be improvised):
    a. General physical and mental condition of patients, signs and symptoms which may be indicative of change.
    b. Stresses in human relationships between patients and patients' families, visitors and personnel.
 3. Performing nursing procedures within the framework of a disaster situation by utilizing skill and judgment for the good of the greatest number of people, for example:
    a. Administering medications and treatments as directed.
    b. Improvising supplies, equipment and techniques as necessary.
    c. Carrying out precautionary measures, including the maintenance of a safe and sanitary environment and the separation of patients with communicable diseases.
    d. Performing emergency aid measures.
    e. Utilizing improvised supplies and observing aseptic techniques, including sterilization.
 4. Working toward restoration of community and family life according to available resources by:
    a. Encouraging individual self-help and work therapy.
    b. Encouraging activities of daily living, with adaptations designed to attain and maintain a sanitary and a healthful environment.
    c. Applying the principles of prevention of deformities, using improvised equipment and available resources.
    d. Utilizing existing community facilities and resources, including family and neighbors, for continuing patient care.
B. Promoting the effectiveness of the employing health service agency in disaster preparedness through:
 1. Knowing and interpreting the disaster plan of the employing health agency.
 2. Understanding the relationship between the agency plan, the local government plan, and the local Red Cross plan.
 3. Promoting maintenance and restoration of community health by participating in the control of environmental health hazards.

"Knowledge replaces fear," states the bulletin, *Medical Self-Help Training—For You and Your Community*. "Medical Self-Help is a program designed to provide information and training to the people of the United States that will prepare them for survival in a time of national disaster when the services of a physician or other allied health personnel are not available."* The goal? To train at least one member in every family through a 16-hour course that covers radioactive fallout and shelter, healthful living in

---

Medical Self-Help Training—For You and Your Community. U. S. Department of Defense and U. S. Department of Health, Education, and Welfare, Public Health Service Publication No. 1042, 1963, p. 4.

emergencies, artificial respiration, bleeding and bandaging, fractures and splinting, transportation of the injured, burns, shock, nursing care of the sick and the injured, infant and child care, and emergency childbirth.

If this course is available to you, you should take it. The State Health Department or the State Civil Defense Office can provide you with specific information about when and where it is offered. If you take it, you will see many relationships between that course and the background information and skills you already have concerning emergency care.

As you continue to practice as an LPN, it will be your responsibility to take such courses and keep yourself up-to-date if you are to be an able community member during a disaster.

SUMMARY

The person who gives first aid has an obligation to summon needed help. Some states have laws that require a person involved in an automobile accident to give aid to any other person in the accident. The "Good Samaritan Act" (a law in some states) permits a person to render first aid treatment without the fear of a possible lawsuit.

Furnish the physician with enough information by telephone or messenger to permit him to give directions for immediate care and to know how many people are involved and the exact location of the accident.

The firsts in emergency action are: Never move patient unless necessary. Stop any bleeding. Start artificial respiration if breathing has stopped. Be ready to position for shock. Summon help as soon as possible.

Fast, sensible action is needed in any emergency situation. It can save lives and prevent serious disabilities.

GUIDES FOR STUDY AND DISCUSSION

1. Where do accidents rank among the top ten causes of death? Make a list of things that produce accidental death.
2. What is *first* aid? Who renders it? What responsibilities does this person assume?
3. In case of an accident, there are four things to do to help the physician when he is called. Use each one for a group discussion on why it is essential.
4. You are alone and the first person to arrive at the scene of a one-car highway accident involving two victims. What are the first sensible actions to take?
5. What first aid measures should one take to treat the following victims: in shock; bleeding; not breathing; drowning; has fractured spine; poisoned; burned?
6. What must you remember about using a tourniquet?
7. Under what circumstances (poisoning) would you use the universal antidote? When should you induce vomiting? When should you not induce vomiting?

8. What is meant by a "hidden medical problem"? How could such a problem be dangerous to a person when he is an emergency victim? What is the Medic-Alert project?

9. What types of responsibilities might you have to carry as an LPN during a community-wide disaster situation?

SUGGESTED SITUATIONS AND ACTIVITIES

1. Prepare a bulletin board display of news items which proves this statement: "People of all ages are victims of a great variety of life-taking circumstances."

2. Prepare a skit for study guide number 4 which shows you know what to do.

3. Visit a nearby hospital and find out: 1. what provisions they have for the treatment of poison victims. 2. what are their arrangements (plans) in the event of a fire in the hospital. 3. what provisions they have made in the event of a community disaster.

NURSING THE MOTHER, NEWBORN, CHILD, AND ADOLESCENT

The purpose of Unit XI is to relate the daily living needs of patients to the particular needs of the mother, during pregnancy and labor and following delivery, and to the unique needs of the newborn, the child, and the adolescent.

The content in this unit is directly related to knowledge of the normal reproductive functions of the female and all aspects of human development related to the age groups included here (See Unit IV).

Knowledge concerned with medical-surgical nursing of children and adolescents is found in Unit X and is not repeated here. Chapter 54 provides you with an opportunity to discover many of the similarities and differences between medical-surgical nursing for adult and for the younger patient.

NURSING THE MOTHER

OBJECTIVES FOR THE STUDENT: Be able to:

1. Locate the gross parts of the female reproductive system on an anatomical chart.
2. Explain why pregnancy is called a normal process.
3. Tell how conception takes place.
4. List some positive signs of pregnancy.
5. Describe the function of the placenta during pregnancy.
6. Name some benefits of early prenatal care.
7. Identify three changes that take place in the body during pregnancy other than in the uterus.
8. Name the three stages of labor.
9. Name five things that should guide nursing action during puerperium.
10. Describe a well-balanced diet for the expectant mother.

SUGGESTED STUDY VOCABULARY*

mortality	primipara	umbilical cord
pregnancy	multipara	postpartum
fetus	dilatation	puerperium
prenatal	effacement	perineum
dysfunction	engagement	lochia
fetal heart sounds	lightening	abortion
striae	false labor	ectopic pregnancy
mammary glands	true labor	toxemia
trimester	uterine contractions	mastitis
	amniotic fluid	neonatal

*Look for any terms you already know.

INTRODUCTION

While there has been a decline in the infant death rates in the United States and in Canada over the past years, both countries have higher death rates than several developed countries, chiefly some in Europe. According to the United Nations's 1968 Demographic Yearbook, the United States ranked 13th and Canada 14th in the number of infant deaths for every 1000 live births.

The problems of infant mortality and mental retardation are receiving emphasis through federal government urging and financial support to states. Both levels of government are sharing the costs in bringing prenatal care to the "local level" of the city, the county, or a group of counties. The focus is "local community action" to meet the needs of socioeconomically deprived people found in areas of dense population as well as in rural areas.

The key to success depends upon getting the help to the people who need it. Health personnel are raising questions about why more people are not reached: "Are clinics, public health departments, and hospitals so busy; personnel so rushed or too few; waiting periods so long; or transportation to the center impossible; that the would-be patients give up and just stay away?"

The purpose of this chapter is to acquaint you with the needs of the mother throughout pregnancy, labor, delivery, and postpartum. Restudy Chapter 13, The Structure and Function of the Reproductive System; Chapter 18, Life before Birth as Part of Human Development; and Table 31–14, Drugs which Affect the Uterus.

SIGNS OF PREGNANCY

The pregnant woman is often alerted to her condition before she seeks the physician's diagnosis. Signs of pregnancy fall into three groups: *presumptive, probable,* and *positive.*

PRESUMPTIVE — EARLIEST INDICATIONS. Menstruation ceases, but this by itself is not always an absolute predictor. The breasts become more firm and feel full and tender; the nipples are firmer and dark colored. Nausea and vomiting are not always present. If they are they usually occur in the morning ("morning sickness"). The enlarging uterus presses on the bladder early in pregnancy, causing frequency of urination. As the uterus rises in abdomen, frequency ceases until close to time of delivery.

PROBABLE — LIKELY. The abdomen increases in size and shape as the uterus enlarges and rises above the pelvic rim. After about four weeks, the uterus becomes more round and soft. The cervix becomes less rigid and more soft. Pregnancy tests may be used. Many of these tests use pregnancy urine because it contains a specific hormone coming from the implanted ovum. The urine is used in one of two ways: 1. injected into an animal (e.g., rat, mouse, rabbit, frog) which reacts in certain ways — called *biologic test.* 2. injected into an animal causing it to produce specific antibodies. Serum from this animal is in turn used with the patient's urine to see if it contains the specific hormone coming from an implanted ovum — called *immunologic test.* This test is faster than the biologic test. None is 100 per cent accurate, hence a positive test result is called "a probable sign."

POSITIVE — CERTAIN. Fetal heart sounds are heard and can be counted with the aid of a stethoscope. Their rate is usually about twice as fast as those of the mother. The fetus kicks; it can be felt by the physician. Mother may feel "life" earlier. The fetal skeleton can be observed by x-ray.

Length of Pregnancy

Calculating the expected date of delivery is a medical responsibility. The length of pregnancy is inexact, but it ranges from about 267 to 280 days. Full-term births may occur two weeks ahead or two weeks after the date determined by the physician. Outside that range, a baby is considered pre- or postmature.

At best, calculation of the date of delivery is only an estimate, because only about 50 per cent of all babies are born on or near the due date.

NEEDS AND CARE DURING PREGNANCY

Importance of Early Care

A new speciality in medicine is perinatal pathology, the study of the causes of deaths of babies during pregnancy, delivery, and the early days of life. There are many unanswered questions about mental retardation and infant mortality. The answers, when they are found, are bound to influence many aspects of prenatal care.

A drug with the trade name RhoGAM Rh$_o$ (D) Immune Globulin (Human) is used as a vaccine to prevent Rh hemolytic disease among babies. It is injected intramuscularly into the unsensitized Rh negative mother within 72 hours after her delivery of an Rh positive baby. RhoGAM contains passive antibodies which prevent the mother from building active immunity against the Rh positive fetal cells. In this way, the drug prevents Rh hemolytic disease of future newborn. If the Rh negative mother has been previously sensitized by a previous pregnancy, a transfusion of Rh positive blood by mistake or by a miscarriage, the drug is not helpful.

As pointed out earlier, the emphasis in prenatal care is to have the mother seen regularly so that *all* aspects of her well-being and of the fetus may be safeguarded throughout pregnancy. This type of prenatal care reduces complications.

Regular visits to the clinic provide opportunity for the patient to get answers to her questions and to be guided by the instructions of the physician and staff members. The mother is more apt to go through her pregnancy with minimum discomfort, both physical and emotional, and will deliver a healthier baby when she has this type of care throughout pregnancy.

From the First Medical Visit on

During the first visit, the physician gives the patient a thorough examination. The nurse who assists is in a particularly good position to reassure the anxious patient (especially if it is her first experience) by providing privacy while she is undressing, by making it easy for her to ask questions, and by telling her what to expect during the examination.

A medical history is taken. Besides the usual types of questions asked during a regular medical examination, information on the patient's menstrual history is sought (e.g., onset, frequency, and duration of periods), along with the history of any previous pregnancies. General state of health information includes:

1. Body build, size, structure, and weight.

2. Condition of breasts.

3. State of circulatory, respiratory, and urinary systems; chest x-ray; blood pressure; blood tests; syphilis (in some states), hemoglobin, cell count, Rh factor and blood type; urinalysis for sugar, casts, and albumin.

4. State of nourishment—undernourished, overweight, and causes of vitamin deficiency.

5. Condition of teeth, nose, and throat.

6. Presence of dysfunctions, such as of thyroid, or diabetes.

7. Condition of pelvis, vagina, cervix, and abdomen, pelvic measurement, and presence of scars, tumors, hernias, tenderness, and enlarged lymphatics.

8. Presence of fetal heart tones.

Physiological Changes

During pregnancy certain changes take place in the mother's body, other than the growth of the fetus.

WEIGHT. Weight gain can be rapid after the first three months, owing to the growth of the fetus, the placenta, the amniotic fluid, and the weight of the uterus. Water is retained by the body, and fat and proteins are stored as the body makes hormonal adjustments to provide an increased blood supply and meet the patient's need for more protein during pregnancy, labor, and lactation. The average weight gain during pregnancy is between 20 and 25 pounds. Excessive weight gain is a matter of concern to the physician. Likewise, he is concerned about patients who are undernourished from the start.

BREASTS. An increase in the size and feeling of fullness is noticed shortly after the first period is missed. This is due to an increased blood supply and enlargement of the secreting glands. Gradually the breasts become larger and more prominent; the nipple and surrounding area are darker.

URINATION. The muscle tone of the kidneys and ureters decreases after the fourth month. The ureters enlarge and peristalsis is less active. The flow of urine from the kidneys to the bladder is slowed. The change may be due to hormones. This situation is corrected about eight weeks after the birth of the infant.

CIRCULATION. The increased amount of fluid retained by the body tissues results in an increase in circulation. The parts of the circulating blood are not increased in the same proportions; there is a larger increase in plasma than in red corpuscles which results in slight anemia. The increase in volume of blood is made necessary by the various demands of the fetus and the mother and is thought to be controlled by the hormonal glands. Also, it provides an excess of fluid which may be reduced in the placental stage of delivery by hemorrhage. Blood pressure levels change little during a normal pregnancy.

HEART. Upward pressure of the uterus on the diaphragm causes pressure on the heart. It is thought by some that the heart may enlarge somewhat to accommodate the increased blood volume. The pulse rate is slightly more rapid but within normal limits.

DIGESTION. "Morning sickness" was mentioned earlier as a presumptive sign and is very common during the first few months. If vomiting persists, it becomes a serious problem and can lead to loss of fluids and electrolytes or starvation.

Distorted senses of smell and taste account for a dislike of odors and some foods. Heartburn and dyspepsia are common complaints during the last three months.

Constipation occurs frequently, even in women who have had no such previous problem.

In general, common digestive tract disturbances are thought to be due to alterations in its functions. Stomach acid and pepsin are decreased; the stomach empties more slowly as its muscle tone diminishes and its position is altered.

ENDOCRINE GLANDS. Many ductless glands increase in size, and all increase in activity during pregnancy. They supply additional secretions to meet growth demands of the fetus, and supply reserves for the mother. The metabolic rate is lower during the first three months but it increases with time. Patients often mention feeling tired at first; extreme fatigue may be a sign of some type of gland dysfunction.

SKIN. The skin stretches to accommodate the increase in body size. Reddish lines (striae) may appear on the abdomen and thighs, owing to splitting or tearing of the elastic fibers below the skin, and may fade to whitish lines; but they do not disappear after the birth of the child.

There is an increase in the amount of pigment deposited around the nipple and in a line up the mid-center of the abdomen. Some faint brownish color may appear on the cheeks, forehead, and bridge of the nose.

Physical Needs

The pregnant woman should see that her physical needs are met as normally and as safely as possible. In many ways the nurse helps her to understand why the physician counsels her as he does, so that she will use better judgment.

DIET. What the patient eats is important to herself and to the fetus. Faulty nutrition contributes to pregnancy problems so the patient receives diet instructions concerning the proper kinds and amounts of food. If the patient is a growing adolescent, she will need additional nourishment to allow for her growth and that of the fetus. The lack of this is thought to be responsible for increased premature births and more cases of toxemia in this age group. Diet during the first trimester should be sufficient to provide some reserves needed during the last two trimesters when nourishment demands increase due to uterine and mammary gland growth.

A well-balanced diet including meat, eggs, milk, other fresh dairy products, fresh fruits, and fresh vegetables generally is sufficient for the mother and the fetus. If for any reason the mother starts her pregnancy with too little food reserve or for some other reason is not able to take in sufficient calcium, iron, and vitamin B to meet all requirements, supplementary vitamin and mineral preparations are ordered. Eating bizarre foods, as discussed in Chapter 26, is a practice that prenatal clinics try to eliminate. Pica is the medical term for a distorted appetite or a craving for something unusual.

Carbohydrates and fats are balanced with protein intake and in sufficient amounts to permit reserves to be stored for later use. Proteins are increased to meet the demands for new tissue growth for the mother and for fetal development.

Sufficient iron is needed to create more hemoglobin for the increased blood supply. Calcium is needed by both the mother and the fetus, so that a calcium supplement may be prescribed. To insure adequate nutrients for both the mother and the fetus, a list of basic foods which should be included in the daily diet is provided.

CLOTHING. Loose-fitting clothing prevents constriction about the waist. Maternity dresses are comfortable and reveal less of the silhouette. Girdle wearing or the use of an abdominal support is discussed with the physician; their use varies according to the patient, time, and physician. Generally speaking, low-heeled walking shoes (with support for the arches) should be worn to provide comfort and support.

Table 52–1 includes some additional general living needs according to trimesters.

Table 52–2 lists some complications during the prenatal period.

Emotional Needs

The prospect of adding a new member to the family is accompanied by varied feelings on the part of the mother, father, and older children. Sometimes these are feelings of joy and elation; the family is happy about the pregnancy. Other times emotional distress is present because of the adjustments that will have to be made in finances, housing, delayed plans, and the mother's quitting work.

The more expectant parents know and understand about normal pregnancy, the less anxious they will be about the coming event. A good many old wives' tales have made people fearful of what might happen; it can be a relief to them to know that the handed-down tales are not true.

Classes for Expectant Parents

Having a baby is a family affair. The addition of a new family member affects the lives of all other members, whether it is the first child or the fifth. Parents can help older children understand and accept the new infant if they themselves understand what to expect in normal pregnancy, labor, and delivery and know the proper care of the newborn.

Expectant parent classes are conducted for husbands and wives to help prepare them for their parent roles. Any number of community agencies sponsor these classes (e.g., Red Cross, public school adult education programs) at times convenient for both parents to attend. All types of visual aids are used—films, models, charts, and equipment. The classes include a discussion of natural childbirth, what it is and what it is not; a tour of hospital facilities, if possible; a discussion of what a new baby is like, how he acts, how

he should be handled, what to have ready when the infant is taken home, and how to care for him; a discussion of the needs of the mother during pregnancy, her diet, exercise, body mechanics, rest, and emotional support; and a discussion of the feelings of both husband and wife, superstitions, and old wives' tales.

Family-centered maternity care is the name commonly given to one way of meeting the needs of parents and children during and following pregnancy. The idea behind it is to make it a family affair by keeping the family together as much as possible. It includes education of the expectant parents, couples about to be married, and high school and college students; prenatal clinics; home visits; and family member experiences in the hospital's obstetric department. This approach to maternity care means that the policies and rules for the obstetric department are changed to provide opportunity for father participation, and that all personnel in the obstetric department function in behalf of this approach.

At present, many hospitals follow a specialized pattern of care in the obstetric department. There are three separate units, each with its special functions: labor and delivery, nursery, and postpartum. At times the patient (and the husband) may wish it were less specialized and perhaps more humanized as she moves through the process. There has been (and still is) good reason for developing and maintaining this pattern of care. It is more successful from the patient's point of view when personnel from these three units make provisions for her and her husband to live this experience in an environment of real emotional support from admission to discharge.

NEEDS AND CARE DURING NORMAL LABOR AND DELIVERY

Labor is the word used for the process by which the fetus and placenta are expelled from the uterus. There is still uncertainty about what starts it, but it is felt that body hormones play an important role in it. Labor is commonly divided into three stages. The first stage is dilatation of the cervix—stretching and thinning of the cervix as it pulls itself back (*efface-*

TABLE 52–1. SOME GENERAL LIVING NEEDS DURING EACH TRIMESTER

LIVING NEED	FIRST TRIMESTER	SECOND TRIMESTER	THIRD TRIMESTER
Sleep and rest	Easily fatigued. Needs 8 – 10 hours sleep and rest during the day.		More sleep required. Daily rest periods with feet elevated.
Bathing	Ordinary habits may be followed. Avoid extremely hot or cold water. Daily bathing necessary due to increased skin secretions.		Shower baths to prevent unclean water from entering vagina.
Care of teeth and mouth	Visit dentist; cavities are treated and infected teeth removed. Mouth wash soothing in case of increased salivation.	Teeth are observed for new caries, inquiry is made regarding toothache. May need to revisit dentist.	Observation continued by the physician.
Care of breasts	Adequate support to prevent loss of tissue tone following pregnancy. Gentle washing necessary.	Expose nipples to air to harden skin.	Wash with mild soap and warm water. Cover nipple with clean gauze if secretions soil clothing. When possible expose nipples to air to further harden skin.
Bowels	Daily movement needed. Physician inquires about habits and orders corrective measures.	Physician continues to observe patient's needs.	Constipation may increase. Enemas are avoided.
Exercise and activities	Usual activities of work and exercise unless arduous and fatigue causing. Heavy lifting, etc., avoided. Fresh air and outdoor exercise needed.		Less physical work, slower movements, and less mental strain and nervous tension required. Moderate daily outdoor exercise and fresh air.
Coitus	Generally permitted unless history of abortions.		Generally not permitted for several weeks before labor.
Travel	Permitted, but fatigue to be avoided. Subject to motion sickness.	Fatigue may come more easily, thus length of trip may need to be shortened.	Usually not advised after the 36th week.
Smoking and alcohol	If used, only in moderation. Alcohol adds unwanted calories.		Restricted as delivery approaches.
Visits to physician	Usually every 3 weeks.		Every 2 weeks.

TABLE 52–2. COMPLICATIONS DURING PREGNANCY

CONDITION/DISEASE	SIGNS AND SYMPTOMS	MEASURES TAKEN
I. *Bleeding — of serious importance. Can be caused by: A. Abortion — the interruption of pregnancy prior to fetal viability (before 28th week) Types: 1. Spontaneous — occur by themselves without outside interference. 2. Induced — occur due to outside interference. a. Therapeutic† — performed by the physician when mother's life or health is in danger. b. Criminal — pregnancy terminated without legal or medical sanction.	Vaginal bleeding, backache, mild abdominal cramps. Early abortion signs occur before 20th week. Late abortion signs occur between 20th and 28th weeks. Patient frequently hemorrhages and develops infection.	Patient instructed to report to physician at once. The physician usually orders increased bed rest, less activity, coital abstinence, drug therapy. Reassurance is needed. Hospitalization may or may not be required. Preventive measures to control hemorrhage, restore fluids. Surgical procedure with legal sanction. Life-saving measures used to combat shock and infection.
B. Ectopic pregnancy — the implantation of fertilized ovum occurs in a place other than the normal location (inside or outside of the uterus). Locations include: 1. Abnormal location in uterus itself, i.e., cervical canal. 2. Uterine tube. 3. Ovary. 4. Abdomen. 5. Broad ligament.	Pain, hemorrhage, shock.	Surgical removal almost always required. There is serious danger to the mother if pregnancy allowed to terminate. Fetal death almost always occurs.
C. Placenta praevia — the implantation of fertilized ovum at such a low uterine level that the placenta is near to or covers the cervix.	Scanty vaginal bright red bleeding, at first. Seeping may continue or stop for a while. Painless bleeding becomes more severe when it recurs, usually during the last trimester.	Patient is immediately hospitalized. Measures are taken to save the baby and the mother.
D. Premature separation of the placenta (abruptio placentae) — occurs during last half of pregnancy or during first two stages of labor.	Slight degree of separation produces sudden abdominal pain, moderate vaginal bleeding, a tender uterus. Extensive separation produces sudden, severe abdominal pain with profuse external bleeding.	This complication often threatens the life of mother and baby. Immediate hospitalization with transfusion to replace blood and treat for shock. Cesarean section may be indicated.
II. Hyperemesis gravidarum — excessive nausea and vomiting during pregnancy. The cause is unknown but seems to include a disturbance of the nervous system, changes in gastric function, abnormal production of some hormones.	Repeated loss of food intake, weight loss.	Hospitalization required. Bed rest, quiet environment, no visitors (usually). Fluids and food carefully controlled. Firm, understanding kindness is used by staff. Sedation is ordered, intake and output recorded. Urine and blood tests

Table continued on the opposite page.

TABLE 52–2.   COMPLICATIONS DURING PREGNANCY (Continued)

CONDITION/DISEASE	SIGNS AND SYMPTOMS	MEASURES TAKEN
		done regularly. I.V. fluids administered to overcome fluid loss and electrolyte imbalance and to provide vitamins and nutrients.
III. Toxemia of pregnancy — a general reaction due to unknown causes. Terms used: **preeclampsia** — without convulsions. **eclampsia** — includes convulsions.	Hypertension, edema, protein in the urine, convulsions, and coma. There may be disturbances including visual, renal, cardiac, respiratory, and gastrointestinal. Patient is asked to report such symptoms as edema of hands and feet, dizziness, headaches, blurred vision, vomiting, decreased urinary output, and rapid weight gain.	Observant prenatal care recognizes early symptoms and treatment includes bed rest, salt restrictions, diuretics to relieve edema, proper diet, sedation. Pregnancy is terminated if patient's condition does not improve. When convulsions are involved, they are treated first and the treatment of pregnancy follows.

*Special nursing measures would be in keeping with medical or surgical management to control hemorrhage, combat shock, and give reassuring support to the patient.

†Legal controls vary among states ranging from abortion only to save the life of the would-be mother to no restrictions at all.

---

ment), opening to permit the fetus to come through. The second stage is the expulsion of the fetus (the birth of the baby). The third stage is the separation and expulsion of the placenta. While each stage produces certain changes and leads to the next, it sometimes happens that one stage leads into the next so rapidly that it is difficult to say where one begins and the other ends.

A number of factors can influence the length of time a patient is in labor, including whether it is the first labor. This usually takes longer, about 12 to 16 hours. *Primipara* is the term used to denote a patient bearing a first child. *Multipara* is the term used to denote a patient who has had a child before. Labor for this patient usually lasts from eight to 12 hours. The position of the fetus in the uterus, the size and shape of the pelvis, the patient's anxiety or tenseness, the shape and structure of the uterus, and the ability of the cervix to undergo dilatation also influence the length of labor.

The Patient's Body Gets Ready

The body of the mother prepares itself for labor several days to several weeks ahead of time. The abdomen distends because of the continued increase in the weight and size of the fetus in the uterus. This affects breathing, walking, and posture. Vaginal secretions increase. The fetus positions itself as it descends into the pelvis (called *engagement*); in the primipara it occurs well ahead of time. The downward position of the fetus (called *lightening*) usually makes the patient more comfortable because of decreased pressure on the heart, stomach, and lungs. Irregular uterine movements are sensed by the patient. These contractions are painless (called false labor) but are often mistaken by the patient for true labor contractions.

Labor Begins

The body shows some definite signs when it is ready or about ready to begin to move the fetus out of the uterus. The patient has what is called "bloody show"; this is a vaginal discharge of bloody mucus and fluid from the blood-tinged mucus plug that has filled the cervix during pregnancy. Or, the patient may have recurrent pains in the back or abdomen that become increasingly more severe and more frequent. The membranes (bag of waters) rupture, releasing the amniotic fluid that has provided the "watery climate" for the fetus.

Labor pains are the rhythmical, recurring, and painful contractions of the uterus. At first they are slight, lasting a few seconds and recurring about every 15 minutes. As labor goes on, the pains become stronger, are more frequent, and last longer. By the time the cervix is all but fully dilated, the pain is very intense, coming on every two or three minutes and lasting well over a minute. A labor pain has been described as having three phases: a slow onset, a gradual increase in strength, and a gradual decrease in strength. Knowing this will help you understand the patient's behavior during labor. Likewise, you can see and feel the gradual rise and the gradual fall of the uterus. The patient often cries out as the pain becomes intense; she twists and turns and her face reddens. As the pain subsides, she breaks out in a profuse sweat and is very tired from exertion. The patient rests between contractions and may even fall asleep. Figure 52–1 shows a piece of equipment that helps to reduce discomfort during labor pains.

First Needs Upon Admission

Certain things must be done as soon as the patient is admitted to the maternity unit. If the physician is present he will carry out certain parts of the observation and treatment process; if he is not, the registered nurse will proceed to examine the patient to determine the stage of the labor progress and will notify the physician. Initial measures usually carried out include preparing the patient, putting her in bed, securing a urine specimen, and taking and recording TPR and blood pressure.

The patient is examined. The physician goes over the chest and abdomen and listens to the fetal heart sounds. A rectal examination is done to determine how far the cervix is dilated. Sometimes the registered nurse does the rectal examination. A cleansing enema is usually ordered. One needs to determine whether bedpan or bathroom is to be used, depending on the patient's condition. The pubic area and perineum are shaved and washed thoroughly. Again, fetal heart sounds are checked. The patient is questioned about the time that her contractions began and their duration and intensity. Contractions are timed.

Prior to and following the administration of any drug, check fetal heart sounds, contractions, pulse and blood pressure. Sometimes hospitals have special regulations about this.

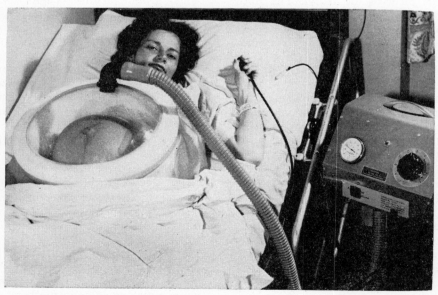

FIGURE 52–1 The patient operates this "decompression chamber" herself. As can be seen, the dome or chamber fits over the abdomen. When a pain starts, the patient presses the switch and the machine draws the air out of the chamber, automatically pulling and raising the abdomen as it does; this movement helps the muscles to contract. (Stryker: Back to Nursing, 2nd Ed.)

Observe vaginal discharges (amount and character). Have the patient void often enough to prevent bladder distention. Stay with the patient. As far as the patient is concerned, the continued presence of the nurse may be the most comforting thing that happens to her. The patient in labor does not want to be alone. Tell her what to expect and explain how she can help. If the husband is present, he is less apt to be anxious than if he is pacing the floor somewhere else. He can be supportive to his wife and help position her and coach her about how to breathe properly to aid labor, if he is so informed. Hospitals vary in their policies about the role of the husband during labor, but there is never a question about the need for the nurse to be present and supportive to the patient in labor.

The Second Stage of Labor

This is the expulsion of the fetus from the uterus — the birth of the baby. In working up to this point, uterine contractions have become very strong and occur about every two minutes. The cervix is fully dilated and the patient senses the need to bear down hard and complete the birth process; in fact, she is totally involved mentally and physically in accomplishing this.

The patient is moved to the delivery room, where she is positioned and draped. Any intact membranes are ruptured, anesthesia is administered, and an incision may be made to increase the size of the vulvar opening (called *episiotomy*) to make delivery safer for mother and baby.

The nurse in the delivery room not only assists the physician but is aware that the patient needs to feel that she is getting assistance too. As stated earlier, the patient's only concern now is to carry through the delivery process and give birth to her baby.

After guiding the baby out of the birth canal, the physician holds the newborn securely as shown in Figure 52–2 to help drain mucus from the mouth, nose, and throat. Breathing is established and the umbilical cord is clamped and cut. Several different types of materials are used to tie off the cord, such as cotton or linen tape, plastic tubing, or an aluminum disposable clamp. The physician pays particular attention to the infant's breathing, color, and general condition, including obser-

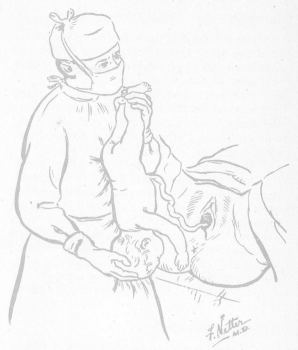

FIGURE 52–2 Physician supporting newborn baby immediately after delivery, before severing cord. (Bookmiller et al.: Textbook of Obstetrics and Obstetric Nursing, 5th Ed.)

vation for any abnormalities; the baby is then given to the nurse.

The Third Stage of Labor

During this period, the placenta separates from the uterine wall and is expelled from the body. The physician examines it to be sure it is intact and that all of it has been expelled.

For an hour or so following delivery, careful observation for possible postpartum hemorrhage continues. To emphasize the importance of this critical period, it has been called by some the "fourth stage of labor." A rapid pulse at this time would be a sign of possible hidden hemorrhage.

The role of the delivery room nurse requires judgment and skills that take more understanding than it is usually possible to gain in a practical nursing program. Additional learning and guided experience may make it possible for an LPN to become skillful enough to function safely in Role II in the delivery room. This is determined by hospital policy as well as by individual abilities.

Immediate Care of the Newborn

After receiving the infant from the physician, the nurse places it in a warm bassinet or incubator and again observes breathing, color, and general condition.

All state laws require that the eyes of the newborn be treated to prevent blindness from the gonorrhea organism. If specified, a 1 per cent solution of silver nitrate is dropped into each eye; if not, an antibiotic is used.

Before removal from the delivery room, the baby and mother are properly identified; generally some type of wrist or ankle band, or both, is used, giving the necessary identifying information (See Fig. 52–3). Footprints also are used for this purpose. The baby is weighed and measured and the mother told the size and sex of her baby. After these necessary procedures, the infant is moved to the nursery. See Figure 52–4 for a copy of a birth certificate.

The Premature Infant

This term applies to the newborn who is not full term or who weighs less than five and one-half pounds. Based upon this definition, about one out of every 10 babies born is premature. Prematurity accounts for one-half or more of newborn deaths.

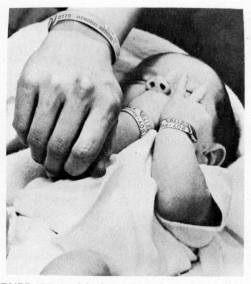

FIGURE 52–3 Mother-infant Ident-A-Band are applied in the delivery room. (Hollister, Inc.) (Stryker: Back to Nursing, 2nd Ed.)

Because of the many limitations of this newborn, expert nursing care is required. The matter of providing nourishment, warmth, and conserving the energy of the infant in all that is done for him demands special skills and knowledge which must be gained through additional study and experience.

NEEDS AND CARE DURING PUERPERIUM

Puerperium or postpartum is the period of six to eight weeks following delivery when the uterus returns to normal size and function and menstruation is re-established. The mother loses weight, and the abdominal muscles regain their tone.

Nursing Care During Hospitalization

While the patient has the same daily living needs as other patients, certain nursing measures are necessary to help her meet her particular needs at this time. She may be discharged earlier in some instances than in others; this depends upon the physician and the hospital policy. Generally, the period of hospitalization extends to several days.

The emphasis in caring for the postpartum patient should be to prevent infection of the breasts or pelvis, to help her handle any feelings of depression, to see that she gets needed rest and adequate food, to watch for normal elimination, and to help her to get acquainted with her new baby. Give her all needed instruction and assistance to aid her return to self-care; encourage ambulation to promote regular body processes if the doctor permits it.

Physical Needs and Care

Soon after delivery the mother should receive a cleansing bath. It will be refreshing and it affords you an opportunity to listen to the patient who may wish to talk about "her delivery." In addition, she can be instructed about how to bathe herself, including breast and perineal care.

Bathing involves the same principles for this patient as for others. An exception in the

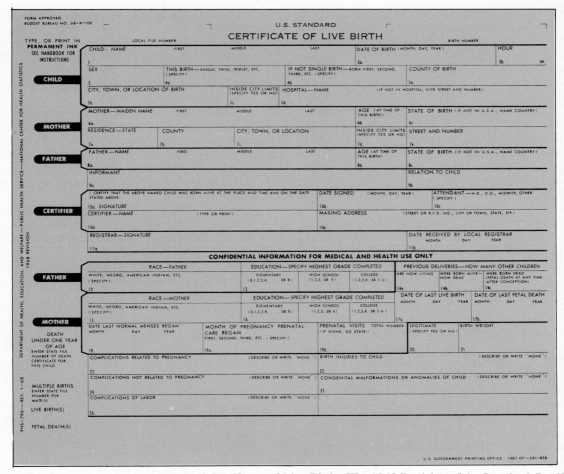

FIGURE 52–4 United States Standard Certificate of Live Birth. (The 1968 Revision of the Standard Certificates, U.S. Dept. Health, Education, and Welfare. Public Health Services Publication.)

procedure is that the breasts are bathed first and special instructions are given for perineal care. The patient is taught how to care for herself, observing the use of any special materials or methods to be followed to guard against infection.

By the second day, the patient is usually ambulatory, and takes a shower bath. Tub baths may or may not be recommended for several weeks following delivery.

Being up and about or sitting up in bed helps to restore body processes and aids drainage.

PERINEAL CARE. A nurse's respect for asepsis shows by her manner and action when she teaches the patient how to carry out perin-

eal care and how to be careful not to introduce microorganisms into the vaginal area. While the procedure for carrying it out may vary from hospital to hospital, the purposes for doing it are always the same: cleanliness and comfort, promotion of healing, and prevention of infection. Closeness to the rectum makes it extremely important to avoid contaminating the vaginal area from that source.

LOCHIA. Lochia is the term for the vaginal discharge that takes place during the first week or two following delivery. This discharge comes from the inner wall of the uterus as it heals itself. At first the fluid is bright red, but in a few days it becomes brownish-red and finally yellowish white as the uterine healing process becomes complete. Note and record the amount and color of the lochia. The patient may express concern about the bright red discharge when she first gets out of bed. Watch to see if it persists; usually it does not continue beyond a spurt or small gush.

ELIMINATION. The patient may experience some early difficulty voiding. Bathroom privileges generally are allowed (patient should be assisted at first) several hours after delivery. Observation can help prevent a distended bladder. Failure to void sufficient amounts within a reasonable time should be reported.

Constipation often persists early in recuperation. This can be due to lack of bowel tone, some dehydration, a predelivery enema that emptied the lower bowel, or some dysfunction of the anal muscle as a result of pressure during labor. Then, too, there can be anal discomfort due to an episiotomy or to lacerations. Generally a mild cathartic or a cleansing enema is ordered within a day or two. In giving an enema, use care in inserting the enema tube to avoid injury to or contamination of the perineum. The patient is reminded how to care for herself following a bowel movement to avoid contamination of the perineal area.

DIET. At first the patient may be on a light diet with extra fluids. After that she will have a general diet with high protein and vitamin content. The at-home diet for the mother nursing her baby should contain approximately 2500 calories and continue to be high in proteins and vitamins. Additional calcium and iron may be needed during lactation. A mother breast-feeding her baby should drink at least 3 pints of milk a day.

AFTER-PAINS. For a while during puerperium, uterine contractions continue, sometimes causing considerable discomfort. Explain that the uterus is contracting and returning to normal size and that the pain gradually will disappear. If the pain becomes too severe the physician usually orders a mild medication.

SLEEP AND REST. During her recuperation from labor and delivery, the mother needs and should be permitted to rest. Plan nursing care activities to allow time for rest and the environment conducive to sleep. Too many visitors can prevent proper rest and for that reason, among others, many hospitals have rules limiting the number of visitors allowed at one time.

BREAST CARE. The chief things to remember about breast care are the need for adequate breast support, for protection from breast infection, and for prevention of trauma to the nipples.

The breasts are bathed first when the bath is given. With a clean washcloth, warm water, and soap, wash one breast with gentle circular movements, starting with the nipple and working outward. Dry with a clean towel. Using another clean washcloth and towel, repeat the process for the second breast.

Breast binders should support engorged breasts and be comfortable for the patient. Tighter fitting binders are used when lactation is to be discontinued.

Mothers are encouraged to nurse their babies if they are able, as nursing is good for both the mother and the baby (Fig. 52–5). However, this does not mean that it is the place of the nurse to urge her if she does not choose to do so, nor to cause her to feel guilty about her decision.

Emotional upset can interfere with lactation; when such is observed it should be reported. Pain from sore or cracked nipples will interfere with the release of milk; the breast may be full but the milk refuses to "come down."

Emotional Needs

During the postpartum period the mother begins to regain her strength and to think about the days and months ahead. The birth process is over and the realization that a new baby brings new responsibilities sometimes creates nervous tension and worry. The patient may need or want to talk about this; report any such observations. There are ways to help the mother handle her worries; the registered nurse should be involved to see that help is given. The physician will need to know about it too because, while it usually passes, the patient's reactions might result in a serious psychiatric disturbance.

Rooming-in

The rooming-in service of some hospitals permits the mother to have her infant in her

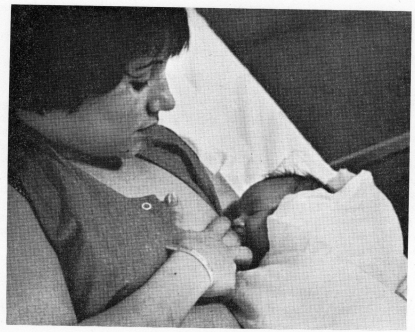

FIGURE 52–5 Mother-baby contact is a satisfying experience for both. (Bookmiller et al.: Textbook of Obstetrics and Obstetric Nursing, 5th Ed.).

room or in an adjacent room where she can be with and care for him. She is able to observe his activities and participate in his care under the supervision of a nurse. The mother learns her child's schedule for care while still in the hospital and in this way has less worry about how to proceed at home. Such an arrangement is especially good for the husband, who can also participate in the care of his child by learning to diaper the baby and to burp him after a feeding.

Rooming-in service varies with hospitals and the facilities the hospitals use. Most babies spend the night in a large nursery and are taken to the mother's rooms as early as the mothers want them in the morning. It is a training period for the mother and prepares her gradually for the care of her child. There are some disadvantages to the rooming-in practice. Visitors are not allowed except for the father, who must be properly gowned to prevent infection. Some mothers are not ready to assume such responsibility at this point in their recuperation. Still, it has the advantage of having the mother near the baby for whatever emotional comfort it brings.

Teaching Mothers

As pointed out, the mother is taught how to care for herself (bath, breasts, perineal care). She also has opportunity to learn how to care for her infant. Nursing care today includes mothers' classes to teach bathing the baby and preparing the formula (if needed). There is no better way for the new mother to learn how to handle her baby and give him a bath than to see the nurse demonstrate this procedure, using equipment generally available in the home situation. If the mother has opportunity to bathe her own baby under supervision, it will help to dispel uncertainty when she goes home.

Getting Ready to go Home

Present-day obstetrics is concerned with the patient until she is fully recovered and physically normal. Prior to her discharge, the intern or the physician completes a partial examination. He weighs the patient, takes the blood pressure, and observes the condition of her breasts, abdomen, and perineal and vaginal areas. Findings are recorded on the patient's chart. The physician requests that the patient call at his office for a final examination in about eight weeks.

Final Examination

The physician's office nurse will probably send an appointment card to the patient, scheduling the date and time of an appointment.

The office examination will include those areas observed on the patient's leaving the hospital, to be sure involution and the discharge have ceased. The physician needs to be sure that the lacerations are healed, that the breasts are healthy, and that the patient is in good physical condition. He will ask about the baby and arrange to place him under the care of a pediatrician if necessary.

COMPLICATIONS

Thus far, only normal pregnancy, labor, delivery, and puerperium care have been discussed. Each of these periods can have its accompanying disorders and diseases. Tables 52–2, 52–3, and 52–4 list the more common conditions associated with each. Disorders commonly called medical-surgical diseases, when present during pregnancy and following, require additional medical and nursing measures appropriate to each such patient and are not repeated here.

TABLE 52–3.   COMPLICATIONS DURING LABOR AND DELIVERY

CONDITION/DISEASE	SIGNS AND SYMPTOMS	MEASURES TAKEN
The fetus presents itself for delivery in a variety of positions. The details of the difficulties encountered by the patient and the physician may be found in a reliable textbook on maternity nursing if such information is sought.		
I. Bleeding during labor.		
A. As discussed in previous table under placenta praevia and premature separation of the placenta.		
B. Rupture of the uterus — long, difficult labor may aggravate a previous operation (i.e., cesarean section) on the uterus and cause it to rupture.	Increased tenderness at the site of the scar progresses until uterine wall opens with excruciating pain. Patient collapses and goes into shock. The fetus is expelled into the abdominal cavity.	Life-saving measures are used to replace blood and surgically remove the uterus. Death almost always follows for the fetus and very often for the mother.
C. Inversion of uterus — uterus turns inside out following delivery.	Hemorrhage and shock.	A surgical procedure is necessary to replace it.
II. Pelvic contractions and pelvic tumors — may obstruct the birth canal or alter it.	Labor is prolonged and difficult.	A vaginal delivery may or may not be possible.

TABLE 52–4.   COMPLICATIONS DURING PUERPERIUM

CONDITION/DISEASE	*SIGNS AND SYMPTOMS*	*MEASURES TAKEN*
I. Hemorrhage — caused by portions of the placenta clinging to the uterine wall, failure of uterus to contract after placenta is expelled, injury to the uterus, or some abnormal function during the third stage of labor.	When postpartum bleeding exceeds a pint of blood it is considered serious. Bleeding may occur at any time postpartum, but frequently is seen between the 6th and 10th day when it occurs.	Source of bleeding is determined and hemorrhage stopped at the earliest possible time. Fluids and blood are replaced as patient is treated for shock and possible infection.
II. Mastitis — infection of the breast more often than not due to poor habits of cleanliness (patient or personnel) which have permitted organisms to enter the breasts through the nipples.	Painful, inflamed breasts, cracked nipples, chills and fever.	The best measures are those used to prevent its occurrence: proper cleansing of breasts prior to and after nursing, safe technique to prevent spread of organisms to breast area, proper care of nipples. Antibiotics are used to combat the infection. Compresses may be ordered.
III. Infections — may be directly related to the puerperium or be otherwise present in the patient.	Chills, fever, lassitude.	Here again the best treatment is prevention by having a safe environment and using unquestionably safe techniques. The patient is isolated and the infant is not brought to the area. Antibiotics are given and strict measures are used to curb the infection and prevent its spread.
IV. Puerperal thrombosis — blood clots in the legs or pelvis. The chief danger is that the clot, or part of of it, may break off and be carried to the lungs (embolism).	Elevated temperature, painful swollen leg. Skin is tightly drawn over area which is white and very tender.	Anticoagulant drugs are used. Bed rest, leg elevated, heat lamp for warmth, and relieve pressure of bed covers.

SUMMARY

Facts prove that early and continuous prenatal care can produce healthier mothers and babies. Presently, more efforts are being made to provide prenatal care at the community level to try to reduce the rates of infant mortality and mental retardation in this country.

Modern care emphasizes education for parenthood, regular medical examination, proper diet, exercise, and preventive measures, as well as follow-up supervision of the mother and the baby.

Pregnancy is a normal process and produces certain changes in the mother as the fetus continues development to full term. Medical science is concerning itself with the reasons that babies die during pregnancy, delivery, and the early days of life. They are likewise concerned with early detection of mental retardation and ways to prevent its occurrence.

The mother during labor, delivery, and puerperium has need for special attention to certain aspects of her physical care, and likewise has a pronounced need for emotional support as well. You can be a valuable team member in helping to meet this need.

GUIDES FOR STUDY AND DISCUSSION

1. Why is prenatal care valuable? How does it help the patient? Why do not all patients receive it?

2. Why should the pregnant adolescent consume extra nourishment? Why should food reserves be stored during the first trimester?

3. What is the function of the placenta? What happens to it after the baby is born?

4. Signs of pregnancy are listed as presumptive, probable, and positive. What are some examples of each?

5. Pregnancy is divided into trimesters. How do living needs change from the first to the second to the third?

6. How does the body adjust to pregnancy? How do these adjustments influence the mother?

7. The mother in labor needs emotional support. How can you help provide it?

8. What are the three stages of labor? As a practical nurse, which ones are you apt to be involved in?

9. Patient teaching is a part of postpartum care. What is the mother taught?

10. How do you, as a practical nurse, guard against infection while giving postpartum care?

11. What factors should guide nursing action during postpartum care?

12. How does the bath for this patient differ from the bath for an adult on a medical-surgical unit? How is it similar?

13. What precautions are taken in providing breast care?

SUGGESTED SITUATIONS AND ACTIVITIES

1. Be ready to express and support your opinion: Is a mother who is experiencing normal labor sick?

2. Imagine yourself employed in the nursery caring for newborns who are separated from their mothers except at feeding time. You want to "humanize" the part you play in the life of the mother as much as possible. What things must you consider? What things can you do?

3. Locate recent articles in the news media that discuss efforts to improve prenatal care or the problems faced in infant mortality and retardation, or that praise or criticize present maternity care.

4. Examine the list of health information gathered during the first prenatal clinic visit. Visit a clinic and find out how this information is gathered. See who is involved besides the physician.

5. Why is a birth certificate necessary? Examine Figure 52–4 and note the types of information called for. How might it be used? How does it take care of multiple births?

CHAPTER 53

NURSING THE NEWBORN

TOPICAL HEADINGS

Introduction
The Normal Newborn
Needs and Care of
    the Newborn

Some Disorders and
    Disabilities of the
    Newborn
Summary

Guides for Study and
    Discussion
Suggested Situations
    and Activities

OBJECTIVES FOR THE STUDENT: Be able to:

1. Describe the appearance of the normal newborn.
2. Compare the vital signs of the normal newborn with those of an adult.
3. Describe two body functions that are not fully developed at birth.
4. Tell how to protect the newborn from infection during the bath.
5. Compare the aseptic practices of the nurse in the regular nursery with those in the isolation nursery.
6. Demonstrate how to hold an infant safely and securely.
7. Describe the characteristics of an adequately nourished infant.
8. Name the chief causes of newborn respiratory difficulties.
9. Describe four signs of possible brain hemorrhage in the newborn.

SUGGESTED STUDY VOCABULARY*

infant mortality
newborn
neonatal period
fetus
infant
fontanel

meconium
congenital
regurgitate
cleft lip
anoxia
pallor
asphyxia

cleft palate
isolation
asepsis
vernix caseosa
reflexes
anomaly
atelectasis

---

*Look for any terms you already know.

INTRODUCTION

Chapter 18, Life before Birth and during the First Year, describes the appearance, activities, and abilities of the newborn. All that is included here is a listing of the chief characteristics.

The newborn is completely dependent upon others for meeting his daily living needs.

Due to his size, his "unsettled" body heat regulation, his brand new digestive and urinary tracts, his limited ability to communicate, and his inability to ambulate, the newborn's well-being depends upon a person who knows how to assist him safely.

The main emphasis in this chapter is to identify and describe the needs of the normal newborn and care; the last portion includes some problems that are encountered in newborns.

THE NORMAL NEWBORN

Newborn usually means an infant from birth to two months of age. The neonatal period is the first four weeks after birth. The child is called an infant until he assumes an upright position (12 to 14 months).

Appearance of the Newborn (See Chapter 18)

1. Weight usually ranges from five and one-half pounds to nine or 10 pounds (average is about 7½ pounds).

2. Length is about 20 inches; boys are slightly longer than girls.

3. Head is longer from front to back than from top to chin and is large in comparison to the rest of the body. It may be molded (Fig. 53–1).

4. The fontanel (anterior) is a diamond-shaped "soft-spot" at the top of the head where the skull bones have not yet grown together. It takes about 18 months for fusion of the bones.

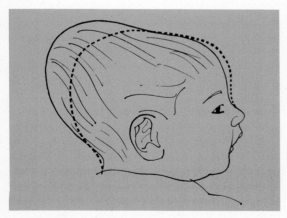

FIGURE 53–1 Molding of the head occurs as a result of the ovverriding of the parietal bones as the head passes through the birth canal. The head appears longer than normal. This condition disappears without treatment within a few weeks. The dotted lines show the normal contour of the head as compared with the molded head of a newborn. (Leifer: Principles and Techniques in Pediatric Nursing, 2nd Ed.)

5. Facial features are small. The eyes are closed most of the time. The lower jaw is set back and the chin seems to rest on the chest because the neck is short.

6. Extremities: The hands are held in fists; the legs are often pulled up onto abdomen, which protrudes somewhat.

7. The skin is dusky red with slightly blue-tinged extremities. If the skin is light it becomes slightly pink as circulation improves and vivid red when crying. The nonwhite newborn may have dark bluish areas on the lower back and buttocks that later disappear. *Vernix caseosa,* a protective white cheesy material ("cheesy varnish") may cover parts of the body.

Reactions of the Newborn (See Chapter 18)

The infant displays disorganized movement of extremities. His reflexes are present; his muscles have tone. He can suck, breathe while sucking, swallow, sneeze, cough, yawn, hiccough, vomit, sigh, grunt, cry, smile after a fashion, and hear. He responds with a jerk or a cry to loud noises. He has a sense of balance and he responds to love and body contact. He urinates frequently and passes meconium stools at first.

Normal Vital Signs and Blood Pressure of the Newborn

The numbers indicate *average or approximate rates only.*

About eight hours after birth, the newborn's temperature returns to normal if adequate protection is provided. Heat and cold affect the newborn's temperature because his control center is unstable or not fully developed; he is unable to perspire or shiver. Heat causes a rash. If he becomes uncomfortably warm he fusses, and he also dislikes the sensation of cold (i.e., a wet diaper).

The infant's pulse is 100 (sleeping) to 150 (awake and active); it is irregular and influenced by respirations.

His respirations are 40 to 60 and somewhat irregular—a group of short breaths followed by a long pause.

The blood pressure reading varies with the weight of newborn. For example, for an 8-pound baby, 75/50 is normal, for a 10-pound baby, it's 90/60.

NEEDS AND CARE OF THE NORMAL NEWBORN

Each newborn is an individual with unique needs that are related to his individual growth and development. Because he sleeps more than he is awake, he needs to have his own feeding schedule plus suitable amounts and kinds of food. His environment makes a difference to him—he prefers reasonable quiet, comfortable warmth, and being dry. The newborn will exercise himself if his movements are not restricted; in fact, he seems to feel this need and fusses when he cannot move freely. Equally important to the newborn is receiving love and affection; he does not thrive without it.

The gene code established certain things about the newborn at the time of conception, and these work together with his surroundings to influence his growth and behavior patterns. Very early he begins to show his individuality. Any mother who has had more than one child will soon tell you how different one baby was from the others. If you observe him for awhile you can soon know what to expect under certain circumstances. For example, you can just about tell how he will behave when he is left alone, when he is hungry, and when he is taken from his mother's arms or from the breast at feeding time if he has not satisfied his desire to suck.

The newborn finds his own comfortable position for sleeping, a way of waking up, and ways of demanding food and seeking attention. It does not take him long to sense his mother's voice and her way of providing affection; these seem to have their own special meaning for him and he responds in his own individual way.

Physical Needs and Care

The infant's body soon adjusts to life outside the uterus and he begins to desire being comfortable, having enough to eat, a good place to sleep, clean, dry skin, and freedom to move his arms and legs.

HOSPITAL ENVIRONMENT. Here personnel wear special garb and carry out rigid aseptic practices to maintain an infection-free nursery, because infection for a newborn is a most dangerous condition. The environment of the newborn in the hospital nursery is a protected climate that is designed to prevent infections and to maintain a constant comfortable temperature (65 to 75° F.).

BATHING. Opinions vary as to whether or not the new infant should be bathed. Some say that no water or oil baths should be given; others argue that the skin should be cleansed. In some instances, only the face and hands are washed and the rest of the body is carefully wiped with sterile cotton to remove wastes (blood and meconium) and to spread the vernix caseosa. Whatever the established procedure, these points are to be kept in mind from the first bath on:

1. *Prevent infections.* Use every safety means, proper handwashing techniques, proper handling of supplies, and proper disposal of used materials.

2. *Maintain a safe, comfortable environment.* Avoid drafts and keep the temperature between 65 and 75° F.

3. *Handle and hold the infant with care.* Provide adequate back and head support (see Fig. 53–2).

4. *Assemble needed materials ahead of time.* If water is used, its temperature should be 100 to 105° F. Soap is not often used until the child is older. Determine what, if any, solution may be used for special areas or purposes.

5. *Cleanse female genitalia observing this rule:* wipe from front to back to avoid bringing contaminating material from the anal region to the vaginal and urethral area.

6. *Use extraordinary care in cleaning the mouth, nose, and ears.* The tissues are very thin and are easily traumatized. Cleanse these parts first. Wipe the eyes from inner cannula outward.

7. *Observe for any untoward signs or abnormalities.*

8. *Stay with the infant all the time.*

The daily bath serves several purposes. It stimulates circulation, provides exercise, guards against infections, cleans the skin for comfort, provides time for affection and attention, and provides opportunity to observe for abnormal conditions.

The postpartum mother needs to be taught how to bathe her baby if she does not already know. Even then, a demonstration bath, using the type of equipment found in the home, may furnish her with some new ideas. One thing that should be pointed out is *infant safety from start to finish.*

Since 1913, the Children's Bureau of the

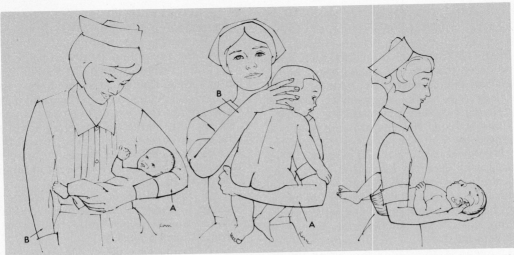

FIGURE 53-2   Three ways to hold an infant. 1, The cradle position. 2, The upright position. 3, The football hold. 1 and 3 allow the use of the free arm for other purposes. (Leifer: Principles and Techniques in Pediatric Nursing, 2nd Ed.)

United States government has provided a booklet called *Infant Care** that has been a "best seller" through the years. It not only discusses equipment for bathing, things to observe, and the precautions to take while bathing the baby, but it covers every aspect of daily care during the first year of life.

CLOTHING.   The most important item is the diaper, and the supply should be generous. Other items include cotton shirts, loose jackets or "sacks," sweaters, and cotton blankets. The amount of clothing worn depends upon the temperature. Ordinarily, a 70° F. temperature is suitable and comfortable. Freedom from excessive clothing is enjoyed by the infant. Some type of outdoor garment is needed for cold weather.

FEEDING.   The newborn loses some weight during the first few days. Breast fluids contain very little nourishment at this time; the infant needs water and may be given a weak formula (every three to four hours) to satisfy him and prevent dehydration. Following the initial weight loss the first week, and for three or four months, the infant gains about an ounce per day.

---

*U. S. Department of Health, Education, and Welfare, Children's Bureau: *Infant Care*, Children's Bureau Publication Number 8, 1963. Superintendent of Documents, U. S. Government Printing Office, Washington, D.C.

When breast milk is available, additional feedings are used to supplement his needs if the supply is somewhat lacking. However, if the supply of breast milk is very scanty (less than one-half of the infant's needs), the infant is weaned and given formula feedings.

Breast feeding the baby is desirable if this is the mother's choice. Human milk has the following advantages: it is a natural infant food, free from possible contamination; the temperature is even; the supply generally increases to meet the infant's demand, and it is available.

Whether to breast feed or not is up to the mother, unless otherwise indicated by the physician. She has to decide this question and should not be unduly influenced by others. When there is appropriate opportunity, the nurse can help her to understand the advantages and the disadvantages, without casting doubt or making the mother feel guilty if she decides not to breast feed her baby.

Common judgment now states that the baby should be fed when he is hungry. In this way he establishes his own schedule. Active nursing for 15 to 20 minutes is usually sufficient. Beyond that, the mother and the baby get tired. Between nursings, feedings of warm water are given.

Prior to leaving the hospital, the mother will have an opportunity to become familiar with breast feeding her baby. She should know how to hold and position the infant, how long to let him nurse, how he should grasp the nipple, and how to burp him, and she should be instructed in how to care for her breasts.

The nursing mother needs an adequate, nourishing diet. It should be well balanced and include increased amounts of some protective foods such as milk, lean meats, citrus fruits, green leafy vegetables, and more liquids. See Table 53–1 for a daily food guide.

Bottle feeding is often necessary and has its advantages. For any number of reasons, the baby is given formula instead of being breast fed. The reasons include failure of the baby to grow and gain weight normally or inability of the baby to get the milk, lack of sufficient breast milk, underdeveloped breasts, a poor state of health of the mother or the presence of a specific illness (e.g., tuberculosis or syphilis), or the need of the mother to be away from home at feeding time (if she works, for instance).

Formula is a term given to the milk preparation for artificial feeding. Any special ingredients are ordered by the physician if the routine formula of the institution needs to be modified for an infant. Procedures for preparing formula feedings observe strict asepsis practices to avoid possible contamination.

Other Nourishment Needs. Milk (human and cow's) does not supply enough vitamin C and vitamin D. Evaporated milk has been enriched with vitamin D but lacks vitamin C. These vitamins are added to the diet

TABLE 53–1. DAILY FOOD PATTERN FOR THE NURSING MOTHER*

GROUP	TYPE of FOOD	EACH DAY
Milk group	Milk	4-6 cups (to drink and in foods)
	Dairy products such as cheddar cheese, cottage cheese, and ice cream	May sometimes be used in place of milk
Vegetable — fruit group	Select from those rich in vitamin C Grapefruit, orange, tomato, (whole or as juice, canned, or fresh), raw cabbage, green or sweet red pepper, broccoli, fresh strawberries, guava, mango, papaya, cantaloupe	2 servings
	Select from those rich in vitamin A Can be judged fairly well by color — dark green and deep yellow: apricots, broccoli, cantaloupe, carrots, greens, pumpkin, sweet potatoes, winter squash	1 or more servings
	Others, including potatoes	2 or more servings
Meat group	Meat, poultry, or fish	1-2 servings
	Dry beans, peas, peanut butter	Occasionally in place of meat
	Eggs	1 serving
Bread and cereal group	Whole grain or enriched bread; restored breakfast cereals; and other grain products, such as cornmeal, grits, macaroni, spaghetti, and rice	3-4 servings
Other foods	Foods such as sugars, oils, margarine, butter, and other fats which may be used in cooking and to complete meals, provide additional food energy and other food values. Vitamin D in some form, if diet does not provide an adequate amount	According to doctor's instructions

* U.S. Department of Health, Education, and Welfare, Children's Bureau: *Infant Care*, Children's Bureau Publication Number 8, 1963. Superintendent of Documents, U.S. Government Printing Office, Washington, D.C.

under the direction of the pediatrician, who determines the best sources of them and what will be adequate amounts for the individual baby. Small amounts of water are also provided.

Holding the baby while he nurses is more satisfying to him and is safer. The mother can enjoy this contact with her baby, too. The bottle is tipped so that the neck and nipple are full of milk before the nipple is put into the infant's mouth, which prevents his sucking air into his stomach. In his eagerness, the baby often swallows some air, and during his feeding he will need to be "burped" or "bubbled" (Fig. 53–3).

Whatever his schedule or means of being fed, if the infant is satisfied, contented, and growing normally, he is adequately nourished.

SLEEPING. Sleeping is an individual matter with infants. Ideally, they should sleep about 20 hours a day during the first month or two, and wake only when they are hungry. Some babies do this; others are awake early in the morning and late at night. They fight to keep awake during the day and sleep only in naps. These babies are not ill and seem to grow and develop as normally as the more sleepy baby.

The baby should be encouraged to sleep and rest as much as possible during the first growing months. Gradually he will be awake longer during the day but should sleep most of the night after his evening feeding. He may even sleep until bath time after an early morning feeding. By the end of the first year the baby should have two long naps in the daytime and should sleep all night.

Sleeping Position. Most babies seem to sleep on their stomachs with the legs drawn up to the side or under the abdomen; they seem to be more comfortable this way. Some authorities say that there are two reasons why a baby is not encouraged to sleep on his back. The more important one is that if the baby regurgitates food or vomits, this material may choke him. Also, his bones are somewhat soft, and the back of his head may be flattened slightly from constant pressure. If the baby persists in sleeping on one side of his head, the bed might be turned around to encourage him to turn his head. Changing the position of the bed or putting the baby's head to the foot of the bed every other night or so will prevent his sleeping constantly on one side of his head.

If possible, the baby should sleep in a room of his own from the time he returns from the hospital but be near enough to the parents that they will hear prolonged crying.

ELIMINATION. The infant's first stools (meconium) are a sticky greenish-black solid material. Gradually they become lighter in color. The number of stools per day varies. Some babies have a stool during or after feeding, others have two or three during 24 hours. The number or timing is unimportant if the stools are normal in appearance. Any evidence of change in consistency and odor is reason for concern if it persists. Such observations in the nursery are reported at once.

The small intestine of the infant is easily upset by bacteria and by some foods. Diarrhea is a serious condition for an infant if it goes unchecked, and can be fatal. Extreme measures are taken in the nursery when there is the earliest evidence of diarrhea.

EXERCISE. While it is true that the infant needs and gets a great deal of sleep during his early life, he needs exercise as well. He provides some of this for himself as he waves his

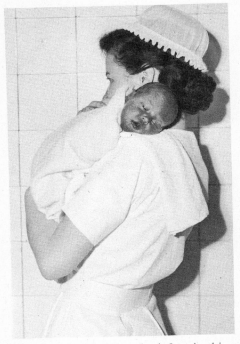

FIGURE 53–3 By holding the infant in this position after eating, the baby can easily be "burped." Notice the protection under the head to prevent contamination. (Bookmiller et al.: Textbook of Obstetrics and Obstetric Nursing, 5th Ed.)

arms and kicks his legs about all at once. He soon tries to lift his head, and will grasp a rattle, shaking it vigorously. He also gets exercise during his bath and when he is picked up for feeding or for any other purposes. If the new mother is hesitant about holding her baby, help her by showing how the head and back are supported and the body is securely held.

A baby is born with a sense of balance and a need to feel secure and safe; he soon becomes accustomed to the hands and holding movements of the person who gives him care.

Emotional Needs and Care

One cannot really separate the infant's emotional needs from his physical needs, except to discuss them under two separate headings. This is only a convenient way to emphasize their importance.

The infant's future well-being is as closely related to feelings of love, security, and affection as to an adequate diet and a comfortable crib. He responds to his parents' affection and especially does he come to feel his mother's presence very early in life. By the time he is a few weeks old his eyes follow her as she moves about within range, and he is fully capable of reminding her that he is present.

The infant needs the people around him and he soon knows who feeds him, holds him, and otherwise makes him feel comfortable and secure. Parents, brothers and sisters, and grandparents all become a part of his life.

SOME DISORDERS AND DISABILITIES OF THE NEWBORN

A large proportion of neonatal deaths are due to disorders peculiar to infancy and immaturity, namely: *congenital deformities, birth injuries, postnatal asphyxia,* and *atelectasis.*

Congenital Deformities

When the disability makes it impossible for the baby to live very long, steps are taken at once to correct it surgically. All members of this team are highly skilled and the newborn's postoperative care is provided by highly skilled personnel. Some examples of conditions that require surgical treatment are hernias of abdominal viscera, absence of an anal opening, an esophagus that does not lead into the stomach, and a bowel obstruction.

Any deformity that exists at the time of birth is called a congenital deformity or an anomaly. Sometimes the physician can determine deformity before birth. The cause of congenital anomalies is not known and at present there is no known way to prevent them. The new efforts in perinatal pathology mentioned in the previous chapter may help find some answers.

One problem related to the birth of an imperfect or deformed newborn is the parent's feelings; they are apt to think that possibly it was their fault. This, of course, is not true. The genetic code sometimes gets mixed or scrambled and the result is abnormality. Any body system can be involved and the list of anomalies is very long.

The delivery room examinations by the obstetrician and the nurse are to find out what, if any, abnormal conditions are present. Some do not show up until later, in the nursery. This means that nursery personnel likewise are observing for any apparent malfunctions or deformities. The presence of one anomaly suggests that others might be present too.

One sign that indicates that there is possibility of a malformation someplace is the newborn's cry. If it is not full and lusty, the obstetrician recognizes it as a sign to look for the reasons. The cry sign ranges from absence of any sound to weak, hoarse, harsh, or high-pitched cries.

CLEFT LIP AND CLEFT PALATE (Fig. 53–4). Often these two deformities accompany each other. Both are the result of the failure of the upper mouth structure to fuse or join together properly. The cleft lip is visible, and is detected at once, whether it is slight or extreme. The cleft palate is not visible; it must be located by examination.

These deformities are surgically corrected as soon as the physician decides that the baby is able to undergo the operation. The sooner it is corrected, the sooner the infant can suck in a normal way and avoid possible malnutrition.

Feeding the newborn with a cleft lip or a cleft palate requires skill to see that sufficient nourishment is taken but that it does not get into nasal passages. Regurgitation is a prob-

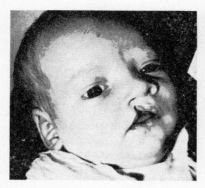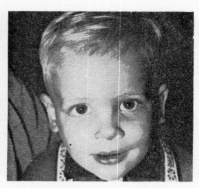

FIGURE 53-4 Cleft lip. A, Before operation. B, After operation. (McDonald: *Bright Promise*. National Society for Crippled Children and Adults, Inc.)

lem if care is not used. Sometimes a special plate device is used in the roof of the mouth during feeding until the repair is made. Mouth breathing dries out membranes and cracks can occur if meticulous mouth care is not performed.

Postoperative nursing concerns with the infant who has had a surgical repair of a cleft lip or cleft palate are:

1. Prevent crying by holding and cuddling him as often as necessary and by feeding him on time so that he does not get hungry. Crying puts strain on the sutures.

2. Feed him with a rubber-tipped medicine dropper, and direct the feeding away from both the operative area and the sutures.

3. Use arm restraints to prevent rubbing or scratching of the face. Remove them periodically to permit movement and exercise.

Release one arm at a time and hold the infant so that his movements can be controlled.

The object of the infant's care is the same as that for any normal infant (keep him clean, dry, comfortable, and well-fed) plus the need to prevent crying and to keep the operative site clean. Mouth breathing continues to be a skin and membrane care problem.

Vomiting is a sign that should not be ignored. It signifies that, for some reason, the stomach cannot retain the feeding. Observe the manner in which it occurs. The physician needs to know when it occurs—at a specific time, right after eating, in the morning? Did the vomitus come out with force (projectile)? What was the appearance of it?

CLUBFOOT (Fig. 53–5). The cause of true clubfoot comes from some defect in the development of the part in the uterus. The

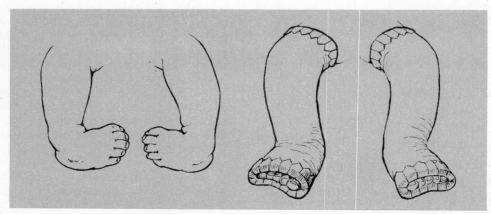

FIGURE 53-5 There are several types of clubfoot. Here both feet are involved, but this is not always the case. Notice one type of cast used to correct the deformity. (Marlow: Textbook of Pediatric Nursing, 4th Ed.)

clubfoot should be corrected at the earliest possible time to prevent any undue posture or muscle developments. The infant may not even be hospitalized. Appliances and corrective devices can be applied while the baby stays at home. Regular outpatient visits follow.

Congenital Disease

Infants can be born with disease. One of the more frequently mentioned disorders is the blood disease known as *erythroblastosis fetalis* (Rh factor disorder). The newborn's erythrocytes are damaged and destroyed because his Rh positive blood factor is incompatible with his mother's Rh negative blood factor. Up to now, immediate exchange transfusions have been used to replace most of the infant's blood with Rh negative blood. The use of the new vaccine RhoGam may make such exchange transfusions unnecessary in time to come.

Congenital heart disease is due to some malformation in the heart or the blood vessels close to the heart. It may be an inherited weakness or it may be caused by some type of infection or by malnutrition experienced by the mother during pregnancy. Nursing these infants requires professional skill in detecting the signs and symptoms associated with the condition and in carrying out or assisting with special therapies ordered by the physician.

If the practical nurse is involved, it should be in a Role II capacity, performing selected tasks assigned to her such as securing equipment and positioning and restraining the patient.

Birth Injuries

Birth injuries may cause permanent damage (even death) or temporary injury; they may require treatment or disappear by themselves. Some causative factors include the position of the fetus in the uterus, the part of the body presented first in delivery, excessive size of the fetus, prolonged labor, and abnormal uterine contractions. Not all injuries are apparent at birth but show up hours later.

Brain hemorrhage (intracranial hemorrhage) is a serious complication often due to prolonged labor and difficult delivery by forceps. Excessive pressure on the fetal skull causes such extreme overlapping of the cranial bones that underlying brain tissues are torn rupturing the blood vessels.

SIGNS AND SYMPTOMS. Any of the following signs indicate possible brain hemorrhage and should be reported at once.

1. cyanosis — may come and go or be constant.
2. abnormal respirations — grunting sounds, irregular, noisy (Cheyne-Stokes), slow, shallow, rapid. Very slow breathing is a critical sign.
3. convulsions — twitching of the lower jaw (with or without salivation), mild somewhat local twitching to spasms of the entire body.
4. cry — weak, shrill, or sharp.
5. spasticity — may be generalized to include backward arching of the neck and head with the legs extended.

MEDICAL TREATMENT AND NURSING CARE. The extent of damage determines how effective curative treatment will be. The focus of nursing care is to not move/handle the infant anymore than is absolutely needed. This means that feeding is done with the least possible movement; no breast feeding, weighing or bathing. The head is slightly elevated above the level of the hips. Sedatives may be ordered as well as oxygen and antibiotics.

Other birth injuries include facial and arm paralysis, fracture of bones, dislocation of joints and pronounced moulding of the head.

Respiratory Distress

Postnatal asphyxia. Asphyxia means too little oxygen (anoxia) and too much carbon dioxide in the blood and tissues due to respiratory difficulties. The newborn should cry at once after birth to start his lung expansion. A brief pause of 30 seconds or so causes the infant to turn bright red and to resist having his mouth opened. Longer periods of no breathing produce skin pallor and the body is limp. Anoxia can occur in the uterus, and it accounts for many fetal deaths as well as permanent brain damage. Failure to breathe may be due to mucus obstructing air passages, an overdrugged mother, a congenital defect of the heart/lungs, or a cerebral injury, or a combination of these.

Failure of the newborn (or the mother) to breathe gets immediate action from delivery room personnel. Resuscitation equipment should be at hand and in working order for immediate use to save life—the infant's and the mother's, if needed. The baby should be kept as warm as possible while receiving treatment (heated crib, warm blankets, etc.) and the naked body protected when handled.

Atelectasis. This condition means a collapsed or airless state of the lungs. In the uterus, the lungs are collapsed and hold no air. The first lusty cry after birth starts lung expansion (which is gradually completed in several days). Factors which can prevent full lung expansion are blockage of the small air passages (e.g., mucus, deformity) and/or partial lung development.

Treatment includes: a clear airway, oxygen, high humidity, antibiotics (to prevent infections), position changes and sniffs of carbon dioxide to stimulate respirations.

Infections

The prevention of infection is uppermost in the mind of nursery personnel. Strict aseptic practices must be followed at all times to avoid infections and there must be continuous observation for any possible indication of infection in an infant.

If there is *any* sign of infection, the infant is removed from the regular nursery and is placed in strict isolation. The remaining babies are observed closely and new infants are not placed in the regular nursery, but are set apart in another room. This requires three sets of personnel because each group stays within its environment to prevent any cross-contamination and to prevent the spread of airborne organisms.

All personnel—in each of the three areas—observe strict aseptic practices as to clothing, gown and mask techniques, handwashing, handling of equipment, and disposal of wastes; they make close observations of the infants under their care to detect any change that might indicate the spread of the infection.

Infections may attack the skin, the gastrointestinal tract, the respiratory tract, or the nervous system. In the newborn, infection fast becomes an over-all debilitating condition. Fluid balance is of serious concern. Even mild diarrhea can, in a short time, dehydrate the infant, robbing tissue cells of the electrolytes and fluids needed to function properly. The heat regulating center is easily thrown off balance, creating fever problems which add to the dehydration problem. The newborn has little reserve with which to fight infection; his assistance must come from additional fluids, drugs, and nourishment and from equipment in the hands of skillful personnel.

Personnel with any type of infection, respiratory or otherwise, should not work in the nursery. Organisms can be airborne as well as spread by direct contact. The newborn is unable to cope with infections; his care and treatment become critical to saving his life.

SUMMARY

The newborn has some built-in capacities to help him get started. He can suck and swallow to get nourishment, and can sneeze, cough, and cry to call attention to himself. He learns almost at once who feeds, protects, and loves him and thus feels safe in her presence.

Safe care for the newborn includes strict aseptic practices and techniques that protect his health and provide for his safety and well-being.

A great proportion of all neonatal deaths is due to congenital deformities, birth injuries, postnatal asphyxia, and atelectasis.

GUIDES FOR STUDY AND DISCUSSION

1. What abilities does a normal newborn possess?
2. How do his vital signs compare with those of an adult?
3. What does a newborn "ask" out of life to start with?
4. When giving an infant a bath, what precautions are taken to prevent infection? to provide safety?

5. How can you tell when an infant is adequately nourished?

6. What are the advantages of breast feeding?

7. Why are some babies bottle fed?

8. What is lacking in both human and cow's milk that the infant needs? How does he get it?

9. What is the feeding problem with a newborn having a cleft lip and cleft palate?

10. What are the signs of possible brain hemorrhage in the newborn?

SUGGESTED SITUATIONS AND ACTIVITIES

1. Using Table 53–1 as a guide, prepare some type of visual aid that will show an adequate diet for a nursing mother for one day. Show costs for each meal. Would this food be obtainable on a low-cost food budget?

2. Make a list of the questions postpartum mothers ask you. Keep track of your answers. Be ready to compare these questions and answers with your classmates. See how many are similar.

3. What would you do if:

    a. You noticed a sign of diarrhea in the nursery?

    b. An infant insisted on sleeping on the same side all of the time?

    c. A newborn suddenly had a shrill, weak cry?

4. Visit the delivery room and view the resuscitation equipment. Who is responsible for its working order? Who uses it?

CHAPTER 54

NURSING THE CHILD AND THE ADOLESCENT

TOPICAL HEADINGS

Introduction
Essential Needs and
　Special Considera-
　tions
Admitting the Child
　to the Hospital
Nursing Problems
Adaptation of Nur-
　sing Measures

Signs and Symptoms
　of Illness
Reasons for Hos-
　pitalizing Children
Communicable Dis-
　eases Common to
　Childhood

Other Infectious Dis-
　eases of Children
Summary
Guides for Study and
　Discussion
Suggested Situations
　and Activities

OBJECTIVES FOR THE STUDENT: Be able to:

1. Name five factors which make nursing a child different from nursing an adult.
2. Describe two normal development patterns of the adolescent that may influence his nursing care.
3. Given a negative child-patient reaction situation, tell how to proceed to establish improved relationships.
4. Tell how providing safety for the ill child differs from that of the adult patient.
5. Compare the techniques for taking the temperature, pulse and respirations of a child with those for the adult.
6. Tell how communicable diseases are spread.
7. Distinguish between the purpose of isolation technique and that of surgical asepsis.
8. Give two reasons why immunization is a good health practice.
9. Name ten conditions/diseases common to both children and adults.
10. Name five conditions/diseases more common among children than adults.
11. Describe two differences between making observations of a sick child and of an adult patient.

SUGGESTED STUDY VOCABULARY*

adaptation	confidence	convulsion
foot drop	temporal artery	jaundice
stressful situation	carotid artery	obstruction
rehabilitation	injection sites	postnatal asphyxia
physical therapy	rectum	suicide
dependence	colon	laceration
independence	cyanotic	isolation technique
restraint	congenital deformities	communicable disease
fatigue		asepsis

---

*Look for any terms you already know.

INTRODUCTION

The nursing measures used for adult patients are useful (sometimes with adaptations) in caring for children and adolescents. The purposes, safety factors, and principles or facts that guide your action are the same. Body diseases and disorders are common to young and old; it is difficult to name diseases that attack only one or the other. Apply this same reasoning to signs and symptoms. Turn to Chapter 41 and examine the many signs and symptoms of illness listed there that are found among all ages.

What, then, makes the difference between nursing the child and the adult? Several important factors stand out. His size requires greater care in handling, smaller equipment, and smaller drug dosages. His social adjustment is family-centered, and being hospitalized takes him away from his family, so he has to adjust to strangers if he is to feel secure. His need for physical safety is greater because his environment is different. One of his greatest problems may be loneliness and inability to communicate with or relate to others. Being ill is something he may not be able to understand. He is fretful and restless, or he finds it difficult to follow directions about eating, resting, taking medicine, and receiving treatments. In contrast to that of the mature adult, the general management of a child calls for ability to help him feel secure and accept, as much as possible, his surroundings and what is happening to him.

To make meaningful observations and to understand the child's behavior, you must associate him with what is normal for a person his age. Unit IV in general and Chapters 19 and 20 in particular are good back-up content. Chapter 41 has already been mentioned for signs and symptoms, observations, and nursing care. Unit IX is the "patient-needs" structure for learning to assist all patients with their daily living essentials. Appendix III shows what adaptations in nursing procedures must be considered when they are used with children.

This chapter does not attempt to repeat diseases and disorders included in Unit X. Children and adolescents are included in much of that discussion. The focus here is upon special considerations—the precautions, adjustments, and adaptations that are necessary for this patient because of his age, size, and emotional and social behavior.

ESSENTIAL NEEDS AND SPECIAL CONSIDERATIONS

Keep in mind that the severity of the patient's condition has everything to do with how and how much personal care should or will be provided. His state of dependence or independence and his ability to move, take nourishment, and generally tolerate or participate in his daily care will all influence his need for assistance.

Bath and Personal Hygiene

Most children require the assistance of a nurse for some or all personal hygiene. The infants and very young children are bathed by the nurse. Older children may be able to attend to some or all of their personal hygiene themselves, relying on the nurse to assist them with the difficult things and to assemble their materials and equipment. The adolescent will appreciate privacy, whether he participates in self-care or is assisted by the nurse. He is likely to be particular about his appearance, and will not want to be rushed if he is involved in self-care activities. Young patients can be helped to clean their teeth and nails and to comb their hair, and they may be taught new health habits. They respond to a bath and personal care in much the same way as adults do; they like it and show that they do, especially if it resembles their home habits of care or they feel secure and friendly with the nurse.

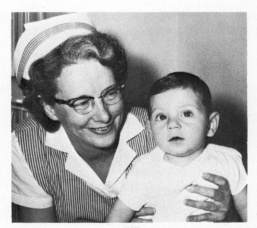

FIGURE 54–1 This young patient seems satisfied with his nurse. (Courtesy Polk County Practical Nursing Program. Bartow, Florida.)

Personal care time is observation time. During the bath there is opportunity to note such things as the condition of the skin, discolored areas, swelling, restriction of motion in any part, evidence of discomfort, and general well-being. He may furnish some clues, subjective or objective, about how he feels. During personal care you have an opportunity to improve relationships and to help the patient feel secure and cooperative (Fig. 54–1).

Clothing for the bed patient is lightweight and comfortably loose to allow freedom of movement and to permit easy access to the body for treatments and care. Robes, slippers, or street clothes are worn by ambulatory patients, depending on what is available and what the patient needs. Whatever he wears should fit him so that he does not feel out of place, or trip and fall because it is too large.

Rest and Sleep

Children require more sleep and rest than adults; this is true in both health and illness. The amount of sleep varies with the age of the child and his condition. If he is in traction or otherwise inhibited (i.e., respirator, casts, I.V. fluid injection) his position will have to remain fairly constant. Sometimes it is necessary to restrain certain parts of the body. These factors may make him restless and wakeful. A clean dry bed and gown contribute to his comfort; a glass of milk or other nourishment may help. If the patient is young, your presence may help quiet him.

Find out from the parents if the child has sleeping habits at home that might be upset by being in the hospital. The child himself may furnish clues that can be helpful at bedtime.

The room should be dimly lighted, reasonably cool, and quiet. When children of varying ages are in the same room it may be difficult to maintain quiet. Provide quiet bedtime diversion. Taking a favorite toy to bed should be possible in the hospital as well as at home.

During the evening and night observe children frequently; they do not use the same means to make their needs known. If treatments are being carried out (e.g., I.V. fluids, steam inhalation) observation should be more frequent than it is for adults who might be able to call if they need help.

Nutrition and Fluids

The sick child may be put on special diets, just as adults are, when they are needed. The child and adolescent need nourishment to promote growth as well as body repair; this makes it essential to see that diets are consumed. This may be a challenge to you.

Adolescents in particular are apt to consume restricted foods or to refuse to eat a prescribed diet. When this occurs, try to determine what, if any, variation may be allowed and let them help decide what to order.

Ambulatory patients should eat together if there are facilities for this. Assist those who need help and encourage all who can to help themselves. Stay with them if at all possible and help make mealtime a pleasant experience (See Fig. 54–2).

The bed patient needs to have his tray conveniently located and as securely placed as possible to avoid spilling mishaps. When a child is upset or refuses to eat for some reason, the nurse should take time and use patience in trying to help him. If the problem persists, discuss it with the charge nurse. The nutritionist may be able to make some helpful suggestions.

The habit of washing the hands before and after meals should be observed. Likewise, it is a nursing responsibility to observe appetites and whether or not the patient eats his food.

Elimination

Children void more frequently than adults; this means that the bed patient will need the bedpan more often. Stay with the child using the bedpan if there is any question of his safety or his needing assistance. Do not keep him waiting too long for the bedpan or for having it removed. If the child was a bed wetter before being hospitalized, he no doubt will continue as a patient. It is not very realistic to try to break him of this habit while he is away from home in strange surroundings.

Hand washing should follow the use of the bedpan or toilet.

Body Alignment and Activity

Good posture and proper body alignment are encouraged whether the patient is prone in bed, up on a back rest, or walking around the

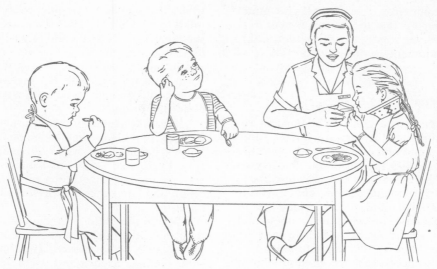

FIGURE 54–2   Mealtime is a convenient time to further develop good relationships with children.

ward. The body not only needs every assistance to re-establish proper functions, but proper alignment prevents deformity. The upright position or the straight relaxed position in bed contributes to good body functioning. Changing the position of the infant and young child frequently during the day helps to prevent fatigue, stimulates good circulation, and contributes to general comfort. Moving about in bed during the day is a form of exercise. This is important to relieve muscle strain and prevent deformities. A foot rest properly placed in bed permits the child to press his feet against something firm. This, too, is a form of exercise and will prevent foot drop.

If the child's body is to be held in one position, pillows or sandbags against both sides of the part will keep it in place. The weight of the bed clothing may be kept off the legs and feet or a part of the body by placing a cradle over the part and making the bed over his support. Diversional activities help to relieve the monotony of long hours in restricted positions.

Keep in mind that children like to move about by nature. If the patient's condition requires that he remain in bed, but he is not otherwise restricted or immobile, find out if he may be allowed to dangle his feet over the side of the bed, flex his knees onto his stomach, do low bicycle motions on his back, or raise and lower his arms while he counts slowly. Hand,

arm, and leg exercises can relieve body strain and, perhaps more important, can provide fun for the patient. Any such activity should have the approval of the physician. Discuss this with the charge nurse to be sure that any such activity is within the physician's order of treatment.

Environment

Young patients enjoy a pleasant, cheerful environment. Decorations should be something they can understand, such as well-known storybook and cartoon characters.

Pediatric departments often have playrooms into which patients are wheeled in chairs or cribs to join in activities with ambulatory children. Food trays may be served there as well as between-meal nourishment. Volunteer workers frequently are assigned to escort patients to this area and remain with them as nursing personnel are seldom free enough of other responsibilities to give constant attention to the activities and the safety of the patients.

An adolescent may be sharing a room with older patients. Some feel that this arrangement is good for both age groups. Just remember that the adolescent wants privacy and personal possessions in his environment.

While the housekeeping department is responsible for daily cleaning, see that the patient's environment is clean and safe at all times. This means that the floor is free of hazards, surfaces are kept free of dirt and litter, and unit equipment is properly cleaned and stored.

Medical Treatment and Care

It is obvious the child or adolescent receives medicines and treatments for the same reasons that adults receive them, and that the same safety factors are observed in carrying them out. The difference in providing these services to the young patient concerns his development, size, and possible inability to cooperate because he does not understand what is wrong or why he is ill. He may be frightened or just obstinate and stubborn.

The nurse needs to have an approach to sick children that makes her acceptable to them and make them, in turn, feel friendly toward her. The same can be said for all other members of the team too. Sick children are dependent upon medical and nursing personnel in ways that adults are not. Children need obvious tenderness and caring. They respond to this and come to feel secure even when treatments are provided. Not all health personnel are able to extend overt understanding and caring to children.

Emotional Adjustments

Often hospitalization of the child is more difficult for the parents than for the patient. The mother in particular, when she visits or remains with the child, is quite alert to the manner and approach of the nurse (e.g., how she relates to and communicates with the child, how the child responds, how she handles him if he cries or is shy).

Parents can be helpful, and they deserve to feel welcome, because they in turn can help their children. It is an improvement in today's hospitals to see mothers staying with their children. To make his experience as meaningful and bearable as possible for the mother, who quite naturally is worried and concerned, offer to let her assist with her child's care if this is possible. She may be better able to get the child to eat than anyone else; she knows how to entertain him or divert his attention because she knows his habits and interests. You may be able to learn things about the patient from her that will help you when the mother is not present (e.g.,

toilet, eating, and sleeping habits). Keep in mind that, while it is not the chief purpose of the hospital to train a child in his living habits, he may learn some health habits such as washing his hands at certain times, brushing his teeth, and helping with his personal hygiene if he is old enough to be interested and if his condition permits.

Show consideration for parents who stay for long periods of time by being certain they know what facilities are available for food and rest. Prolonged stays are usually due to the serious state or uncertainty of the child's condition and can be very stressful situations for parents.

When the child is hospitalized for a long time, his relationship with the nurse and the physician is strengthened. He comes to consider them as friends and is comfortable with them, if their approach warrants it. The mother usually finds after a few days that she is unable to stay for long periods, so the child begins to adjust to new faces and to make new friends.

The adolescent may or may not adjust rapidly to long-term illness. He may be so anxious about what he is missing on the outside that he will pretend he is not sick, and his behavior is a challenge to any nurse. This is more apt to be true if the nurse and patient are near the same age.

Answering parents' questions about specific progress of the child or the probable outcome of the disease is the responsibility of the doctor. While you may be the convenient one to secure information from, use good judgment and a friendly manner in offering to secure someone to help them.

Diversional Activities and Rehabilitation

Toys are an important part of a child's life. He may not be permitted to take his own toys into the ward, but hospital toys may be satisfactory substitutes.

During the acute stage of illness a child may need little diversion. As he recovers he will become acquainted with his surroundings and the other patients. Toys and books within his reading ability help him pass the time, and parents may read to their child when they come to visit him. If you can find time to play with the patient, it may be easier to establish good relationships. Volunteer workers often read to groups of children. Children are curious about what is happening, and will talk with the nurse and others as they go by the cubicle doors or the foot of the bed. The radio, television, and record player afford diversional activity. They usually are in the playroom for small children. Adolescents may have their own radio or may be in a room where it and television are available. Volunteer workers may bring books to the patients on a regular schedule.

Certain children will require additional therapy, which will be carried out by specially trained personnel. Sometimes the patient is taken to a special department for physical therapy; sometimes the staff member works with the patient in his room. When a patient is receiving special therapy, find out what you should be aware of and what you should and should not do when you are caring for him so that your care is in keeping with the rehabilitation plan.

Children who are physically handicapped and who must exercise to regain strength and body movement will need help and encouragement from the nurse. Involve the patient in as much self-help activity as permitted; help him maintain as much independence as possible.

Long-term patients of school age have a problem (Fig. 54–3). Making up schoolwork with the help of a tutor or of the teacher will keep the child busy and will prevent his falling behind the rest of his classmates.

ADMITTING THE CHILD TO THE HOSPITAL

There are many ways to prepare a child for leaving home, being with strangers, and being hospitalized. Children learn to be with others through many experiences (i.e., baby sitters, nursery school, and school). If parents take time to determine that such experiences, especially for the young child, are satisfying and leave the child with a feeling of security, being a patient in a hospital need not be as much of an adjustment for him.

A visit to a hospital when the child is well so that he comes to accept it on a friendly basis is a good practice. In this way his first association with it is not related to something that "hurts." He comes to know it as a place to go when one is sick. Very often children play doctor and nurse, and this play helps them to feel that hospital personnel are friendly people who want to help sick people get well.

The child's adjustment to his hospitalization depends upon his age and how accustomed he is to having "outsiders" with him. The very young child does not understand needed changes; his greatest help will come from being cared for by people who make him feel secure and loved. No one in the hospital plays a more important role in this than the nurse.

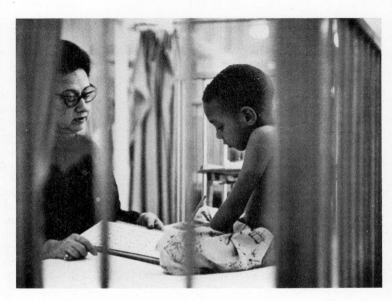

FIGURE 54–3 This child is on bedrest and cannot be taken to the classroom in the hospital with other children. The schoolteacher therefore visits him in his room and helps him gain the satisfaction of keeping up with his class. (Courtesy of Children's Hospital of Philadelphia, Public Relations Department.)

Each hospital has its own procedure for admitting a patient. The admitting officer secures information (personal history of child's likes, habits, and any allergies may be supplied then or later) from the parent, and the patient is examined in the emergency room, an examining room or taken to his room and examined there. Depending upon the circumstances (e.g., child's condition, parent's condition, hospital policies) the parents may or may not be present while the doctor examines the child (see Chapter 28). The nurse assists, perhaps as much by comforting the patient (or parents) and making it possible for the doctor to proceed as in any other way. If the child needs to be restrained, it should be done as gently and quickly as possible. Resistance to restrained movements comes soon for the young patient; he does not like being forcibly held.

Putting the Child to Bed

Whether the patient's bed or crib is alone in a room or one of several, it should be the proper size for his comfort and equipped for his protection. High side rails are standard equipment for children's beds to prevent falls and discourage climbers. Crib-net restraints are commonly used to keep children in bed (Fig. 54–4).

Personal clothing is cared for by parents or stored. The bedside table is equipped with necessary articles for personal hygiene. While the doctor makes his initial observations during the examination, the nurse has responsibility to continue observing for anything that may have been overlooked or that develops as she prepares the child for his bed.

NURSING PROBLEMS

Behavior

Much has already been said about helping the child to adjust to and cooperate in his care. As with any person, the child brings his behavior with him. What he does outside the sickroom to meet his needs, he will do in the sickroom as well—but to a greater degree. In many ways no patient has more need for kindness than the sick child. He has little or no ability to understand why he is sick or what it means. Firm, gentle kindness must be used with good judgment in providing his care; it stands to reason he cannot have his own way about everything. But it is important for the child to experience a warm, friendly person in the nurse who cares for him.

Signs and Symptoms

Sometimes symptoms are not readily apparent; they cannot be seen and the child either cannot or does not tell how he feels. Signs of illness in children tend to appear rapidly, especially in young children. It is not uncommon for a temperature to be elevated very fast, or vomiting to develop suddenly.

Observation for pain requires more than having the patient tell about it; he may not be able to. Facial expressions, body posture, restlessness, and crying may be the most direct evidence of pain.

Signs and symptoms of bladder and bowel difficulties are detected more often by the appearance and the amount of elimination than any other way.

Evidence of appetite or lack of it can be seen, as well as some of the apparent reasons, if the patient is observed during the day.

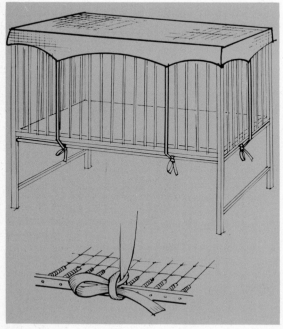

FIGURE 54–4 The crib-net restraint. (Leifer: Principles and Techniques in Pediatric Nursing.)

Obtaining Urine Specimens

When collecting a regular or routine specimen of urine, carefully wash the genitalia and give the child a drink of water. If he is an older child, place him on a bedpan or chamber and he will usually void. If the patient is an infant the problem is more difficult. Figure 54–5 shows how this can be done for both male and female babies. Another method is to use a piece of plastic in place of the regular diaper. After the infant voids, carefully remove the plastic diaper and pour the contents into the

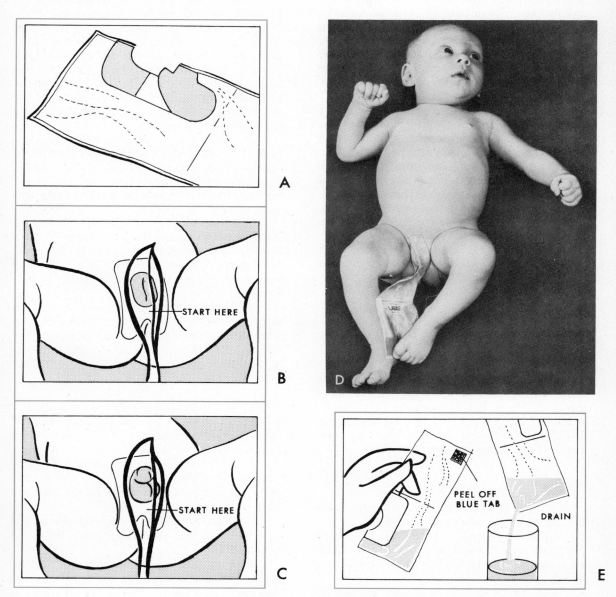

FIGURE 54–5 Hollister's pediatric urine collector for use with both sexes. *A,* Remove protective paper, exposing hypoallergenic adhesive. *B, For girls:* Stretch perineum to remove skin all around the vagina. Be sure to start at the bridge of skin separating the rectum from the vagina and work upward. *C, For boys:* Fit bag over penis and press flaps firmly to perineum, making sure entire adhesive coating is firmly attached to skin with no puckering of adhesive. *D,* Hollister bag in place. *E, To drain:* Hold bag in left hand. Tilt bag so urine is away from blue tab. Remove tab and drain in clean receptacle. (Courtesy Hollister, Chicago, Illinois.)

specimen bottle. A sterile specimen is taken with a catheter in much the same way as for adult patients. See Appendix III — 24 hour urine specimen.

Feeding

Food selection should be within the child's likes (consult child's personal history). New foods can be introduced in small portions without a long discussion over whether or not he will like it. Studies show that children do have preferences for certain foods such as plain meat, ice cream, bread, raw fruit, cereals, and milk.

When a child refuses to eat there is a reason. The problem is to try to learn the reason. Factors such as fatigue, discomfort, an overanxious mother close at hand, a means for getting attention, and no appetite may account for it. While the patient needs nourishment, he should not be forced to eat. After a reasonable time, the tray should be removed and the patient served at the next regular eating time. Parents deserve an explanation of why the tray was removed, and their cooperation should be sought if they can help with the problem.

ADAPTATION OF NURSING MEASURES

Appendix III includes several commonly used nursing procedures, each with a stated purpose. Many list adaptations that can be made for children. The following discussion points out particular considerations in addition to the content in Appendix III.

The Bath

The purpose of the bath is the same for the infant, child, adolescent, or adult.

Smaller children will require full assistance and so will older children if their condition requires it. Encourage any who can to assist.

The room should be warm enough to prevent chilling and the bath materials at hand before starting.

Be sure to use gentle strokes about the eyes, nose, mouth, and ears to prevent injury. Wash body creases, genitalia, and buttocks well, and dry them thoroughly, especially when bathing an infant. Give any needed attention to skin care. Observe safety factors.

Taking the Temperature

In addition to the technique for using the thermometer and taking the temperature, the following points should be emphasized:

1. A rectal thermometer is used, unless contraindicated, because it is more accurate and safe. It is difficult for a child to keep a mouth thermometer in place with the lips closed to obtain an accurate reading. There is also danger that a child may bite and break the thermometer, chewing and even swallowing the glass and mercury.

2. Remain with the child while the thermometer is inserted. The child usually will not remain in position without moving or turning. The thermometer may break, slip out of the rectum, or even slip beyond reach into the rectum.

3. Most children are accustomed to having their temperatures taken at home by their mothers. If the experience is new to the child, or if he is frightened, secure his confidence before starting the procedure, in order to prevent injury.

4. Temperatures are usually not taken during the night or when the child is sleeping. They are taken at stated intervals during the day except when indicated or specially ordered by the physician.

Pulse and Respiration

It is difficult to take an accurate count of the pulse and respiration of a very young child but certain points are important:

1. Observe the type and character of respiration. Any change from the normal or any apparent difficulty should be noted and reported at once.

2. Pulse and respiration are more accurately counted and observed if the young child is asleep.

3. Respiration may be counted during the rise and fall of the abdomen and may be easier and more accurate to observe than that of the chest.

4. Pulse of the young child may be counted by gently placing the finger tips over the temporal artery or the carotid artery at the side of the neck. For babies the hand may be

placed lightly over the fontanel. The radial pulse is usually taken in older children, the same as for adults.

5. Often the type and character of the pulse and respiration are more important to observe than the count.

Taking the Blood Pressure

Specific adaptations for this procedure are included in Appendix III (see Blood Pressure).

Giving Medications

The basic principles for the preparation and administration of medications for children are the same as for adults (see Chapter 30). Other points regarding the giving of medications to the sick child include:

1. The reaction and behavior of the child are often due to the attitude and approach of the nurse. If you use a friendly and kind but firm manner the child will usually accept and follow your directions.

2. Some medications may be diluted or mixed with drink or food to disguise the taste. Often this method is used to be certain the child has taken all of the medication.

3. The capsule may be emptied or the tablet powdered if the child is too young or has difficulty swallowing either. The medication is then mixed with a small amount of food or drink for swallowing. The older child should be taught how to swallow a tablet or capsule of medication.

4. Any medication that is lost or vomited will probably be repeated. The time and way this is done should be determined by the charge nurse or physician.

5. A favorite cup or a straw may be more acceptable to a child for taking fluids.

6. Care must be taken to avoid breaking the needle when an injection is given. Restrain the child securely. See Figure 54–6 for cases in which only one nurse is involved; a second nurse may be necessary under difficult circumstances. Holding a favorite toy, assuming a certain position, or giving a "count down" are examples of how the child may have his attention diverted.

7. Because of the muscular development of small children, the sites for administering intramuscular injections differ from those for older children and adults (Fig. 54–7).

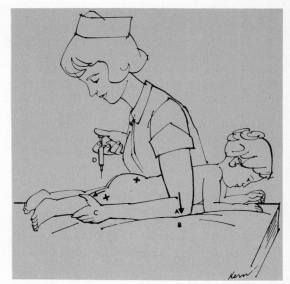

FIGURE 54–6 Restraining a child for the administration of an intramuscular injection. (Leifer: Principles and Techniques in Pediatric Nursing, 2nd Ed.)

Giving an Enema

Specific adaptations for this procedure are included in Appendix III (see Enemata).

Reducing an Elevated Temperature

See Appendix III (Baths-Therapeutic) for adaptations.

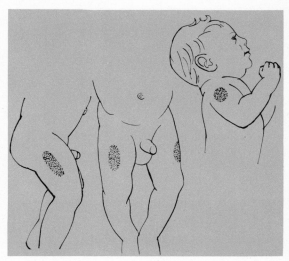

FIGURE 54–7 The shaded areas show appropriate sites for intramuscular injection for the young infant. (Leifer: Principles and Techniques in Pediatric Nursing, 2nd Ed.)

The physician may order one of several methods to help reduce a high temperature. Cool water given by rectum is one method used. A certain amount of water may be ordered. If the body temperature has not decreased after a certain period of time, the treatment may be repeated. It may be continuous until the temperature is reduced to a certain degree. Before beginning this treatment, know the amount and temperature of water to be used, the degree of body temperature to reach, the length of time the irrigation is to continue, and results which might be expected. The points listed regarding the enema also apply to this method of injecting cool water into the rectum and lower colon.

A tepid sponge bath (cool water or cool water and alcohol) is another measure used to reduce body temperature.

If the child becomes chilled or cyanotic during any of these procedures, the treatment should be stopped. Avoid exposure or prolonged treatment. Usually the temperature of the water ordered is two degrees below body temperature. Observe closely to avoid untoward results.

SIGNS AND SYMPTOMS OF ILLNESS

The child may or may not be able to tell exactly how he feels or where he hurts. Observation must include any and all evidence. Use Chapter 41 along with the following description* of symptoms and indicated abnormal conditions to help you understand what to observe and report.

*Adapted from Lyon and Wallinger: Nursing of Children, 5th Ed.

SYMPTOM	ABNORMAL CONDITION INDICATED
General Appearance	
a. Below normal weight and height	a. Poor nutrition
b. Abnormally thin with the appearance of general fatigue.	b. Some chronic illness, i.e., tuberculosis
c. Overly fat or extremely thin	c. Endocrine disorder, poor nutrition
d. Abnormal bone structure, walk, or posture	d. Congenital deformities
Skin	
a. Flushed, hot skin, dry or with profuse perspiration; dry lips; sleepiness or nervousness; upset disposition.	a. Elevated temperature, infection
b. Rash or vesicles	b. Communicable disease
c. Blisters which become pus pimples and sores on face, hands, and body	c. Impetigo
d. Scratches on neck and back and itching in the hairy areas	d. Lice—body, head, and pubic areas
e. Swelling; edema	e. Kidney condition
f. Enlarged glands and lymph nodes	f. Infection
g. Pallor and cold extremities	g. Possible shock
h. Cyanotic coloring	h. Lack of oxygen
i. Yellowish tinge to whites of eyes and skin	i. Possible jaundice
j. Clammy, cold	j. Subnormal temperature
Facial Expression	
Anxious, drawn, worried	Troubled mentally
Chest	
a. Cough; grunting and wheezing sounds when breathing	a. Infection of the chest or nasopharyngeal passages
b. Retraction of the ribs; neck above the sternum or abdomen below the sternum	b. Obstruction of the larynx
Abdomen	
Hard and rigid, distended, painful when palpated	Infection of the appendix or peritoneum
Stomach	
Nausea and vomiting	Overeating; indigestible food; irritation from some drug; pressure on the brain; toxemia from kidney condition; early indication of some communicable disease; obstruction of the intestine; etc.

Intestines
  a. Diarrhea

  b. Constipation

a. Onset of an illness; bacterial infection; uremia; extreme excitement
b. Poor eating habits; poor health habits; lack of bulk in the diet; poor muscle tone in the intestine

Nervous System
  Convulsions, twitching of all or a part of the body
Crying

Brain injury; acute infection; lack of vitamin D and calcium
Loud—general discomfort, pain
Fretful—hungry
Sharp and high—indigestion, pain

REASONS FOR HOSPITALIZING CHILDREN

Children are hospitalized for many of the reasons which cause adults to be hospitalized; they are exposed to the same general causes of illness, namely: *microorganisms, body deformities and abnormal functions, improper nourishment, accidents, poisons and poisoning, housing as related to health and disease, and heredity.*

Each chapter of Unit X includes general disease conditions found among all age groups. Use that material for reference. See also Chapter 43, Patients with Cancer, and Chapter 53, Nursing the Newborn.

The leading causes of death among children and adolescents indicate the reasons why many children are hospitalized.

The infant under one year: post natal asphyxia, immaturity, congenital malformation, pneumonia, birth injuries and accidents (e.g., mechanical suffocation).

The child from one to four years: accidents, burns, pneumonia, and congenital malformations.

The child from five to 14 years: accidents (e.g., motor vehicle), drowning, cancer, and congenital deformities.

The adolescent to adult years: accidents (majority are motor vehicle), cancer, and suicides.

Illness among infants is often related to some type of malfunction in the body. Because of his size and his limited function in breathing, circulation, or digestion, his condition is questionable. He has very little physical reserve. Improved diagnostic techniques, therapeutic equipment, and surgical procedures have benefitted this age group.

Among all children from over one year old through adolescence, motor vehicle accidents account for the greatest number of deaths. Many children are hospitalized because of fractures, lacerations, internal injuries, bruises, and head and neck injuries.

Burns account for many long-term pediatric patients. Children are curious. They need to see things and to imitate the actions of parents. Lighting matches, poking in an open fire, pulling kettles of hot water or food from the stove, and playing around an open tub of hot water are common causes of burns. Another cause of burns is electricity—playing with electrical outlets and appliances. Experiments with homemade power devices and chemistry sets are responsible for many serious accidents among older children.

Poisoning also accounts for many long-term patients, especially among young children who swallow caustic materials. The average home has dozens of toxic substances (e.g., detergents, insect spray, furniture polish, paints, drugs, and cosmetics) that curious small children will consume if they have access to them.

Cancer is the number one killer of children from age three to 15. Leukemia accounts for about one-half of these deaths; others include cancer of the brain, kidneys, bone, and so on.

Tumors are comparatively rare among children. Children are less able to clearly express their complaints. Diagnosis is often made only when the tumor is big enough to be noticed, which may be too late. They include eye tumors (retinal glioma), which usually at-

(*Text continues on page 704.*)

TABLE 54-1. COMMUNICABLE DISEASES (See Table 27-2 Plan for Routine Protective Immunization)

DISEASE: METHOD OF SPREAD	PREVENTION	INCUBATION	SIGNS AND SYMPTOMS	LENGTH OF CONTAGIOUSNESS	SPECIAL NURSING PROBLEMS AND COMPLICATIONS
Chickenpox Airborne droplets.	None. Immune after one attack.	2-3 weeks; usually 14-16 days.	Mild fever, general malaise, headache, successive crops of small raised areas filled with clear fluid that go on to form crusts. Itching of the skin.	6 days after appearance of rash.	Prevent scratching. Trim finger nails and keep them clean. Ease itching with soothing lotion. Secondary infection may result.
Diphtheria Droplets from respiratory tract of person with disease or carrier.	Active immunization – usually given with whooping cough and tetanus immunization.	1-7 days or longer.	Grayish membrane in throat, nasal discharge irritating to nose and upper lip, fever, harsh cough, nose stopped up, malaise.	Until causative organism disappears from the respiratory tract.	Isolation by aseptic technique. Omit daily bath if patient is very sick; good mouth care. Skin around nares and upper lip cleaned often. Throat irrigations often ordered. Omit all but essential personal hygiene measures if patient is seriously ill. Complications may include: bronchopneumonia, cardiac failure, kidney changes.
Epidemic influenza Airborne droplets.	Active immunization vaccines.	24-72 hours.	Sudden chills, fever, cough, muscle ache.	Not known.	Bed rest, increased fluids. Complications – secondary infection of respiratory tract. Allergic responses may occur if allergic to egg or chicken.
German measles (3-day measles) Direct contact and airborne.	A new vaccine has been prepared	2-3 weeks; usually 18 days.	Cold symptoms, mild fever, pale red rash that fades in 3 days. Enlarged glands at back of neck and behind the ears.	Not known.	Bed rest until fever is gone. Avoid exposing any pregnant woman especially during first trimester; it causes such birth defects as brain damage, blindness, congenital deformities.
Measles Direct contact and airborne.	Passive immunization lasts about 2-3 weeks. Active immunization is now available.	1-2 weeks; usually 10 or 11 days.	Dry cough with cold symptoms, red eyes before rash appears. Koplik spots (red with white centers) in mouth,	Until 5 days after appearance of rash.	Room dimly lighted; protect eyes from hands and relieve itching with eye irrigations. Relieve body itching by tepid bath and lotion. Force fluids

(Table continued on the opposite page.)

TABLE 54-1. COMMUNICABLE DISEASES (Continued)

Disease / Transmission	Prevention	Incubation period	Symptoms	Period communicable	Treatment and nursing care
			high fever, rash, enlarged lymph nodes.		during fever. Complications — middle ear infection, pneumonia, bronchitis, nephritis, encephalitis.
Mumps Contact with salivary secretions.	A new vaccine has been prepared.	14-28 days; usually about 18 days.	Fever, headache. Salivary glands develop painful swelling, as well as other nearby glands. Swelling may occur in one or both sides of face.	Until swelling disappears.	Local heat or cold to swollen glands. Liquid or soft foods. Bed rest until swelling is gone. May be serious for adult patients.
Poliomyelitis (Infantile paralysis) Contamination by nose and throat secretions, intestinal excretions.	Complete the series of one or the other types of vaccine.	5-35 days.	Early signs — slight fever, headache, vomiting. Later signs — intense headache, nausea, vomiting, muscular soreness, stiff neck, and back rigidity.	As long as fever persists.	Hospitalization. See Chapter 49 for nursing care.
Scarlet fever Droplet infection, direct or indirect transmission.	Active immunization — series of injections.	2-3 days.	Headache, rapid pulse, fever, vomiting, rash, red-strawberry tongue, middle and inner ear infections.	From onset to recovery.	Drug treatment to counteract toxins and organisms. Emphasize fluids, pain relief, mouth care, bed rest. Complications — kidney disease and rheumatic fever.
Whooping cough (Pertussis) Airborne.	Active immunization. Given as part of diphtheria, pertussis, tetanus immunization.	5-21 days; usually within 10 days.	Cold symptoms, dry cough in spells (worse at night), with noisy whooping gasp for air. Dyspnea and vomiting may occur.	4-6 weeks.	Provide rest to prevent coughing; warm humid air; avoid chilling. Small feedings; feed again after vomiting. Sedation may be used to quiet patient. Serious illness for small infants. Complications — bronchopneumonia, middle ear infection, hemorrhage during coughing, encephalitis.

tack children under four years of age; brain tumors, some common symptoms of which are blurred and double vision, interference with muscular coordination, vomiting without nausea, drowsiness, headaches, and convulsions; and abdominal tumors, frequently of the kidney, which are usually seen in children under eight years of age.

COMMUNICABLE DISEASES COMMON TO CHILDHOOD

A disease is called communicable when it is spread by direct contact with the infectious means which causes it; they are spread by: 1. Direct contact with body discharges. 2. Open sores and ulcers. 3. Using contaminated objects such as drinking glasses, toys, and clothing—called indirect contact. 4. Some living thing that carries the infectious agent from place to place such as flies or mosquitoes.

Table 54–1 lists some of the more common communicable diseases either prevented by immunization or occurring today.

General Principles of Nursing Care

The patient with a communicable disease must be set apart from other patients to prevent the spread of his disease. Special techniques used to confine the organisms within the patient's unit are called *isolation techniques*.

Isolation is required for most communicable diseases from the first day of infection to the last day on which the patient may be dangerous to others.

The nurse wears a mask and gown while giving nursing care and washes her hands carefully with a brush, a mild soap, and, if possible, in warm running water each time she has cared for the patient, before and after using the gown, and before she eats food. The mask and gown may or may not be disposable. In either case, putting on and removing the gown is done in such a way as to protect the nurse and her uniform and confine the organisms to the patient's unit (medical asepsis).

The patient may be isolated in a special part of the hospital set aside for that purpose or in a hospital for communicable diseases. He may be given care in his own home. Wherever he is, the idea back of his care is to take all precautions in handling body discharges, equipment, and unit refuse that will prevent the spread of organisms.

Nursing Care for the Isolated Patient

Special skin care is usually needed to prevent/relieve itching. Medical orders may include special baths, oiling the body or the use of some ointment; alcohol rubs are not used when a skin rash is present because they are drying and irritating.

The secretions from the eyes, ears, nose, and throat should be removed with tissues or gauze and these soiled tissues put into a paper bag attached to the side of the bed and discarded as required. If nasal discharges irritate the nostrils or the upper lip, this area should be lubricated with petrolatum or some special ointment.

Mouth care helps to prevent or eliminate the unpleasant taste which so often accompanies these diseases. An elevated temperature and mouth breathing cause the lips to parch and crack and require lubrication. Small patients frequently need help with mouth care. Use gentle strokes and movements when cleansing around the eyes, nose, and ears and when giving mouth care.

DIET. The diet and fluids are ordered to prevent loss of weight, to preserve the fluid balance of the body, and to supply an abundance of repair material. Forced liquids and water may be ordered to bring down the temperature and to maintain body nutrition. Fluid intake and output should be measured and recorded on the patient's chart. Regular elimination, bladder and bowel, is essential. Specimens of the urine and the stool may be sent to the laboratory for examination on the physician's order.

The patient in isolation has no visitors except parents and then only under strict rules of conduct to prevent the spread of the disease. Help parents to understand their role in visiting the child who is isolated; they deserve an explanation of what they may and may not do in this situation.

TERMINAL DISINFECTION. When the patient recovers sufficiently to be discharged, he is given a bath, a shampoo, and clean clothing, and is transferred to a clean room or discharged from the hospital.

The hospital unit is cleaned thoroughly. Reuseable equipment must be washed carefully and boiled (if possible) for at least 10 minutes or sterilized in an autoclave to make it safe for use again. Hospital policy governs terminal disinfection and the reuse or discard of articles.

ASEPTIC METHODS IN ISOLATION. To prevent infection for herself and to prevent the spread of disease to others, the nurse follows certain practices of general cleanliness when caring for a patient with a communicable disease.

Hands. Keep your hands clean, soft, and free of cuts and abrasions. This includes scrubbing under running water, whenever they are soiled, especially before eating and after each patient contact. A hand lotion or cream will prevent chapping and cracking of the skin. Cuts and abrasions should receive care at once as broken skin may be the port of entry for organisms which cause an infection.

Secretions (eyes, nose, throat) and excretions (feces and urine) are disposed of in the manner prescribed by the board of health or by hospital policy.

MASK AND GOWN TECHNIQUE. A mask is worn to protect the wearer from the coughs and sneezes of her patient; it is changed when damp.

The gown is a large cover-all with short or long sleeves. In isolation it is worn to protect the wearer's clothing. The nurse wears a gown to protect her uniform from contamination so that when she removes it (according to procedure), she leaves the contamination in the patient's room and avoids transporting it to others.

To Put on a Gown. The hands are scrubbed clean; the dry hands and arms are slipped through the sleeves of the gown without touching the outside. It is fastened at the neck with strings and at the waist with strings that cross at the back and tie in the front. The hands are washed again.

To Remove the Gown. The strings at the waist are untied, the hands are washed. The strings at the neck are untied, brought to the front, and tied loosely together. The hands are slipped out of the sleeves to the shoulders of the gown. The one shoulder of the gown is turned over the other to fold the gown in half with the outside turned inward. The shoulder seams are held together. The gown is hung on a hook on a clean wall by the tied neck strings of the gown. The hands are scrubbed a second time. This is one way to safely use a gown. There are others, all based upon the same need to keep the contamination confined to the patient's unit. If the gown is disposable, it is put into a container designated for that purpose.

OTHER INFECTIOUS DISEASES OF CHILDREN

While the following diseases are found in all age groups, they do occur most frequently among infants and children and present particular nursing problems.

Impetigo occurs more readily among infants than among older children and adults because infants lack resistance. It is caused by an organism that invades the outer layers of the skin and is readily transmitted from one child to another, for example, in the nursery. Strict isolation technique is required for the care of this patient; antibiotic ointments and drugs are most often used under a specific plan of medical management.

Scabies is caused by the female itch mite that burrows under the skin and deposits eggs. The areas most frequently involved are those between the toes and fingers, on the wrists, in the axillae, on the abdomen, and around the genitals. The mite is easily transferred from one person to another.

The disease is cured when the mite is killed, but this involves treating every infected person in the household at the same time. All bed linen and clothing must be boiled or dry cleaned. Treatment includes relieving the itching.

Ringworm is a fungus infection that affects the scalp, skin, and feet. Ringworm of the scalp is slow to respond to treatment; treatment includes shaving the head, thoroughly washing each area daily, and applying some type of fungicide. Ringworm of the feet is picked up at swimming pools and in public shower stalls.

Pinworms are parasites that invade the large intestine, cause infection, lay thousands of eggs in the area of the anus, and cause severe itching. The eggs are spread from one person to another, especially when groups live in close contact and hygiene habits are poor. Contamination (eggs) is carried on hands from scratching, on soiled clothing, soiled bedding, or on contaminated objects put to the mouth, and the cycle starts over again.

The treatment involves the use of drugs (anthelmintics) which in themselves are dangerous and must be given exactly as ordered. If the child is being treated at home, the mother needs to thoroughly understand the exact dosage of the drug and adhere to strict hand hygiene for the child. All articles (e.g., clothing, towels, bed linen, toilet seat) should be thoroughly cleaned daily. Clothes are boiled to kill the eggs; objects are scrubbed.

In the hospital the child is kept apart from others and strict measures are used to sterilize the bedpan and handle the linen.

SUMMARY

There is much that is the same in caring for a sick adult and caring for a sick child. They have the same diseases and disorders, show the same signs and symptoms, need many of the same treatments, and have the same essential daily needs.

The differences in providing effective, safe care for the child arise from his size and state of physical development, his state of social development, and his limitation in communicating. He is not capable of understanding why he is sick or what is happening to him. One of the main qualities of effective nursing care is the expression of caring as well as providing the care. The sick child needs to feel secure when he is hospitalized and the nurse can be a most important person in providing this feeling of security.

Nursing measures are adjusted to the patient's size and physical development. Observations are more difficult when the patient cannot tell how he feels or what he is experiencing.

Visting parents need consideration when their children are ill; they are concerned and anxious and should be provided every possible thoughtful consideration.

GUIDES FOR STUDY AND DISCUSSION

1. What are the main characteristics of the adolescent? How might these qualities influence his behavior when he is a patient?

2. In your opinion, what are the most outstanding differences between caring for an ill child and caring for an adult?

3. What personal capacities do you possess that can be used to strengthen your relationships with a sick child? What capacities do you need to improve?

4. What is similar about immobilizing a body part of a child and one of an adult? What factors may differ?

5. What are the benefits of frequent changes of bed position?

6. Why are nursing personnel especially aware of the child's safety?

7. What adaptations are made for the toddler when carrying out the following nursing measures: taking the temperature, taking the pulse, counting the respirations, administering an intramuscular injection, giving an enema?

8. Why is making subjective observations of a child different from that of an adult? How can you tell a toddler is having pain? What kind of pain?

9. Why is immunization important? Why are not all children immunized as recommended?

10. What is the purpose(s) behind isolation technique?

11. The diet of the patient with a communicable disease is expected to serve several useful purposes. What are they?

12. Using Unit X as source material, complete this chart in your notebook. Be ready to compare your list with others.

Ten Medical-Surgical Conditions Common to Children/Adolescents			
Conditions/ Diseases	Signs/ Symptoms	Treatment/ Care	Adaptations in Nursing Care

SUGGESTED SITUATIONS AND ACTIVITIES

1. In each of the following situations, decide how you would proceed. Be ready to explain what you would do.

     a. The physician has just ordered a tepid sponge for a six-year-old who has a high temperature. You are to give it. The mother is present and is very anxious about her child and about what you are going to do.

     b. An 18-year-old boy refuses to take his medicine.

     c. A two-year-old child is awake and crying at 2 A.M.

     d. An eight-year-old girl refuses to eat her lunch because her mother did not stay to feed her.

2. There are advantages and disadvantages in having an adolescent patient share a room with an elderly patient. Be ready to argue either for or against the idea.

member of the mental health team giving direct assistance to these patients. There are many employment opportunities for the LPN in this field and your basic program provides an excellent foundation for future skill development in this field.

There is no accurate way to know how far-reaching are the three health problems of mental illness, alcoholism, and mental retardation. As yet people are not as free to face them as they are to face physical health problems, but this aspect of the situation is showing improvement in our society. Wide-spread efforts on the part of government, voluntary agencies, news media, and concerned citizens are bringing the problems into the open. Any disgrace attached to these problems is gradually being replaced with understanding. Newer treatments and attitudes have unlocked the doors of many institutions where, in the past, patients were held apart from society with little or no help to rejoin it.

Change in attitudes unfolds slowly and there is a distance to go in helping family members and society in general to dispel their fear and prejudice and accept the fact that mental and behavioral problems are not shameful occurrences but disorders which can and do happen.

MENTAL ILLNESS

Man's mind and body influence each other as they work together. The mind has the ability to become excited and to set off a variety of emotions. In turn, mind and emotions influence the physical body. Recall an instance when you were excited, perhaps waiting for something unusual to happen and the palms of your hands were moist or your heart beat faster than usual. Everyone experiences emotions and could not exist without them. The person who is able to keep his emotions within normal bounds is able to behave accordingly.

Each individual is surrounded by sights, sounds, objects, and people, all of which make up his environment and he reacts to them. People are a particularly important part of that environment. Man is involved with and dependent upon others. He must find his place among his fellow men, or life becomes meaningless and he loses his place in the scheme of things.

When a person is unable to cope with his environment, or feels he cannot find meaning in his relationships with other people, he feels threatened. His self-esteem and self-confidence are harmed, and he tries to protect them. He withdraws from the environment that threatens him and tries to remake it so that he is comfortable in it. A person who is mentally ill acts in ways that have meaning for him and that safeguard his image of himself and his self-esteem, but to other people, who do not know what he feels threatened by, his behavior, moods, interests, habits, and speech do not seem normal or meaningful. This individual is helped only when his environment is made less threatening to him.

Terms for Mental Disorders

In mental illness, as in physical illness, there are different conditions, bearing different names.

INSANITY. The term insanity is a legal one, used by the courts and meaning unsoundness of mind. It indicates that the person is not capable of being at liberty or free to act on his own. Insanity is defined by law in different ways in the various states; its basis in law makes it a legal rather than a medical term. Medical personnel choose medical terms rather than legal ones in referring to these patients.

PSYCHOSIS. This is a medical term for prolonged thought and behavior disorders, such as paranoid and schizophrenic psychoses.

PSYCHONEUROSIS. This term includes a variety of feelings that in part overwhelm the patient (e.g., anxiety, inadequacy, inability to handle a situation). He is in touch with life as it is lived, but does not feel equal to its demands. The personality remains more or less intact, but anxiety is high.

PERSONALITY DISORDERS. This is a broad term including such things as chronic alcoholism and psychopathic personality—lack of emotional maturity, unwillingness to take responsibility, and possibly lying or stealing, or addiction to narcotics. This individual does not grow up in thought and action, and he gets into trouble because of his immaturity.

CHANGE IN BRAIN FUNCTION. When changes in brain tissue occur they can produce changes in personality and behavior. Things that damage the brain and change its function are injury, arteriosclerosis, alcoholism, and central nervous system diseases. Noticeable changes are seen in relation to judgment, memory, learning, and orientation as to time and place.

MENTAL ILLNESS AND THE EFFORTS OF SOCIETY

World War II caused us to take a hard look at mental illness because so many men were rejected for military service because of mental instability. What were the causes and what was being done for patients? How were they cared for? The Mental Health Act passed in 1946 led the way for improvements which have been slowly coming ever since. A boost to these efforts came in 1963 when Congress passed a law (Community Mental Health Centers Act) that provided for community-based facilities and programs (prevention, treatment, rehabilitation) within reach of large numbers of local people rather than a limited few as in the past when most mentally ill persons were "sent away" to large institutions behind locked doors for years and perhaps for life.

Moving mental health facilities to more local communities has another distinct advantage. The attitude of the general public toward mental illness changes as people see that it is treatable (and no disgrace) and that, through rehabilitative programs, many people are gainfully returned to society. The general public is asked to support local efforts and, in turn, the public calls upon the community mental health team to help with local problems (e.g., drug abuse, juvenile delinquency).

In brief, the improvements in the field of mental health/illness over the past 25 years include: bringing mental health facilities closer to the people (e.g., clinics, local hospital facilities, area services), stressing prevention and rehabilitation as well as treatment, protecting patients without barring windows and locking "cell doors," educating the public to accept mental illness without feeling disgraced by it or fearful of it, and training all types of personnel.

TREATMENT TODAY

One of the most noticeable differences in treatment today is the fact that treatment is more apt to be short-term than long-term. Drugs have been contributing to this change since about 1953. While the drugs do not cure mental illness, they do help to control such symptoms as purposeless overactivity, destructive behavior, confusion, hallucinations, and delusions. Two such drugs are Thorazine and Serpasil; the dosage and the length of time the drug is taken varies considerably from one patient to another. Each patient's symptoms are assessed before drugs are prescribed so that he will get the right amount of relief. The patient has to understand the necessity for taking the drugs as prescribed so that his symptoms are controlled in the proper way. Even then it is possible for some unwanted side effects to appear.

The community mental health center is equipped to provide inpatient services, outpatient services, emergency services, partial hospitalization, and consultation and education. These five types of service in a community represent a tremendous improvement over the past, when deviant behavior (e.g., threatened suicide, alcoholism, destructive acts) put the patient in jail (it still does, if there is no provision in the local hospital for caring for these patients).

Another noticeable change in treatment is the emphasis on rehabilitation, which is "retraining to live in society." In addition to drug therapy, the patient is helped to develop work skills, work habits, proper attitudes toward work, counselling, and work placement. He is not left on his own to make the adjustment or fail to make it; he receives assistance. Rehabilitation is also coming to include social rehabilitation (e.g., personal hygiene, daily grooming, and taking responsibility for home and living needs).

Three factors that limit progress are a serious lack of trained personnel in the mental health field, a lack of time and money to study the problems and find solutions, and the fact that the public is still unaware of the needs of these discharged patients and is not always willing to aid them or accept them back into the home and community and on the job.

ALCOHOLISM

"An alcoholic is a person who drinks when he does not want to drink and this interferes with his way of life. He uses alcohol as a tranquilizer to calm feelings of anxiety, to fight feelings of depression, or to avoid facing problems directly. The use of alcohol . . . interferes with his interpersonal relationships."* Alcoholism is a serious health problem in this country. It reaches into all parts of society, affecting men and women of all ages and from all types of home situations. In addition to the alcoholic himself, the family and community are deeply involved.

From the standpoint of just dollars and cents alone, each year almost half a billion dollars are lost because of absenteeism from work. Another two billion dollars are used for treatment. Business and industry have joined hands with medical science and government to help find ways to assist alcoholics.

From the standpoint of human misery, the individual and his family members suffer endlessly unless they are helped to understand the nature of alcoholism. The alcoholic drinks to cover up his feelings of insecurity and depression; he seems incapable of facing problems and carrying responsibilities. The family is apt to feel that he could stop drinking if he just wanted to; this leads to extreme frustration for all concerned. They also feel that the problem is a disgrace and try to hide it from others. Obviously, the family members need assistance as well as the patient. They need to understand that the compulsive drinker can do little under his own power and that all the scolding and shaming in the world is not going to change him. The alcoholic's first step is to admit to himself and others that he has a problem of drinking when he does not want to and that he needs help to cope with it. He can seldom manage the problem alone because the underlying problems that cause his drinking are beyond him to figure out and to handle.

The effects of alcoholism are serious; they account for more deaths, both directly and indirectly, than do all other long-term or chronic illnesses. Not only are body tissues affected directly, but malnutrition results from drinking instead of eating and the body is an easy target for illness.

Some of the signs and symptoms of alcoholism are as follows. The alcoholic suffers

a kind of alcoholic amnesia, he has blackouts during which he can't remember a thing. He sneaks drinks, drinks alone, and hides the amount he drinks. He clings to the alibi, "I can quit anytime I want to." He begins early morning drinking, an "eye-opener" to start the day, and may go on prolonged drinking bouts, called benders. He protects his liquor supply (Fig. 55–1). He has tremors and shakes, has all sorts of anxieties and fears, is unreasonable, and may lose his friends and his job.

There is no known cure for alcoholism, nor any one remedy useful to every victim. What is known, however, is that it is never safe for an alcoholic to take "just one drink," because he cannot stop with one. He has no control over his drinking. Help must be directed by a physician who makes a complete study of the individual's difficulties. Sometimes drugs help to ease the alcoholic's misery so that he can benefit from further treatment, which hopefully will help him to understand why he drinks when he does not want to. One such drug is Antabuse. Treatment also includes psychotherapy on an in- or an outpatient basis.

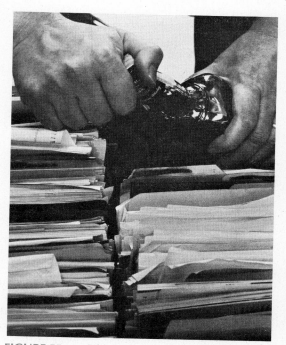

FIGURE 55–1 This man has a serious problem; he is unable to work without drinking so he uses the filing cabinet to protect his supply. (Courtesy of *STEELWAYS*, publication of American Iron and Steel Institute.)

*Travis: Alcoholism. *In* Crawford, A. K., ed.: *Mental Health and Psychiatric Nursing in Practical Nurse Education*. U. S. Dept. of Health, Education, and Welfare—Southern Regional Education Board, 1967, p. 38.

One organization that helps a small number of alcoholics is Alcoholics Anonymous (A.A.). Each member is an alcoholic who has faced up to his problem. Through fellowship, these members support each other by being available when needed and meeting regularly to enjoy the success of staying sober.

As pointed out, the family members need assistance to help them understand the nature of uncontrolled drinking. They can talk with the family physician, a religious counselor, and other persons involved with a like problem. One organization, Al-Anon Family Groups, is a local group made up of relatives and family members of alcoholics; they share common problems in the hope that this will enable them to understand how they can be helpful to the alcoholic in their respective families.

As a practical nurse, you will become more directly acquainted with alcoholism as you care for alcoholics who are admitted to the general hospital when their needs are acute and they are unmanageable. In many cases, within a few days the patient seems to have recovered and appears quite normal. You may feel that recovery was a miracle (and maybe it was), but unless this patient is helped to understand that he has a problem and he needs help, chances are very high that alcoholism will again send him back to the hospital or to jail.

MENTAL RETARDATION

Mental retardation is a condition (not a disease) whereby the nervous system does not develop in the usual way or is damaged early in life causing the person (retardate) difficulty in learning and in using what has been learned. This incomplete mental development can make life adjustments difficult, often leading to personality and behavior problems.

There is a wide range in the extent of disability among the mentally retarded; it extends from *mild* to *moderate* to *severe*. About 80 out of 100 retardates are mildly disabled and are educable or able to learn (at a slower rate); some 16 or so are moderately retarded but can be trained while the remaining three/four are so severely retarded they require constant, life time care.

The causes of mental retardation are many; we know about only a few. To date, scientists can point to about 100 different causes, but they also know that these causes only account for one out of every four cases of mental retardation. Among the identified causes are injury during the birth process, infections of the mother during early pregnancy, disorder in the genes, abnormal chromosomes, and disorders of metabolism. The reason(s) for a much higher death rate among retardates is not clear.

Serious efforts are now made to help educable retardates. Many public school systems have special classes with teachers trained to bring out the best efforts of the retardate. This is hopeful because it permits many of them to live at home within the family circle. They can learn a skill and earn a living rather than be placed in an institution. Community mental health resources help parents to cope with their anxiety and concern. They evaluate the capacities of retardates so they can reach toward their highest possible abilities.

SUMMARY

A society is faced with many types of public health problems that touch and influence the well-being of its citizens. Three of these problems—mental illness, alcoholism, and mental retardation—account for half of the patients who are in hospitals in this country. We are beginning to search for answers to these health problems. We realize that efforts must be made to help restore all patients who can be helped and to prevent the problems in the first place.

A person who is mentally ill behaves in a manner that protects himself and his self-esteem. Often this behavior is meaningless and senseless to others, but it has meaning for the patient. Treatment includes trying to determine what environmental factors are threatening to the patient.

Treatment of mental disorders today is apt to be short-term rather than long-term. Drug therapy enables patients to live more normal lives away from institutions while receiving further treatment.

Community mental health centers bring at least five types of patient services to the community: inpatient, outpatient, emergency, partial hospitalization, and consultation and education. Rehabilitation is a new and a growing effort in the field of mental health; its purpose is "retraining to live in society."

Alcoholism costs this country about two and a half billion dollars a year in work absenteeism and treatment. This problem reaches into all parts of society. While there is no known cure for alcoholism, the physician should guide whatever treatment is used. It may involve the clergy or a fellowship group such as the A.A. and it may help the family members. Alcoholism accounts for more deaths than do all other long-term and chronic disorders.

About eight out of every 10 mentally retarded persons can be trained to lead purposeful lives and be self-supporting. The public school system and community mental health centers are helping retardates and parents cope with these needs.

GUIDES FOR STUDY AND DISCUSSION

1. What does it mean to say "man must have a place in the scheme of things or his life becomes meaningless"?
2. What happens when a person is unable to cope with happenings and people? What does he try to do about his environment? What are the results?
3. What is the difference between psychosis and psychoneurosis?
4. What is meant by personality disorder?
5. How has the mental illness picture changed in the past 25 years? In your opinion, what is the most hopeful part of this?
6. What problems still exist in the field of mental health?
7. Who is the alcoholic? What help does he need? his family need?
8. What are some signs of problem drinking?
9. What is the difference between mental illness and mental retardation?
10. Many mental retardates are educable. What does this mean? What is being done for them?

SUGGESTED SITUATIONS AND ACTIVITIES

1. Prepare an exhibit of materials for classroom purposes. Gather any type of news articles, pamphlets, or visual aids (including student-made ones) that tell something about the nature of mental illness, alcoholism, or mental retardation, and what is being done to meet these problems. When the exhibit is complete, review it and see if you can raise one question you would like to have answered. Figure out where you might search for or get this answer.
2. Find out what your community does for: mental retardates, alcoholics, and the mentally ill.
3. Be prepared to discuss this topic with your classmates: The alcoholic cannot be cured. What should this tell the nurse who cares for him?

NURSING THE MENTALLY ILL

TOPICAL HEADINGS

OBJECTIVES FOR THE STUDENT: Be able to:

1. Describe two main differences between mentally ill patients and physically ill patients.
2. Compare nursing a mentally ill patient with nursing a physically ill patient by citing three differences.
3. Explain how anxiety can be detrimental.
4. Name five ways mentally ill patients communicate with others.
5. Describe an open door therapeutic environment.
6. Defend the statement: helpful and supportive relationships with patients are the heart of therapy in psychiatry.
7. Identify something about nursing the psychiatric patient that will be useful in nursing the patient with physical illness.

SUGGESTED STUDY VOCABULARY*

behavior
tension
anxiety
communication
reminisce
bewildering
terror

panic
aggressive
supportive
evasion
dehydration
constipation

delusion
manipulate
depressed
therapeutic environment
sociopath
custodial care

---

*Look for any terms you already know.

INTRODUCTION

The mentally ill person is not a different being; he too is a person, and he has needs to be met. He needs help to organize his strengths so he can react to his environment in a more purposeful way and without so much tension. His built-up, long-standing tension has caused him to behave in exaggerated ways that appear meaningless to those who do not understand the reasons for it. Everything about his care should be directed toward helping him see his environment as nonthreatening and supportive.

The skills that are so commonly used in the care of the physically ill patient are used less often in caring for the mentally ill patient. However, there are similarities between these two types of patients. The purpose of this chapter is to discuss behavior patterns and show how tension dictates behavior in all persons. In addition, it points out what must be taken into account to help this patient meet his unique needs.

As you proceed, notice what things about the mentally ill patient seem quite like the physically ill patient. Likewise, make note of differences and how these differences change your nursing action.

THE MENTALLY ILL PERSON

Psychiatric hospitals are places where anxiety and tension operate at high levels, not only in the individual patient and patient groups, but often in personnel as well. It would seem reasonable, then, to examine what is involved in the concept of anxiety, first by exploring it in its lesser degrees in normal situations, by reviewing what has already been observed by you in your general hospital experience and finally, using this information as a broad base, coming to a better understanding of the difficulties of the psychiatric patient. This method of approaching the problem depends on two assumptions:

1. That all humans behave quite alike generally. The only major differences are in degree and kinds of behavior.

2. That much of the apparently disturbed behavior in the psychiatric patient is his effort to deal with a much larger, longer-persisting amount of tension than some of the other patients you encounter.

THE CONCEPT OF ANXIETY

One of the most important things necessary to understanding human behavior is the concept of *anxiety*. In the hospital there is no way for the nurse to escape contact with the anxious patient; in life there is no way for any of us to escape the anxious person. It is simply a question of whether we meet the situation well, resort to evasion, delay, or flight, or become anxious ourselves. The body reacts to anxiety in many ways (Fig. 56–1).

ANXIETY CAN BUILD UP. There are certain phases or stages which are identifiable in the development of anxiety. First, there are the mild degrees of tension that are signals

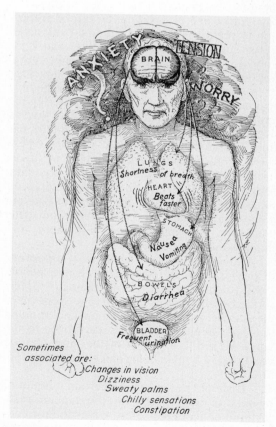

FIGURE 56–1 Anxiety. (Dowling and Jones: That the Patient May Know.)

that we need to become more aware of what is going on in a situation. For example, if students were not slightly concerned about a coming examination, it is doubtful if they would exert much energy studying. The announcement of the scheduled date, then, alerts them to the situation.

Once alerted, the next activity is to investigate the problem. This is done by requesting information from the instructor, by talking to students who have previously taken the course and, by various other means, expanding awareness of what the examination will involve.

Then comes a certain gathering of forces and a narrowing down to a part of the situation. One student becomes aware that she has only a weak understanding of a part of the material and begins to concentrate on that area. This is helpful, but, it tends to shut out other vital areas if her anxiety continues to rise.

What happens, if tension continues to mount? The student takes a part of this very small piece and blows it up, far out of proportion to reality. She goes back and back again to reassure herself that she knows what is involved, let us say, in taking a temperature. Suppose, by this time, her concern develops even more. Quite clearly, she will not be able to operate much longer at this rate. During the examination, her anxiety has risen to such a degree that her mind is emptied of all information. The anxiety has reached a degree where the student is temporarily crippled as far as useful activity is concerned. Most students, fortunately, reorganize themselves and go on to cope successfully. If they were to become panic-stricken and run from the room, this would be the final degree of anxiety that humans can experience.

Panic might be defined as a temporary disorganization of personality, since people cannot sustain a nonthinking, nonhearing, terrorized state for any length of time. Some people handle panic by screaming and running aimlessly about; still others are frozen to the spot. All in all, it is one of the most chaotic conditions a human being can experience (Fig. 56-2).

It should be said that a certain amount of anxiety is very useful to the human race. Without concern for safety we might not consult a physician when we are ill. It also should be said that, at a certain point, anxiety may become a powerful interference in happy, pro-

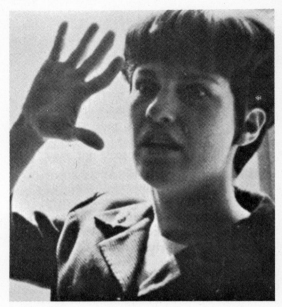

FIGURE 56-2   Fear and panic are expressed in this face. This person seems frozen to the spot. (Schifferes: Essentials of Healthier Living, 3rd Ed., John Wiley and Sons, Inc.)

ductive living. If we are too anxious to use the physician's help, once sought, then this is detrimental to our welfare.

Nurses quite frequently sense or automatically know that a patient is disturbed and take effective steps to reduce his tension. Sometimes, however, strong signals or cues are missed, to the patient's discomfort and the nurse's regret.

Here is an illustration: A patient sometimes comes into a hospital for a complete health examination and, on the surface, this appears to be nothing which should cause undue concern. Inwardly, however, he is frightened that he might have cancer, and he might try asking a series of roundabout questions in order to find out if he has. Unaware that these questions indicated difficulty, the nurse could answer in a way that increases the patient's anxiety, through all of the phases discussed, to an apparently sudden eruption of panic-stricken behavior. This has been known to include walking out of the hospital without a physician's sanction.

From the worried student to the patient afraid of dying to the psychiatric patient seems a long road. Actually, it is part and parcel of the same behavior. The difference is in degree.

Psychiatric patients are not different; they are simply more worried, less able to use their capacities to deal with life. Their need for help in organizing their strengths to get well is greater.

Much of the behavior that can be observed in psychiatric wards is the end result of a chronic, long-standing anxiety. Much of the nurse's work on a day-to-day basis with psychiatric patients is dealing with the tensions that develop from within the patient and which almost always are involved with the small society in which the patient lives 24 hours a day. Thus we must consider both the broad reasons for psychiatric disorders and individual variations.

LONG-TERM ANXIETY. First, the long-term uneasiness, fear, and anxiety which persist in the life situations of many people lead, in some, to mental illness. The reason some individuals can meet disaster after personal disaster and maintain their stability is composed of many factors. Most psychiatrists would agree, however, that the way a person is accepted by those about him when he is very young has a great deal to do with it. If one has been loved and respected as a child, then one will generally grow to see himself as a person who can deal with life as competently as the next fellow. He feels a sense of worth and dignity which cannot be shaken. If, on the other hand, one has been exposed to frequent situations where disrespect, rejection, and unconcern have operated, the end result will be a person who is convinced that he is essentially worthless. This appears most clearly in a disorder called schizophrenia. Made anxious for so many years, these persons reach a point where they can no longer deal with the world. They build a world of fantasy and delusion which relieves them of the necessity of coping with a threatening environment.

A basic feeling of worthlessness or anxiety takes other forms familiar to everyone. Alcoholism is one example. Many alcoholics will tell you that they drink to relieve anxiety. Depressed patients clearly show a sense of despair and anxiety about life. These are but two of the many broader patterns of behavior seen in psychiatric patients which are related to chronic, long-term anxiety.

Going back to our concept of anxiety in its varying degrees, let us visualize a sample situation in a psychiatric patient. Quite frequently, and naturally enough, patients exhibit concern about the date they will be released to go home. A patient, hearing the head nurse tell the doctor that Mr. Jones is going home, is alerted to his own hospitalized situation. His concern moves him to approach one of the personnel about the matter. The person approached states that he does not know when the patient will be able to go home. The patient, becoming more anxious, begins to think of nothing else. All of the pleasant morning bustle of the ward is shut out of his attention. He paces the hall muttering about going home. His anxiety is swiftly becoming greater. He then takes a piece of the whole situation and blows it up quite unrealistically. He begins to say loudly, "I'll never go home; I'll die here," and this is repeated over and over, ever more loudly. Suddenly he screams, runs to the door, and begins to beat on it in a state of panic. If he had been assisted earlier, perhaps as he paced, the anxiety might not have moved to panic. If, for example, his growing tension had been noted as he walked and muttered, a nurse might have fallen into step with him, perhaps walking quietly along, perhaps answering questions, but conveying a sense of someone's being there to support him.

These are the central and essential factors in work with psychiatric patients: 1. recognition of the varying degrees of anxiety that develop in the everyday situation, 2. the information that today's anxiety is built on yesterday's experience with people, and 3. the knowledge that simply conveying a sense that you are there to help and listen will reduce anxiety enough so that the patient can begin to look at the situation as it really is.

MENTAL ILLNESS IS LARGELY A PROBLEM OF COMMUNICATION

At first glance, it does not strike most people that the ability to talk to others, or the lack of it, has anything to do with the large numbers of patients in our mental hospitals today. Yet close examination of the problems of these patients indicates that this is the case. Almost everyone knows that persons who express to others ideas that are false beliefs and that cannot be corrected by reason (called delusions) are sick. If they kept these ideas to themselves, no one would suspect that they were viewing the world in a distorted way. It is in the process of communicating these notions to others that these people run afoul of the social concept of mental illness.

A deeply depressed person is so ill that he cannot break through his misery and despair to communicate with others. When he is able to talk again, we say he is "getting better." In contrast, there are smooth-spoken persons in mental hospitals who are extremely glib with words. They use words to manipulate situations and very frequently personnel get so caught up in these networks of words that they are in considerable difficulty before they know it.

The Overtalkative Patient

Everyone knows people who talk more than the average. A steady flow of words may indicate a lively, intelligent interest in the world around the individual, or it may serve as a smoke screen for many difficulties. There are mentally ill persons who talk under tremendous pressure, jumping from one topic to another with such speed that it is difficult to follow them. This is an indication of their inner anxiety and tension. Your chief role might well be that of a listener in this case. It is safe to assume that most overtalkative patients are not, at the moment, as interested in the conversation of others as they are in their own. Since the attention of such persons is quickly diverted, they are likely to be in constant physical motion, attending to the affairs of the unit. Their bright, often entertaining chatter makes them well accepted by most personnel who often fail to realize that they are covering an often massive anxiety.

The Patient who Manipulates Others with Words

There are certain persons in our society whose skill in using words carries them a long way in social relationships. Often they are found engineering rather questionable transactions wherein the key factor is the ability to convince the other fellow that he ought to part with a sum of money. This person, commonly called the *sociopath*, is frequently found in a psychiatric hospital. Here his activities, at first so innocent and acceptable, generally become an upsetting factor in the hospital community. He does not learn from experience, psychiatrists say, but there is one thing he has learned too well: that magic words like "I like you" bring forth certain responses from others that generally bring pleasure to him. The words that, in a sense, hold our society together, he uses for his own selfish ends. It is best when dealing with this individual to remember his ability to charm and flatter and also to recall that he may deviate from the truth if it will serve his purpose.

The Confused and Reminiscing Aged Patient

The physical damage in the brain which affects some of our population as they grow older creates a problem in communication. Some talk in pieces of sentences that do not make sense to the listener. It requires patience to perceive the meaning of such jumbled fragments. Others communicate quite clearly, indeed, but would rather talk about the past, and most of their conversation centers about events in their more productive years. The pleasure that it gives these patients when they find a warm and responsive person to listen is great indeed.

The Patient who Develops his own Private Language

There are many young patients in the psychiatric group who, when their ability to deal with their fellow man and reality becomes disturbed, develop a private language of their own. They take a word that has an understood meaning and put their own interpretation on it. Thus, although it means something to them, the listener may not understand at all. Or perhaps they will take parts of two words and make a third word which is new, again bewildering to the nurse for a while. Maybe they will be conversing and jumble a sentence. Remember that these communications have meaning for the patient and cannot be treated lightly.

The Silent Patient

Some psychiatric patients present a rather difficult problem. The depth of their difficulty with people is so great that they have stopped trying to get in touch with their fellow human beings, at least with words. Silence is a very effective way of controlling a situation, expressing anger, or acting out hopelessness, and it generally makes the person who is trying to establish relationships quite uneasy. In fact, it is a very effective way of getting rid of people. Understanding something of the way that silence may be used makes it easier to sit with a silent patient and so indicate that he is not alone.

Nonverbal Communication

The other important part of getting our feelings across to others consists not of the things we say, but of the things we do or perhaps fail to do. A patient walking angrily up and down the hall communicates anger by walking heavily, by the expression on his face, and perhaps by a clenched fist. A patient who spits may be communicating contempt and disrespect for others. The tremendous anxiety of the patient with an ashen face, a racing pulse, and a terrorized look is unmistakable. The message is clear without a spoken word.

Some of the broader and unspoken communications need consideration. The patient's very presence in the hospital tells you quite a few things. Whether he is depressed, overactive, or aggressive tells you that he has chosen (or has been forced into) a certain pattern of acting in life, even though it has not worked too well. You then will want to consider the many aspects of nonverbal communications.

NURSE-PATIENT RELATIONSHIPS

Chapter 34 points out the importance of relationships between the nurse and any patient. The same general factors are important in the care of the mentally ill person, but more emphasis is placed on some particular ones.

Establishing relationships with the mentally ill patient requires awareness of your own behavior to avoid using any threatening remarks or mannerisms. He does not respond in the usual way so you have to be careful not to let this influence your attitude toward him and his needs. From time to time it may be necessary to seek guidance in handling your feelings so that your influence continues to be supportive.

With this patient it is quickly noticeable that it is most often the nurse who initiates and maintains the patient relationship. Many times this is done in the face of apparent or actual disinterest on the part of the patient. In the general hospital, unless the patient is very ill, an attempt will be made to maintain the social conventions. While it is true that such a patient might express irritation and hostility, it is usually not as exaggerated as the behavior of some psychiatric patients at times. The establishment of helpful and supportive relationships with the patient is the heart of therapy in psychiatry. There are many medications and treatments which are used in the treatment of the mentally ill, but it is generally agreed that they are more effective as devices to reach the patient than they are as cures in themselves. For example, electroconvulsive therapy might relieve a deep depression, making it easier for the members of the psychiatric team to establish relationships with the patient. It is from this point that much of the helpful work is done; hence, it is called the heart of therapy in psychiatry. Drug therapy likewise is used to hold exaggerated behavior under control in order to permit the establishment of supportive relationships.

Important Factors in Establishing Relationships

The following qualities are necessary in all effective nursing, but their purposes need special emphasis here.

ACCEPTANCE. Understanding that a person with mental illness has intelligence, even though he is less able to use his capacities to deal with life, that the psychiatric patient is not different, and that mental disorder is illness the same as physical infirmity. This includes being nonjudgmental and without prejudice.

FRIENDLINESS. Extending genuine warmth to another. It is a "climate"; it can be felt by others. This must come, not as something turned on and off, but in a natural, sincere way if the patient is to believe in it and trust it. Friendliness is supportive to him.

SINCERITY AND HONESTY. These two factors go hand in hand. The patient needs to know that those who are with him, trying to help him, are truthful and genuine and that he can trust them. One way to encourage this trust is to show respect for the patient. Another way is to let him know, in a sincere way, that you approve of something he has done well.

TACTFULNESS. This factor has been mentioned in relation to dealing with any patient, but the emphasis here is even stronger. The patient may put an unusual degree of emphasis on something said or done. He may refuse to do something simply because it takes on different meaning for him. Appropriateness in handling the situation so it is acceptable (nonthreatening) to the patient can be called tactfulness.

TOLERANCE. This includes the ability to not "lash out" at another even though his (or her) behavior may not seem to be acceptable. Tolerance has its place in effective nursing care as well as in living in general.

SELF-CONTROL. Self-control deals with self-confidence, mental calmness, and poise, among other things. To have poise and calmness when patients show upset emotions or lash out either physically or verbally is essential in establishing good relationships. The patient senses this acceptance—this lack of anger—and feels more secure.

LISTENING. Listening is an essential communication skill. For this patient, "full stop listening attention" is most necessary, and he can sense whether you are listening or not. Then, too, you need to be very much aware of what he is saying; it has meaning for him and you need to try to understand what he is expressing.

Many types of people work together in planning and carrying out each patient's care program. It is developed around his needs and geared to help him make necessary behavioral adjustments in handling his tensions and feelings.

In trying to set up good nurse-patient relationships remember that the patient might very well resent a person who represents authority. The nurse's uniform may stand for just that unless the person wearing it is careful not to convey feelings of superiority in what she says or does. Mentally ill adults should be treated as adults, with respect shown for them and their intelligence. These patients are more sensitive and quicker to understand than one might think. Regardless of age, actions and words have meaning for them, and nothing about your relationships with them should convey any type of threat or disregard for their worth and dignity.

Conversation with Patients

As stated earlier, mental illness is largely a problem of communications. Patients run the gamut, from overtalkativeness to word manipulation to the use of confused pieces of sentences and silence. Sometimes the nurse talks, sometimes she listens, and sometimes she too is silent along with the patient. Understanding what to say (if anything) and how to listen or just be with a patient is gained through study, practice, and observation of those skilled in the art. While friendliness has been pointed out as a factor in good nurse-patient relationships, a word should be said about personal friendships. The patient's feelings about a friendly nurse can be quite different from his feelings about a nurse who is a personal friend.

OBSERVING THE PATIENT

Because the psychiatrist must necessarily use many different means of getting facts and information to help him to determine the underlying factors and treatment, those who work with patients observe patient behavior to help supply pertinent information. Gathering objective behavioral information is different from gathering objective information such as noting the amount and character of drainage on a dressing. It is a learnable skill concerned with noticing and describing meaningful facts about such things as facial expressions, body mannerisms, how the patient communicates, general conduct as a member of the hospital family, hygiene habits, and sleep and rest patterns. It is true that appetite, elimination, temperature, pulse, respiration, and other more familiar observations are made, but they are not the chief focus of attention unless responsible for some factor in his illness.

Factors that can Influence Observations

Certain things may affect one's ability to observe objectively and from time to time it may be necessary to discuss personal feelings and reactions with appropriate personnel so that patient relationships are supportive rather than threatening. It is not unusual for an LPN to have mixed feelings about caring for the mentally ill patient (at least at first). For one thing, from a physical point of view many patients look normal and healthy. This makes it hard to believe that they are ill; and this can be disturbing because the person in uniform, "ready to care for the sick," may not know how to act. She is used to doing things for someone with needs she can see, but here there may be no apparent evidence of need.

When a patient's behavior seems normal it may be difficult to realize he is ill and needs to be hospitalized. It can be frustrating when he expresses hostile feelings and sarcastically calls the nurse "stupid" or otherwise ridicules her. It is essential that the nurse's behavior be directed toward helping the patient use his capacities to deal with his inner tensions and conflicts in a constructive way; this may require appropriate staff help.

Another feeling factor which may influence observation is one which can come from caring for the patient who is withdrawn. He wants to be by himself and talk with no one. This situation may cause you to feel useless and even helpless to the point that you try to avoid this patient. However, your silent presence may be very supportive to him.

Recording Observations

From one general hospital to another the form of the patient's chart itself may vary; the same is true for mental hospitals, and possibly more so. Policies regarding the types of information to be included are not the same, by any means. Because the mentally ill patient is usually hospitalized for a longer period of time, steps are taken by each institution to cut down on "routine" charting to keep the chart within a reasonable size for use and storage.

Graphs may be used for recording more than the usual observations. Charting can be only as accurate as the person making the observations. Whatever the method used, it is necessary that there be common understanding among the personnel about what is important to observe and how it is to be recorded.

PROVIDING FOR DAILY NEEDS

The mentally ill patient has the same daily living needs as other patients. Due to his pattern of communication and behavior, it is ob-

vious that meeting his needs requires the assistance of a personnel team that is well aware of any special emphasis needed to help him back to independence.

One factor related to all aspects of patient care is safety. Anyone who is entirely unable to control his behavior must be protected from harming himself or others. This factor is handled in many different ways today. Some institutions have very strict rules and keep all potentially dangerous instruments under lock and key; others allow almost everything to be available to patients, except for razor blades. The degree of such freedom is determined by the patient's needs as well as the policies of the hospital.

Personal Care and Hygiene

This is as important for the mentally ill patient as for any other patient. He may not be interested in his personal hygiene for any number of reasons, such as lack of previous hygiene habits, or seeming lack of energy as well as interest to do anything for himself.

Some patients need continued encouragement and motivation to keep clean. Telling them that they "should" does little good if they get no further encouragement. Personnel can set a first-class example in their own grooming habits. Perhaps the most important thing in getting the patient involved is to encourage him when he makes ever so slight an effort to take care of himself. Any small success can be mentioned. Fellow patients can help one another in this respect too.

Patients may or may not be permitted to keep certain daily grooming aids in their rooms. When they are not allowed to, provisions are made for the safe storage of their possessions.

Some mentally ill patients will not be ambulatory and their daily needs will be met with assistance from the nurse or the attendant. Keep in mind the necessity for a safe environment and the need for all possible self-assistance.

Sleep and Rest

Illness changes patterns of sleep and rest; medications influence these patterns. The mentally ill patient may be so upset and disturbed that his sleep habits are quite different than usual. Nighttime may increase his anxiety. If it does, this would be a meaningful observation, as would the fact that he appears to sleep easily in the daytime. The disturbed patient needs help and encouragement to relax and regain his normal habits. Sometimes a *sedative tub bath* is given. For about 20 to 30 minutes, the patient is kept in a bathtub about half full of water (tested temperature 94 to 98° F.). No soap is used; the purpose is not cleansing but rather quieting the patient.

Nutrition and Fluids

It is easy for this patient to get insufficient fluids. Look for these signs of dehydration—dry, cracked lips, skin wrinkled and lacking tone, dryness of the mouth. Frequent suggestions about drinking water and providing between-meal liquids help encourage the patient to consume more normal amounts.

Personnel often eat with the patients, which provides opportunity to converse with them and observe their behavior in this group situation. Very often interest in food and self-appearance are early signs of improvement. Any sign of improvement in a patient's behavior during mealtime, whether alone or with others, should be mentioned to him because this kind of recognition can serve to motivate and encourage him.

Elimination

Observing the function of the bowels cannot be left to chance. Staff may need to determine this through direct observation if indicated.

Mental disorders can have a slowing effect on some physical body processes. Digestion and elimination are two such examples.

Some patients become very anxious about their bowels and continuously communicate this anxiety by requesting treatments and medications. Others pay no attention at all and, unless watched, easily become constipated.

Regular exercise (outdoors when weather permits), plenty of fluids, and a balanced diet help to maintain normal digestion and elimination.

Environment

It is now realized that being hospitalized in and of itself can be a disturbing factor in the life of this patient. The trend today is toward an "open door" therapeutic environment. The climate is informal and friendly. Most staff members wear street clothes, as do the patients. Doors are seldom locked and patients are on their honor to a great extent. Each patient is helped to realize that he has the responsibility of helping other patients abide by their privileges.

Privileges of movement or freedom outside of the hospital environment are prescribed, like any other good medicine, according to the patient's ability to handle them. As he becomes more independent in his behavior, privileges allow him more independence.

Another feature of this therapeutic environment is the patient's participation in selecting his room and taking responsibility for keeping it presentable. He is also expected to help others (patients and staff) in caring for the appearance of the unit as a whole and shares in decisions about this.

Living in an "open door" environment provides for the usual needs a patient has under ordinary living conditions. Provisions are made for selecting menus or preparing one's own food, eating with others, doing personal laundry, having access to a telephone, receiving and sending mail without having it censored, pursuing study and craft skills, taking part in athletic activities, enjoying conversation with others, and asking for conferences when wanted.

Patient safety is a concern in "open door" therapy too, but every effort is made to make it as unobvious as possible. About the only thing withheld from the patient is a razor blade. To know of the patient's whereabouts when he leaves the unit, he is asked to sign out and in and observe his prescribed privileges.

The therapeutic use of environment in helping the mentally ill is beginning to bring changes to the traditional "closed door" hospitals too. As yet, it is far from being a universal or common approach, but its influence is seen in small ways in many facilities.

Treatment

Today many patients still receive custodial or guardian care because of the lack of sufficient numbers of trained personnel. It is being recognized that the mental health team can be made up of persons such as LPN's who do not have professional training plus personnel who do. This fact has brought into focus the need for ongoing educational programs for all involved.

The object of treatment today is to provide a therapeutic environment in all aspects of the patient's living. Due to the shortage of highly trained psychiatric personnel, the staff on the units or wards must be taught how to maintain a supportive and friendly environment for patients.

At best, in large mental hospitals, psychiatrists conduct group therapy sessions, but these can be of little lasting value to the patient if he must return to "guardian protection." These sessions provide opportunity for patients and staff to discuss all types of things, including their shared responsibilities in living together and their feelings.

Individual patient therapeutic needs are assessed by the psychiatrist with help from staff members, and an individual plan of action is developed accordingly. Therefore, all personnel who share in the life of a particular patient need to be familiar with his plan so they can support rather than destroy its value.

Especially is this true for personnel who are in direct and daily contact with patients, such as the LPN.

To give you an idea of the wide range of personnel who share in patient care and the therapeutic environment, the list includes psychiatrists, psychologists, social service workers, registered and practical nurses, occupational therapists, recreational therapists, attendants, aides, vocational rehabilitation workers, volunteer workers, and aspects of community life such as local industry. The length of the list alone points up the importance for in-service and out-service educational programs so that *all* concerned know what their contribution must be.

Treatment today involves short-term, intensive therapy in order to reach more patients, even if the level of effectiveness is not ideal. Communities are beginning to provide a variety of supportive services, as pointed out in the previous chapter, so that help can be available on a more flexible basis. The use of drug therapy has previously been described to show how it fits into the changing patterns of patient care.

SUMMARY

Care of the mentally ill is undergoing far-reaching changes today. The emphasis is on providing a therapeutic environment—a climate that is non-threatening and supportive to the patient's efforts to organize his strengths to control his behavior. This effort requires that all personnel who share in providing this helpful climate understand the meaning and purpose of their individual contributions.

In great measure, mental illness is a matter of patient communication in dealing with his internal conflicts and anxieties. He must preserve self and self-esteem and he manipulates himself (e.g., his language, motions, and posture) in order to do this.

Anxiety within bounds is a part of life and can be useful. It can spiral out of bounds, however, and be a destructive force that completely disorganizes human behavior.

GUIDES FOR STUDY AND DISCUSSION

1. In what ways is caring for a mentally ill patient similar to caring for a patient with physical illness? How is it different?

2. Name some skills that you gained in taking care of physically ill patients that may not be used as much with mentally ill patients.

3. In your opinion, what new or different skills do you imagine you might need to be a member of the mental health team? If you were employed in a mental hospital, where and how would you expect to gain these skills?

4. What are the stages of anxiety build-up? Under what circumstances is anxiety useful? detrimental?

5. How does a panic-stricken person behave?

6. What does it mean to say that mental illness is largely a problem of communications?

7. What is meant by exaggerated behavior?

8. How can you show a patient that you are listening to what he is saying?

9. Personnel must be careful not to convey threat or disregard for the mental patient. Why is this so?

10. What is meant by an open door therapeutic environment?

11. Why is the nurse rather than the patient so often the one to initiate and maintain relationships?

12. Why are helpful and supportive relationships with the patient called the heart of therapy in psychiatry?

SUGGESTED SITUATION AND ACTIVITY

1. Complete this form.

Type of Communication	Characteristics of the Patient	What the Nurse Should Keep in Mind
Overtalkativeness		
Manipulating others with words		
Confused and reminiscent		
Private language		
Silence		
Nonverbal communication		

APPENDICES

APPENDIX I

COMMON ABBREVIATIONS USED IN RELATION TO MEDICATIONS AND TREATMENTS

According to Time and Hour of Administration

Abbreviation	Meaning	Abbreviation	Meaning
a.c.	before meals	A.M.	before noon
p.c.	after meals	P.M.	after noon
		m. et n.	morning and night
q.h.	every hour	m/n	midnight
q.2h.	every 2 hours (use with any number)	n. or noct.	night
q.i.d.	four times a day	h.	hour
q.d.	every day	h.s.	at bedtime, hour of sleep
alt. dieb.	alternate days	ad lib.	as desired
alt. hor.	alternate hours	p.r.n.	as necessary, as required
alt. noct.	alternate nights	s.o.s.	if necessary (i.e., one dose)
b.i.d.	twice a day	stat.	at once, immediately
t.i.d.	three times a day		

According to Preparation and Administration

Abbreviation	Meaning	Abbreviation	Meaning
aa	of each	liq.	liquid
ad.	up to	lot.	lotion
aq.	water	m.	minim
C.	centigrade	n.b.	note well
c	with	no.	number
cap.	capsule	O.	pint
cc.	cubic centimeter	ol.	oil
comp.	compound	os	mouth
D.	give	oz. ℥	ounce
dil.	dilute	per	by
dim.	one-half	pil.	pill
div.	divide	pulv.	a powder
Dx	diagnosis	q.s.	a sufficient quantity
elix.	elixir	Rx	treatment
et	and	s	without
ext.	extract	ss	one-half
F.	Fahrenheit	sat.	saturate
fld., fl.	fluid	s. fr.	whiskey
Gm.	gram or grams	sol.	solution
gr.	grain or grains	sp., spt.	spirit
gtt., gtts.	drop, drops	subq.	subcutaneous
garg.	gargle	syr.	syrup
hypo., H.	hypodermically	tab.	tablet
I.M.	intramuscularly	tr., tinct.	tincture
inf.	infusion	tbsp.	tablespoonful
I.V.	intravenously	tsp.	teaspoonful
lb.	pound	ung.	ointment
lin.	liniment	℥	dram

MEDICAL TERMINOLOGY*

SOME FREQUENTLY USED WORD-FORMS, PREFIXES AND SUFFIXES

Combining Form	Pertaining to, relationship to, meaning	Example
aden-, adeno-	gland	adenoma, adenotomy
algesi-	pain	algesia
arthro-, arthr-	joint	arthropyosis, arthritis
bi-	two, twice	bilateral
bili-	bile	biliuria
bio-	life	biology
brachi-	arm	brachialgia
brachy-	short	brachycardia
brady-	slow	bradycardia
broncho-	bronchi	bronchoscope
caco-, cac-	bad, ill	cacostomia, cachexia
cardia-, cardio-	heart	cardialgia, cardiogram
celio-	abdomen	celioma
chole-	bile	cholecyst
cleido-	clavicle	cleidocranial
colpo-, colp-	vagina	colporrhaphy, colpotomy
costo-	rib	costo-inferior
cranio-	cranium, skull	craniotomy
cyano-	denoting blue	cyanosis
cyst-, cysto-	sac, cyst, bladder	cystectomy, cystocele
dent-, dento-	tooth	dentalgia, dentoid
dermato-, derma-, dermat-, dermo-	skin	dermatoid, dermatome dermatoma, dermovascular
dorso-, dorsi-	back	dorsolateral, dorsiflexion
dys-	difficult, painful	dysmenorrhea
electro-	electricity	electrocardiogram
encephalo-	brain	encephalogram
entero-	intestine	enterocolitis
erythro-	red	erythroderma
eu-	well, easily, good	euphoria
fibro-	fibers	fibroid
galacto-, galact-	milk	galactophlebitis, galactoma
gastro-, gastr-	stomach	gastroenteritis, gastrectomy
gero-, geronto-	old age, aged	geratic, gerontology
glosso-, gloss-	tongue	glossocele, glossitis
glyco-	sugar	glycosuria
gyneco-, gyn-	woman	gynecology, gyniatrics

*Dorland's Illustrated Medical Dictionary, 25th Ed.

Combining Form	Pertaining to, relation-ship to, meaning	Example
hemo-, hem-, hemato-	blood	hemophobia, hemuresis, hematoma
hepato-, hepat-	liver	hepatoma, hepatitis
histo-, hist-	tissue	histoma, histic
homo-	same	homogeneous
hydro-, hydr-	water	hydrocele, hydruria
hystero-	uterus, or hysteria	hysterotomy, hysteropia
ileo-	ileum	ileotomy
lacto-	milk	lactose
laparo-	loin, or flank	laparorrhaphy
laryngo-	larynx	laryngoscopy
lepto-	slender, thin, delicate	leptodermic
leuko-, leuco-	white	leukocytosis, leucocyte
lipo-	fat	lipoma
litho-	stone	lithogenesis
masto-, mast-	breast	mastoplasty, mastitis
mega-, megalo-	great, huge	megacardia, megalogastria
meningo-	membranes covering the brain and/or spinal cord	meningocele
meno-	menses	menorrhea
metro-, metra-	uterus	metrorrhagia, metralgia
mono-	one, single	monophobia
multi-	many, much	multiform
myelo-, myel-	marrow	myelosarcoma, myeloma
myo-, my-	muscle	myocardial, myoma
narco-	stupor or stuporous state	narcosis
necro-	death, dead	necropsy
neo-	new or strange	neoplasm
nephro-, nephr-	kidney	nephroma, nephrectomy
neuro-, neur-	nerve, nervous system	neurology, neuralgia
oligo-	little, scanty, few	oliguria
oophoro-, oophor-	ovary	oophorocystectomy, oophoritis
ophthalmo-, ophthalm-	eye	ophthalmology, ophthalmic
oro-	mouth	oronasal
ortho-	straight, normal, correct	orthopedic
osteo-	bone or bones	osteomyelitis
oto-, ot-	ear	otoscope, otitis
patho-	disease	pathology
pedia-, pedo-	child or foot	pediatrics, pedodontics
pharyngo-	pharynx	pharyngocele
phlebo-, phleb-	vein or veins	phlebotomy, phlebitis
photo-, phot-	light	photophobia, photic
phren-	mind or diaphragm	phrenic
pneo-	breath, breathing	pneograph
pneumo-	lungs, breath	pneumopexy
poly-	many, much	polyuria
procto-, proct-	rectum	proctoscope, proctitis
pseudo-, pseud-	false	pseudopregnancy, pseudaphia
psycho-, psych-	mind	psychotherapy, psychiatric
pyelo-, pyel-	pelvis of kidney	pyelogram, pyelitis

Suffix	Meaning, Pertaining to	Example
-odynia	pain, distress	gastrodynia
-oid	likeness, form	bronchoid
-oma	tumor	myoma
-osis	process, a disease	nephrosis
-ous	full of, pertaining to	menstruous
-pathy	a morbid condition, disease	osteopathy
-pexy	surgical fixation	oophoropexy
-phobia	fear	photophobia
-plasty	shaping, or surgical formation	oophoroplasty
-plegia	paralysis, or a stroke	hemiplegia
-rrhage	excessive flow	hemorrhage
-rrhaphy	suture of	oophororrhaphy
-rrhea	flow, or discharge	menorrhea, diarrhea
-scope	instrument for examining	stethoscope
-scopy	act of examining	cystoscopy
-sis	state, or condition	varicosis
-stomy	creation of an opening into, or between	gastrostomy
-tome	an instrument for cutting	dermatome
-tomy	the operation of cutting	herniotomy

NURSING PROCEDURES

CONTENTS

Several essential factors are a part of each of the following 26 procedures and are not repeated each time: *Ready the environment; ready the patient; provide for patient privacy; observe safety precautions; exercise good judgment; observe, report and chart results; observe strict surgical aseptic practices and/or medical aseptic practices as each instance may require.*

Each procedure includes: Statement of Purpose; equipment; supplies; materials needed; and the course of action to follow. When pertinent, common variations and adaptations (e.g., due to age of patient) are included at the end of each procedure.

For your convenience, the 11 rules to guide action in practicing sterile technique are listed here in brief form. (See Chapter 42 for a full discussion.)

1. Start with clean hands.

2. Handle sterile equipment only with sterile equipment.

3. Establish a sterile field to receive sterile supplies.

4. Keep the field sterile.

5. Keep the inside of a sterile package sterile when it is opened.

6. Do not open a sterile package until ready to use the contents.

7. Use sterile lifting forceps according to prescribed practice.

8. Use only a sterile instrument to remove a sterile object from a sterile container.

9. Open a sterile container according to prescribed practice.

10. Discard any contaminated equipment or supplies during a procedure.

11. Finish with clean hands.

HANDWASHING

Purpose

Helps prevent and limit the spread of microorganisms from one person to another; helps keep hands free from infection and the skin in good condition; provides a practice in the promotion of health in daily living.

Equipment, Supplies, Materials

Running water, soap (bar or liquid) or detergent, disposable wood sticks, hand and nail brush, towels or paper, and hand lotion.

Course of Action

1. Select lavatory or a deep sink with a temperature mixer and with foot, knee, or elbow-control faucets, if possible; consider foot and knee-controls as contaminated.

2. Know if hand or elbow-controlled faucets are considered clean or contaminated. Use paper towel to *open* faucet, if considered "clean." Use paper towel to *close* faucet, if considered contaminated ("dirty"). Consider the faucets dirty if not certain whether dirty or clean.

3. Open faucets to provide continuously running water with regulated flow and temperature.

4. Clean hands carefully with wood stick and nail brush as necessary.

5. Wet hands and apply cleansing agent to both surfaces of hands and between the fingers. If using bar soap: Pick up bar of soap and lather hands and wrists. Hold soap on back of brush when using brush. Rinse bar and brush thoroughly when washing is completed and drop into proper container. If using liquid soap or detergent: Dispense the liquid soap or powder from container with appropriate technique, obtaining more from time to time as needed.

6. Wash hands thoroughly, using a rotary motion, and rinse well; reapply cleansing agent and extend to wrists and forearms. Repeat washing and rinsing for at least one minute, or longer as may be necessary. (See Fig. A-1).

7. Keep hands and forearms lower than elbows when washing and rinsing.

8. Repeat and continue the washing and rinsing procedure, if hands become contaminated or there is any break in the technique before washing is completed.

9. Use paper towels to dry hands thoroughly.

10. Use a clean, dry, paper towel to close a faucet by hand. (See Fig. A-2).

11. Use a hand lotion or cream after each washing, or as often as possible; rub in lotion until absorbed, giving attention especially to cuticles.

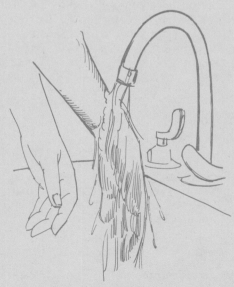

FIGURE A-1

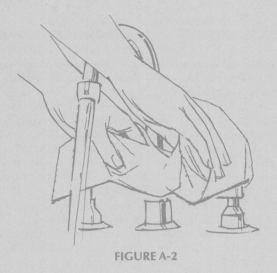

FIGURE A-2

SOME COMMON VARIATIONS AND ADAPTATIONS

1. Roll long sleeves of uniform well above wrists, or above elbows, if conditions indicate, before starting to wash hands; remove wrist watch and place on a clean surface.

2. Wash wrists and area covered by cuffs if a long sleeved gown has been worn.

3. Use cleansing agent if there has been contact with pathogenic organisms and wash for at least two minutes.

4. Soak hands and forearms in specified solution, if required, for as long as indicated.

5. Hold hands higher than elbows when washing and rinsing to provide for *surgical asepsis.* Follow the procedure for the length of time required by the policy of the institution or agency.

BEDMAKING

Purpose

Prepare an unoccupied bed to receive the patient. A closed bed is for a patient newly assigned to the bed. An open bed is for a patient who is out of bed.

Equipment, Supplies, Material

Mattress protector and pad, plastic or rubber draw sheet, blanket, spread, two large cotton sheets (contour or straight, as provided), cotton drawsheet, and pillow case.

Course of Action

1. Make certain bed has been cleaned; use *only* clean linen and bedding to make a closed bed.

2. Adjust bed to flat position; lock casters.

3. Straighten mattress with top end to top of bed.

4. Cover mattress with protector and close zipper or fasten ties; place protector so that opened side is on the far side of the bed or at the foot.

5. Place the folded mattress pad at top of mattress and unfold from top to bottom; adjust placement and remove wrinkles.

6. Place bottom sheet on mattress. If using a contour or fitted sheet: Place folded sheet to center top of mattress. Unfold carefully, from top to bottom, next, the far side and then the near side; center and straighten sheet. Lift corner of mattress and cover first top corner and then bottom corner with sheet corners; straighten and place edge of linen under side of mattress.

If using a straight sheet: Place folded sheet to center top of mattress with wide hem at the top; unfold carefully, first from top to bottom, then the far side, and then the near side; center and straighten sheet. Provide for 18 to 20 inches of sheet at top of mattress; if possible, place bottom hem even with edge of mattress at the foot. Stand facing side of mattress at top corner. Use hand toward foot of bed to lift corner of mattress and pull sheet over top end of mattress with other hand. Pull linen on the straight, working from the center toward the outer edge of the mattress. Make fitted, square, or mitered corner, as shown in the steps in Figure A-3. Grasp sheet with fingers, palms downward; place sheet under side of mattress, working toward foot of bed. Keep back straight, knees flexed, and feet separated slightly.

7. Place folded or rolled waterproof drawsheet in center of bed with top edge about 15 inches from top of mattress; unfold near side; cover with cotton drawsheet and turn about three inches over top edge.

8. Grasp ends of both drawsheets to place under side of mattress; work from

center toward top edge of drawsheets, then center toward bottom. Avoid moving or shifting mattress.

9. Move to the top of the bed on the opposite side to finish making bottom part of bed. Proceed as on the first side, pulling the linen smooth and taut and working toward the foot of the bed.

10. Remain at second side of bed to make top of bed if it has been possible for top linen to be conveniently placed.

11. Place folded top sheet to center top of mattress and unfold carefully in the same way as for the bottom sheet. Place wide hem wrong side up with the upper edge even with the mattress; center and straighten sheet. Cover bottom end of mattress with top sheet and make fitted corner.

12. Place folded blanket at center of mattress with the upper edge of blanket about six or eight inches from top edge of mattress; unfold carefully in the same way as the sheets. Center and straighten blanket; cover bottom end of mattress and make fitted corner.

13. Place folded spread at center of mattress with the hem even across the top edge of mattress. Make certain right side of spread is turned up. Unfold carefully in the same way as the sheets; center and straighten spread; cover end of mattress and make fitted corner, omitting last fold (Fig. A-3D) for spread to hang straight along side of bed.

14. Return to first side of bed to complete top of bed; straighten top bedding and move to bottom corner; place one piece

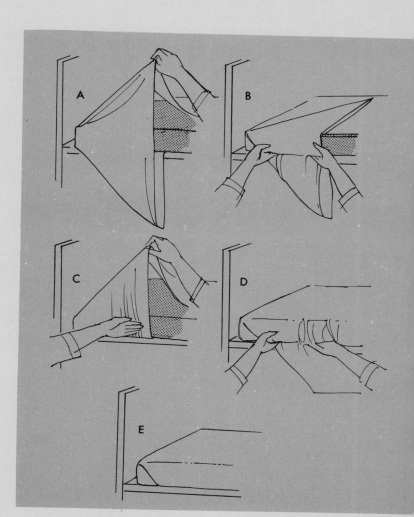

FIGURE A-3 (Monteg and Swenson: Fundamentals in Nursing Care, 3rd. Ed.)

at a time over end of mattress and make a fitted corner for each.

15. Place pillow on bed and unfold pillow case; keep pillow on bed and pull pillow into case. Pull corner of pillow into corner of case on the smooth (without the seam) side; fold or pleat linen on the seam side of the pillow case.

Closed Bed

1. Put pillow at top of bed with seam side of case toward top and the open end away from door.

2. Turn spread over pillow if length is sufficient; otherwise, place pillow over spread.

Opening Closed Bed

1. Place pillow at foot of bed.

2. Turn top of spread over edge of blanket.

3. Turn top sheet over blanket and spread to make cuff.

4. Fan-fold top bedding for desired or convenient use: Stand at side of bed, facing the foot. Using both hands to grasp across cuffed bedding, fan-fold bedding, as you walk toward foot of bed.

5. Replace pillow at top of bed.

Open Bed

1. Remove all linen from bed, even if some is to be used to remake bed. Remove each piece separately, folding from top to bottom.

2. Use clean linen if possible.

3. Follow steps 3 to 14 given previously.

4. Cuff top bedding as it is placed. Turn top of spread over edge of blanket; then turn top sheet back over blanket and spread to make cuff.

5. Fan-fold top bedding as described for opening the closed bed.

6. Place pillow in pillow case and place on bed (step 15).

TAKING TEMPERATURE

Purpose

Determine the temperature of the body heat as an observation of the patient.

Equipment, Supplies, Materials

Clinical thermometer, tissues or cotton pledgets, lubricant (water-soluble), paper and pencil, and watch with second hand.

Course of Action

1. Select type of thermometer according to method of taking temperature. Use a thermometer with a slender bulb or stubby bulb for an oral or mouth temperature, a thermometer with a pear-shaped bulb for a rectal temperature, and a thermometer with a stubby bulb for an axillary temperature.

2. Grasp plain end of the clean thermometer. Use tissue or cotton to wipe off the antiseptic solution with a firm, spiral motion from the plain tip over the bulb.

3. Examine thermometer for breakage or imperfection.

4. Stand with back to light, hold thermometer at eye level and read the mercury level.

5. Shake thermometer until the mercury level reaches at least 95° F. (35° C.).

Oral Temperature

1. Make certain patient is in a comfortable position, either sitting or lying down.

2. Place bulb end of the thermometer under the patient's tongue. Ask patient to keep lips closed and see that he does not talk, bite the thermometer, or remove it.

3. Leave thermometer in place for three to five minutes.

4. Remove thermometer and wipe with a firm, spiral motion from tip to over bulb.

5. Read thermometer. Shake mercury down; place thermometer in antiseptic solution. Record reading.

Rectal Temperature

1. Turn or ask patient to turn on side, if possible.

2. Use tissue to lubricate bulb end of thermometer to about one inch above bulb.

3. Turn linen back from buttocks; lift upper buttocks until anus is seen clearly.

4. Insert thermometer into rectum from 1 to 2 inches.

5. Hold in place for three to five minutes.

6. Remove thermometer; wipe with a firm, spiral motion from tip to over bulb.

7. Read thermometer and record. Shake mercury down. Wash thermometer in cold soapy water and rinse before placing in antiseptic solution.

Axillary Temperature

1. Ask or assist patient to turn on back; remove sleeve of gown from one arm.

2. Dry axilla with bath towel, patting gently (avoid friction) — do not wash.

3. Place bulb end of thermometer high in axilla with the plain tip pointing toward the head; bring arm across chest and ask patient to grasp his shoulder. (See Fig. A-4.)

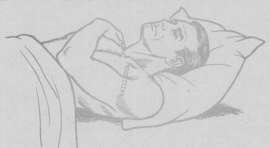

FIGURE A-4 (Kozier and DuGas: Introduction to Patient Care, 2nd Ed.)

4. Hold thermometer firmly in place for 10 minutes.

5. Remove thermometer; wipe with a firm, spiral motion from tip to over bulb.

6. Read thermometer and record. Shake mercury down. Wash thermometer in cold soapy water and rinse before placing in antiseptic solution.

SOME COMMON VARIATIONS AND ADAPTATIONS FOR INFANTS AND CHILDREN

1. Place and hold child in a comfortable position. Use rectal method. Insert thermometer about one inch and hold it securely in place.

2. Use position and method of holding infant or young child according to age and conditions:

  a. Place infant on back. Put index finger between infant's ankles and grasp legs firmly; flex back on abdomen and hold. (See Fig. A-5).

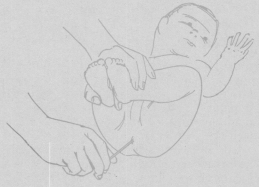

FIGURE A-5

  b. Place infant or young child on his abdomen across your lap, with his legs hanging toward the floor.

  c. Place older child in the prone position in bed or on an examination table.

TAKING PULSE

RADIAL

Purpose

Determine the pulse rate; obtain an estimate of the character (rhythm, quality) of the pulse; aid in making observations.

Equipment, Supplies, Materials

Watch with second hand and paper and pencil.

Course of Action

1. Make certain patient is in a comfortable position, either sitting or lying down. Ask patient to remain quiet.

2. Provide support for patient's arm. You may bring patient's arm across his chest, place it alongside his body, if he is in a lying position, or place it on arm of chair, side of bed, or table, if he is sitting in a chair. Turn palm of hand down.

3. Use tips of first three fingers, locate radial artery and press gently against radius.

4. Count the number of pulsations (beats) for one minute; observe the quality, any irregularities of the pulse.

5. Repeat the count if unsure of accuracy of observations.

6. Record rate and observations.

SOME COMMON VARIATIONS AND ADAPTATIONS

1. Count pulse rate at another site if radial pulse is not detectable, if condition(s) prevent, or to check against radial count. Other sites are the temporal, facial, femoral, and dorsalis pedis arteries.

2. For infants and young children: Use the temporal area, if possible, or place the hand over the heart region.

3. Count the pulse when the patient is asleep if wakeful conditions affect the pulse rate.

APICAL — RADIAL

Purpose

Determine if there is a pulse deficit.

Equipment, Supplies, Materials

Stethoscope, watch with second hand, and paper and pencil.

Course of Action

1. Obtain second nurse to take radial pulse.
2. Place fingertips near the left nipple (under the left breast of a mature woman) and locate the apex of the heart.
3. Place tips of the stethoscope in ears and the bell over region of the apex; listen for heart sounds.
4. Use the same watch; decide when to start counting at the same time.
5. Count the radial pulse and the heart beats during exactly the same period of time for one minute. Repeat count for accuracy and to note quality of pulse.
6. Record rates and observations; chart both counts according to policy of institution.

TAKING RESPIRATIONS

Purpose

Determine the rate of respirations; observe the quality and characteristics of the respirations.

Equipment, Supplies, Materials

Watch with second hand and paper and pencil.

Course of Action

1. Make certain patient is in a comfortable position, either sitting or lying down.
2. Count and observe the respirations after or before taking the pulse, while fingertips are on pulse.
3. Count the rise and fall of the chest as one respiration.
4. Count the respirations for one minute; repeat count and observations if in doubt.
5. Observe for sounds accompanying breathing.
6. Record.
SOME COMMON VARIATIONS AND ADAPTATIONS
1. Watch the rise and fall of the chest or the upper abdomen while the patient is asleep to count and observe respirations of certain patients.

2. Place fingertips on patient's radial pulse and bring his hand and forearm across his chest to help detect respirations, if there is difficulty in seeing the chest rise and fall. Or place hand directly on patient's chest.

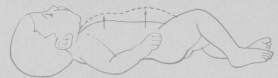

FIGURE A-6 (Leifer: Principles and Techniques in Pediatric Nursing, 2nd Ed.)

3. Seek assistance to check accuracy of count and observations of respirations.
4. Watch the movements of the abdomen when taking the respirations of an infant or a young child. (See Fig. A–6.) Note if chest and abdomen rise together, with no retractions. Observe for lagging of the chin and any grunts or other sounds while breathing.

TAKING BLOOD PRESSURE

Purpose

Determine the arterial pressure of blood by measuring the systolic and diastolic arterial pressures.

Equipment, Supplies, Materials

Sphygmomanometer (mercury manometer or aneroid type), stethoscope, and paper and pencil.

Course of Action

1. Select a cuff with width appropriate to size of upper arm and age of patient.
2. Cleanse the ear tips of the stethoscope.
3. Open the mercury manometer and place conveniently at eye level on a firm, level surface.
4. Check the manometer for leakage of air.
5. Make certain patient is sitting or lying in a comfortable position. Support the forearm of arm to be used at heart level with the palm of the hand turned up. Support the forearm on a hard surface, like a table top, if the patient is sitting.
6. Remove sleeve from arm unless sleeve is loose enough to turn up to at least 5 inches above elbow.
7. Make certain cuff is deflated entirely.

8. Wrap cuff evenly and securely around the upper arm with tubing toward the upper side. Make sure lower edge of cuff is one inch above space at bend of elbow. Tuck end of cuff under edge of last turn. (See Fig. A-7.)

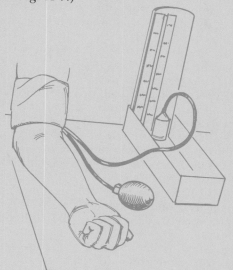

FIGURE A-7 (Hughes: Pediatric Procedures.)

9. Fasten hooks of the gauge (dial) to an upper edge of cuff, if aneroid type is being used; make certain gauge is placed for an accurate reading.

10. Place ear tips of the stethoscope into ears.

11. Close the valve on the rubber bulb.

12. Use fingertips to locate the strongest pulsation of the brachial artery and gently position the bell of stethoscope over this spot. Make certain the entire end of the bell is on bare skin and not touching the cuff.

13. Squeeze the bulb quickly; inflate the cuff until the pulsations of the artery can no longer be heard.

14. Keep eye on column of mercury or the dial.

15. Open the valve on the rubber bulb slowly.

16. Listen for the *first sharp, clear, rhythmic sound and note the number* on the scale or the dial for the *systolic pressure* reading.

17. Allow the cuff to deflate slowly; listen for a *sudden change in sound to a soft or muffled thump and note the number* on the scale or the dial for the *diastolic pressure* reading.

18. Open valve to expel all air in cuff; allow the mercury to fall to "0" in the mercury manometer.

19. Wait at least one minute before repeating process to check for accuracy; follow steps 11 through 18 above.

20. Remove cuff from arm and fold or roll to place in case. Cleanse ear tips of the stethoscope.

21. Record both readings according to policy of institution.

SOME COMMON VARIATIONS AND ADAPTATIONS FOR CHILDREN

1. Remove sleeve from arm if *brachial artery* is to be used. Use cuff the width appropriate to size and age of child. Cuff should cover about two-thirds of upper arm. Generally, use a 3-inch cuff for two- to eight-year-old child, a 4-inch cuff for eight- to 12-year-old child.

2. Remove clothing from lower extremity if *femoral artery* is to be used.
   a. Place child in prone position.
   b. Use cuff the width of about two-thirds the length of the thigh.
   c. Wrap cuff smoothly and snugly around the thigh; place cuff so that lower edge is about one inch above the popliteal space.
   d. Flex the leg slightly.
   e. Place the bell of the stethoscope over the popliteal artery.
   f. Follow procedure given for using the brachial artery.

3. Record site and artery used, systolic and diastolic readings, and observations of physical and emotional state of child, especially before and during time that reading was taken.

COLLECTION OF URINE SPECIMEN

Purpose

Aids in diagnosis and determination of treatment and progress of patient.

Equipment, Supplies, Materials

Specimen container for urine (single or gallon [calibrated], clean or sterile, as needed) specimen label, bedpan or urinal, and graduate, if needed.

Course of Action

Clean Single

1. Have patient void in a clean bedpan or urinal; or, if possible and appropriate, have patient void directly into the specimen container.

2. Measure amount of urine voided or being sent as a specimen, if required.

3. Send at least 4 ounces, unless orders state otherwise.

"Clean Catch," "Clean Voided," "Midstream," "Sterile Voided," "Sterile"

1. Instruct patient to drink several glasses of water or other fluids at least 30 to 60 minutes before specimen is to be collected.

2. Instruct patient *not* to void and to notify nurse if a desire to void occurs.

3. Wash, or instruct patient to wash, vulva or glans penis with warm water and soap. Use materials and solution designated by institution or physician to cleanse further. For female: Cleanse downward, from anterior to posterior. Use one swab for each stroke, then discard. Hold labia apart when patient voids and to collect specimen. For male: Cleanse from distal tip of the glans to the base of the penis. Use one swab for each stroke, then discard. Retract foreskin for thorough cleansing and keep retracted when patient voids and to collect specimen.

4. Have patient void small amount, (about 2 ounces). If possible, have patient stand to use bedpan or the toilet in the bathroom; make certain patient does not touch bedpan or urinal. Ask female patient to spread and hold labia apart. Then have patient void rest of urine directly into the sterile specimen container. Use a sterile pitcher to catch urine, if more convenient with some patients; then transfer to specimen container.

5. Obtain a "sterile" specimen of urine by catheterization only if ordered by the physician.

6. Send specimen to the laboratory at once, or refrigerate if a culture is to be taken.

Timed

1. Instruct patient about voiding to collect specimens at certain times.

2. Use the appropriate technique to collect the type of urine specimen required.

3. Collect the necessary amount of urine at the specified times.

24-hour, Single or Cumulative

1. Start collection of urine according to the 24-hour cycle used by the physician or the hospital, or at a time specified.

2. Prepare containers; label fully (name, date, time) and place in a cool, appropriate location.

3. Have patient void at time collection is to start; discard urine.

4. Collect all urine voided during the next 24 hours; have patient void at the end of the 24-hour period and add urine to the collection.

5. Measure urine, if required; measure during collection to total, or measure the entire amount at the close of the 24-hour period, if calibrated container is not available for collection.

6. Send the entire specimen or a portion of it to the laboratory, as ordered.

24-hour, Fractional

1. Start collection of urine at the time specified and use the four-, six-, or 12-hour intervals specified by the physician.

2. Prepare containers; label fully and place in a cool, appropriate location.

3. Have patient void at time collection is to start; discard urine.

4. Collect all urine during one time interval into one container; measure, if required, each voiding during the collection, and total.

5. Have patient void at the end of the 24-hour period and add urine to the collection.

6. Send collection of urine to the laboratory at the end of each time interval, or send collections for all of the time intervals when the 24-hour cycle is completed.

SOME COMMON VARIATIONS AND ADAPTATIONS FOR INFANTS AND CHILDREN

1. Elevate head of bed or the head and shoulders.

2. Collect specimen in appropriate container if child is old enough to co-operate.

3. Assist child to stand, if permissible and if child is old enough.

4. Use suitable restraints only as necessary.

5. Use the disposable plastic collectors (diaper, bag, tube), if available; follow directions specific for each to apply and use. See Figure A-8 for one type of plastic collector available to collect a single specimen.

6. Collect a single urine specimen using the method described and shown in Figure 54–5 for the female, or for the male.

7. Collect a 24-hour urine specimen. One method is shown in Figure A-9.

8. Remove the collector as soon as the urine has been voided, or the time interval has passed, and transfer the urine to the proper specimen container.

9. Protect infant's skin from coming

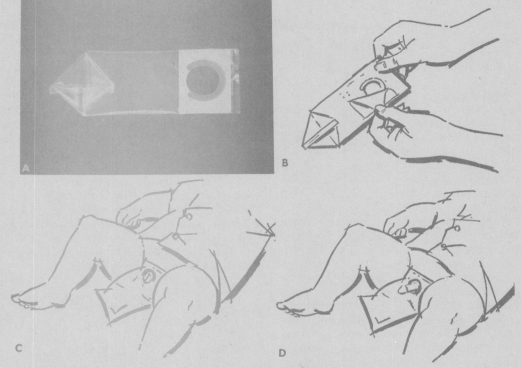

FIGURE A-8   (Bookmiller, et al.: Textbook of Obstetrics and Obstetric Nursing, 5th Ed.)

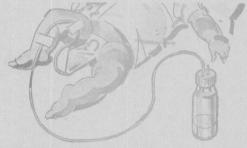

FIGURE A-9   (Sterilon corporation, Buffalo, New York.)

in contact with glass or the edge of container by covering it with one-inch wide adhesive tape.

10. Take care with use of adhesive tape. Use as little as possible and remove skin from tape rather than the tape from skin.

COLLECTION OF STOOL SPECIMEN

Purpose

Aids in diagnosis and determination of treatment and progress of patient.

Equipment, Supplies, Materials

Specimen container for stool, specimen label, two tongue blades, bedpan with cover, toilet tissue, and urinal.

Course of Action

1. Obtain stool in a clean bedpan; instruct an ambulatory patient to use bedpan placed on toilet or on chair in bathroom.

2. Keep stool specimen free from urine and toilet tissue, if possible; ask patient to void before having stool.

3. Inspect stool for any unusual appearance; look for and include with the specimen any portions of fresh or old blood, pus, or mucus.

4. Prepare specimen at once. Lift about 2 or 3 tablespoons of stool into the specimen container with the two tongue blades. Cover securely.

5. Use a warmed bedpan to collect stool for a *warm stool specimen*. Prepare specimen at once in a warmed container; cover container, place on a covered warm water

bottle, and cover both to take to the laboratory.

6. Send or take any stool specimen to the laboratory as soon as obtained. Give specimen directly to technician or make certain specimen is placed in the correct location.

SOME COMMON VARIATIONS OR
ADAPTATIONS

1. Collection of stool specimen following an enema: Let bedpan with contents stand for five to 10 minutes, then pour off top fluid to discard. Use the tongue blades to lift stool into the specimen container. Make certain container is leak-proof and is capped securely.

2. Collection of a liquid stool specimen: Let bedpan with contents stand for five to 10 minutes, then pour off top fluid to discard. Pour about 2 ounces of the liquid stool into a safe specimen container and cap securely.

3. Collection of stool specimen from an infant or a small child: Use tongue blades to transfer sufficient portion of stool from the diaper to the specimen container (use sterile tongue blades and a sterile specimen container if a stool culture is ordered). Give enema to obtain stool specimen *only upon written order* of the physician. Make certain order is specific as to type and amount.

COLLECTION OF SPUTUM SPECIMEN

Purpose

Aids in diagnosis and determination of treatment and progress of patient.

Equipment, Supplies, Materials

Specimen container for sputum, such as wide mouth jar, plastic-coated container, or Petri dish, specimen label, and mouth tissues.

Course of Action

1. Use a sterile container to collect sputum if a culture is to be made.

2. Collect specimen early in the morning, before mouth care or breakfast. Permit patient to rinse mouth with water and to swallow a drink of water before coughing to raise the sputum.

3. Collect a 24-hour sputum specimen during any one 24-hour time interval, usually from 7:00 or 8:00 in the morning until the same time the next morning. Provide containers at bedside and instruct patient to save all sputum in the specimen container(s).

4. Ask patient to cough deeply to bring material from the lungs (not the back of the nose or throat). Have patient use tissues to cover mouth when coughing. Ask patient to hold container, if possible, and to expectorate directly into container.

5. Avoid contamination with sputum; watch carefully to keep outside of container and hands free of sputum during collection of the specimen and its transportation to the laboratory.

6. Provide an appropriate outside cover for the specimen container when the specimen is being collected and when the specimen is being taken to the laboratory.

7. Send the specimen to the laboratory at once, or as ordered; place in refrigerator if there is any delay in sending it.

COLLECTION OF VOMITUS SPECIMEN

Purpose

Aids in diagnosis and determination of treatment.

Equipment, Supplies, Materials

Specimen container, specimen labels, mouth tissues, and emesis basin.

Course of Action

1. Use a clean or sterile emesis basin and specimen container, as ordered, to collect vomitus specimen.

2. Provide emesis basin to collect vomitus.

3. Pour 1 to 2 ounces of vomitus in watertight specimen container and cap securely.

4. Measure portion for specimen as well as the entire amount of vomitus, if intake and output are being measured.

5. Collect vomitus as a single specimen, or as an accumulated specimen for a specific time interval, as ordered.

6. Send vomitus specimen to laboratory or keep for observation by the physician, as ordered.

GIVING AND REMOVING BEDPAN AND URINAL

Purpose

Furnish the means for bladder or bowel elimination for the bed patient.

Equipment, Supplies, Materials

Bedpan with cover, urinal with cover, toilet tissue, wash basin with warm water and soap, and washcloth and towel.

Course of Action

Bedpan

1. Provide a clean, warm, dry, covered bedpan. Warm bedpan with warm running water on the inside; make certain outside is dry.

2. Make adjustments with bed and position of patient. If possible, bring bed to level position with head elevated slightly and place patient in the dorsal position.

3. Turn upper side and corner of top bedding onto patient; protect patient from exposure. Free gown or pajamas from area for bedpan.

4. Place bedpan. Ask patient to flex knees, to place forearms on bed with palms turned down, and to press with heels and palms to raise buttocks. Slip upper hand and forearm under the lower part of patient's back. Use lower hand to grasp side of bedpan, slip bedpan under buttocks, adjust placement for use, safety, and comfort.

5. Elevate the back and knees, unless contraindicated. Make certain body is in good alignment and supported with pillows. Stay with patient, if necessary.

6. Place signal cord and roll of toilet tissue within reach of patient; ask patient to put on signal light when finished. Assure patient of return. Leave the room and close the door; return to check if signal light is not on within five to 10 minutes.

7. Remove bedpan and cover at once. Ask patient to raise buttocks as before. Support patient and remove bedpan carefully.

8. Cleanse the patient if he is unable to care for himself; turn him on his side and use toilet tissue. If necessary, wash perineum with warm water and soap, rinse and dry well.

9. Adjust position of patient and arrange top bedding.

10. Provide the means for patient to wash hands with warm water and soap.

11. Observe contents of bedpan before discarding. Measure or take specimen, if indicated; record and report, as necessary.

12. Take urinal with bedpan to a male patient when a bedpan is needed.

Urinal

1. Provide a clean, warm, dry, covered urinal. Warm urinal with warm running water on the inside. Make certain outside is dry.

2. Place patient in the dorsal position and elevate head of bed slightly, if permissible.

3. Lift top bedding at the side and place urinal on side of bed within reach of patient's hand.

4. Assist patient, as needed. Place urinal for the helpless patient with as little exposure as possible. Stay with the patient, if necessary.

5. Place signal cord within reach; ask patient to put on signal light when finished. Assure patient of return. Leave the room and close the door; return to check if signal light is not on within five to ten minutes.

6. Remove urinal and cover at once; hold and carry carefully.

7. Provide the means for patient to wash hands with warm water and soap.

8. Observe contents of urinal before discarding. Measure or take specimen, if indicated; record and report, as necessary.

Some Common Variations and Adaptations

1. Cover or pad seat (the flat, back portion) of bedpan when condition of patient indicates.

2. Ask patient to use trapeze, if available, to lift buttocks when bedpan is placed and removed.

3. Obtain assistance to place and to remove bedpan for a helpless patient or a patient who cannot help lift buttocks: Turn or roll patient on side toward raised side rails, the assistant, or pillows placed on side of bed. Place and hold bedpan against buttocks as patient is turned back upon it. Adjust placement of patient on bedpan for use and comfort. Reverse actions to remove bedpan. Cleanse patient when turned to remove bedpan.

4. Obtain a male nurse or attendant, if available, to assist with urinal for a helpless male patient.

ASSISTING PATIENT TO BECOME AMBULATORY

Purpose

Provision of some exercise, physical activity, and physical and mental comfort, prevention of fatigue and complications, maintenance of normal body functions and processes, rehabilitation, and regaining independence.

Equipment, Supplies, Materials

Patient's bathrobe and slippers or street clothes and shoes (low heels), footstool, walker, and straight chair.

Course of Action

1. Obtain assistance, if needed.
2. Adjust upper and lower parts of bed to level position; lower height of bed, if possible.
3. Place footstool at center side of bed and either cover with a paper towel or place patient's bed slippers on it.
4. Instruct patient what to expect, how to help himself, and the safety precautions to take.
5. Fan-fold or turn down top bedding.
6. Assist patient (according to his needs) to get out of bed, dress, and walk.

Assisting out of and into bed

1. Stand at side of bed with foot toward head of bed placed slightly forward.
2. Bring patient to a sitting position on side of bed. Take pulse and note his color.
3. Instruct patient who is able to help self to:
   a. Flex knees and hips; turn on side bringing knees near edge of bed.
   b. Place hand of upper arm on bed in front; leave under arm at side.
   c. Turn and bring body to upright position and, at the same time, swing legs over side of the bed.
   d. Support self with both hands on bed, one on either side with palms down; place feet on footstool or into slippers.
4. Assist patient who needs help.
   a. Bring patient close to near side of bed.
   b. Place hand toward head of bed well under the upper part of patient's back; place other hand well under both thighs of patient; ask patient to place his near hand across top of your shoulder that is toward head of bed.
   c. Ask patient to flex knees slightly, to push on bed with his far hand, palm down, and to swing legs over side of bed.
   d. Support patient and bring to sitting position on side of bed; place feet on footstool or into slippers.

5. Allow time for patient to become adjusted to upright position; make observations (reactions, color, pulse).
6. Continue to support patient. Stand facing patient with one leg between patient's knees; hold hands on sides of chest or below axillary region with thumbs pointing upward. Ask patient to keep both hands on side of bed or to place them on your shoulders.
7. Assist patient (as needed) with bathrobe or to dress partially or fully and to walk.
8. Instruct and assist patient into bed by reversing these steps.

Walking with Nurse

1. Provide reassurance, support, and instructions needed.
2. Use proper body mechanics and maintain body alignment for patient and self.
3. Maintain type of support as needed by using one of the following means:
   a. Stand near patient's side, hold near arm under forearm and grasp hand.
   b. Stand near patient's side, hold near arm around patient's waist, and with other hand hold patient's hand or forearm (See Fig. A-10).

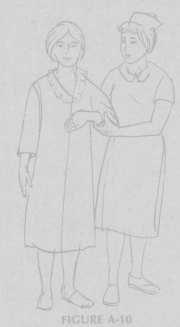

FIGURE A-10

   c. Stand in back of patient; grasp clothing, a belt, or a folded towel around patient's waist at center back.

4. Arrange with co-worker on the opposite side of patient to use the same means to help support and walk with patient.

5. Instruct patient in the normal pattern of walking: Move opposite arm and leg forward, then the other opposite arm and leg; as the right arm and left leg, then the left arm and right leg.

6. Walk in step with patient.

7. Make observations (color, respirations, skin, remarks) and prevent fatigue.

8. Assist into chair or back into bed following period of ambulation. Make observations again.

Walking with Walker

1. Instruct patient in proper use of a particular type of walker. You may have to demonstrate.

2. Make necessary adjustments with hand bars, armpit extensions, seat, or other parts according to needs of patient and type of walker.

3. Make certain patient knows how to enter and leave the walker, manipulate seat for use, and bear weight on hands, not the axillae. (See Fig. A-11.)

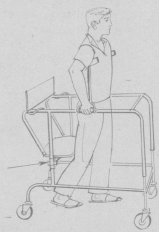

FIGURE A-11   (Sutton: Bedside Nursing Techniques, 2nd Ed.)

4. Furnish support as needed.

5. Caution patient to use safety factors and to avoid fatigue.

Walking with Chair

1. Instruct patient in how to walk with one or two straight chairs for support; demonstrate.

2. Place back of one chair directly in front of patient; have patient place hands on back of chair, press down to push chair ahead, and start to walk slowly.

3. Place backs of two chairs with space for patient to stand between. Have patient place hands on back of chair on either side, push chairs, and start to walk slowly. (See Fig. A-12.)

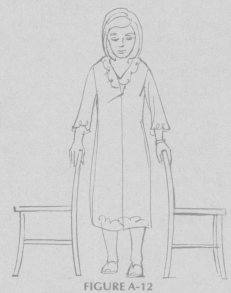

FIGURE A-12

4. Furnish support as needed.

5. Caution patient to use safety factors and to avoid fatigue.

ORAL HYGIENE

Purpose

Provide for clean teeth and mouth; help to maintain a healthy condition of mouth.

Equipment, Supplies, Materials

Toothbrush or denture brush, dentifrice, paste or powder, mouthwash solution, mouth care cup, denture cup, curved basin, water, and face towel. May need straw or drinking tube, tongue depressor, cotton applicators, dental floss, small bulb syringe, paper wipes, gauze squares, lubricant, and waste container.

Course of Action

1. Furnish assistance and adapt mouth care according to state of dependency, age, limitations, and mouth problems of the patient.

2. Supply and arrange articles needed for care.

3. Provide a safe, convenient, comfortable position for the patient.

4. Respect patients' preferences and

habits regarding privacy, temperature of water, use of mouthwash, and time, if possible.

5. Instruct the patient, if necessary, regarding oral hygiene (e.g., when and how to brush teeth, rinse the teeth and mouth, use mouthwash).

6. Observe condition of mouth and gums.

Self-Care

1. Have the ambulatory patient brush teeth at the lavatory or at the bedside; provide chair next to lavatory or the bedside table if needed.

2. Elevate head of bed for the bed patient; bring over-bed or bedside table into convenient placement.

3. Instruct and assist either patient only as needed or requested.

Partial Care

1. Provide the means necessary for the patient to give as much care to self as possible.

2. Give assistance as needed. Some examples: Give support and prevent fatigue. Protect top bedding and patient's clothing with towel. Put dentifrice on brush; hold brush; rinse brush. Hold curved basin; turn faucets on and off if at lavatory. Hold mouth cup with water for rinsing mouth and for use of mouthwash. Clean or assist with cleaning of dentures. Provide for after-care and storage of articles.

Complete Care

1. Adjust patient's position, perhaps turn him onto his side. Elevate his head and shoulders with back rest or pillows. Turn head to one side if patient is unconscious or must remain flat in bed. Provide chair or stool at bedside or lavatory for patient who is able to be out of bed or is ambulatory.

2. Protect top bedding and patient's clothing with towel; place face towel across pillow under face.

3. Use a well-covered tongue depressor to gently hold the mouth open and to press against the tongue; *do not put fingers into mouth.*

4. Make several swabs: Cover 2 to 3 inches of the end of a narrow tongue depressor with gauze; wrap and fasten gauze tightly.

5. Use gauze swabs to clean teeth and tongue; use cotton applicators to wipe gums and inside of mouth. Use toothbrush only if permitted and with great care. Use caution to avoid injury to tissues.

6. Moisten swab or applicator with solution. Avoid soaking or dripping with excess solution. Paste or powder should *not* be used if patient is seriously ill, unconscious, or not responsible.

7. Wipe teeth with stroke toward cutting edge of teeth; clean outer and then inner surfaces of teeth.

8. Discard or remoisten swabs as necessary.

9. Rinse teeth and mouth with fresh swab or applicator moistened with water.

10. Wash and dry face. Use plain tongue depressor to apply lubricant to lips if needed or desired.

Cleaning and Care of Dentures

1. Ask patient to take out dentures, if able; if unable, remove dentures. Use paper wipes to carefully remove first the lower plate and then the upper.

2. Take dentures in denture cup or curved basin to a lavatory or other suitable place to clean.

3. Use great care to prevent chipping, breakage, or loss. Cover bottom of small, clean basin with gauze squares. Use tepid water to partially fill basin; hot or cold water should *not* be used either to wash or to rinse dentures. Hold dentures low over basin to wash or rinse; running water from a faucet should *not* be used. Use gauze piece to hold denture while washing and rinsing.

4. Clean dentures: Rinse with plain water; brush well with dentifrice; rinse well with plain water.

5. Place dentures in a clean denture cup, cover with plain water, and return to bedside.

6. Have patient clean and rinse mouth, if able; if necessary, carefully clean tongue with gauze swab and gums with cotton applicator.

7. Have patient replace dentures, if able; if unable, replace dentures: Hold denture plate with paper wipes and replace first the upper and then the lower plate.

8. Protect dentures from loss or breakage when not in patient's mouth: Place in denture cup, cover with water, place cover on cup securely; mark cup with full identification and place in a safe place. Caution patient to use denture cup, *not* to wrap dentures in paper tissue or linen or to place loose in bedside table.

SOME COMMON VARIATIONS AND ADAPTATIONS

1. Make certain patient rinses mouth

well. Pay particular attention to such patients as those wearing dental braces or on liquid diets. Ask patient to *force* the liquid (water or mouthwash) between teeth and about gums.

2. Use a small bulb syringe to help clean and rinse mouth *only* if patient is conscious, responsible, and old enough to follow directions.

3. Use dental floss *only* when indicated or ordered. Instruct, demonstrate, or assist patient with correct use: Pull a short length of floss carefully between two teeth. Pull down against the side of one tooth, then against the side of other tooth; pull out floss without cutting across gum.

4. If a dentifrice is not available, use water or a weak solution of salt or sodium bicarbonate, if patient prefers.

5. Stay with a child or elderly person to assist with self or partial care.

6. Provide special mouth care according to patient's condition and needs, policy of nursing care, or physician's orders. The measures may include specified, frequent intervals for attention and care, use of mouthwash or irrigating solutions, use of certain equipment and methods, and use of a certain lubricant or a medicated preparation on the lips or in the mouth.

BACK RUB

Purpose

Help stimulate circulation to promote relaxation and comfort; provide for observation of skin condition; help keep skin in good condition; prevent decubitus ulcers and relieve pressure areas.

Equipment, Supplies, Materials

Skin lotion or solution, talcum powder, and bath towel.

Course of Action

1. Warm solution by placing container in warm water bath.

2. Put bed in level position.

3. Remove pillows; leave one pillow under head if requested.

4. Ask or assist patient to move to near side of bed and lie on abdomen (prone position) or on side (Sim's position).

5. Fan-fold or turn bed linen to expose area from neck to buttocks.

6. Place bath towel lengthwise on bed next to body.

7. Bathe entire area if necessary or bath time; rinse and dry well.

8. Make certain hands are warm. Warm hands under running water, if necessary.

9. Shake back lotion well. Pour small portion into palm of one hand, then bring palms together to spread lotion to other hand.

10. Rub the patient's back:
   a. Keep fingers together; use palms of both hands for strokes.
   b. Begin at the sacrum and move slowly up to the neck.
   c. Use firm, rhythmic strokes; move inward, upward, and outward in circular motions (Fig. 35–1).
   d. Rub the buttocks, back, and shoulders.
   e. Give particular attention to bony prominences, reddened areas, and folds in skin.
   f. Reapply lotion to palms as necessary, but avoid excessive use.
   g. Take at least three minutes to give a back rub, longer if necessary.

11. Apply talcum powder, if to be used. Sprinkle powder on hands and apply gently in same manner as the lotion. Avoid using too much powder.

BED BATH

Purpose

Provide the means for a patient who must remain in bed to have a bath; give the nurse a good chance to make observations, especially about the condition of the skin, and to find out the needs of the patient; help the patient to have some movement and exercise and to feel refreshed and comfortable; provide the opportunity for some self-care when the patient is able to bathe himself partially.

Equipment, Supplies, Materials

Two bath towels, face towel, washcloth, bath blanket, bath basin, soap in soap dish, rubbing alcohol or skin lotion, talcum powder, and deodorant. You may need bed linen, laundry bag or hamper, clean gown or pajamas, bedpan or urinal, and articles for care of teeth and mouth, nails and hair.

Course of Action

1. Prepare the environment: Check room temperature; clear and place bedside and over-bed tables for convenience; close door to room and screen bed unit.

2. Remove head pillows and lower back rest according to condition and comfort of patient.

3. Loosen and remove spread, then blanket; next, cover patient with bath blanket as top sheet is removed. Fold each piece as removed for reuse or discard for laundry.

4. Place face towel under head and neck; place bath towel across chest and top of bath blanket.

5. Provide for oral hygiene.

6. Provide bedpan or urinal.

7. Fill bath basin about two-thirds full with water 105° to 115° F.

8. Bring patient to near side of bed, if possible; remove gown from under bath blanket.

9. Keep the following in mind in giving the bath:

    a. Use firm, gentle strokes to wash, rinse, and dry.

    b. Change the water at least twice, and more often if necessary.

    c. Bathe one part or area of the body at a time, and in the order one usually follows for bathing oneself: First, face, neck, and ears; arms and hands; chest and abdomen. Change water and wash legs, groin, and feet. Change water again and wash back and buttocks; pubic and perineal areas.

10. Wet washcloth and squeeze out excess water. Wrap washcloth around palm and fingers of hand to form a "mitten"; apply soap. Keep bar of soap in soap dish. (See Fig. A-13).

11. Bathe face, neck, and ears; use only clear water to wash ear canals.

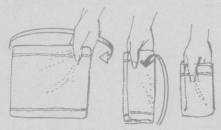

FIGURE A-13

12. Bathe arms and hands: Place bath towel lengthwise under arm to bathe. Wash the arm on far side, then the near side. Lift and support arm to bathe it, paying particular attention to axilla. Place basin on towel on near side of bed to wash hands in water. Give attention to fingernails and apply deodorant.

13. Bathe chest and abdomen: Use bath towel to cover chest as bath blanket is fan-folded to waist. Bathe chest and breasts, paying particular attention to area beneath breasts. Leave towel over chest and fan-fold bath blanket to groin. Bathe abdomen, paying attention to umbilicus and skin folds. Pull bath blanket up over chest and remove towel. Change water.

14. Bathe legs, groin and feet: Expose thigh, leg and foot on far side. Flex knee and place bath towel lengthwise under entire leg. Secure bath blanket at top near groin. Support leg and bathe thigh and leg. Lift foot with heel in palm of hand, place bath basin on towel, then lower foot into water to bathe; bathe well between toes. Remove bath basin; dry and cover entire leg with bath blanket. Repeat to bathe thigh, leg, and foot on near side. Give needed attention to toenails. Change water. (See Fig. A-14).

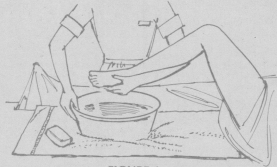

FIGURE A-14

15. Bathe back and buttocks: Ask or assist patient to turn on abdomen or side close to near side of bed. Spread bath towel lengthwise on bed next to body; turn bath blanket to expose neck, back, and buttocks and bathe entire area. Give back rub unless contraindicated (see back rub).

16. Bathe pubic and perineal areas: Ask or assist patient to turn on back; spread bath towel under buttocks. Place bedside table with bath basin and soap, washcloth, and towel within easy reach of patient and ask patient to finish bath. Bathe patient, if necessary; obtain a male nurse or attendant, if possible, to bathe a male patient.

17. Provide clean gown.

18. Give or assist with hair care (see Hair, Daily Care.)

The Partial Bath

According to the purpose, the time of day, and the agency, a "partial bath" may be called a sponge bath or A.M. or P.M. care. It is a bath given for the same purposes as those listed for the complete bath, but includes only selected parts of the body (e.g., face, hands, and arms; or back and perineum; or mouth and hair care.

Chapter 54 includes additional comments about bathing children.

BATHING

TUB BATH (CLEANSING)

Purpose

Allow the patient who is able and permitted to bathe in a tub; provide the opportunity for self-care, motion and exercise, and increased circulation, which promote relaxation, refreshment, comfort, and a feeling of accomplishment and of independence.

Equipment, Supplies, Materials

Bath towel and washcloth, bath mat, rubber mat (non-skid), bathroom stool or chair, and bath blanket, if necessary. Soap, back lotion, talcum powder, deodorant, robe, slippers, and gown or clothes for dressing.

Course of Action

1. Make certain bathroom and tub are clean and that temperature of room will be comfortable and safe.

2. Place supplies and linen near tub for convenience.

3. Place rubber mat on bottom of tub. Use a folded bath towel if rubber mat is not available.

4. Fill tub about one-third with water at 105° F., unless otherwise ordered.

5. Place bath mat on floor next to tub.

6. Provide assistance to patient, as necessary, to get to and from the bathroom, to dress and undress, and to get into and out of the tub.

7. Instruct patient regarding safety precautions:

    a. Use grab bars or rails in getting in and out of tub.

    b. Sit in tub with the feet toward the water faucets.

    c. Drain water from tub before getting out of tub.

    d. Do not add cold or hot water.

    e. Call nurse (or assistant) for any help.

    f. Leave door unlocked.

    g. Get out of tub before starting to dry self; stand on bath mat or sit on stool or chair.

8. Provide privacy and prevent chilling: Use bath blanket, gown, or bath towel when getting in or out of tub or dressing or undressing; keep door closed.

9. Permit and encourage patient to bathe self, if possible; wash and dry back for him.

10. Remain in or near bathroom while patient bathes; check frequently if not in constant attendance.

11. Allow the patient to remain in tub no longer than 10 minutes for a cleansing bath unless time is otherwise ordered or permitted by physician.

12. Provide for back care according to the needs, wishes, and convenience of patient.

13. Furnish any needed assistance before or after the bath for personal hygiene (mouth and teeth, hair, elimination).

SOME COMMON VARIATIONS AND ADAPTATIONS

1. Adjust the amount and temperature of water according to the age and size of the patient as well as his needs and personal desires, if possible.

2. Place a low, suitable stool or seat in tub for patient to sit on if condition of patient or circumstances warrant it.

3. Stay with a child or elderly person during entire bath. Allow him to bathe self but assist as necessary. Expect and plan to take more time with this patient.

4. Obtain sufficient help to lift a patient who becomes unable to get out of tub without full help.

5. Dry patient as much as possible before attempting to lift or to assist a patient out of tub.

6. Obtain a male nurse or attendant, if possible, to assist with a male patient.

SHOWER BATH (CLEANSING)

Purpose

Allow the patient who is able and permitted to bathe in a shower; provide the opportunity for self-care, motion and exercise, and increased circulation, which promote relaxation, refreshment, comfort, and a feeling of accomplishment and independence.

Equipment, Supplies, Materials

Bath towel and washcloth, bath mat, rubber mat (non-skid), soap, back lotion, talcum powder, deodorant, robe, slippers, and gown or clothes for dressing, bathroom stool or chair, and bath blanket and shower cap if necessary.

Course of Action

1. Make certain bathroom and shower are clean and that temperature of room will be comfortable and safe.

2. Place supplies and linen near shower for convenience.

3. Place rubber mat on floor of shower; use a folded bath towel if rubber mat is not available.

4. Place bath mat on floor next to shower.

5. Provide assistance to patient to and from the shower, to dress and undress, and to get into and out of the shower as necessary.

6. Place stool or chair in the shower if one is to be used.

7. Turn on the hot water first, then the cold. Adjust temperature, force, and direction of water for safety and needs of patient before patient enters shower stall.

8. Instruct patient regarding safety precautions:
   a. Use grab bars in getting in and out of shower stall.
   b. Leave door unlocked.
   c. Call for nurse or assistant for any help.
   d. Do *not* adjust temperature or flow of water.
   e. Step out of shower stall *before* turning off water (if patient is able and responsible for self-care).
   f. Turn off the hot water first, then the cold.

9. Provide privacy and prevent chilling: use bath blanket, gown, or bath towel when getting in or out of shower and dressing or undressing. Keep door closed.

10. Permit and encourage patient to bathe self; assist, as necessary, as with washing the back or feet.

11. Remain in bathroom or near shower.

12. Allow the patient to remain in the shower no longer than 10 minutes for a cleansing bath.

13. Provide for back care according to needs, wishes, and convenience of patient.

14. Furnish any needed assistance before or after the shower for patient's personal hygiene (mouth, teeth, and hair care and elimination).

15. Turn off water if patient falls or becomes faint. Dry patient as quickly and as much as possible. Obtain sufficient help to lift patient or to assist with a patient who needs full help to leave the shower stall.

16. Obtain a male nurse or attendant, if possible, to assist a male patient.

SPONGE BATHS (ALCOHOL, COLD, TEPID)

Purpose

Decrease an elevated body temperature; produce relaxation, sleep, and cleanliness.

Equipment, Supplies, Materials

Bath basin, two bath towels, three washcloths, bath thermometer, rectal thermometer, covered ice cap, filled, hot water bag filled with water at 105° F. and covered, a small basin with cracked ice, protective pillow cover, protective drawsheet, two bath blankets, and paper and pencil. Ethyl alcohol, 70 per cent (usually one part alcohol to three parts water, or one part alcohol to one part water), isopropyl alcohol (rubbing alcohol compound) may be ordered.

Course of Action

1. Know the purpose of the sponge bath and the specific directions given in the physician's order, such as the solution to be used, the temperature of the solution, the duration of the bath or the body temperature to be reached, whether the bath is to be continuous or repeated after a certain lapse of time, the results to be obtained, the specific observations to make, and the precautions to take.

2. Have patient empty bladder.

3. Lower or adjust bed to a flat position, if possible or permissible.

4. Use bath blanket to cover patient as top bedding is fan-folded to foot of bed. Place protective drawsheet covered with bath blanket under patient; place protective cover on pillow and replace linen pillow case.

5. Prepare the water or the solution ordered in a bath basin. Use bath thermometer to measure the temperature; adjust temperature as ordered by the physician or follow the policy of the agency.

6. Move patient to near side of bed; remove gown.

7. Take temperature, pulse, and respirations.

8. Apply hot water bag to feet and ice cap to top of head (as ordered or permitted).

9. Maintain desired temperature of water or solution during the sponge bath, according to the physician's order. Keep bath thermometer in the bath basin of water. Use ice as needed to keep water cooled to a constant temperature, or to gradually cool the water to a lower temperature as the bath is given.

10. Unfold the washcloths and place in the basin of water. Use washcloths alternately, leaving one in the water to cool as the other two are being used. Exchange washcloths frequently to keep cool.

11. Place one towel over top of bath blanket and chest; place one towel under the arms and legs as they are sponged.

12. Use long, smooth, light strokes to sponge. Dry with light patting *only* if necessary to remove excessive moisture.

13. Sponge the face with plain water. Sponge the arm on the far side, then the arm on the near side; sponge the leg on the far side, then the leg on the near side; sponge the back. Omit sponging the abdomen.

   a. Stroke arm from neck over upper shoulder to axilla and inner part of arm down to palm of hand.

   b. Stroke leg from top of hip over outer and inner surfaces of thigh and leg to the feet. Pay extra attention to groin and popliteal areas.

   c. Keep cooled, moist washcloth in the axilla as the arms and legs are sponged.

   d. Continue to sponge each arm and each leg as described above for five minutes.

   e. Stroke back from neck over buttocks for five to ten minutes.

14. Take the temperature during the bath and the pulse and respirations frequently.

15. Observe the patient closely during the bath for unfavorable signs and symptoms, such as cyanosis, chilliness, and weak pulse; discontinue bath, apply warmth to body; and report if these or other unfavorable signs appear.

16. Put gown on patient. Change bedding if needed. Provide for rest and comfort of patient.

17. Leave patient between bath blankets if sponge bath is to be repeated; repeat *only* if ordered and according to specific directions.

18. Take temperature, pulse, and respirations 20 to 30 minutes after completing the bath; take more often, if indicated, to observe results obtained.

SOME COMMON VARIATIONS AND ADAPTATIONS

1. Various terms may be used to describe the temperature of the bath. The following range of temperatures* is given frequently:

   lukewarm, 94° F. to 96° F.
   tepid, 85° F. to 92° F.
   temperate, 75° F. to 85° F.
   cool, 60° F. to 75° F.
   cold, 32° F. to 70° F.

2. Use a large bath basin or the bath tub, according to the age and size of the patient, *if the physician orders* the body or a part to be immersed or soaked.

3. Place a bath blanket over a protective drawsheet and cover self to hold a small child in lap to sponge, if necessary or more convenient.

4. Take 15 to 20 minutes to give sponge bath to a child.

5. Know whether alcohol rubbing compound may be used after sponging the back with water or used as a substitute for the water to stroke the back.

6. Obtain specific directions, and follow the physician's order or the policy of the agency, to carry out any similar method ordered to reduce body temperature, e.g., immersion in a tub, cold water mattress, cold wet sheets, cold pack, or ice or ice water.

7. Know the amount and kind of fluids to give the patient during or following the bath, if ordered.

COLLOIDAL AND MEDICATED BATHS

Purpose

Provide relief from burning or itching discomfort; apply a medication; cleanse skin with a disease, an infection, or disorder.

---

*Dorland's Illustrated Medical Dictionary, 24th Ed., p. 187.

Equipment, Supplies, Materials

Two or three soft bath towels, washcloth, bath blanket, bath mat, clean gown, rubber bath mat, portable tub, basin, or container of appropriate size for use when a part is to be soaked, bath thermometer, and ingredients as ordered for preparation of bath.

Course of Action

1. Know the purpose of the bath and the specific directions given in the physician's order, such as ingredients to be used, temperature of solution (may need to alternate, using one temperature and then another), duration of the bath, specific observations to make, and precautions to take.

2. Have patient empty bladder.

3. Prepare solution.

4. Follow orders regarding use of sponging, soaking, jet force, and vapor (enclosed in cabinet).

    a. Cereal tub bath: Boil and stir 2 cups of cereal (oatmeal, bran, or soybean) with 2 quarts of water for five minutes. Pour into mesh bag. Fill bath tub about three-fourths full with tepid water (95° F. - 35° C). Stir mesh bag of cereal around in tub for several minutes to mix thoroughly. Prepackaged cereal preparations give directions on the package (e.g., Aveeno, Soyaloid).

    b. Starch bath: Pour 2 quarts boiling water over one cup of starch (laundry starch or cornstarch). Add this solution directly to tub three-fourths filled with tepid water. Uncooked starch paste may be added to the tub.

    c. Medications may include potassium permanganate, peroxide, or detergent.

5. Allow patient to stay in tub about 20 to 30 minutes. If permitted or ordered longer, add hot water in small amounts as needed to maintain desired temperature.

6. Provide for safety and comfort:

    a. Place rubber mat in the tub (cereal may make tub surface slippery).

    b. Observe for signs of fatigue, overexertion, chilling.

    c. Remain with patient if necessary.

    d. Prevent chilling; use bath blanket across shoulders if needed.

    e. Pat rather than rub skin areas during and following bath.

    f. Soak or sponge crusts or exudates from skin; use gauze cereal for this purpose if part of the procedure.

    g. Ask ambulatory patient to rest in bed for at least 30 minutes following bath; provide rest and needed warmth following treatment.

7. Observe condition of the skin and pertinent patient remarks following treatment.

SOME COMMON VARIATIONS AND ADAPTATIONS

1. Restrain extremities of child during bath to keep him from scratching.

2. Divert small child's attention during tub treatment if needed to complete it.

3. Apply oil (if ordered) with a piece of cotton rather than gauze; pat on rather than rub.

4. Soak a local area for 15 to 20 minutes.

5. Use sterile materials and supplies when surgical asepsis required. *Apply aseptic practices in any event.*

SITZ BATH

Purpose

Provide relief from pain; cleanse anal and perineal area; promote healing by soaking the pelvic region.

Equipment, Supplies, Materials

Bath tub, portable sitz bath or chair, inflated rubber ring, linens as for a tub bath, and footstool.

Course of Action

1. Prepare the environment and equipment before patient is involved.

2. Fill tub with sufficient water to reach umbilicus. Water temperature 110° F. to 115° F. if purpose is to apply heat to area; 94° F. to 98° F. if for cleansing purposes. Check temperature often to keep it constant.

3. Treatment lasts from 15 to 30 minutes or as indicated by the physician.

4. Have patient sit on rubber ring. Ask him to flex his knees to keep extremities out of water as much as possible.

5. Check for pressure areas against thighs if patient is using a sitz chair. Provide stool for feet to relieve pressure on thighs.

6. Cover patient with bath blanket to prevent chilling.

7. Insure privacy. This may require posting a notice on bathroom door.

8. Remain with patient.

9. Observe for signs of faintness or fatigue. Fifteen to 30 minutes can be tiring and cause position discomfort.

10. Ask patient to remain in bed for awhile after treatment.

ENEMAS

Purpose

Inject a liquid substance into the rectum to be retained or expelled, according to the specific results desired as, for example, to remove feces or flatus, soften feces, coat and soothe mucous membranes, or provide a therapeutic or systemic effect.

Equipment, Supplies, Materials

Disposable container with solution and rectal tip, or disposable or nondisposable irrigation can or funnel, tubing, clamp, connector, rectal tube (No. 22 to No. 32 Fr. for adults; No. 10 to No. 12 Fr. catheter for child), and small basin, paper towel or toilet tissue, lubricant (water soluble), tissue squares, solution in pitcher or large graduate, kind and amount as ordered, at temperature about 105° F. or as ordered (use bath thermometer to take temperature), and small plastic or rubber protector with cover. Have bedpan with cover, roll of toilet tissue, and bath blanket at bedside. A standard may or may not be needed.

Course of Action

1. Select equipment according to the patient's age, size, and condition, the type and amount of solution, and the purpose (retention, nonretention).

2. Use a funnel or small container for small amount of solution, oil, or solution of thicker consistency, solution to be given very slowly and under low pressure, retention enema, or child.

3. Know the purpose of the enema and any specific directions given in the physician's order.

4. Have patient empty bladder.

5. Have patient in bed, *not* sitting on a commode or toilet stool in bathroom.

6. Lower or adjust bed to a flat position, if possible and permissible.

7. Use bath blanket to cover patient as top bedding is fan-folded to foot of bed.

8. Ask or assist patient to turn to left lateral position with knees flexed (left Sim's), if possible, with buttocks close to near side of bed.

9. Place covered bed protector under buttocks and over side of bed; drape patient with bath blanket.

10. Lubricate 2 inches of tip of rectal tube with tissue; stroke toward top to avoid filling side or end openings in tube.

11. Pour solution into container and expel air from tubing and tube. Allow solution to flow to tip of rectal tube; close clamp on tubing or pinch tube a few inches from tip and hold closed.

12. Raise upper buttock to expose anus; hold lifted buttock until after rectal tube is inserted.

13. Insert tip of rectal tube. Ask patient to take a deep breath. Rotate tip slowly to insert. Insert slowly and gently to about 3 to 4 inches (adult), just beyond the internal sphincter.

14. Release flow of solution and allow solution to enter rectum slowly, under low

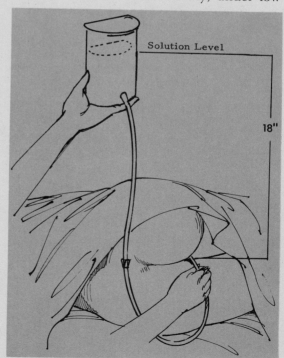

Solution Level

18"

FIGURE A-15

pressure; hold container so that level of solution is not over 18 inches above rectum. (See Fig. A-15.)

15. Adjust flow of solution for patient's comfort and until sufficient or required amount of solution has been taken:

    a. Lower height of container to lower pressure and to slow the rate of flow.

    b. Pinch or clamp tubing to stop flow of solution for a few minutes.

    c. Ask patient to take deep breaths through the mouth.

    d. Apply pressure over anus while solution is being given, if necessary.

    e. Encourage patient.

    f. Discontinue enema at once and report if difficulty occurs, e.g., if solution does not flow in readily and easily, or if patient has severe pain or a reaction.

16. Prevent funnel or container becoming empty before all of solution has been given; pour solution from pitcher or graduate to keep refilled until required amount has been taken.

17. Pinch rectal tube close to anus as last of solution enters rectum.

18. Withdraw rectal tube, rotating slowly and gently; place rectal tip on the paper towel.

19. Instruct and assist patient to obtain desired results from enema.

Nonretention Type

1. Apply slight pressure over anal region; hold or press buttocks together.

2. Ask patient to remain in same position for five to 10 minutes to retain solution as long as possible.

3. Place patient on bedpan; raise backrest or support patient in upright position. If possible, help patient to toilet in bathroom.

4. Make certain call signal and roll of toilet tissue are placed for convenient use; ask patient to turn on call signal when enema has been expelled.

5. Leave patient alone to expel the enema unless he must be assisted or supported because of age or condition.

6. Return to check on patient in about five to 10 minutes.

7. Caution patient using bathroom not to flush toilet until results have been observed.

8. Observe results and note especially, according to purpose of enema, the amount,

consistency, and color of feces; presence and estimated amount of flatulence; presence of foreign materials or mucus; unusual odor or appearance of returns; comments and reactions of patient, if any (e.g., "I feel better," "I'm all worn out," presence of pain or straining). Obtain specimen if ordered or pertinent. Ask charge nurse to observe results if unsure of results obtained.

9. Report at once to charge nurse or physician if no solution or fecal material can be expelled, or if desired results have not been obtained; obtain order and directions for further action, which may include:

    a. Allow more time for patient to expel solution.

    b. Massage abdomen lightly toward the left side and down.

    c. Turn patient from side to side; walk with patient; take patient to toilet in bathroom; place patient in knee-chest position.

    d. Siphon enema: Have patient lie on right side with knees flexed. Place bedpan or other container suitable to receive solution on a chair or stool at side of bed so that it is lower than patient's hips. Connect rectal tube to a small funnel and lubricate the tip. Pinch tube and fill funnel with tap water (105° F.). Insert tip of rectal tube 3 to 4 inches. Invert funnel quickly and lower over the bedpan to receive the enema fluid as it is drawn from the patient's colon; repeat, if necessary, to start siphonage. Measure amount withdrawn.

Retention Type

1. Apply light pressure over anal region; hold or press buttocks together.

2. Ask patient to stay quiet and to remain in same position for as long as possible.

3. Reassure patient. Return as necessary to check on condition of patient.

4. Observe results and note especially according to purpose of enema: duration of retention (e.g., complete, none, or partial, how much solution expelled, after what length of time), reaction and comfort of patient.

5. Report to charge nurse if solution is retained for desired length of time or the desired results or purpose of the enema are not achieved.

6. Observe expelled returns as to the

amount, color, and consistency of solution or fecal material; note specific discomforts or difficulties.

SOME COMMON VARIATIONS AND ADAPTATIONS

1. Use a commercial enema according to the physician's order, the policy of the agency, or the directions given on the set; usually given at room temperature.

2. Place patient in the right lateral, dorsal, or knee-chest position.

3. Make necessary arrangements and take precautions to give an enema to an incontinent or an unconscious patient:

   a. Use large covered protective draw-sheet to protect bed from leakage during the enema.

   b. Place patient on bedpan before starting enema.

   c. Obtain assistance to turn an unconscious patient onto bedpan.

   d. Use care and the means necessary to support back and to prevent pressure or damage to skin; use firm pillows with protective coverings.

   e. Wear rubber gloves if it is necessary to hold rectal tube in rectum or there is leakage during the enema.

4. Use sterile equipment and supplies and sterile technique if an order is to give a "sterile" enema.

5. Repeat an enema *only* when there is a written order to do so; check specific directions regarding:

   a. When the repeat enema is to be given (e.g., immediately, after an interval of one hour).

   b. How many enemas are to be given (e.g., once, for 4 hours, or until certain results are obtained).

   c. How much solution to be given, and whether at one time or over a certain period of time.

   d. When order reads for enema to be given "until returns are clear" or "until temperature reduced," know the specific directions to follow.

   e. What precautions to take and observations to make to avoid fatigue, dehydration, injury (e.g., irritation to anus, rectum, and bowel mucosa), distention, and discomfort.

   f. What after-care is to be given (in addition to making certain the patient and bed are clean and dry,

applying a lubricant to anus, if permitted, and providing for rest).

For Infant and Child

1. Know the directions specified in the physician's *written* order for the type, amount, and temperature of solution to be used, as well as the precautions to take and the observations to make *before* giving any enema.

2. Use a No. 10 to No. 12 Fr. catheter, or the size specified. Insert catheter very carefully (never with force or difficulty) from 1½ to 3 inches, according to size of child. Expect to hold the catheter in place during the entire enema.

3. Prepare the crib or bed with an extra, covered protective drawsheet over bed. Use covered protective covers on pillows.

4. Place child on appropriate size bedpan. Fold diaper or small sheet to pad bedpan under the buttocks. Position and support body for proper alignment; place pillows under head and back.

5. Use restraint to hold legs in position over sides of bedpan with the use of a diaper. (See Fig. A-16.)

6. Use the left lateral or Sim's position for an older child.

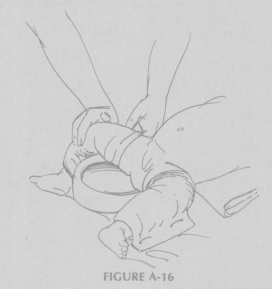

FIGURE A-16

7. Hold container no higher than 4 inches above rectum. Give any type enema very slowly. Use pressure over the anus during the enema and for a few minutes following to help obtain the results desired.

8. Watch for signs or symptoms of distress; discontinue at once at first appearance and report to nurse in charge.

9. *Stay* with the child until the enema

A SUMMARY OF THE SEVERAL TYPES OF ENEMA

Type	Purpose	Solution
Nonretention		
*1. Cleansing	To cleanse of fecal material	Normal saline, soapsuds, tap water
*2. Carminative	To expel flatus	Parts of magnesium sulfate, glycerin, and water; milk and molasses
3. Antihelmintic (can be retention)	To expel worms	Drug specified
4. Astringent	To contract tissues	Alum in water
Retention		
*1. Lubricating	To soften feces	Vegetable oils (olive, cottonseed)
2. Emollient	To coat and soothe mucous membranes	Vegetable oils, starch
3. Nutrient	To provide nourishment	Dextrose
4. Sedative	To induce sleep	Paraldehyde or chloral hydrate in saline or oil
5. Stimulating	To stimulate body processes	Normal saline, black coffee, water

*Types of enema given most frequently.

is fully expelled or until the results are obtained; place an older child on toilet to expel a nonretention type enema, if permissible and possible.

10. Observe and record with exactness.

URINARY BLADDER TREATMENTS

CATHETERIZATION

Purpose

Empty bladder to relieve pressure and retention; secure specimen; determine amount of residual urine; protect perineum from urine.

Equipment, Supplies, Materials

Sterile:
Catheter: Child, No. 8 or No. 10 French; Female, No. 14 or No. 16 French; Male, No. 20 or No. 22 French.

Basin for solution and cotton balls, water soluble lubricant, towel, gloves, and specimen bottle (if necessary).

Non-Sterile:
Drape sheet or bath blanket, container for urine, bed protector, waste container, and light.

Course of Action for Female

1. Position and drape patient in dorsal recumbent position.

2. Protect bed linen under patient's buttocks with covered waterproof material.

3. Focus light on perineum.

4. Wash and rinse the genital area thoroughly.

5. Arrange the sterile field, providing all needed supplies.

6. Wash hands and put on sterile gloves or finger cots, if available; otherwise use cotton balls to expose the meatus.

7. Separate the labia minora with protected thumb and index finger to expose the meatus and hold until procedure is completed. (See Fig. A-17.)

8. Cleanse the exposed area using cotton balls and solution; cleansing strokes move from top toward the vagina. Use fresh cotton ball for each downward stroke.

9. Lubricate the catheter tip for about 1½ inches; avoid clogging tip eye. Place open end of catheter in basin to catch the urine.

10. Insert catheter gently into meatus until urine begins to flow, usually 2 to 3 inches. Avoid forcing catheter or inserting beyond usual length.

11. Collect any required specimen.

12. Hold catheter in place until urine

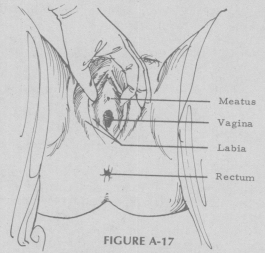

FIGURE A-17

ceases to flow, unless the amount seems excessive (more than 1000 cc.).

13. Pinch off catheter and gently remove.

14. Report observation if bladder did not appear to be empty when procedure was terminated.

Course of Action for Male

1. Observe steps 1 through 6 for female patient.

2. Retract foreskin of penis and hold back.

3. Cleanse the exposed area using solution and one cotton ball for each stroke, working from distal toward proximal position. Place cleansed portion on sterile field.

4. Lubricate catheter tip about 1½ to 2 inches; lubricate meatus with one or two drops of lubricant. Place open end of catheter in basin to catch urine.

5. Position the penis at about a 60° to 90° angle in relation to the body and gently insert catheter about 6 to 8 inches until urine flows. Proceed slowly and gently with catheter insertion, lowering the penis slightly after the catheter is about 5 inches in place. A slight rolling movement of catheter may be helpful during insertion.

6. Collect any required specimen.

7. Pinch off catheter and gently remove when urine ceases to flow or the amount of urine seems excessive (more than 1000 cc.).

8. Report observation if bladder did not appear to be empty when procedure was terminated.

SOME VARIATIONS AND ADAPTATIONS

1. Use same procedure for older child as for the adult. Be sure to let the child know what is to be done. It will help to let him see the equipment ahead of time.

2. Have a very good light when catheterizing an infant because the meatus is very small. Locate it without probing for it. Secure assistance to position infant if needed.

INDWELLING CATHETER (FOLEY)

Purposes

Provide a continuing means for emptying the bladder to prevent infection; allow healing to take place; keep incontinent patient dry; restore normal bladder function; keep accurate record of urine output.

Equipment, Supplies, Materials

Foley catheter (sterile), Asepto syringe (sterile), solution (normal saline-sterile), drainage tubing (with clamp and connecting rod), drainage container (sterile), and container holder.

Course of Action

1. Secure proper size Foley catheter. if not specified by physician, ask him. Commonly used size for adults is No. 18, 5 cc.

2. Observe technique for regular catheterization when inserting the deflated Foley catheter. Empty the bladder.

3. Inject the amount of solution specified on the catheter into the proper lumen (leading to the balloon) with the Asepto syringe. Clamp off or seal off end of tube. If using self-sealing lumen, introduce solution with sterile syringe and needle (No. 20).

4. Connect catheter to tubing with connecting rod. Have clamp closed.

5. Place free end of tubing in container.

6. Suspend container in holder and open clamp.

7. Anchor tubing securely to thigh; allow some curvature in tubing between anchor point and the point of insertion. (See Fig. A-18.)

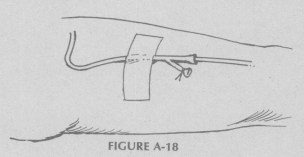

FIGURE A-18

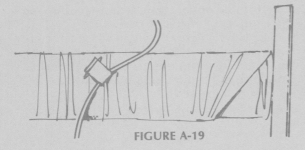

FIGURE A-19

8. Anchor tubing to bottom sheet, again allowing some curvature in tubing. (See Fig. A-19.)

9. Check the complete length of tubing to be sure there are no twists or kinks.

SOME COMMON VARIATIONS AND ADAPTATIONS FOR INFANT

1. Select appropriate size Foley catheter. Trauma can result from inserting one that is too large. Ask, if size is not specified.

2. Observe the amount of fluid needed to inflate the balloon.

INSTILLATION OF DRUGS

Purpose

Place a drug in the bladder.

Equipment, Supplies, Materials

Catheterization set, needed equipment, medication as ordered (sterile container), and syringe barrel or funnel (sterile).

Course of Action

1. Prepare medication as ordered (amount, temperature).

2. Catheterize patient; leave catheter in place.

3. Insert funnel or syringe barrel into free end of catheter.

4. Pour medication into funnel or syringe slowly.

5. Remove catheter.

IRRIGATION

Purpose

Apply heat; apply medication; cleanse; prevent infection.

Equipment, Supplies, Materials

Catheterization set, needed equipment, solution as ordered (sterile container), Asepto syringe, large syringe barrel, funnel (sterile), and basin (sterile).

Course of Action

1. Position and drape patient.

2. Prepare solution; determine proper temperature.

3. Catheterize patient; leave catheter in place.

4. Insert funnel or syringe barrel into free end of catheter.

5. Pour (or introduce with Asepto syringe) about 50 cc. to 100 cc. of solution slowly into catheter. Keep funnel low; pinch off catheter just before funnel empties.

6. Tip funnel or syringe barrel over basin to permit solution to return from bladder.

7. Repeat steps 5 and 6, using all solution or amount indicated by the physician.

8. Remove catheter.

SOME COMMON VARIATIONS AND ADAPTATIONS FOR INDWELLING CATHETER

1. Disconnect catheter from tubing and place free end of catheter in sterile basin.

2. Place free end of tubing on a sterile field.

3. Introduce small amount (15 to 30 cc.) of solution with Asepto syringe.

4. Withdraw syringe and allow solution to drain into basin.

5. Repeat steps 3 and 4 until solution has been used or the return is clear.

6. Reconnect catheter and tubing. Check to see that tubing has no twists or kinks.

COLOSTOMY

Purposes

Cleanse the bowel; aid proper functioning of colostomy; relieve distention; maintain normal skin condition of the area.

Equipment, Supplies, Materials

Irrigation equipment; can or container, tubing with clamp and glass connector, catheter (whistle tip No. 16 or No. 18 French commonly used), and pole standard; solution (100° to 105° F.) as ordered (e.g., 1000 to 2000 cc. water or normal saline), container for pouring, lubricant (water soluble), two large curved basins, bedpan, bed protective materials, toilet tissue, waste container, bath basin, towel, washcloth, soap or prescribed cleansing material, water, dressings, plastic bag, and adhesive material.

Course of Action

Determine first if patient has double-barreled colostomy, whether the distal loop or the proximal loop is to be irrigated. Proceed as follows with a single opening or a proximal opening:

1. Position patient close to edge of bed in sitting (dangling) or Fowler's position.

2. Cover bed area involved with protective material; be sure side of bed is well covered.

3. Provide means for bowel drainage to run off into bedpan or pail by arranging plastic trough between patient and bedpan, or use curved basins for bowel drainage and empty into bedpan.

4. Remove dressings or disposable colostomy bag and discard.

5. Cleanse surrounding skin area and stoma (opening) and position curved basin against abdomen.

6. Position irrigating container (with tubing and attached catheter) about 2 feet above level of stoma so that solution level will be about 18 inches above stoma. (See Fig. A-20.)

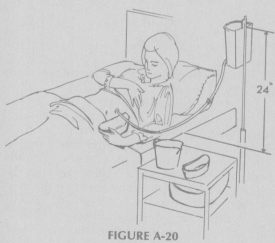

24"

FIGURE A-20

7. Open clamp and expel air from tubing; close. Lubricate catheter tip.

8. Insert catheter tip into stoma about 4 inches with gentle rolling motion.

9. Introduce about 500 cc. of solution slowly into the bowel. Halt the flow momentarily if patient complains of discomfort.

10. Remove catheter to permit drainage of feces into curved basin or through trough into bedpan.

11. Repeat process until return flow is clear (may take from 30 minutes to an hour or longer).

12. Find out if special precautions are needed for distal loop irrigation. Above procedure might be used or patient may be placed directly on bedpan or toilet. Protect bed well if a bed procedure.

13. Use same process for irrigating colostomy with irrigating dome, except that patient is seated on the toilet. (See Fig. A-21.)

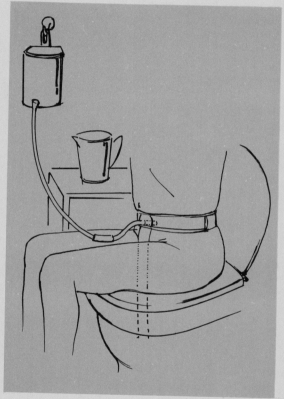

FIGURE A-21

14. Position the rubber or plastic dome or cup directly over stoma so that hole in the dome is in line with stoma. Secure it in position by waistline belt.

15. Drop the plastic drainage tube between patient's legs into toilet bowl.

16. Proceed (or have patient proceed) until return flow is clear.

17. Cleanse stomal area thoroughly; dry well.

18. Apply any medication to skin area as may be ordered; apply ample dressings around and over stoma.

19. Secure plastic disposable bag to area if this is used instead of dressings.

TRACHEOSTOMY CARE

Purpose

Provide clear passageway for breathing by suctioning, by wiping away any mucus coughed up, and by cleaning inner cannula.

Equipment, Supplies, Materials

Suction equipment, including Y-tube inserted in the tubing, extra tracheostomy set (same size and complete in all respects), sterile catheters (whistle tip with additional holes along side), sterile gauze squares, small bottle brush, pipestem cleaners, and gauze.

Course of Action

To Suction
1. Use Y-tube to control amount of suction. Taking thumb off the free arm of the Y-tube stops the suction. (Fig. A-22.)

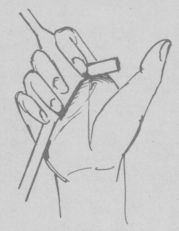

FIGURE A-22

2. Insert catheter the length of inner cannula (only) with thumb off the Y-tube.

3. Start suction; regulate with thumb over free end of Y-tube. Continue about 10 to 15 seconds. (See Fig. A-23.)

4. Resume after three or four minutes. Repeat only until cannula is clear; avoid "oversuctioning."

5. Rotate catheter while withdrawing it; release thumb on Y-tube if suction pulls against side of tube. (See Fig. A-24.)

6. Clean catheter after each use; wipe and flush with water or normal saline. Have it clean and in working order at all times.

To Keep Opening Clear
1. Wipe mucus from opening with cellulose tissues (avoid getting lint into opening).

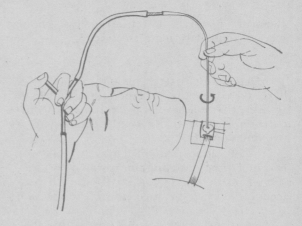

FIGURE A-23 (Sutton: Bedside Nursing Techniques, 2nd Ed.)

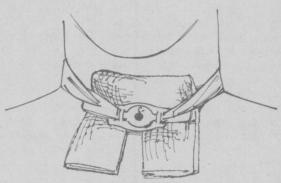

FIGURE A-24

2. Use suction after coughing to clear out mucus.

3. Teach patient to wipe mucus from opening (if possible).

To Clean Inner Cannula
1. Unlock and remove the inner cannula. *Never* remove outer cannula.

2. Wash thoroughly under cold running water, using a pipe stem cleaner, a bottle brush, or piece of gauze pulled through the lumen. Be sure lumen is thoroughly clear of mucus and crusts.

3. Rinse and dry thoroughly.

4. Suction outer cannula before inserting inner tube.

5. Replace inner cannula and lock into position.

6. Change gauze squares and check neck tapes to see that tube is securely in position. (See Fig. A-24.)

NOTE: The outer cannula is not removed by the LPN; neck tapes are not changed by the LPN. A spare inner cannula should be at hand (and used if necessary) when removing and cleaning the inner tube.

NOTES

NOTES

GLOSSARY
AND INDEX

This list of words represents some common terms which may or may not be in the text proper. Reference should be made to a medical dictionary for more specific information. See Appendix II for word prefixes and suffixes.

Sources: Dorland's Illustrated Dictionary, 24th edition and Miller and Keane: Encyclopedia and Dictionary of Medicine and Nursing, 1972.

A

Abnormal (ab-nor'mal). Contrary to the usual structure, position, or condition.

Abscess (ab'ses). A localized collection of pus in a cavity formed by disintegration of tissue.

Absorption (ab-sorp'shun). The act of taking up liquids as a sponge takes up water.

Accelerate (ak-sel'er-at). To speed up, quicken.

Acidosis (as″i-do'sis). The depletion of the alkaline reserve in the body.

Acute (a-kūt). Sharp. Acute illness: having severe symptoms and a short course.

Addiction (ah-dik'shun). The state of being given up to some habit, as a drug habit.

Adolescence (ad″o-les'ens). The period of change between childhood and adulthood.

Adrenal gland (ad-re'nal). A ductless gland at upper end of kidney.

Alignment (ah-līn'ment). The state of being arranged in a line.

Allergy (al'er-je). An exaggerated sensitiveness of an individual to a substance.

Alveoli (al-ve'o-lī). Air cells of the lungs.

Alveolus (al-ve'o-lus). A cavity in the maxillary process of the jaw in which the root of the tooth is fixed.

Ambulatory (am'bu-lah-to-re). Able to walk.

Amnesia (am-nē'ze-ah). Loss of memory.

Amputation (am″pu-ta'shun). The surgical cutting off of a limb or other part.

Anabolism. See Metabolism.

Analgesic (an″al-je'sik). A drug which relieves pain; relieving pain.

Anemia (ah-ne'me-ah). Deficient quantity or quality of the blood.

Anomaly (ah-nom'ah-le). A deviation from the normal standard.

Anorexia (an″o-rek'se-ah). Lack or loss of appetite for food.

Anoxia (an-ok'se-ah). Lack of sufficient oxygen in body tissues.

Antibodies (an'te-bod-ēz). Substances in the blood which act to overcome a specific foreign substance.

Antiemetic (an-te-e-met'ik). Preventing or arresting vomiting.

Antiseptic (an-te-sep'tik). That which retards or prevents the growth of bacteria.

Antitoxin (an″te-tok'sin). Any substance developed in the body to neutralize a poison.

Anuria (ah-nu're-ah). The suppression of urinary secretion; without urine.

Anus (a'nus). The distal or terminal outlet of the alimentary canal.

Apathy (ap'ah-the). Indifference; lack of feeling or emotion.

Apex (ā'peks). The tip, point, or end of anything.

Aphagia (ah-fa'je-ah). Refraining from eating.

Aqueous humor (a'kwē-us). The watery fluid filling the anterior and posterior chambers of the eye.

Articulation (ar-tik″u-la'shun). The junction between two or more bones of the skeleton.

Ascites (ah-si'tēz). Escape of serous fluid into the abdominal cavity.

Asepsis (ah-sep'sis). Freedom from microbes and their products.

Asphyxia (as-fik'se-ah). Suffocation.

Assimilation (ah-sim″i-la'shun). The transformation of food into living tissue.

Asthma (az'mah). A disease characterized by difficulty in breathing.

Astringents (as-trin'jents). Agents which cause contraction and arrest discharges.

Atrophy (at'ro-fe). A wasting or diminution of size.

Axilla (ak-sil'ah). The armpit.

Axon (ak'son). The extension of a nerve cell which conducts impulses away from the nerve body.

B

Bacteria (bak-tē're-ah). Microorganisms; vegetable bodies.

Benign (be-nīn'). Not malignant; favorable for recovery.

Beriberi (ber″e-ber'e). A disease caused by the lack of antineuritic vitamin.

Bichloride of mercury (bi-klo'rid of mer'ku-re). A germicide.

Bicuspid (bi-kus'pid). Having two cusps or points.

Biopsy (bi'op-se). The removal and examination, usually microscopic, of tissue or other material from the living body for purposes of diagnosis.

Buccal (buk'al). Pertaining to the mouth.

Buttocks (but'oks). The muscular prominences covering the hip joint; rump.

C

Calcium (kal'se-um). A basic element of lime.

Callus (kal'us). A thickening of the skin due to pressure.

Calorie (kal'o-re). The amount of heat required to raise a gram of water 1 degree Centigrade.

Cancer (kan'ser). An exceedingly harmful, usually rapid growth of body cells.

Canine (ka'nin). A single cuspid tooth.

Carbon dioxide (kar'bon di-ox'ide). A pungent asphyxiant gas, the waste product of respiration.

Cardiac (kar'de-ak). Pertaining to the heart.

Cardiograph (kar'de-o-graf). An instrument for recording the heart movements.

Caries (ka'rēz). (Dental) Decay of tooth structure.

Cartilage (kar'tĭ-lĭj). The gristle or white elastic substance attached to bone surfaces at the joints.

Catabolism. See Metabolism.

Cathartic (kah-thar'tik). A drug which stimulates the evacuation of intestinal waste; purgative.

Cephalic (sĕ-fal'ik). Pertaining to the head.

Cerumen (sĕ-roo'men). Earwax.

Cervical (ser'vi-kal). Pertaining to the neck.

Cervix (ser'viks). The narrow lower end of the uterus.

Chancre (shang'ker). A primary lesion of syphilis.

Chyle (kīl). A fluid consisting of lymph and emulsified fats which is the result of digestion in the intestine.

Chyme (kīm). A thick grayish liquid which is the result of digestion in the stomach.

Ciliated (sil'e-āt-ed). Provided with a fringe of fine hairs.

Clitoris (kli'to-rus). A small sensitive organ located at the upper part of the vulva.

Colitis (ko-li'tis). Inflammation of the colon.

Collapse (ko-laps'). Marked depression of vital activities of the body.

Colostomy (ko-los'to-me). The formation of a permanent artificial opening into the colon.

Coma (kō'mah). A loss of consciousness.

Communicable (ko-mu'ni-ka-bl). Passing from one to another.

Complication (kom'pli-ka'shun). Associated with another disease.

Congenital (kon-jen'i-tal). Existing at, and usually before, birth.

Conscious (kon'shus). Being aware of one's own existence; mentally responsive.

Contagious (kon-ta'jus). Spreading by direct contact with the sick person or objects he has handled.

Contaminate (kŏn-tăm'ĭ-nāt). To soil or stain by contact; to pollute.

Contracture (kon-trak'tur). A state of permanent contraction of the muscle; a drawing together.

Contraindication (kon"trah-in"dĭ-ka'shun). Any condition, especially any condition of disease, which renders some particular line of treatment undesirable.

Contusion (kon-tu'zhun). A bruise.

Convalescence (kon"vah-les'ens). The stage of recovery after an illness.

Convulsion (kon-vul'shun). A violent involuntary contraction or series of contractions of the voluntary muscles.

Copulation (kop"u-la'shun). A sexual union in which the penis of the male is introduced into the reproductive tract of the female.

Corrosive (ko-ro'siv). Destructive to the tissue.

Coryza (kŏ-ri'zah). Cold in the head.

Creatine (kre'-ah-tin). A constituent of muscle tissue.

Creatinine (kre-at'i-nin). A basic substance of blood and urine.

Crusts. Scabs on the skin.

Culture (kul'tūr). A production of micro-organisms on some nutrient substance.

Cyanosis (si"ah-no'sis). Bluish discoloration of the skin due to lack of oxygen.

Cyst (sist). A sac containing a liquid.

Cystitis (sis-ti'tis). Inflammation of the bladder.

Cytoplasm (si'to-plazm). The protoplasm surrounding the nucleus of a cell.

D

Debilitate (de-bil'i-tāt). To lose strength.

Decidua (de-sid'u-ah). A membrane formed during pregnancy and discarded after birth.

Defecation (def-e-ka'shun). Passing of feces.

Dehydrate (de-hi'drāt). To remove or pull the fluid from.

Delirium (de-lir'e-um). An excited mental state in which the patient talks irrationally.

Delusion (de-lu'zhun). A false belief or fancy.

Dendron (den′dron). A branch of a nerve cell.

Denture (den′tur). A manufactured set of teeth. May be partial or complete.

Deodorant (de-ō′dor-ant). An agent which corrects offensive odors.

Depressant (de-pres′ant). A medicine which reduces body activity.

Dermis (der′mis). The true skin.

Dextrin (deks′trin). A soluble carbohydrate.

Dextrose (deks-trōs). A fruit sugar.

Diagnosis (di-ag-nō′sis). The act of recognizing a disease from its symptoms.

Diagnostician (diag-nos-tish′an). One skilled in recognizing diseases.

Diaphragm (di′ah-fram). A dome-shaped muscle which separates the thoracic and abdominal cavities.

Diarrhea (di″ah-re′ah). Frequent evacuation of the bowels.

Diathermy (di′ah-ther″me). The generation of heat in the body tissues due to resistance by the tissues to high frequency electric currents forced through them.

Dilatation (dil-ah-ta′shun). The condition of being stretched beyond the normal dimensions.

Diphtheria (dif-the′re-ah). An acute infectious disease caused by the Klebs-Löffler bacillus developing in the mucous membranes of the throat.

Disinfectant (dis-in-fek′tant). An agent which destroys infection-producing organisms.

Disorientation (dis-o″rē-en-ta′shun). A state of mental confusion as to time, place, or identity.

Distal (dis′tal). Farther from point of attachment.

Distention (dis-ten′shun). The state of being enlarged.

Diversional (di-vur′zhun-al). Something which distracts.

Dorsal (dor′sal). Pertaining to the back.

Duct (dukt). A canal or passage for fluids.

Ductless (dukt′les). Having no definite outlet.

Duodenum (du-o-dē′num). The first 10 inches of the small intestine.

Dysentery (dis′en-ter-e). A condition of the colon marked by inflammation, pain in the abdomen, and frequent stools.

Dysmenorrhea (dis-men-o-re′ah). Painful menstruation.

Dyspepsia (dis-pep′se-ah). Indigestion.

Dyspnea (disp-ne′ah). Difficulty in breathing.

Dysuria (dis-u′re-ah). Painful or difficult urination.

E

Edema (e-dē′mah). An accumulation of fluid in the tissues.

Electrocardiogram (e-lek″tro-kar′de-o-gram). A graphic tracing of an electric current produced by the contractions of the heart.

Emaciation (e-mā-se-a′shun). A wasted condition of the body; excessive leanness.

Embolism (em′bo-lizm). An obstruction of a blood vessel by a clot of blood.

Embolus (em′bo-lus). Any abnormal particle carried by the blood stream from its point of origin to a different site, as a blood clot or an air bubble.

Embryo (em′bre-o). A term applied to the unborn child from conception to about the third month of pregnancy.

Emesis (em′e-sis). Vomiting.

Emetic (e-met′ik). A drug which will cause vomiting.

Emollient (e-mol′e-ent). A soothing medicine.

Endocrine glands (en′dō-krin). Ductless glands; glands of internal secretion.

Enuresis (en″u-re′sis). Involuntary discharge of the urine during sleep.

Epidemic (ep-i-dem′ik). A disease spreading to many persons at the same time.

Epiglottis (ep-e-glot′is). A thin plate of yellow elastic cartilage which closes to protect the larynx during swallowing.

Epinephrine (ep-ĭ-nef′rin). The active principle of the medulla of the adrenal bodies. It acts to slow the heart and increase blood pressure.

Epistaxis (ep-i-stak′sis). Nosebleed.

Equilibrium (ē-kwi-lib′re-um). A state of balance.

Erythrocytes (e-rith′ro-sīts). Yellowish, circular, biconcave disks, found in the blood, which contain hemoglobin and carry oxygen.

Ethmoid (eth′moid). Sievelike.

Eustachian tube (u-stā′ke-an). An opening from the nasopharynx to the middle ear.

Excoriation (eks-ko″re-a′shun). Any superficial loss of substance, such as that produced on the skin by scratching.

Excreta (eks-kre′tah). Any waste or fecal matter discharged from the intestine.

Expectoration (eks-pek″to-ra′shun). Coughing up sputum from the air passages; also the matter expectorated.

Extension (eks-ten′shun). Pulling two ends of a part, one from the other.

Exudate (eks′u-dāt). The discharge through pores, such as sweat.

F

Febrile (feb′ril). Pertaining to fever; feverish.

Feces (fe′sēz). Discharge from the rectum; stool.

Fetid (fe′tid). Having an unpleasant odor.

Fetus (fe′tus). A term applied to the unborn child after the third month of pregnancy.

Fimbriated (fim′bre-at-ed). Fringed.

Flaccid (flak′sid). Weak, lax, and soft.

Flatulence (flat′u-lens). Excessive gas in the stomach or intestine.

Flexion (flek′shun). The act of bending or condition of being bent.

Fluoroscope (floo-o′ro-skōp). A device used for examining deep structures by means of the roentgen rays.

Forceps (for′seps). A two-blade instrument with handles used to grasp and pull small objects.

Functional (funk′shun-al). Pertaining to the special action or function of an organ.

G

Gangrene (gang′grēn). Death of tissue.

Gastrointestinal (gas″tro-in-tes′tĭ-nal. Pertaining to stomach and intestine.

Gavage (gah-vahzh″). Forced feeding by means of a tube passed directly through the mouth down to the stomach.

Genes (jēnz). Factors in the chromosomes which determine hereditary characteristics.

Genitalia (jen″i-ta′le-ah). The reproductive organs.

Germicide (jer′mi-sid). An agent that kills germs.

Gestation (jes-ta′shun). Pregnancy.

Glucose (gloo′kos). A sugar.

Gluteus (gloo-te′us). Buttocks.

Glutin (gloo′tin). A sticky substance from the protein of wheat.

Glycogen (gli′ko-jen). A white, tasteless carbohydrate.

Gonorrhea (gon-o-re′ah). A contagious inflammatory condition of the genital mucous membrane.

Green soap. A liniment of soft soap.

Gynecological (jin″ĕ-ko-loj′ek′l). Pertaining to the science of diseases of the genital tract in women.

H

Habit (hab′it). A fixed practice established by repetition.

Hallucination (hah-lu″sĭ-na′shun). A sense of perception not founded upon objective reality, such as the hearing of unreal sounds.

Hematemesis (hem-at-em′e-sis). Vomiting of blood.

Hematuria (hem″ah-tu′rē-ah). The discharge of blood in the urine.

Hemiplegia (hem-e-ple′je-ah). Paralysis of one side of the body.

Hemophilia (he-mo-fil′e-ah). A congenital condition characterized by delayed clotting of blood.

Hemoptysis (hem-op′ti-sis). The spitting of blood.

Hemorrhoids (hem′o-roids). Enlarged veins in the lower rectum; piles.

Heredity (he-red′it-e). Transmission of characters from parents or other ancestor to offspring.

Hernia (her′ne-ah). The protrusion of a loop or knuckle of an organ or tissue through an abnormal opening.

Herpes (her′pēz). A cluster of water blisters, usually on the face and mouth.

Hormones (hor′mōnz). A chemical substance produced in an organ, which, carried to an associated organ by the blood stream, influences its functional activity.

Humidity (hu-mid′ĭ-te). The percentage of water vapor in the air to the total amount possible at the same temperature.

Hydrotherapy (hi-dro-ther′ah-pe). Treatment of disease by baths and mineral water.

Hygiene (hi′je-ēn). The science of health and its preservation.

Hymen (hi′men). A membranous fold which partially or wholly covers the external opening of the vagina.

Hyperglycemia (hy″per-gli-se′me-ah). Excessive sugar in the blood.

Hyperventilation (hy″per-ven″ti-la′shun). 1. More than the normal amount of air in the lungs. 2. Abnormally deep and excessive breathing.

Hypnotic (hip-not′ik). An agent that produces sleep.

Hypodermoclysis (hi-po-der-mok′li-sis). Injection of fluids into the tissues under the skin.

Hypothyroidism (hi-po-thi′roid-izm). An abnormal condition caused by deficient activity of the thyroid gland.

Hysteria (his-tēr′e-ah). Lack of control over emotions or acts.

I

Immobilize (im-mo′bil-iz). To render incapable of being moved.

Immune (i-mūn′). Protected against a disease, as by inoculation.

Immunize (im′u-nīz). To render safe from disease.

Impaction (im-pak′shun). The condition of being firmly lodged or wedged.

Incisor (in-ci′zer). A tooth which is adapted for cutting.

Incontinence (in-kon′ti-nens). The inability to control elimination of urine or feces.

Incubation (in-ku-ba'shun). The period during which bacteria develop in the body and before which the symptoms of the disease are apparent.

Incus (ing'kus). One of the small bones of the middle ear.

Infection (in-fek'shun). The invasion of the body by microorganisms.

Inflammation (in"fla-ma'shun). The reaction of tissue to irritation which is characterized by redness, heat, swelling, pain, and loss of function.

Inoculation (in-ok"u-la'shun). The injection of viruses into the skin or flesh to obtain immunity against certain diseases.

Insecticide (in-sek'tĭ-sīd). A substance which kills insects.

Insidious (in-sid'e-us). Coming on in a stealthy manner.

Insomnia (in-som'ne-ah). Inability to sleep; abnormal wakefulness.

Insulin (in'su-lin). Substance produced by the pancreas.

Intercellular (in-ter-sel'u-lar). Between the cells of any structure.

Intern (in'tern). A resident or indoor physician or surgeon in a hospital.

Intravenous (in-trah-vē'nus). Situated within a vein.

Isolate (i'so-lāt). To separate from other people.

L

Labyrinth (lab'i-rinth). The internal ear.

Laceration (las"er-a'shun). The act of tearing. A wound made by tearing.

Lacteals (lak'tē-alz). Lymph vessels in the intestine.

Lanolin (lan'o-lin). Wool fat.

Laryngitis (lar-in-jī'tis). Inflammation of the larynx.

Lateral (lat'er-al). Denoting a position more toward the side. Pertaining to a side.

Lavage (lah-vahzh'). An irrigation; washing out the stomach, for example.

Lens (lenz). A structure in the eye which changes shape to focus images on the retina.

Lesion (le'zhun). An opening into the tissue; a wound, cut, or sore.

Lethargy (leth'ar-je). A state of stupor, dullness, indifference, lacking of feeling.

Ligament (lig'a-ment). A tough, fibrous band binding together bones or supporting internal organs.

Ligate (li'gāt). To tie or bind with a ligature.

Ligature (lig'ah-tūr). A thread or wire for tying a vessel or strangulating a part.

Lumen (lu'men). The cavity or channel within a tube or tubular organ.

Lymphocytes (lim'fo-sīts). Lymph cells, a variety of leukocyte.

M

Malaise (mal-āz'). A vague feeling of bodily discomfort.

Malfunction (mal-funk'shun). Impaired or faulty functioning.

Malignant (mah-lig'nant). Tending to go from bad to worse. Progressively worse.

Malocclusion (mal"o-kloo'shun). Irregular teeth.

Matrix (ma'triks). The groundwork in which something is cast. The uterus.

Meatus (me-a'tus). An opening to some passageway in the body.

Medial (me'de-al). Midline of the body or nearest that midline.

Membrane (mem'brān). A thin layer of tissue which covers a surface or divides an organ.

Menopause (men'o-pawz). The time of life when women cease to menstruate.

Menses (men'sēz). The monthly menstrual flow in women.

Metabolism (me-tab'o-lizm). The sum of all of the physical and chemical processes by which living organized substance is produced and maintained (anabolism) and the change by which energy is made available for the uses of the organism (catabolism).

Micturition (mik-tu-rish'un). The passing of urine.

Mitosis (mi-to'sis). The process of cell division by which two new daughter cells are formed each with the same number and type of chromosomes as the parent cell.

Mobilize (mo'bi-liz). To make movable.

Mucus (mu'kus). A sticky watery fluid secreted by the glands of the mucous membranes.

Muscles (mus'elz). Bundles of elastic fibers which by contraction produce movement.

N

Nausea (naw'se-ah). An unpleasant sensation, vaguely referred to the stomach and often culminating in vomiting.

Necrosis (ne-kro'sis). Death of a portion of tissue.

Negative (neg'ah-tiv). Not positive; without result.

Neonatal (ne"o-na'tal). Pertaining to the first four weeks after birth.

Neoplasm (ne′o-plazm). A new tissue mass (tumor).

Nephritis (ne-fri′tis). Inflammation of the kidney.

Neuron (nu′ron). A nerve cell with all its processes.

Neurotic (nu-rot′ik). A nervous person, one who is ill without cause.

Nocturia (nok-tu′re-ah). Excessive urination at night.

Nomenclature (no′men-kla-tūr). A system of names used in a science or group.

Nutrient (nu′tre-ent). A substance which affects the metabolic processes of the body; nourishing.

O

Obese (o-bēs′). Excessively fat.

Obstetrics (ob-stet′riks). The branch of medicine dealing with pregnancy, labor, and the puerperium.

Occupational therapist (ok″u-pa′shun-al ther′-ah-pist). One who treats physical and mental disabilities by means of work adapted to speed up recovery.

Oculist (ok′u-list). One skilled in treating diseases of the eye.

Oliguria (ol-i-gu′re-ah). Scanty secretion of urine.

Onset. The period during which the first symptoms of a disease develop.

Optician (op-tish′an). One who makes glasses.

Oral (o′ral). Pertaining to the mouth.

Orifice (or′ĭ-fis). The entrance or outlet of any body cavity.

Orthopedics (or-tho-pe′diks). That branch of surgery which deals with the correction of deformities and chronic diseases of joints and the spine.

Orthopnea (or″thop-ne′ah). Inability to breathe except in an upright position.

Oxidation (ok″sĭ-da′shun). The act of taking up oxygen.

P

Pallor (pal′or). Paleness; absence of the skin coloration.

Palpitation (pal″pi-ta′shun). An abnormally rapid and fluttering heart beat felt by the patient.

Palsy (pawl′ze). Loss of motion or sensation in a part or limb.

Papules (pap′ūlz). Small nipple-shaped elevations; pimples.

Paraplegia (par″ah-plē′jē-ah). Paralysis of the legs and lower part of the body.

Parenteral (par-en′ter-al). Not through the alimentary canal, e.g., by intravenous injection.

Parietal (pah-ri′ĕ-tal). Wall of a cavity. Parietal bones are those of the upper sides of the skull.

Parturition (par-tu-rish′un). The act of giving birth to a child.

Pasteurization (pas″tūr-i-za′shun). The use of heat by which pathogenic bacteria are killed and other bacterial development is considerably delayed.

Patella (pah-tel′ah). The knee cap.

Pellagra (pel-lag′rah). A disease due to insufficient B complex vitamin.

Pericardium (per-e-kar′dē-um). The double membrane which envelops the heart.

Periosteum (per-e-os′te-um). The tough, fibrous membrane surrounding a bone.

Peripheral (pe-rif′er-al). Pertaining to an outward part or surface.

Peritoneum (per-i-to-ne′um). The membrane lining the abdominal cavity.

Permeable (per′me-ah-bl). A membrane through which certain liquids may pass.

Petrolatum (pet-ro-la′tum). An ointment-like substance used as a base for other salves and as a soothing application to the skin.

Phagocytes (fag′o-sits). All cells which destroy microorganisms or harmful cells by surrounding them and absorbing them.

Pharmaceutical (fahr-mah-su′ti-kal). Pertaining to drugs and a pharmacy.

Pharmacologist (fahr-mah-kol′o-jist). One who makes a study of drugs.

Phobia (fō′be-ah). A continued abnormal fear.

Podiatrist (po-di′ah-trist). One who treats diseases of the foot.

Polyuria (pol″e-u′re-ah). Excessive urination.

Posterior (pos-te′re-or). Situated in the rear.

Postpartum (pōst-par′tum). After delivery.

Pregnancy (preg′nan-se). The period when the fertilized egg is developing in the uterus.

Premature (pre-mah-tur′). Occurring before the proper time.

Prenatal (pre-na′tal). Existing or occurring before birth.

Procedure (pro-se′dur). A series of steps by which a desired result is accomplished.

Process (pros′es). A projecting point or prominence.

Prognosis (prog-nō′sis). A statement of the probable outcome of the disease.

Prophylaxis (pro″fi-lak′sis). Prevention of disease.

Prosthesis (pros-the′sis). The replacement of an absent part by an artificial one, such as an eye, leg, or arm.

Prostration (pros-tra′shun). Extreme exhaustion.

Prothrombin (pro-throm′bin). A substance

thought to exist in the blood which can be changed to thrombin.

Psychiatry (sī-kī′ah-tre). The treatment of mental disorders.

Psychosis (sī-kō′sis). Mental disease.

Puncture (punk′tūr). A deep wound made by a sharp pointed instrument.

Purulent (pu′roo-lent). Consisting of or containing pus.

Pus. An inflammation product made up of tissue debris, bacteria, leukocytes, and serum.

Pustule (pus′tūl). An elevation on the skin filled with pus or lymph.

Pyloric (pi-lor′ik). Pertaining to the opening of the stomach into the duodenal portion of the intestines.

Pyogenic (pi-o-jen′ik). Producing pus.

Pyrosis (pi-ro′sis). A burning sensation; heartburn.

Q

Quarantine (kwor′an-tēn). To detain or isolate because of suspected contagion.

Quadriplegia (kwod″rĭ-ple′je-ah). Paralysis of all four limbs.

R

Recumbent (re-kum′bent). Lying down.

Recuperate (re-ku′per-āt). To recover from an illness; to gain strength.

Reflex (re′fleks). An automatic response to a given stimulus.

Regurgitate (re-gur′ji-tāt). To throw up undigested food.

Rehabilitation (re″ha-bil″ĭ-ta′shun). The restoration of an ill or injured patient to self-sufficiency or to gainful employment at his highest attainable skill in the shortest possible time.

Relapse (re-laps′). The return of a disease after its apparent cessation.

Relaxation (re-lak-sa′shun). A lessening of tension. A mitigation of pain.

Remission (re-mish′un). The abatement or subsiding of the symptoms of a disease.

Resuscitation (re-sus″ĭ-ta′shun). The restoration to life or consciousness of one apparently dead.

Retention (re-ten′shun). Abnormal holding back of matter normally excreted.

Rickets (rik′ets). A disease due to a vitamin D deficiency in the diet.

Rigor (ri′gor). Stiffness; rigor mortis—stiffness of body after death.

S

Sacrum (sā′krum). Triangular bone of the lower spine.

Salivary gland (sal′ĭ-ver-e). Gland secreting a digestive juice at the angle of the jaw.

Sanatorium (san″ah-to′re-um). A hospital for convalescents, especially one for the treatment of the tubercular.

Saturated (sat′u-rāt-ed). Unable to hold in a solution any more of a given substance.

Sclerotic (skle-rot′ik). Hard, or hardening.

Scoliosis (sko-le-o′sis). An abnormal curvature of the spinal column, especially laterally.

Scurvy (skur′ve). A nutritional disease caused by an insufficient amount of fruits and vegetables in the diet.

Sebaceous (se-ba′shus). Secreting a greasy lubricating substance.

Secretion (se-kre′shun). 1. The process of the giving off of a specific product as a result of the activity of a gland. 2. Any substance produced by the process of secretion.

Sedative (sed′ah-tiv). A drug or other agent which allays activity and excitement.

Segmentation (seg-men-ta′shun). The division into similar parts; for example, that which takes place in the fertilized ovum.

Senile (se′nil) A progressive feebleness of body and mind generally associated with aging.

Sera (se′rah). The plural of serum, the clear portion of the blood.

Serum (se′rum). A clear portion of any animal fluid separated from its more solid portion; especially the clear liquid which separates in the clotting of blood from the clot and the corpuscles.

Shock (shok). Depression of body functions usually associated with lowering blood volume and sometimes leading to death.

Sinus (si′nus). A cavity.

Sitz (sitz′). A bath in which the patient sits in the tub, the hips and buttocks being immersed.

Smear (smēr). A specimen for microscopic study prepared by spreading the material across the glass slide.

Somatic (so-mat′ik). Pertaining to the body.

Somnolence (som′no-lens). Sleepiness; also unnatural drowsiness.

Specialist (spesh′al-ist). A doctor who has had postgraduate study in a certain special class of disease and devotes himself to this area.

Sphincter (sfingk′ter). A circular muscle which closes a natural entrance or outlet to a cavity.

Sputum (spu′tum). Material discharged from throat and respiratory passages and ejected from the mouth.

Stasis (sta′sis). A stoppage of the flow of blood or other body fluid in any part.

Sterilize (ster'i-līz). To destroy all micro-organisms.

Stethoscope (steth'o-skōp). An instrument by means of which internal body sounds may be heard.

Stimulant (stim'u-lant). A drug or other agent which increases the activity of a part.

Strabismus (strah-biz'mus). A squint; cross-eye.

Stupor (stu'por). Partial or nearly complete unconsciousness.

Suppository (sŭ-poz'ĭ-to-re). A medicated solid mass of suitable size and substance for insertion into the vagina or rectum.

Suppression (su-presh'un). A sudden stoppage of a secretion.

Suture (su'tūr). A surgical stitch or seam; also the line of junction of cranial bones.

T

Tactile (tak'til). Pertaining to touch.

Technique (tek'nēk). A method of procedure; details of a mechanical process.

Technician (tek-nish'an). One who is well trained in technical procedures.

Tenesmus (tĕ-nez'mus). Straining at stool or in urination, often painful and ineffectual.

Tetanus (tet'a-nus). Lockjaw, an acute infectious disease producing a toxin which causes persistent spasm of the voluntary muscles.

Tetany (tet'a-ne). A condition of muscular spasm due to disturbed calcium metabolism.

Therapeutic (ther"ah-pu'tik). Pertaining to the treatment of disease.

Thrombin (throm'bin). The fibrin ferment of the blood; an enzyme present in shed blood but not in circulating blood, which converts fibrinogen to fibrin.

Thrombus (throm'bus). A clot in a blood vessel or in a cavity of the heart.

Tonus (to'nus). The slight, continuous contraction of muscle which in skeletal muscles aids in the maintenance of posture and in return of blood to the heart.

Tourniquet (too'nĭ-ket). A special instrument used to compress a blood vessel to control bleeding.

Toxemia (toks-e'me-ah). A general intoxication or poisoning due to absorption of bacterial products (toxins) formed by some local infection.

Toxic (tok'sik). Poisonous; pertaining to poisoning.

Toxin (tok'sin). Any poisonous substance of microbic, vegetable, mineral, or animal origin.

Transfusion (trans-fu'zhun). The introduction of whole blood, plasma substitutes, or other injectable solution directly into the blood stream.

Trauma (traw'mah). A wound or injury.

Tympanites (tim"path-ni'tez). An accumulation of gas in the abdomen.

U

Unconscious (un-kon'shus). Not responding to sensory stimuli.

Urea (u-re'ah). The chief nitrogenous substance of the urine.

Uremia (u-re'me-ah). An accumulation in the blood of substances which should have been eliminated in the urine.

Urinalysis (u"rĭ-nal'ĭ-sis). Analysis of the urine.

Urinate (u'ri-nāt). To pass urine.

Urticaria (ur"tĭ-ka're-ah). A vascular reaction pattern of the skin marked by the transient appearance of smooth, slightly elevated patches which are redder or paler than the surrounding skin and attended by severe itching.

V

Vaccination (vak-si-na'shun). Inoculation with vaccine to protect against disease; in particular, against smallpox.

Valve (valv). A fold in a canal or passage which prevents contents from being forced backward.

Varicose (var'i-kōs). Unnaturally swollen and contorted.

Vertigo (ver'te-go, ver-ti'go). A sensation as if the external world were revolving around the patient or as if he himself were revolving in space.

Vitamins (vi'tah-minz). Substances found in certain foods which are necessary for normal development and absence of which causes deficiency diseases.

Void (void). To cast out as waste matter, especially the urine.

W

Wheal (hwēl). A flat edematous elevation of the skin; a typical lesion of urticaria.

Wound (wo͞ond). An injury to the body caused by physical means.

Page numbers in *italics* refer to tables. **Boldface** numbers indicate pages on which there is an illustration.

A

TABLE OF METRIC AND APOTHECARIES' SYSTEMS

(Approved *approximate* dose equivalents
are enclosed in parentheses.
Use *exact* equivalents in calculations.)